ADMINISTRATION OF

Health and
physical education
programs

INCLUDING ATHLETICS

SIXTH EDITION

ADMINISTRATION OF
Health and physical education programs

INCLUDING ATHLETICS

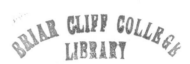
CHARLES A. BUCHER, A.B., M.A., Ed.D.

Professor of Education, New York University, New York, New York

WITH 328 ILLUSTRATIONS

Saint Louis
THE C. V. MOSBY COMPANY
1975

Sixth edition

Copyright © 1975 by The C. V. Mosby Company

All rights reserved. No part of this book may be reproduced in any
manner without written permission of the publisher.

Previous editions copyrighted 1955, 1958, 1963, 1967, 1971

Printed in the United States of America

Distributed in Great Britain by Henry Kimpton, London

Library of Congress Cataloging in Publication Data

Bucher, Charles Augustus
    Administration of health and physical education
programs, including athletics.

    Originally published under title: Administration of
school health and physical education programs.
    1. Health education. 2. Physical education and
training—Administration. I. Title. [DNLM: 1. Physical education and training. 2. School health. WA350
B919a]
LB3405.B83 1975   371.7   74-13260
ISBN 0-8016-0845-7

GW/CB/B   9   8   7   6   5   4   3   2   1

To my wife
JACKIE
and my children
DIANA
RICHARD
NANCY
and JERRY

Preface

Change is characteristic of the times through which we are passing. The energy crisis, ecology, computerization, accountability in government, women's liberation, and other developments are bringing a new way of life to Americans. These societal changes are also having their impact on educational programs. Women are asking to play a more important role in our schools and colleges. Students and faculty are having a say in the formulation of policy. Learning theories embrace self-paced instruction, module scheduling, performance-based learning, and the utilization of community resources. Educators are paying more attention to the handicapped. Planning, programming, and budgeting systems are requiring administrators to justify the expenditures of funds.

The thrust of this revision has been to bring the changes occurring in society and in education to the administration of health and physical education programs, including athletics. Each chapter has been carefully reviewed, evaluated, and revised, incorporating the implications each change has upon the topic being discussed. In addition, current developments, such as innovative ideas and programs in health and physical education and new architectural concepts in the construction and use of facilities, are discussed. All of the component parts of health education and physical education programs are covered.

Another aspect of this revision is that old and outdated illustrations have been removed and replaced with new and relevant photographs, charts, and graphs. As a result, more than 100 new illustrations have been used in further bringing this text up to date.

This revised text enables the student studying for a career in health or physical education, the professor or administrator who teaches and prepares prospective leaders for these fields, and teachers of health and physical education in schools, colleges, and agencies to keep abreast of the changing times and how these changes are affecting their fields of endeavor.

Special thanks are given to those persons and institutions who contributed illustrations and material for this text. Also, thanks are extended to Myra Madnick for all her help.

CHARLES A. BUCHER

Contents

ix

PART ONE

The changing nature of administration

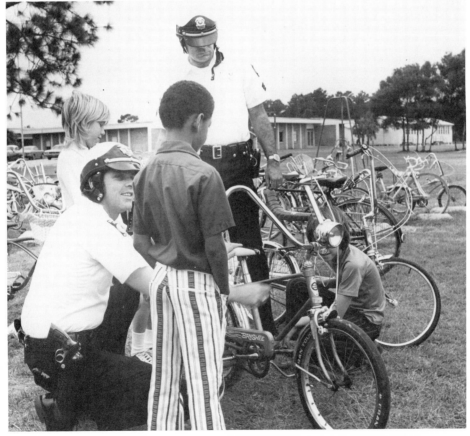

The community and the school ensure a safe bicycling program. (Courtesy AAHPER and The Bicycle Institute of America.)

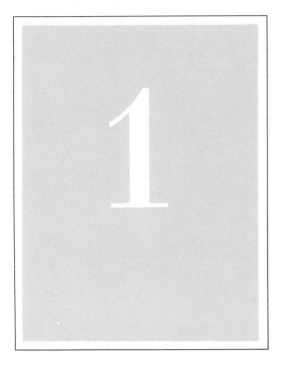

The changing nature of administration

Accountability, performance objectives, school voucher plans, performance based certification, more women administrators, collective bargaining, and the year-round school are only a few of the changes that are being implemented in our school systems. Administrators must be flexible enough to understand, discuss, and be willing to accept change that will better the educational process. Administrative policies must reflect these changes. Education should grow from its own research and applicable research in other fields. Furthermore, open-minded educators and administrators can better help education meet the needs of today's students, parents, and community.

DEFINING ADMINISTRATION

By analyzing several definitions of administration, a reader may be better able to understand what a text in administration is designed to cover. Some of the definitions proposed by experts in this field represent analyses of the administrative process based on research; others have been formulated as a result of experience as an administrator or observation of administrators at work.

Based upon Hemphill, Griffiths, and Frederickson's* research, Jenson and Clark† propose the following as a definition of administration: "The administrative process is the way an organization, through working with people, makes decisions and initiates actions to achieve its purposes and goals." Halpin,‡ after analyzing administration in education, industry, and government, states that administration refers to a human activity involving a minimum of four components: (1) the *functions or tasks* to be performed, (2) the *formal organization* within which administration must operate, (3) the *work group* or groups with which administration must be concerned, and (4) the *leader* or leaders within the organization. Administration has also been defined as a means of bringing about effective cooperative activity to achieve the purposes of an enterprise.

After considerable research and the formulation of a philosophy of administration that is

---

*Hemphill, J., Griffiths, D., and Frederickson, N.: Administrative performance and personality, New York, 1962, Bureau of Publications, Teachers' College, Columbia University. (This study is sometimes referred to as the "Development of Criteria of Success in School Administration" project.)

†Jenson, T. J., and Clark, D. L.: Educational administration, New York, 1964, The Center for Applied Research in Education, Inc. (The Library of Education).

‡Halpin, A. W.: A paradigm for research on administrative behavior. In Campbell, R. F., and Gregg, R. T., editors: Administrative behavior in education, New York, 1957, Harper & Row, Publishers, p. 161.

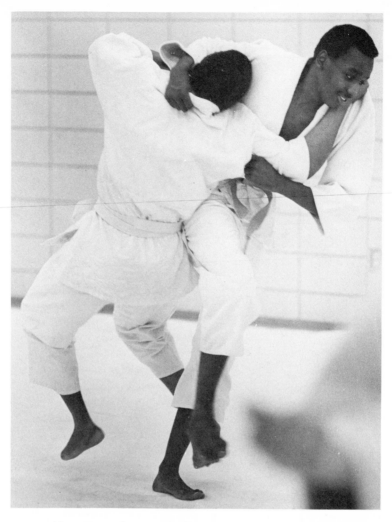

Administrators must provide programs that meet the interests and needs of students. At Florissant Valley Community College in St. Louis the physical education program includes judo as an activity in order to meet student interests and needs. (Photograph by LeMoyne Coates.)

stated later in this chapter, the following definition is proposed: *Administration is concerned with the functions and responsibilities essential to the achievement of established goals through associated effort. It is also concerned with that group of individuals who are responsible for directing, guiding, coordinating, and inspiring the associated efforts of individual members, so that the purposes for which an organization has been established may be accomplished in the most effective and efficient manner possible.*

THE SCOPE OF ADMINISTRATION

It has been estimated that there are more than 5 million individuals in the United States today performing administrative work as their main function. This number is large, but as the technology and the specialized functions of this country advance, there will be an increasing number of individuals needed to perform the myriad administrative duties characteristic of the thousands of organizations in society. There are at least as many administrative positions in physical education and health as there are schools and colleges. This, of course, runs into several thousands of positions. In addition, there are many large educational institutions with several persons who assist in the administrative process concerned with health and physical education programs. Also, there are many

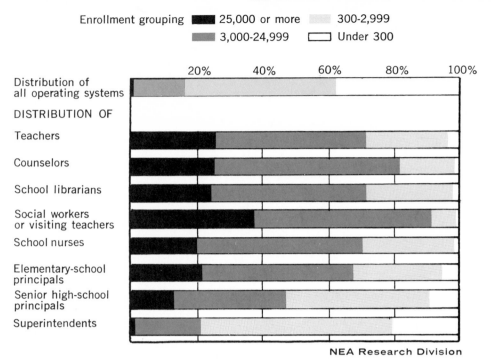

Distribution of personnel by school enrollment, 1968-69. (From Research Division, National Education Association, NEA Research Bulletin **47**:82, 1969.)

agencies such as the YMCAs and Boys' Clubs, who also have administrative positions. Administration offers many career opportunities for both women and men.

It is essential that individuals who perform administrative work know the many aspects of this particular field. If they are not aware of certain basic facts and are not acquainted with acceptable administrative procedures, many errors may be made. This could result in loss of efficiency, production, and staff morale and in poor human relations. Administration is rapidly becoming a science with a body of specialized knowledge that should be known by all who would administer in a wise and effective manner.

A PHILOSOPHY OF ADMINISTRATION

People represent the most important consideration in the world. The real worth of a field of endeavor, organization, or idea is found in what it does for human beings. The most important and worthwhile thing that can be said about a particular vocation, organization, or movement is that it contributes to human betterment.

People have goals that represent a variety of human objectives. They include the need for security for oneself and one's family, the desire to be employed in a worthwhile and gainful occupation, the freedom to worship as one chooses, the enjoyment of recreation, and the desire to obtain an education.

People do not miraculously work together. They do not spontaneously band together and strive to accomplish common objectives. Since many groups of people have common goals, however, they do work together and through associated effort help each other to achieve goals that would be impossible for them to accomplish alone. No one person can establish a school for his children's education, for example, but through the cooperative effort and support of many people a school is made possible. Thus individuals have similar goals that they will work together to attain.

Organizations, in order to function most effectively, must have some type of machinery to help them run efficiently, to organize and execute their affairs, and to keep them operating smoothly, so that the goals for which they have been created will be achieved. This machinery

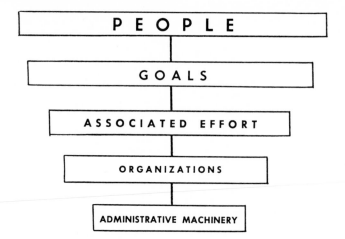

Graphic representation of a philosophy of administration.

is administration. It is the framework of organizations. It is the part that helps organizations implement the purposes for which they have been established.

One method of improving administrative techniques is through a Management Action Program (MAP). MAP combines a preliminary survey of organization function with a group approach to development of specific plans of action that will result in organizational success. There are three basic phases involved in MAP: preliminary survey, action plans, and follow-up procedures.

In the *preliminary survey,* the key people in the organization are interviewed to determine how their operation functions, what problems exist, how these problems are coped with, where the organization is heading, how fast, and what is necessary for success. In the *action plans* phase the key people attend a meeting where each person is expected to be prepared to discuss problems relating to his operations, other operations, and the organization as a whole. In the *follow-up* phase key people are asked to identify unique actions of their organization.

Some of the results of an MAP plan utilized in a school system are as follows:

1. Key administrators participate together in determining and gaining commitment to overall educational objectives.

2. Principals and teachers are involved in specific plans for the educational management of students.

3. Principals aid teachers in meeting mutually committed schedule goals.

Administration, therefore, exists to help people achieve the goals they desire in order to live happy, productive, healthful, and meaningful lives. It is not an end in itself; rather, it is a means to an end—the welfare of the people for whom the organization exists. Administration exists for people, not people for administration. Administration can justify itself only as it serves the people who make up the organization, helping them to achieve the goals they have as human beings.

It can be seen, then, that in an organization, where the associated efforts of many individuals are necessary, there is no spontaneous and automatic working together of the individuals involved. It is not a natural trait of human beings to cooperate and work together in a happy and purposeful manner. This is accomplished through direction, and administration gives this direction.

To a considerable degree, the actions of human beings in society are determined through their association with formal organizations. Formal organizations have leaders and purposes. They depend upon the cooperative efforts of individuals to achieve the objectives that have been set. Many times organizations have failed when their administrators have lacked leadership ability, when there has been a lack of cooperative effort among members, or when the objectives have not been in conformance with what is essential and good for society.

Administration determines in great measure whether an organization is going to progress, operate efficiently, achieve its objectives, and have a group of individuals within its framework who are happy, cooperative, and productive. Administration has to do with directing, guiding, and integrating the efforts of human beings so that specific aims may be accomplished. It refers particularly to a group of individuals, many times called executives, who have as their major responsibility this direction, guidance, integration, and achievement.

Administration is especially concerned with achievement—proof that the organization is producing those things for which it has been established. To be able to achieve these results in a satisfactory manner presupposes an understanding of human relationships and the ability to foresee the future and plan for any eventuality. It demands the capacity to coordinate many different and conflicting types of human personalities. Good administration should ensure that the associated efforts of individuals are productive. To accomplish this, administrators should possess those attributes that are conducive to bringing out the most creative and best efforts on the part of the members of the organization.

Administration also requires close supervision of the facilities, materials, supplies, and equipment essential to the life of the organization. It implies a logical formulation of policies and the effective operation of the organization.

A new concept of administrative philosophy

The traditional concepts of administrative philosophy have usually centered around authoritarian, democratic, or laissez-faire orientations. These philosophies are further discussed in Chapter 5 but will be reviewed briefly here.

1. *Authoritarian.* This philosophy usually implies a one-person leadership with decision-making imposed by the leader upon group members.

2. *Democratic or equalitarian.* This philosophy implies a leader who submits important matters to group discussion and involves group members in decision-making.

3. *Laissez-faire.* This philosophy implies a leader who gives guidance but leaves decision-making to group members.

These orientations may be considered traditional in that they do not allow for the so-called in-between leader, the leader who may be part democratic, part authoritarian, part laissez-faire, depending on the situation. The traditional philosophy views leaders as absolutes, which of course is very unrealistic since the nature of the human personality is usually not so extreme.

Dr. Johnson in her writings has proposed a three-dimensional concept of administrative philosophy that takes into account that a leader may have tendencies toward all three traditional orientations. In illustrating her three-dimensional philosophy she assigns point values to the traditional leadership patterns. The maximum number 5 indicates leadership entirely in one orientation. Thus, a classic authoritarian administrator would be denoted as 5:0:0 (leadership patterns are denoted in alphabetic order from left to right). The democratic leader would be denoted as 0:5:0, and the purely laissez-faire leader would be denoted as 0:0:5.

Since most leadership is not one-sided, an administrator who is strongly authoritarian, but does occasionally utilize democratic procedures, might be denoted by 4:1:0 values. Numerous

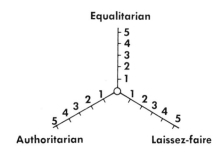

A three-dimensional concept of administrative philosophy. (Courtesy Dr. Marion Lee Johnson, Southeastern Louisiana University and The Physical Educator **28**:39, 1971.)

combinations may be achieved by using a three-dimensional model* (see the accompanying figure).

Leadership orientations will be discussed at length in Chapter 5.

IMPORTANCE OF ADMINISTRATION

A study of administration is important for all teachers of health and physical education. A few of the more significant reasons why teachers should understand administration are discussed in the following paragraphs.

1. *The way in which schools and colleges are administered determines the course of human lives.* The lives of both students and teachers are affected by administration. It affects the type of education offered, the climate in which the education takes place, and the goals that are sought. It vitally affects the happiness and achievement of every teacher.

2. *Administration provides an understanding and appreciation of the underlying principles of the science of this field.* Methods, techniques, devices, and procedures used by the administration can be evaluated more accurately and objectively by faculty and staff if they possess administrative understanding. Also, sound administration will be better appreciated and unsound practices more easily recognized. Human resources will have less chance of being exploited, and efficient management and organization will be furthered through such understanding.

3. *A study of administration will assist in deciding whether a person wishes to select this area on a career basis.* Personal qualifications may be better evaluated and possibilities of success better predicted with increased understanding and appreciation of the administrative process.

4. *Most physical education and health educators perform some types of administrative work and therefore an understanding of administration will contribute to better performance in this area.* Administration is not restricted to one group of individuals. Most teachers and staff members have reports to

*Johnson, M. L.: A three-dimensional concept of administrative philosophy, The Physical Educator **28**:39, 1971.

complete, equipment to order, evaluations to make, and other duties to perform that are administrative in nature. An understanding of the science of administration will assist in carrying out these assignments.

5. *Administration is fundamental to associated effort.* Goals are reached, ideas are implemented, and an esprit de corps is developed with planning and cooperative action. A knowledge of administration facilitates the achievement of such aims.

6. *An understanding of administration helps to assure continuity.* A fundamental purpose of administration is to carry on that which has proved successful rather than to destroy the old and attempt a new and untried path. An appreciation of this concept by all members of an organization will help to ensure the preservation of the best traditional practices that exist in the organization.

7. *A knowledge of administration helps to further good human relations.* An understanding of sound administrative principles will better assure the cooperation of the various members who make up the organization in order that the greatest efficiency and productivity will be assured.

The evidence is ample that administration is rapidly becoming a science and that the study of this science is essential to everyone. A study of administration can result in a better-ordered society through more efficiently run organizations. Every individual belongs to formal organizations. Through a democratic approach to administration the individual can aid in carrying on what has proved to be good in the past and steer a course that will ensure progress in the future.

DEVELOPMENT OF THE THEORY AND PRACTICE OF ADMINISTRATION

It is increasingly being recognized that administration is not something that is hit or miss, trial and error, or a matter of expediency. Instead, there is evidence to show that a theory of administration is emerging. It is recognized that from a study of this administrative theory one will gain the ability to act wisely in specific situations, and since theory is practical, it provides an accurate picture of how human beings work. Administrative theory will also help in the identification of problems that need to be solved if an effective working organization is to exist.

Textbooks and the professional literature on administration indicate a search for a substance of administration and for a framework of theory that would make the substance a meaningful whole. The traditional emphasis has been upon the form rather than upon the substance. Organizations such as the National Conference of Professors of Educational Administration, the Cooperative Program in Educational Administration, and the University Council for Educational Administration are helping to give impetus to this new movement and thereby helping to make administration much more of a science than it has been in the past. Although there are some educators who oppose such a trend, it seems assured that administration is in the process of becoming more scientific and thereby characterized by more objectivity, reliability, and a systematic structure of substance.

The traditional and modern views of administration

The traditional view of administration revolved around the idea that administration existed in order to carry out the policies that had been developed by the duly constituted policy-forming group, such as a board of education. Modern administration not only carries out policy but also plays an important role in the development of policy, utilizing the knowledge and expertise that come from training and experience.

A study of the history of administration shows that policy-forming groups, such as boards of education, were once held accountable for how the schools were administered, whereas the modern approach delegates administrative responsibilities to the trained school administrator. The old concept of leadership in administration was a sort of passive type of leadership that remained in the background while the policy-forming group provided the strength and skill that were needed to run the schools. Under the modern view of administration, however, strong administrative leadership is a requirement so that technical and expert judg-

ments can be made to help the schools to achieve their objectives more effectively. The traditional view of administration claimed the best way to prepare to administer was to practice administering: experience was seen to be the best teacher. The modern view of administration, however, recognizes the value of experience but at the same time maintains that there exists a body of knowledge or theory that, when mastered, can help the administration play a more effective role in the organization with which it is associated.

According to Jenson and Clark,* new perspectives of educational administration are the result of six phenomena:

1. Administration is a science and the administrator is a professional person.
2. An intensive study of administration includes such phenomena as behaviors, social interactions, and human relationships.
3. Application of theory and model constructs are included in the study of administration.
4. Administration is differentiated into two dimensions: content and process.
5. New forces shape new perspectives in administration: new technologies, population trends, value systems, knowledge explosion, ideological conflicts, and so on.
6. Interest of scholars and researchers in the scientific study of the field of administration is increasing.

The preparation of administrators

The modern view of administration is that a professional preparation program for the person who desires to enter the field of administration should include such essentials as: taking foundation work in cognate fields, knowing himself as an individual and as a potential administrator, having competency in administrative skills to be performed, understanding the community, recognizing the importance of instruction, studying and practicing decision making, and realizing the importance of human relations. Finally, there should be on-the-job learning experience that is closely supervised by an experienced professor.

Some universities, as a part of the training and professional preparation of administrators, include a course in Sensitivity Training or Human Awareness. The purpose of these courses is to learn through an analysis of one's own

---

*Jenson and Clark, op. cit., p. 37.

and other people's experiences. In human awareness training, participants work together in small groups in an attempt to better understand themselves and other people. This group is frequently called a *T group,* and the leader is called a trainer. His or her role is to help the group learn from its experiences. The group does not have a definite structure, and the leader initially stresses that the participants themselves will be the forces that determine how individual behavior is influenced. The leader also stresses that the data for learning will be the behavior of the group members.

Several types of content, all of which are pertinent to physical education and health administrators, are suggested by Culbertson* as being needed in the preparation of administrators in order to fulfill the following responsibilities.

----

*Culbertson, J.: The preparation of administrators. In Behavioral science and educational administration, the Sixty-Third Yearbook of the National Society for the Study of Education, Chicago, 1964, University of Chicago Press.

Making decisions. Content should include a study of concept and theories that relate to individual, group, and organization decision making. The relationship of such items as basic research, computer technology, and value systems to decision making would also be considered.

Communication. A study of communication —one-way, two-way, and group, as well as organizational communications—should be included. Mass communications and opinion change should also be considered.

Coping with change. A study of the dynamics of change in relation to individuals, groups, and organizations should be made. A study should also be made of barriers to change, how change can be effected, the leadership needed, conflicts, and related topics. For example, Table 1-1 indicates a number of types of instructional organization and practices. The administration plays a key role in bringing about such changes and practices.

Building morale. Content should include how morale is achieved in a modern organization. Special attention should be given to

Table 1-1. Instructional organization and practices, 154 middle schools in systems enrolling over 12,000 pupils, 1968-69*

Instructional organization and practices	Number and percent of schools by grade level †							
	Grade 5 (20 schools)		Grade 6 (146 schools)		Grade 7 (154 schools)		Grade 8 (148 schools)	
	Number	Percent	Number	Percent	Number	Percent	Number	Percent
Organization								
Self-contained classrooms	10	50.0%	31	21.2%	3	1.9%	3	2.0%
Partial departmentalization	7	35.0	74	50.7	55	35.7	36	24.4
Total departmentalization	3	15.0	35	24.0	91	59.1	105	70.9
No reply	—	—	6	4.1	5	3.3	4	2.7
Practices								
Subject area teams	4	20.0	45	30.8	51	33.1	152	35.1
Interdisciplinary teams	2	10.0	19	13.0	29	18.8	25	16.9
Small group instruction	7	35.0	55	37.7	63	40.9	66	44.6
Large group instruction	4	20.0	35	24.0	45	29.2	47	31.8
Flexible scheduling	5	25.0	39	26.7	44	28.6	43	29.1
Closed-circuit TV	1	5.0	22	15.1	25	15.6	25	16.9
Independent study	3	15.0	30	20.5	39	25.3	40	27.0
Individualized instruction	4	20.0	39	26.7	47	30.5	48	32.4
Tutorial programs	3	15.0	32	21.9	33	21.4	31	20.9

*From NEA Research Bulletin **47:**51, 1969.

†Percentages are based on the total number of middle schools in the survey, which includes each of the grades. The number of schools with each grade is shown in the column headings.

motivation, interpersonal relations, values, organizational loyalty, perception, and so on.

Such content material and preparation, if offered, would produce well-educated administrations, according to the American Association of School Administrators.* The AASA, for example, feels that an administrator (in this case a superintendent of schools, but the points are equally applicable to administrators of physical education and health programs) as a result of his or her professional training should:

1. Have a deep devotion to the human values that are at the heart of America's purpose and upon which her destiny rests and an understanding of the galaxy of relationships and ethical beliefs upon which those values and ethical principles are based.
2. Be able to make wise and sound decisions toward the improvement of teaching and toward more efficient learning.
3. Know laboratory and classroom environments, tools for teaching, and the structural organization for deployment of staff and pupils.
4. Be well schooled in what science and research show about the expectations, drives, fears, interests, and personal diversities that exist in groups of teachers, children, and young people.
5. Understand the American public—what it is, what it wants, how it is organized, how it can make itself felt, and who leads it.
6. Be efficient in using public funds.
7. Have a combination of personal power, insight, and skill that enables him to get a team of associates to work closely and effectively with him. (Some of the most energetic and intellectually astute superintendents—administrators—find themselves carrying more and more burdens because they unknowingly tie in knots the energies and abilities of the men and women closest to them.)
8. Have wisdom and good judgment, as well as skill, in oral and written communication.
9. Possess creative, imaginative, and realistic competence in sensing society's evolutionary and emerging aspirations and needs.
10. Have the vision, courage, and patience needed to plan wisely for the future.
11. Be professionally competent in many areas of evaluation.
12. Comprehend the educational needs of adults, children, and youth.
13. Have an education that feeds upon education, that generates an unquenchable thirst for more understanding, and that keeps him far out in front of the doggedly pursuing menace of obsolescence.

---

*The education of a school superintendent, Washington, D. C., 1963, American Association of School Administrators, pp. 11-12.

Anatomy of administrative leadership

Being the head of a department, division, or school of physical education and health and being the leader of these organizations are two different things. The head can be a person who takes care of the clerical details and occupies the main office in a department or division, but he or she may not necessarily be the leader of the organization. The administrative leader of an organization is one who helps and influences others in a certain direction as problems are solved and goals achieved. In a school, college, or agency situation the persons influenced are teachers, pupils, clerks, parents, custodians, and any person involved with the organization.

The question of what makes a leader is a provocative one. Much research has been done in recent years concerning what constitutes the administrative leader. Years ago it was felt that combinations of personality characteristics or traits were the ingredients that determined who was a leader. However, research such as that of Gouldner,* indicates that: "At this time there is no reliable evidence concerning the existence of universal leadership traits."

Other studies have provided further information in regard to leadership. Stogdill† states as a result of his research that "the qualities, characteristics, and skills required in a leader are determined to a large extent by the demands of the situation in which he is to function as a leader." In other words, a health or physical education administrative leader in one situation may not necessarily be a leader in another situation. Different styles of leadership are needed to meet the needs of different settings and situations. Administration therefore is a social process.

Certain traits and attributes that influence leader behavior have been identified. For example, Pierce and Merrill,‡ in examining re-

---

*Gouldner, A. W., editor: Studies in leadership, New York, 1950, Harper & Row, Publishers, p. 34.
†Stogdill, R. M.: Personal factors associated with leadership: a survey of the literature, Journal of Psychology **25:**63, 1948.
‡Pierce, T. M., and Merrill, E. C., Jr.: The individual and administrative behavior. In Campbell, R. F., and Gregg, R. T., editors: Administrative behavior in education, New York, 1957, Harper & Row, Publishers, p. 331.

search on leadership, found that such qualities as popularity, originality, adaptability, judgment, ambition, persistence, emotional stability social and economic status, and communicative skills were very important for a person to possess if he hoped to lead. The traits that were found to be most significant were popularity, originality, and judgment.

Goldman* examined the research on leadership and suggested that certain factors are significant. When these factors are related to physical education and health administrative leaders, the following guidelines are worth considering:

1. The administrators of physical education and health programs who possess such traits as ambition, ability to relate well to others, emotional stability, communicative skill, and judgment have greater potential for success in leadership than persons who do not possess these traits.
2. The administrators of physical education and health programs who desire to be leaders of their organization must have a clear understanding of the goals of the organization. The direction in which they desire to lead the organization must be within the broad framework of the goals and objectives of the school district and consonant with the needs of the community they serve.
3. The administrators of physical education and health programs who desire to be leaders of their organizations must understand each of the persons who work with them, including their personal and professional needs.
4. The administrators of physical education and health programs who desire to be leaders of their organizations need to establish a climate within which the organization goals, personal needs of each staff member, and their own personality traits can operate harmoniously.

Administrative tasks

Administration is a process involving pertinent tasks that can be performed if an organization is to progress and achieve its goals. These tasks represent the mission of the organization as delineated into subtasks. For example, since the task of the school is to educate, certain subtasks are essential in order to accomplish this mission. Campbell and his associates† analyzed

administrative tasks and came to the conclusion that there were seven operational task areas. These are: (1) school-community relationships, (2) curriculum development, (3) pupil personnel, (4) staff personnel, (5) physical facilities, (6) finance and business management, and (7) organization and structure. In Part Four of this text the following administrative tasks and functions in regard to school health and physical education programs are discussed in detail: the physical education plant, budget making and financial accounting, purchase and care of supplies and equipment, legal liability and insurance management, curriculum planning, professional, school and community relations, office management, measurement of pupil achievement, and teacher and program evaluation. The task of organization and structure is covered in Chapter 3.

Administrative skills

Some administrators are successful and some fail because of the administrative skills they lack. Jenson and Clark,* as a result of their research, have identified three types of administrative skills that are essential: conceptual, technical, and human relations. These skills are necessary for the succesful administration of physical education and health programs.

Conceptual skills include the abilities to see the organization as a whole, to originate ideas, to sense problems, and to work out solutions to these problems that will benefit the organization and establish the right priorities and organizational direction. It reduces the risk factor to a minimum.

Technical skills are the administrative skills that relate to the various tasks that must be performed. For example, such tasks as budgeting, curriculum planning, communication, preparing reports, group dynamics, policy development, and public relations, to name only a few, require certain specialized skills if they are to be performed efficiently and accurately.

The third type of skills, *human relations skills,* refers to the administration's ability to have good working relationships among the

---

*Goldman, S.: The school principal, New York, 1966, The Center for Applied Research in Education, Inc. (The Library of Education), pp. 88-89.

†Campbell, R. F., and others: Introduction to educational administration, ed. 2, Boston, 1962, Allyn and Bacon, Inc.

*Jenson and Clark, op. cit., pp. 56-57.

staff, to get along with people, and to provide a working climate where individuals will not only produce but also grow on the job.

Stages of the administrative process involving decision making

Decision making in the administrative process requires that certain steps be followed. The ordinary problem-solving approach that has been traditionally used includes the recognition of the problem, identifying the alternatives, gathering and organizing facts, weighing alternatives, and finally arriving at a decision. Jenson and Clark,* however, feel that the administration should not stop at the point of arriving at a decision but, instead, feel that it is essential to go on to the stages that involve implementation and assessment. The sequential stages of this process, they feel, are well stated by Burr and his associates:†

1. *Deliberating*. The problem is discussed, facts on the problem are gathered, and the problem is carefully analyzed.

2. *Decision making*. As a result of the deliberation a decision is made. Alternatives are carefully weighed and a choice is made based on the facts.

3. *Programming*. After the decision is made the program is developed so that it is ready for implementation. Questions are asked and actions taken in regard to the resources that are available, the planning that needs to be done, the budget, equipment, and material requirements that exist, and the needs in regard to staff and so on. In other words, information is researched that will provide a successful program and the right direction, in light of the decision that was made.

4. *Stimulating*. After the programming has been developed, it is set into operation. This requires the involvement of people, arousing interest, obtaining commitments, and initiating action. Motivation needs to be encouraged and attitudes developed in this process.

5. *Coordinating*. To effectively implement a program requires the coordination of staff efforts, material resources, proper communication, and other essentials that will assure that the program will be successfully launched.

6. *Appraising*. The last stage in the continuum is evaluating and appraising all stages of the process and the results obtained. It attempts to analyze where the process was successful or where it failed and the reasons for the success or failure. The information gathered will be used in future endeavors.

Rules of administrative organization

Bartholomew* suggests certain rules of organization that he gathered from a study of the field of public and business administration. These have implications for organizing and administering physical education and health programs.

1. *Administrative work may be most efficiently organized by function*. This rule of organization refers to the "doctrine of unity" that holds that all officers engaged in a particular type of work should function under a single authority.

2. *Unified direction should be embodied in the organization*. This refers to the "unity of command," which in essence means that no staff member should be subject to the orders of more than one superior.

3. *Organization may be according to purpose*. Staff, auxiliary, and line activities may be separated.

4. *Organization should be done on a hierarchical basis*. A vertical type of structure that begins at the bottom with production personnel and then goes upward through section heads, division heads, to the organization head should exist. Such units are differentiated on the basis of level of authority and responsibility.

5. *Organization and social purpose cannot be disassociated*. The organization (structure) is a means and not an end in itself.

6. *There is no single correct form of organization*. Such things as size, geography, personnel, and funds available will determine at any given time what is the best organization for a particular situation.

7. *Span of control should be definitely considered in organizational structure*. This rule of organization refers to the number of subordinates who can be adequately supervised by one individual. In other words, the number of communication contacts that can be effectively carried on by an administrative office and subordinates will determine the span of control.

Circular pattern of organizational structure

This pattern of organizational structure is one alternative that has met with great success in

---

*Jenson and Clark, op. cit., pp. 53-55.

†Burr, J. B., and others: Elementary school administration, Boston, 1963, Allyn and Bacon, Inc., pp. 398-402.

*Bartholomew, P. C.: Public administration, Paterson, N. J., 1959, Littlefield, Adams & Co., pp. 4-8.

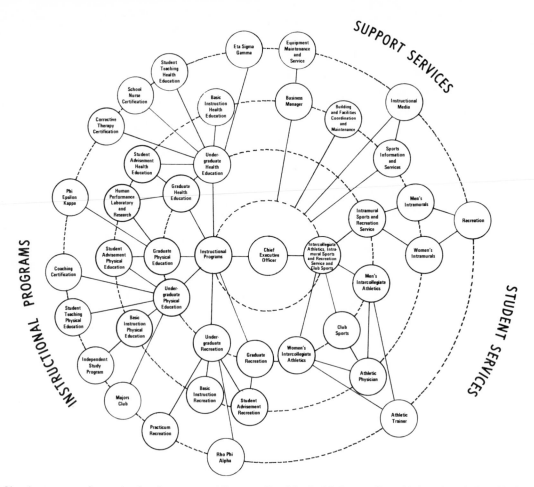

Circular pattern of organizational structure. (Courtesy Dr. Martin McIntyre, State University of New York at Buffalo and AAHPER, Journal of Health, Physical Education, and Recreation **44**:28, 1973.)

recent years. Its basic concepts, however, have not been widely applied in the area of health, physical education, and recreation. The model seen in the accompanying figure can be explained as follows:

1. The innermost circles represent a general function; the functions become more specialized as the circles radiate outwards.
2. The accepted flow of responsibility is indicated by the solid lines.
3. Each program has full access to the resource bank of the organization.
4. The support services contribute to all functions of health, physical education, recreation, and intramural programs.
5. Committees that encompass the total organization should be established in such

areas as curriculum, bylaws, administration, and staff appraisal.

ADMINISTRATION AND POLICY FORMATION

Policies are essential to the efficient administration of any department, school, business, or other organization. Without them, there is little to guide the activities and conduct of the establishment in the pursuit of its goals. With well-thought-through policies the organization can function efficiently and effectively and its members will better understand what is expected of them.

Policies are guides to action. Policies reflect procedures that, when they are adhered to, will fulfill the best interests of the organization and the purposes for which it exists. If properly selected and developed, policies enable each member of an organization to know what duties are to be performed, the the type of behavior that will result in the greatest productivity for the establishment, how best the department goals can be accomplished, and the procedure by which accountability can be established and evaluated.

The efficient administration of a physical education or health education department requires the establishment of sound policies if it is to achieve its goals. During a school survey several years ago the office of a director of physical education was visited. When he was asked to see the policies under which the department was administered, the director replied that no policies existed. Instead, the administrator indicated that he dealt with each problem as it occurred. There were no set guidelines established in advance—no written policies. As a result, chaos reigned in this program. Each faculty member had his own way of handling such things as student excuses from class, testing the skill level of boys and girls, and transporting players to athletic events.

The policies of the federal government are reflected in the laws of the land. They are developed in Congress and, after judicial and executive review and approval, become established policies by which the citizens and organizations of this country are guided. As a result, each person and organization knows whether heroin can be "pushed" or whether people of another color or race can be discriminated against. Just as the national government has policies to guide the actions of its citizens and organizations, so also do the state and municipal divisions of government.

State and local systems of education also have established policies that provide guidelines for such important administrative considerations as the number of days school will be in session, what children and youth must attend school, and for whom educational programs are to be provided. Similarly, just as governmental organizations and their subdivisions establish policies to guide the workings of their organizations, so should physical education and health departments have policies to guide their actions and help in the achievement of their objectives.

Administrative policies imply statements of procedures that will be in force for some period of time. In a sense they represent the legalistic framework under which the organization operates. As such, it is not anticipated they will be changed frequently, but instead will have some sense of permanence. Therefore they are not developed on short notice nor hastily written.

On the other hand, rules and regulations, as compared with policies, are usually more specific in nature and are formulated as a means of carrying out the policy that has been established. For example, an established policy of a school might be that all athletes will be transported to interschool contests by school-owned transportation. Rules and regulations then could be established for such purposes as spelling out the nature and type of such transportation, the students who must comply with the policy, and when and how they will comply. Generally, rules and regulations can be changed much more readily than policies. In fact, some administrators have been known to develop rules and regulations instead of policies so that they can be changed more easily.

Although policies are well thought through and carefully formulated, they should be reviewed periodically in light of any new developments that may occur in the intervening period. For example, at the present time some schools are providing faculty and students with new freedoms, rights, and privileges, which make some existing policies outdated and obsolete. Therefore change is needed.

How policy is developed

Policy emanates as a result of many phenomena. For example, the Constitution of the United States sets forth various conditions that affect policy development in organizations throughout the country. Educators must comply with such conditions as equal rights for all in the public schools, separation of church and state, and various conditions inherent in the democratic process.

Since education is a state responsibility, the state government also issues policies that must be adhered to by local education authorities.

These policies include such items as the number of days schools must be in session; certification qualifications for teachers; subject requirements, and minimum salary schedules for teachers. Within the framework of these policies or guidelines established by federal and state agencies, however, local education authorities, for example, boards of education, are permitted freedom to develop their own policies. Thus, they establish policies on whether students can drive their automobiles to school and whether teachers can have sabbatical leaves. The departments of physical education and health education can develop policies within the framework of the higher echelons of authority previously mentioned. Sometimes local policies conflict with state policies with the result that some of the local policies are declared invalid. For example, in some states where local policies prescribed a certain hair length for students as a graduation requirement, the rule was overturned and declared invalid by the state commissioner of education.

Policy is developed in many ways within a school system and physical education and health education departments. In some school systems and departments it is done autocratically with an administrator or two establishing policy unilaterally. This process is devoid of deliberations and suggestions from the faculty or students. The trend at the present time, however, is toward greater involvement of faculty and students in the development of educational policy. In some colleges and universities, faculty and students are playing a much greater role in determining policies affecting such items as the tenure of professors, grading practices, and school calendars. What is happening at higher education levels is developing in a somewhat slower manner at the public school level.

As a general rule the cliché "many heads are better than one" is true in policy development. Policies must be carefully researched and thought through before being written. Therefore, it is usually much better to involve many people who look at educational problems affecting policies from many different angles.

Although teachers and students may participate in policy development, it should be recognized that the formulation and development of policy is different from the execution of the policy. Execution of policy is usually an administrative responsibility and should be recognized as such.

The writing of policies

Before policies are written, much research must be done to determine what goes into the substance of that policy. This can be done in several ways. One method might be for the director of physical education and health education to appoint a committee to carefully research and recommend policy to the faculty and administration as a whole.

When the committee has been formed, for example, to recommend policy on whether girls should participate on varsity athletic teams with boys, it will want to investigate the facts thoroughly. It may decide to research the state policies regarding this problem, what other school systems are doing in this area, what policies already exist in the school system, the stand taken by selected national professional and athletic associations, views of their superintendent of schools and other administrators, the position of the American Civil Liberties Union, and other sources of information. After gathering all these facts, the committee will want to consider them carefully and then recommend a policy to the faculty and administration. If the recommendation is approved by them, the director of physical education and health education may then recommend it to the superintendent of schools for approval, who in turn, if he or she agrees, may recommend it to the board of education for its final approval as the policy governing the school district.

The policy that finally emanates from the committee should be written in a clear and concise style. There should be no ambiguities or possibilities of misinterpretation of what is intended by the policy statement. The statement of policy formulated by the committee should in turn be carefully reviewed by the department faculty and school administration to further determine that the statement says clearly what the school's position is on this particular issue.

Where policy is needed

It should be recognized that only the most important items facing the departments of physical education and health education should have policy statements. Policies on trivial matters should not be carried on the books since confusion and failure to adhere to many of the policies can result because they are not known or understood. Furthermore, with too many policies the important ones may be obscured by the proliferation of those less important. It is usually better to have only a few carefully researched policies that cover major administrative functions. The other matters, if needing attention, can be covered by rules and regulations or in some other manner.

DEMOCRATIC ADMINISTRATION

The administration should recognize certain steps in the democratic process of a staff and organization working together in order to accomplish group goals. Some of the steps that should be considered are as follows:

1. Goals should be developed through the group process. The goals that are set should be attainable, challenging, and adapted to the capacities of the members.

2. Good morale should be developed among the entire staff. This is essential to constructive group action. A climate of openness must be established in group deliberations. All must feel a sense of belonging and recognize their important contribution in the undertaking. A feeling of oneness should pervade the entire group.

3. Group planning must be accomplished in a clearly defined manner. A stated procedure should be followed. It should be a cooperative undertaking, based upon known needs and flexible enough to allow for unforeseen developments. The fulfillment of plans should bring satisfaction and a feeling of success to all who participated in their formulation and accomplishment. All should share in recognition for a completed job.

4. In staff meetings and other group discussions the administration must encourage the utilization of democratic principles. Each member's contribution must be encouraged and respected. Differences of opinion must be based on principles rather than personalities. The organization's objectives and purposes must be continually kept in mind. All members must be encouraged to facilitate the group process by

accepting responsibility, alleviating conflict, making contributions, respecting the opinions of others, abiding by the will of the majority, and promoting good group morale.

5. There must be periodic evaluation of progress. The group should evaluate itself from time to time on accomplishments in terms of the organization's goals and the effectiveness of the group process. Each individual must evaluate his own role as a member of the organization in respect to contributions made to the group process and the accomplishments of the group.

The problem of divided opinion

In a democratic organization, it is assumed that the wishes of the majority prevail. There is a question that often arises in this connection: Is the majority always right? Very often an important issue will be determined by one vote. Students of history remember that during post-Civil War days one vote kept Andrew Johnson from being removed from office. Every individual can recall similar situations within organizations where like results have occurred. Is this a weakness of democracy? Should important problems, plans, and issues be decided by such a small difference of opinion?

It seems that the reasoning behind such a dilemma is clear. All who believe in democracy recognize the importance of having as much unanimity of thinking as possible. However, they also recognize that it is much better to have a majority make a decision than to have it made by one person who is an autocrat.

The problem of subjective personal opinion as opposed to scientific fact

In many democratic discussions it appears to some individuals that scientific evidence should dictate policies and that personal opinions must not become involved. On complicated issues situations develop where certain individuals are acquainted with scientific data that in themselves define the issue. Therefore, the conclusion is reached that discussion, voting, or other devices are useless since the course of action is very clear as indicated by known fact.

The answer to such a problem seems to be that there will be acceptance if individuals know and recognize the facts. Generally, acceptance fails to materialize when evidence is not conclusive or when it has not been properly publicized. The democratic process can contribute immeasurably to such enlightenment. Through discussion, facts can be presented and understanding reached. Individuals with reasonable intelligence will accept scientific fact against personal opinion, if the presentation is clear and the evidence is convincing. William Gerard Hamilton during the late eighteenth century made a statement which has a bearing on this point: "Two things are always to be observed; whether what is said is true in itself, or being so, is applicable. In general, things are partly true, and partly not; in part applicable, and in part not. You are careful therefore to distinguish; and to show how far this is true and applies, and how far not." The democratic process is the most effective method yet devised to show what is true and applies.

The problem of standards

A question that is often raised in connection with the utilization of the democratic process is: What does it do to standards of performance? There is a belief in some quarters that by allowing majority opinion and decisions to prevail, standards of performance are lowered to a middle level. The individuals who have a low set of standards tend to pull down those with high standards. In effect, this results in a compromise on middle ground. The standards take on mediocrity rather than remain at a high level.

The answer to this problem is difficult. A democracy rests upon the worth of the individual. It has faith in the individual, the goals that he will set, and the standards he wants to follow. The challenge presents itself to those whose standards are high to bring the rest up to their level, rather than to allow themselves to be relegated to a lower one. Such a process may take time. Results are not always immediate in a democracy. Nevertheless, the principles upon which it is based are sound. By utilizing such principles as freedom of discussion and assemblage, it is possible to educate and to elevate standards.

The problem of time

Democratic discussions with their need for deliberation and agreement take time. Such delay often creates problems, sometimes with serious consequences. There is often too much delay between the need for action, decision, and execution. Democracy is based upon the necessity for individuals to see the need for a course of action and then, after seeing this need, deliberate on it, and finally see that the decision that they have made is put into effect.

It is true that this dilemma often works to the disadvantage of many individuals. However, it does not necessarily have to be this way. It has been seen how rapidly the federal government will act in case of emergency. For example, it did not take long for Congress to declare war after the attack on Pearl Harbor or to vote the necessary supplies and help once our country was at war. The delay occurs when there is misunderstanding, when a situation is not meaningful, and when the course of action is confusing. Perhaps it is wise in many cases to have this lag of time. Hasty action also results in many mistakes.

The problem of discussion with uninterested and noninformed individuals

Another problem that frequently arises in democratic deliberations is that some individuals who participate in group discussions are many times not interested or competent to discuss intelligently and constructively the subject at hand. Such a situation may be very helpful as an educational device. As individuals become better informed on various topics, they contribute more. Many minds are better than one or two. Any group should welcome as much help as possible in solving problems.

The problem of authority

Criticism has often been directed against the democratic process from the standpoint that it results in confusion and poor direction. The authority for certain acts is not clearly established. Furthermore, it is conducive to a conflict of ideas, which results in indecisiveness.

It seems important to recognize the part that democratic principles play in such a problem. A democratic organization vests in its members the right to help determine policies, purpose, and methods. They want a "say" in these important factors that vitally affect their lives. At the same time, however, they vest authority for execution of policy and purpose in administrators who are responsible to the group for their actions. Any democratically run organization has to recognize clearly the definite lines that exist between policy formation and execution. If an individual has been placed in an administrative position, the wherewithal to perform his duties effectively must also be granted. In a sense, all individuals have authority in their respective positions. Authority goes with the job and not with the individual. This is true from the top to the bottom of the organization. There is no "final authority" except as it exists in the entire membership. All organizations that are to be efficient and effective must clearly recognize these principles upon which the functioning of an organization rests.

ADMINISTRATION AND THE CHALLENGE OF MODERN EDUCATION

Education is America's largest industry. This country has about 60 million people in classrooms from coast to coast. There are approximately 2 million teachers in the elementary and secondary schools of the nation. More than $50 billion are spent each year on educational programs. The United States government is investing billions of dollars to ensure a quality education for each of its citizens. Educational construction costs more than $5 billion a year. Expenditures on classroom equipment, such as books, audiovisual devices, and desks, amount to $1 billion a year. Certain leading corporations in the United States have linked themselves to the educational business in such areas as copying machines, microfilms, texts and reading material, programmed instruction, electronics, language laboratories, and learning systems.

The growth for education during the last few years has been phenomenal. For example, expenditures in 1950 were about $9.3 billion, or 3.5% of our gross national product (the sum of all goods and services). A rise to more than 8% of the gross national product now exists. Ten years ago school and college enrollments were under 40 million. Enrollments are now in the 60 millions. Textbook sales have risen from about $200 million to $600 million annually in the past decade, or an annual growth of about 12%. Two-year college enrollments have jumped from less than 300,000 students in 1954 to over 1 million today. Also, the last 10 years have seen:

A 71% increase in students getting bachelor's degrees

Almost twice as many persons getting master's degrees

Twice as many persons getting doctoral degrees

An 89% increase in total spending by colleges and universities

A 74% increase in students seeking degrees at colleges and universities

A 13.5% increase in enrollment at public and private elementary and secondary schools

A 25.9% increase in public and private high school graduates

An increase of 507,000 public and private elementary and secondary school teachers

A 47% increase in expenditures for elementary and secondary schools

The projections indicate that the number of high school students has more than doubled, and the number of degree-seeking college students has more than tripled the 1954 totals. A decade from now, an estimated 16.4 million students will be in high school.*

The growth in education during recent years and the future expansion predicted place a heavy responsibility upon those persons who provide leadership in this area to offer a program that will preserve the democratic foundations upon which this nation was built, to help develop the potentials of each young person, and to devise educational programs that keep abreast of the times. This Herculean task falls not only upon those individuals who are labeled administrators but also upon all educators, whatever role they play in the schools. As such, a study of the facts that comprise the components of educational administration is essential to all, teachers and administrators alike.

---

*Projections of educational statistics of 1974-75, Washington, D. C., 1965 edition, U. S. Department of Health, Education and Welfare.

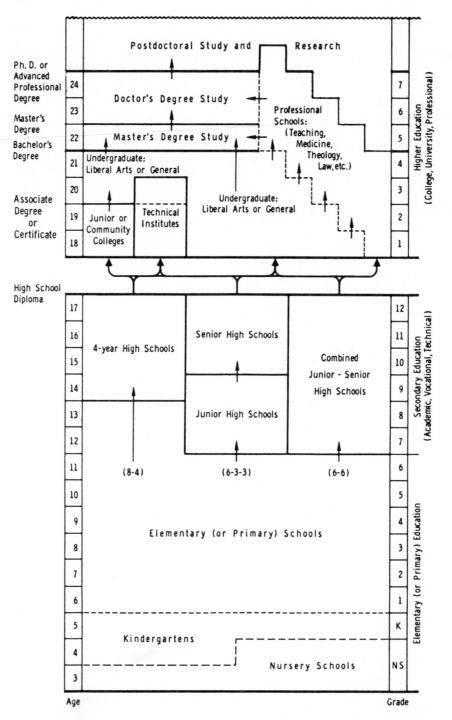

The structure of education in the United States. (From Digest of educational statistics, Washington, D. C., 1972 edition, U. S. Department of Health, Education and Welfare, Office of Education.)

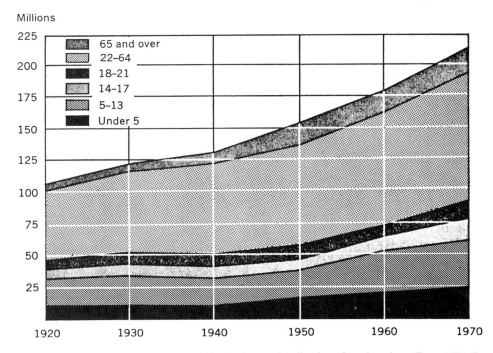

Millions

Fifty years of population growth—1920 to 1970—had many implications for education. (From NEA Research Bulletin **39**:91, 1961.)

THE CHANGING NATURE OF EDUCATION

In addition to the phenomenal growth in enrollments and the cost of running the schools, there have been many significant changes in the manner in which schools and colleges educate our young people. The schools and colleges of America are undergoing a major overhaul. A sampling of some new innovations follows:*

1. The ungraded system in elementary schools that eliminates grade lines in respect to subject matter and student progress
2. Contract grading, a system that permits the students to choose a standard of intended performance established by the leader and to work toward completion of the objectives by satisfying the requirements that comprise the established standard
3. "Shared time" projects in which both public and parochial school students participate
4. Cooperative buying of school supplies and equipment by several school districts
5. Area schools for rural students desiring modern industrial training
6. Individualized approach to learning
7. Foreign languages offered in the elementary grades

8. Project Head Start—a federally aided program to help inner-city youngsters enter school better prepared for their new experience
9. Children taught to read with the assistance of a computerized typewriter
10. The new alphabet (Pitman or Initial Teaching Alphabet) with forty-four symbols that represent various sounds to provide children with their first experience in reading
11. The new mathematics and the new physics
12. The new grammar
13. Greater use of performance or behavioral objectives that contain three basic elements: (1) description of conditions under which students will perform specific tasks or activities, (2) accurate description of the activity to be performed, and (3) statement of the criteria for evaluation of a successful performance
14. Collective bargaining and stronger unions among educators
15. Team teaching—employing two, three, or more teachers
16. Educational television
17. Teaching machines—giving a student knowledge gradually and at his own pace
18. Extension of the school day from 9 A.M. to 5 P.M.
19. The year-round school, such as the 45-15 plan, that breaks the learning sessions into four 45-school-day sessions each followed by a 15-day

*For further discussion of new innovations, see Chapter 3.

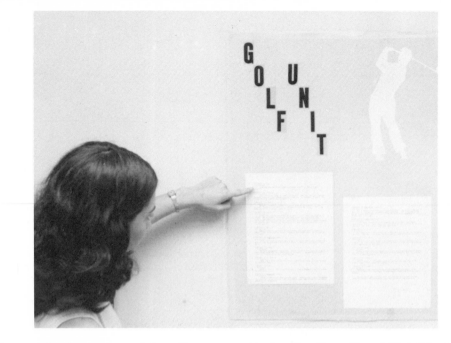

A student examines the requirements for golf on a contract basis at Fort Pierce Central High School in Florida.

student vacation period. Financial savings are realized by a more efficient use of the physical plant and personnel and a more equal distribution of class attendance throughout the entire year
20. Flexible scheduling with class time ranging from 20 minutes to 1½ or 2 hours
21. Independent study to enable students to carry out advanced work
22. Facilities built underground to cut expenses
23. The use of educational parks to bring elementary and secondary schools together on campuses
24. Special programs for the gifted students
25. Aid for inner-city children

Education is on the move. New ways of doing things, new facilities, new programs, and the emphasis on research have become bywords in school systems across the country. Educators need to be aware of the changes taking place in the schools and to adapt their own efforts and special fields accordingly. Administration should help in the evaluation of these innovations, checking the advantages against the disadvantages and weighing their implications for each teacher's field of specialization.

Education exists in and out of the schools

There is an educational revolution going on in education outside the schools. Business organizations have their education departments. Communications media such as television and radio are in the business of education. Youth groups such as the Campfire Girls and Boy Scouts provide educational experiences, and a multitude of other agencies are also involved. It is therefore important to be realistic about education in America and to be concerned with it in its broadest sense—in and out of the schools. This means teachers, administrators, and educators, in general, must prepare themselves to give leadership to out-of-school programs as well as those with which they are directly involved in the schools.

Equality of education for everyone

The civil rights movement, VISTA, and programs for inner-city youth, and other national developments indicate that this country is striving to provide each person, regardless of race, color, creed, or economic means, with a quality education. The implications of such a worthy goal include federal funds, broadened programs, and educational consumers with different needs and interests.

The curriculum reform movement

Knowledge and truth change with history and with the application of the scientific method to

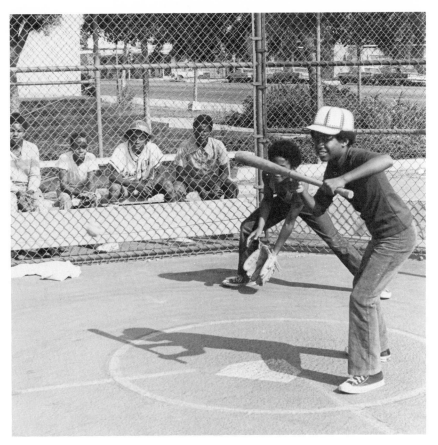

Physical education programs are needed for inner-city youth. A baseball game offered by the Youth Services Section of the Los Angeles City Schools.

social and educational problems. Young people today need to be acquainted with truths that are truths today. The new mathematics and new physics are only a few of the changes in the curriculum reform movement that are taking place in our schools in an attempt to get at the truth. The trivia must be abolished, the overlap and duplication eliminated, and a new look provided where deficiencies and weaknesses exist. There is a need to debate ways of doing this, a need to test results, a need to experiment, a need for new programs, and a need for alternatives.

The systems approach. The systems approach to curriculum development has stemmed from the rapid growth of technology and management in recent years. By borrowing techniques from the business world, educational planners have constructed models that bring together the many facets of the education enterprise: students, parents, school board, teachers, and the community.

The systems approach may be defined as a method designed to collect data on interrelated and interacting components that, when working in an integrated manner, help to accomplish a predetermined goal. The application of this strategy is called a systems approach.

PPBS and PERT. Two specialized management techniques, PPBS (Planning, Programming, Budgeting System) and PERT (Program Evaluation Review Technique), have been used with greater frequency in our schools. PPBS is used to plan goals, programs, assessment, and cost effectiveness, whereas PERT is used to identify the sequence of events and the time necessary to accomplish an objective. In many cases, state and federal granting agencies are requiring these techniques as necessary factors in proposals for new curriculum designs.

The PPBS Cycle begins with an analysis of the overall situation and ranks needs to be met in order of priority. Specific goals are then set in terms of behavioral or performance objectives. Curriculum content of the program is selected to meet the specified objectives. Alternate programs are also delineated. Results must be assessed after the program is implemented in order to ascertain whether initial goals are being met. The cycle may start over again if the program is to be continued.

The scientific study of teaching and learning

There is a realization that the teaching and learning processes can be improved. New techniques can be utilized, new assignments given, and new projects developed. In the preparation of teachers, all parts of a university must work together. Schools of education and the arts and the sciences are both in the business of education whether they like it or not. Learning can be done more efficiently only as constant experimentation takes place and research and testing are done.

The trend toward more public involvement

The increase of state and federal outlays for education means that control is also shifting from local to federal sources. Federal and state grants mean that the conditions under which such monies are expended for educational purposes must meet the approval of the upper echelons of governmental authority.

Accountability. Accountability is a general term that denotes various movements of making persons accountable for their performance. Performance or productivity may be measured by prespecified goals, the outcomes of which must meet certain standards. Accountability in education often includes students as well as teachers and administrators.

School vouchers. This is a relatively new experiment in education where parents are given education voucher certificates to be used at any school within the school system. The schools offer different types of education, some more innovative than others. Some voucher plans include private and parochial schools, and a voucher is applied against the total cost of education at these schools. The voucher system provides parents with more choices, makes schools more accountable to parents, and allows for greater innovation within individual schools of a school system.

The PEPI Project. The PEPI Project (Physical Education Public Information Project) is devoted to inspiring physical education professionals to communicate the worth of their programs to the public. This is done through newspaper articles, appearances on television and radio, films and film strips, and other publicity efforts.

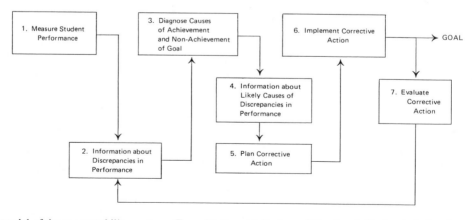

The model of the accountability system. (From McDonald, F. J., and Forehand, G. A.: A design for accountability in education, New York University Education Quarterly 4:7, 1973.)

Closer working relationship among the home, school, and community

The community is voicing increased concern about the education of its children. Parent-teacher organizations, advisory councils, and other lay groups want to have a say about how their educational systems are run. Educators can no longer live a cloistered existence and be oblivious to the public. Avenues of communication must be established if educational problems are to be solved effectively.

The women's movement and administration

The women's movement is primarily responsible for making people aware of the inferior position of women in many areas including civil rights, jobs, and salaries. Women have always been active in the field of education, but a recent survey conducted by the American Council on Education (ACE) indi-

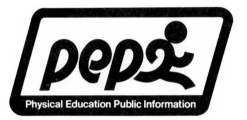

Physical Education Public Information

Physical Education Public Information. (Courtesy AAHPER.)

cates that women have not attained equality in higher education—especially as college teachers and administrators. The ACE study indicates that between 1968 and 1972, female representation on college and university faculties rose less than one percentage point, from 19.1 to 20%. At the University of California at Berkeley there are 58 administrative positions, and at the time of this survey, not one position was occupied by a woman.

Although more teachers are women, statistics show that proportionately more male teachers are selected for administrative positions. A national survey concluded that while 67% of all public school teachers were women, only 15% of principals and .6% of superintendents were female. The same survey showed that in the junior and senior high schools, the percentage of women administrators decreased sharply over the percentage in elementary schools.*

What can be done to correct this discriminatory situation? Some recommendations include:
1. Female applicants for administrative positions should be actively sought.
2. All discriminatory personnel policies should be eliminated.
3. Female students should be encouraged to become professionals and advised of administrative career potential.

*Lyon, C. D., and Saario, T. N.: Women in public education: Sexual discrimination in promotions, Phi Delta Kappan **55:**120, 1973.

Table 1-2. Percentage of women in selected educational positions, New York State, 1970-71/1971-72

Professional field	Percentage 1970-71	Female 1971-72	Percentage change between 1970-1972
Superintendent	0.4	2.6	+2.2
Deputy Superintendent*	11.9	7.1	−4.8
District Principal	1.8	1.8	0
Business Official	10.3	4.3	−6
Administrative Assistant	20.8	12.7	−8.1
Elementary School Principal	21.1	20.1	−1
Middle School Principal	4.6	7.5	+2.9
Junior High School Principal	8.0	7.8	−0.2
Senior High School Principal	2.6	1.7	−0.9
Elementary School Teacher	82.7	82.6	−0.1
Junior and Senior School Teacher	58.3	47.1	−11.2

*This category includes Assistant Superintendents.

From: Public School Professional Personnel Report 1970-71 and 1971-72, the State Education Department, Albany, N. Y.

Table 1-3. Percentage of women among all teachers in selected years

	Elementary	Secondary	Elementary and secondary
1957 to 58	87.2	49.6	73.2
1960 to 61	85.8	47.2	70.7
1963 to 64	85.5	46.1	68.9
1966 to 67	85.4	64.0	68.3
1970 to 71	84.7	45.9	67.2
1971 to 72	84.5	45.8	66.9

From: Estimates of School Statistics, 1971-72, National Education Association, Research Report, 1971-73.

Policy changes must be made at all levels —the local school district, the state department of education, and the federal government—for successful entrance of women into administrative positions.

Competency based or performance based certification and teacher education

A most significant development in education today is competency based certification and teacher education. Competency may be defined as a demonstrated ability that can be required for performance in a specific occupational or professional role. The major purposes of competency based programs are as follows:

1. To identify and state educational goals in terms of the competencies learners should acquire.
2. To develop procedures whereby individuals may be assessed and awarded credentials when these competencies are mastered.
3. To develop educational experiences that will result in the attainment of competencies.

The procedures used to formulate competency objectives should be discussed by groups having a legitimate interest in these objectives. These groups include administrators, trustees, governing boards, public agencies, professional associations, practicing professionals, employers, and representatives of the public interest. Therefore, where pertinent, these groups should be involved in the development of the objectives; in other words, it should be a cooperative undertaking of those groups who

are both internal and external to educational institutions.

Traditionally, learning has been assessed on how persons compare with others in the comprehension of subject matter. Competency based learning, however, stresses the results of the learning rather than the process. It is the competency of each individual that matters, not his or her competency compared to others. Such assessment techniques as standardized instruments, use of external professionals and practitioners, videotape performances, and portfolios of learning experiences may be used to assess competencies.

Different educational experiences will also aid in developing competencies. In addition to classroom learning, clinical experiences, apprenticeships, and individual learning resources will contribute to competency development.

The belief that all problems can be solved through education

The fact that many Americans are killed each year on the nation's highways has resulted in Americans turning to schools for a solution to this problem. The fact that tests have shown that American children are not physically fit has resulted in the public asking the schools to help remedy the problem. Education is increasingly being looked upon as a panacea for many of the problems with which our society is vexed. Consequently, there are pressures for time, personnel, and budget allocations to support the reforms.

The energy crisis and the administration of physical education programs

The shortage of energy sources is affecting each person's lifestyle. The thermostat is lowered, gasoline is in short supply, and travel priorities are established for school busses and school-related trips.

The physical education program is also greatly affected by the energy crisis. In some cases interscholastic athletic programs are being curtailed in order to save gasoline and oil, school schedules are being altered, and new activities are being provided in order to conserve fuel.

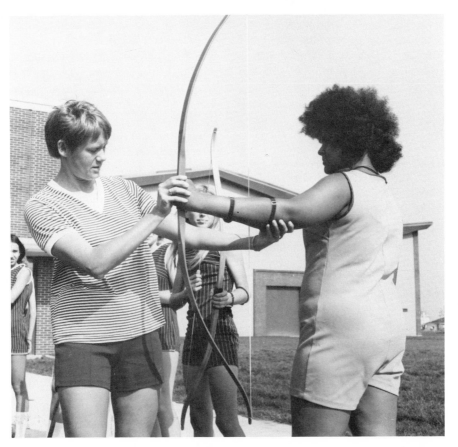

Competency based teacher education is designed to ensure that teachers have the skill, knowledge, and ability to provide excellent instruction for their students. A teacher instructs a student in the use of the bow at Thornwood High School, South Holland, Ill.

A few suggestions that the physical education administration may wish to consider are:

1. Develop an expanded intramural program to accommodate more students if travel is curtailed in the intercollegiate and interscholastic programs.
2. Involve the community, whose limited travel has cut down on their traditional leisure-time activities, in more physical activities conducted during after-school and evening hours.
3. Develop a dynamic physical activity program for the entire community during vacation periods when the gymnasium, playground, swimming pool, and other facilities are more likely to be free.
4. Work closely with the community recreation program in meeting the activity needs of the entire community.
5. Encourage activities that do not require fuel consumption, examples: bicycling and sailing.
6. Lower the thermostat in the gymnasium and other physical education facilities where vigorous activity is taking place.

7. Provide students and adults with a series of warm-up exercises to be engaged in when they get up in the morning. In this way they will not notice the lowered thermostat readings.
8. Where feasible, encourage car pools among students and their parents when young people stay after school and school bus transportation is not provided.
9. Organize a jogging program so that students living within a reasonable distance will use this means of getting to and from school.
10. Develop a publicity program that encourages students to leave their cars at home.

The internationalization of education

The exchange programs involving faculty and students, the increased speed of transportation, the junior-year abroad, the great amount of travel by Americans to other countries, and the creation of international centers and other evidences of cross-cultural intermingling have resulted in educational concern for people and problems outside the continental United States. Americans no longer live by themselves. What they do and how they think affects not only Americans but also other people around the globe. Education is not limited to the United States but involves the entire globe.

THE CHALLENGE OF THE FUTURE AND THE ADMINISTRATION OF HEALTH AND PHYSICAL EDUCATION PROGRAMS

The changes taking place in education and the goals being sought have vital implications for school health and physical education programs.

1. *Health educators and physical educators must be aware of new developments in general education.* There are so many changes taking place in education today that unless a person continually makes a determined effort to keep abreast of these changes, he or she is likely to be out of pace with the times. Each health educator and physical educator should read current literature that concerns itself with new trends and practices in education. There are many excellent publications that cover the latest thinking in education. Keeping abreast of new innovations does not simply mean possessing a superficial knowledge of each development, but, instead, it means being informed of the nature and scope of the innovation, where and why it is being used, its advantages and disadvantages, and its implications for health and physical education programs.

In addition to being knowledgeable about what is happening in education, health and physical educators must be aware that some of the new trends may have special implications for school health and physical education programs. For example, in regard to the nongraded elementary school, one might ask the following questions: Should a student be permitted to proceed at his own rate of speed in areas that have a unique relationship to his physical growth and development in the same way that he would proceed in a course in mathematics where the learning involves primarily mental development? What is the ideal type of schedule for physical education and health education?

Should all class periods be the same length or be of varying lengths? If so, what are they? In what way can programmed instruction be used most effectively in health education and physical education? The answers to such questions will require much thought and investigation, but the end results are very important to the most effective administration of these special fields.

2. *Health educators and physical educators should be continually studying their present programs and practices to determine if they are keeping up with the times.* Just as programs are changing in mathematics, English, and science, so also should programs of school health education and physical education be studied for possible needed changes. Changing for the sake of change itself should not be the case, but sometimes traditional ways of doing things become outmoded and consequently innovations are needed to keep up with the times. For example, such ideas as the following have been suggested and may possibly warrant further study:

a. Physical education classes meeting in the classroom as well as in the gymnasium
b. Health science classes being taught only by teachers trained and interested in this area
c. A textbook in classes of physical education
d. A conceptualized approach to the teaching of health
e. A program of educational athletics
f. A national curriculum in physical education
g. Greater use of performance objectives in curriculum planning
h. A movement education emphasis in physical education
i. Perceptual motor skills as a means of improving reading in the early grades
j. New approaches to the teaching of critical health areas such as alcohol, tobacco, narcotics, and sex education
k. Team teaching
l. Utilization of community resources

3. *Health educators and physical educators should recognize that new challenges to education have administrative implications for their programs.* The tremendous growth and emphasis upon education have special implications for the field of administration. Such factors as policies developed, budgets approved, personnel appointed, facilities and equipment purchased, curricula planned, and special subject matter and activity programs encouraged will determine the direction of school health

and physical education programs in the future. The challenge of the increased role for education in American life, with increased funds, personnel, and facilities to accomplish the objectives that have been established, will be met only as sound administrative practices are followed. The challenge means that all health educators and physical educators should understand what does and does not constitute sound administrative practice.

4. *Health educators and physical educators should place more emphasis on research.* There is an urgent need for more emphasis upon research in the fields of health education and physical education. Research is needed to advance the frontiers of knowledge in regard to these special fields, their contributions to mankind, their role in academic achievement, the function they have in personality development, and the tangible impacts they have on the health, productivity, and leadership of Americans. These are only a few areas that need to be investigated. In addition to more research being conducted, there should be greater emphasis on the training of research workers in professional preparation programs. Also, there should be more outlets for publishing the research findings. At present, the *Research Quarterly* of the American Alliance for Health, Physical Education, and Recreation (about sixty studies a year), *The Journal of School Health,* and *The School Health Review* are the main outlets, although certain psychologic and physiologic publications do provide other means of communication. However, there should be more outlets with greater implementation of findings at the grass roots level.

5. *Health educators and physical educators must become more scholarly.* Excellence in educational undertakings means that the educators involved—the persons who are doing the teaching and administering—must themselves be scholarly individuals. It is important that health education and physical education be able to stand on an equal academic footing with other subject areas and not be found wanting.

6. *Health educators and physical educators must make changes in teacher preparation.* Emphasis should be placed on specialization rather than very general training. One person cannot be expected to teach health, physical education, safety education, and also be a coach. An in-depth study of one subdiscipline of sport and physical education is essential. This is one aspect of *differentiated staffing* that represents a team approach to education to ensure the best possible education for each student.

7. *Health educators and physical educators should endeavor to recruit outstanding students.* Recruitment of talent at the high school and undergraduate level should emphasize the opportunities available to health and physical education college graduates. Many young people are not at all familiar with the career opportunities available in these areas. Promising young people with an interest in physical education should be educated concerning professional preparation programs.

8. *Health educators and physical educators should play an important role in attempting to find solutions to sociopsychologic problems in society.* Many problems exist in the sociopsychologic areas including drug addiction, crime, disintegrating neighborhoods, poor health, poor individual self-concept, and general minority group injustice. All of these problems can be positively affected by health and physical educators.

9. *Health and physical educators should utilize the community agencies to a greater extent.* Specialists in all areas may be just outside the school doors. Educators must learn to develop these resources as an integral part of their programming.

10. *Health and physical educators should emphasize learning, not grading.* In many situations, grading has overshadowed learning, and student accomplishment is judged by test scores rather than by performance objectives. Research into assessment theory is crucial to return learning to its proper place in education.

Questions and exercises

1. Define the term *administration* in your own words. Give illustrations to point out the various facets of your definition.
2. Discuss Management Action Program (MAP), its phases and potential results. Do you think that this is a beneficial administrative technique? Explain your answer.
3. What is human awareness training? How can this

training aid in the administration of health and physical education programs?

4. Write an essay discussing the role of the administrator in achieving cooperation from members of an organization.

5. What are some basic principles that should be observed in respect to channels of communication?

6. Why is a study of administration important to you as a physical educator or health educator?

7. Compare the traditional and the modern views of education. What do we mean by a theory of administration, and how does theory help in the practice of administration?

8. What type of preparation should potential administrators receive according to the administrative theorists?

9. What are the qualities that make for administrative leadership? Will the administrative leader be a success in whatever job he assumes?

10. In respect to policy formation discuss the following: (a) what is policy? (b) why is policy needed? (c) how should policy be developed and written? Prepare a sample policy in physical education.

11. Define the systems approach to curriculum development. In what ways is this approach an effective management technique?

12. What is meant by competency based or performance based certification? Explain this assessment technique in reference to educators and administrators. How do you feel about competency based assessment techniques?

13. What is the current status of women administrators in our school systems? How can this situation be corrected? Do some research at your college or university to determine the administrative positions held by women.

14. Project health education or physical education 20 years into the future and describe the type of program you would like to see.

Reading assignment in *Administrative Dimensions of Health and Physical Education Programs, Including Athletics:* Chapter 1, Selections 1 to 4.

Selected references

American Association of School Administrators: Profiles of the administrative team, Washington, D. C., 1971, The Association.

Brickman, W.: 1972 educational developments and issues, Intellect **101:**217, 1973.

Bucher, C. A.: Foundations of physical education, ed. 7, St. Louis, 1975, The C.V. Mosby Co.

Bucher, C. A., and Koenig, C.: Methods and materials for secondary school physical education, ed. 4, St. Louis, 1974, The C.V. Mosby Co.

Castetter, W. B.: The personnel function in educational administration, New York, 1971, The Macmillan Company.

Center for the Advanced Study of Educational Administration: Perspectives of educational administration and the behavioral sciences, Eugene, 1965, The University of Oregon.

Duryea, E. D., Fisk, R. S., and Associates: Faculty unions and collective bargaining, San Francisco, 1973, Jossey-Bass Publishers.

Field, D.: Accountability for the physical educator, Journal of Health, Physical Education, and Recreation **44:**37, 1973.

Fornia, D.: Signposts for the seventies, Journal of Health, Physical Education, and Recreation **43:**33, 1972.

Glines, Don: Why innovative schools don't remain innovative, NASSP Bulletin **57:**1, 1973.

Goldman, S.: The school principal, New York, 1966, The Center for Applied Research in Education, Inc. (The Library of Education).

Griffiths, D. E.: The school superintendent, New York, 1966, The Center for Applied Research in Education, Inc. (The Library of Education).

Gulick, L., and Urwick, L., editors: Papers on the science of administration, New York, 1937, Institute of Public Administration.

Halpin, A. W., editor: Administrative theory in education, New York, 1958, The Macmillan Company.

Hoffman, J.: Superintendent without a ticket, School Management, **17:**33, 1973.

Jennings, F.: Tomorrow's curriculum: future imperfect, Educational Horizons pp. 34-41, 1972.

Jenson, T. H., and Clark, D. L.: Educational administration, New York, 1964, The Center for Applied Research in Education, Inc. (The Library of Education).

Kerr, Clark: Administration in an era of change and conflict, Educational Record **54:**38, 1973.

Knezevich, S. J.: Administration of public education, New York, 1962, Harper & Row, Publishers, pp. 223-226.

Morphet, E. L., and others: Educational organization and administration, Englewood Cliffs, N. J., 1967, Prentice-Hall, Inc.

Oxendine, J.: Status of general instruction programs of physical education in 4-year colleges and universities, Journal of Health, Physical Education, and Recreation **43:**26, 1972.

Shane, H.: Reassessment of educational issues, Phi Delta Kappa **54:**4, 1973.

Simon, H. A.: Administrative behavior, New York, 1957, The Free Press.

Tead, O.: The art of leadership, New York, 1935, Whittlesey House.

Thompson, J. D., editor: Approaches to organizationl design, Pittsburgh, 1966, University of Pittsburgh Press.

Thomson, S.: Secondary school administration today, The North Central Association Quarterly, pp. 265-269, 1973.

Urwick, L.: The elements of administration, New York, 1943, Harper & Row, Publishers.

Whaling, T.: Managing the school system: a performance improvement approach, NASSP Bulletin **56:**32, 1972.

Willower, D. J., and Culbertson J., editors: The professorship in educational administration, Columbus, Ohio, 1964, The University Council for Educational Administration.

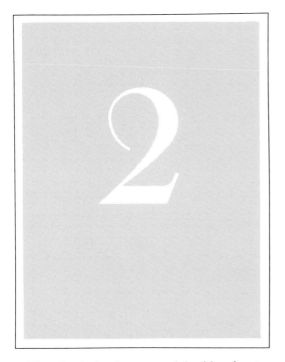

Administrative relationships and objectives

The physical educator and health educator cannot only be concerned with the learning of a skill or a desirable health attitude, but they must also be concerned with an indivdual's emotional, social, physical, and intellectual well-being. One of the most valuable achievements that can be accomplished by educators is instilling in young people a positive self-concept—a good feeling about themselves. This is a valuable objective to work toward, one that will stay with a person throughout life.

A field of endeavor is characterized by the objectives for which it exists. Objectives help the members of a group to know where they are going, what they are striving for, and what they hope to accomplish. Physical educators and health educators have clearly stated objectives toward which they are working. The student preparing for a career in these fields or administrators and leaders working in these fields should understand the objectives and be guided by them. Objectives, therefore, represent the aims, purposes, and outcomes that are derived from participating in physical education and health education programs.

HEALTH EDUCATION AND PHYSICAL EDUCATION DEFINED

The term *health* as defined by the World Health Organization refers to the total health of the person, including mental, emotional, physical, and social health, and not merely the absence of disease and infirmity. The school health program is designed to achieve this objective through a plan of health instruction, health services, and healthful school living. A definition of school health education as included in the report of the Joint Committee on Health Education Terminology,* is: "That health education process associated with health activities planned and conducted under the supervision of school personnel with involvement of appropriate community health personnel and utilization of appropriate community resources."

The term *physical education* as used in this text is defined as follows: *Physical education, an integral part of the total education process, is a program aimed at the development of physically, mentally, emotionally, and socially fit citizens through the medium of physical activities that have been selected with a view to realizing these outcomes.*

---

*Report of the Joint Committee on Health Education Terminology, School Health Review **4**:25, 1973.

31

GENERAL EDUCATION

Since school and college health and physical education should first be viewed within the concept of general education, it is appropriate to first define what is meant by general education and second to delineate the role of health and physical education within general education.

The purposes for which education exists have been set forth by many individuals and many organizations. One group of purposes reflects the socioeconomic goals for education as presented in ten characteristics that are desired for the individual American. These characteristics were stated in 1937 by a committee that included a philosopher, a lawyer, a sociologist, a superintendent of schools, and two secretaries of state education associations: (1) hereditary

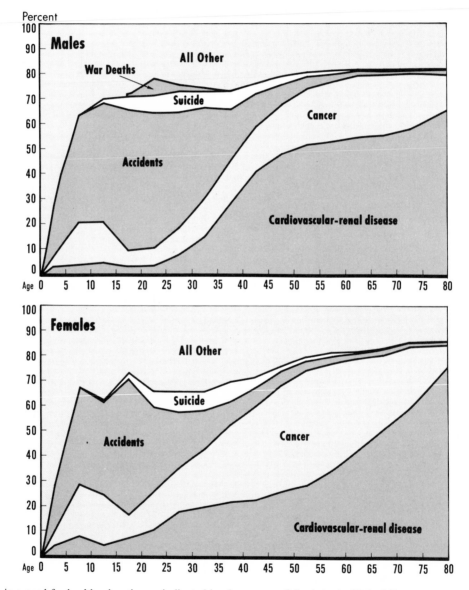

There is a need for health education as indicated by the causes of death in the United States. Percent of death from specified causes by sex and age in 1971. (Courtesy Metropolitan Insurance Company Statistical Bulletin **53**:11, 1972.)

strength, (2) physical security, (3) participation in an evolving culture, (4) an active, flexible personality, (5) suitable occupation (6) economic security, (7) mental security (8) equality of opportunity, (9) freedom, and (10) fair play.

Also included in the report of this committee, which included John Dewey and Willard E. Givens, were statements that "education must be universal in its extent and application, universal in its materials and methods, and universal in its aims and spirit." When analyzing and studying this list, one cannot but realize the great implications each of the items has for the fields of school health and physical education.

In 1938 the Educational Policies Commission also set forth certain purposes of education that they felt included a summarization and enlargement of statements that had been published previously by various committees and individuals representing the National Education Association. These purposes were (1) the objectives of self-realization, which are concerned with developing individuals to their fullest capacity in respect to health, recreation, and philosophy of life, (2) the objectives of human relationship, which refer to relationships among people on the family, group, and society levels, (3) the objectives of economic efficiency, which are concerned with the individual as a producer and a consumer, and (4) the objectives of civic responsibility, which stress the individual's relationship to his local, state, national, and international forms of government.

Today, general education is looked upon as preparing the individual for a meaningful, self-directed existence. For a student to be prepared to accomplish this goal means that he or she must have an understanding of (1) his or her cultural heritage and the ability to evaluate it, (2) the world of nature and the ability to adapt to it, (3) the contemporary social scene and the values and skills necessary for effective participation, (4) the role of communication and skill in communicating, (5) the nature of self and others and growth in capacity for continuing self-development and for relating to others, and (6) the role of esthetic forms in human living and the capacity for self-expres-

sion through them. Thus, the role of general education is a multifaceted undertaking requiring many different experiences and specialties.

HEALTH AND PHYSICAL EDUCATION PROGRAMS CONTRIBUTE TO GENERAL EDUCATION

Health education and physical education are integral parts of general education. Science indicates that these fields of endeavor contribute in many ways.

1. *The mind and body are inseparable.* Physical, mental, social, and emotional development are closely interwoven into the fabric of the human being. A person can think himself or herself into being sick just as sickness can affect one's thinking; therefore, *psychosomatic* has become an important word in our vocabulary. Intellectual, physical, and emotional developments are closely associated. Endocrinology has shown that mentality changes as body chemistry changes. Biology has linked the cell to the learning experience. Psychology points to the fact that the child's earliest learnings are tactual and kinesthetic.

2. *Motor skills contribute to learning.* Intelligence is not the only component of achievement in school. Motor learning is involved in readiness skills that are basic to perception, symbolic manipulation, and concept formation. If motor learning during the early years of childhood is deficient, more complex and advanced learning will be impeded. Psychologists Radler and Kephart* point out that motor activity of some type forms the foundation for all behavior, including the higher thought processes. They further stress that human behavior will function no better than the motor skills that are a part of the individual's makeup.

3. *Health and physical education contribute to academic achievement by developing physical fitness.* Research indicates that students who are achieving academically are also physically above average. It appears that physical fitness,

*Radler, D. H., and Kephart, N. C.: Success through play, New York, 1960, Harper & Row, Publishers.

at least up to a certain minimum level, is essential for good health and necessary for academic achievement.

4. *Health education and physical education contribute to academic achievement through their contribution to social development.* Research shows a relationship between scholastic success and the degree to which a student is accepted by his peer group. Similarly, the boy or girl who learns and applies sound principles of personality development or who is well grounded in motor skills, for example, usually possesses social status among his or her peers.

5. *Health education and physical education contribute to the emotional development of educationally subnormal students.* The value of health and physical education programs for educationally subnormal students may be greater than for average boys and girls. Dr. James N. Oliver, lecturer in education at the University of Birmingham, England, has done much research on educationally subnormal boys

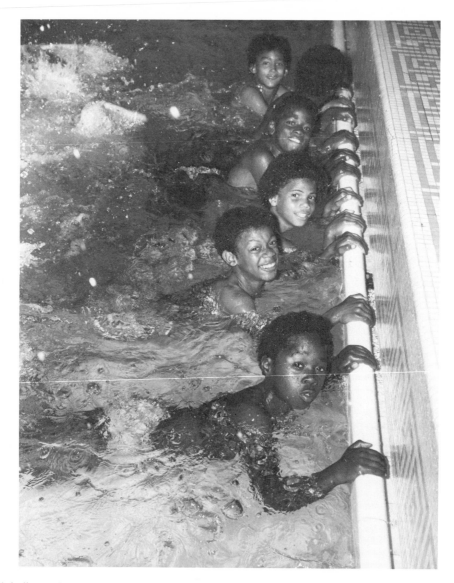

Research indicates that swimming and other physical education activities contribute to academic achievement. This swimming program is provided by the Youth Services Section, Los Angeles City Schools.

and has found that systematic and progressive physical conditioning yields marked mental and physical improvement. He believes much of the improvement results from a boy's feelings of achievement, which have the side effect of influencing his academic work for the better.

6. *Health education and physical education are integral parts of general education since they possess a subject matter essential to human beings.* Just as it is important to teach English so that people can communicate articulately and history so that they will appreciate their cultural heritage, so it is also important to educate people regarding their physical selves so that they may function most efficientlly as human beings. Intelligent young people will by physically active, develop skills, avoid drinking, smoking, and use of narcotics if they are given some good reasons. They are going to have to

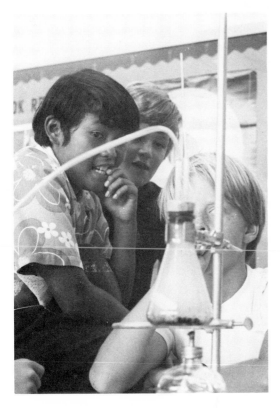

In health education class at Kaiser High School in Honolulu, Hawaii, children of Japanese, Hawaiian, and American backgrounds analyze the effects of smoking. (Courtesy Ed Arrigoni.)

understand and know that the time spent in the pursuit of these goals has its rewards. Thus, facts and subject matter become a necessity.

RELATIONSHIP OF HEALTH EDUCATION AND PHYSICAL EDUCATION

Health education and physical education as professional fields of endeavor are closely allied, especially in respect to their administrative aspects. In many schools and colleges, both come under one administrative head. They are concerned with the accomplishment of similar objectives. In many small communities both health education and physical education, are taught by the same person, although this is not always desirable. Professional preparation institutions usually incorporate both areas in the same schools or departments. In the American Alliance for Health, Physical Education, and Recreation, they are linked together professionally. Individuals working in these specialized areas share facilities, personnel, funds, and other items essential to their programs. General school administrators feel they are closely related.

These are only a few of the reasons why a close administrative relationship should and must exist between these specialized fields. Although professional persons realize the place of each and the need for specialists in each area, at the same time they also recognize the importance of maintaining a close and effective working relationship. The administrator is a key person in seeing that such a relationship is maintained. In some quarters there has been disunity and strained relations between these areas because the administrator did not assume his role of appeaser and unifier.

In recent years educational thinking has been more and more cognizant of the place of health education and physical education in school and college programs. Each is closely related to the other, but at the same time each is distinct. Each area has its own specialized subject matter content, its specialists, and media through which it is striving to better the living standards of human beings. In the larger professional preparation institutions each has its own separate training program. There is continual demand for separate certification of its leaders in the various states. Some sections of the country have recognized this need and have established state certification standards for employment of these specialized workers.

Although many educators and others feel that physical education has traditionally reflected the thinking and work of both areas, this is an erroneous belief. There is a definite need for the specialist in each of the areas of health and physical education. Each can render a service to humanity. Each can make a contribution that is distinct and separate from the other's. Each has its own destiny.

A close relationship among teachers in these areas, however, is evidenced by the fact that, to a great degree, they work on committees together and have professional books and magazines that cover the literature of both fields. Both are concerned with the total health of the individual. Both recognize the importance of activity in developing and maintaining good personal health. Both are concerned with the physical as well as the social, mental, emotional, and spiritual aspects of good health.

Both recognize the importance of developing good human relations as a basis for effective living in a democracy. Both are interested in promoting the total health of the public at large as a means to enriched living, accomplishment of worthy goals, and increased happiness.

The trend at the present time recognizes the close relationship that exists between health education and physical education and at the same time provides for greater autonomy and visibility on the part of each. An example of this is the American Alliance for Health, Physical Education, and Recreation, which has changed to a federation status in order to accomplish this goal.

OBJECTIVES OF HEALTH AND PHYSICAL EDUCATION PROGRAMS

The ultimate objectives of school and college health and physical education programs are similar. The essential difference lies in the fact that each area attempts to achieve its goals by utilizing different skills, media, and approaches. The objectives of each of the two areas are discussed in the pages to follow.

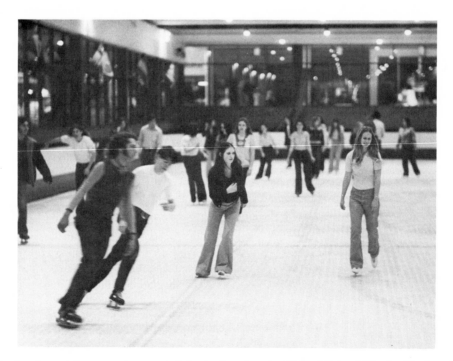

Physical education renders a service to youth in the Los Angeles Unified School District, Student Auxiliary Services Branch. (Courtesy Gwen R. Waters.)

OBJECTIVES OF SCHOOL AND COLLEGE HEALTH EDUCATION PROGRAMS

The long-term, overall objective of a health program is to maintain and improve the health of human beings. This refers to all aspects of health, including physical, mental, emotional, and social. It applies to all individuals, regardless of race, color, economic status, creed, or national origin. Schools and colleges have the responsibility to see that all students achieve and maintain optimal health, not only from a legal point of view but also from the standpoint that the educational experience will be much more meaningful if optimal health exists. A person learns easier and better when in a state of good health.

A synthesis of some of the objectives of the school and college health programs that have been listed by leaders in the field include the following:

1. To teach scientific health knowledge so that the individual can make intelligent health decisions

2. To develop desirable health attitudes in order that the individual will have an interest in applying health knowledge to his own daily regimen of living
3. To convey to the student that health is a three-dimensional entity, embodying social, mental, and physical aspects
4. To contribute to the physical, social, and emotional development of each boy and girl
5. To encourage the student to be a wise consumer and producer with respect to health goods and services
6. To encourage the correction of remediable defects
7. To help students and teachers to live healthfully at school and college
8. To reduce the incidence of communicable disease in the school, college, and community
9. To utilize the many health services available in the school, college, and community
10. To further home-school cooperation in health matters

The commonly mentioned objectives concerned with the development of health knowledge, desirable health attitudes, and desirable health practices deserve further discussion.

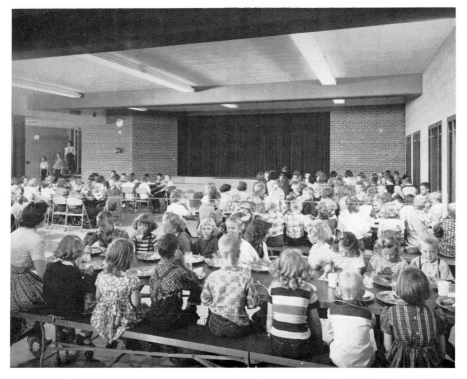

Burnett and Logan, Chicago.

One objective of health education is the cultivation of those habits of living which will promote present and future health. (Washington Irving Elementary School, Waverly, Iowa.)

Development of health knowledge. In order to accomplish the health knowledge objective, health education must present and interpret scientific health data for purposes of personal guidance. Such information will help individuals to recognize health problems and to solve them by utilizing information that is valid and helpful. It also will serve as a basis for the formulation of desirable health attitudes. In the complex society that exists today there are so many choices confronting an individual in regard to factors that affect his health that a reliable store of knowledge is essential.

Individuals should know how their bodies function, causes and methods of preventing disease, factors that contribute to and help to maintain health, and the role of the community in the health program. Such knowledge will aid individuals to live a more healthy life, help protect their bodies against harm and infection, and impress upon them the responsibility for their own health and the health of others.

Knowledge of health will vary with different ages. For younger children there should be an attempt to provide experiences that will teach basic health habits such as cleanliness and the importance of a well-balanced diet. Such settings as the cafeteria, lavatory, and medical examination room offer these opportunities. As the individual grows older, the scientific reasons for following certain health practices can be presented. Some of the areas of health knowledge that should be understood by students and adults include nutrition, the need for rest, sleep, and exercise, protection of the body against changing temperature conditions, contagious disease control, drugs, environmental pollution, family living, human sexuality, the dangers of self-medication, and community resources for health.* If such topics are brought to the attention of persons everywhere and if the proper health attitudes and practices are developed, better health will result.

Knowledge of what constitutes adequate health services should also be understood. Such health services as health appraisal, health counseling, family and marriage counseling, genetic counseling, communicable disease control, education of the handicapped, and emergency care of injuries should be appreciated by all. Only as this knowledge is imparted will the various services be utilized in a manner most conducive to the health of students.

Development of desirable health attitudes. The term *health attitudes* refers to the health interests of the individual or the motives that impel the person to act in a certain way. All the health knowledge that can be accumulated will have little worth unless the individual is interested and motivated to the point that he or she wants to apply this knowledge to everyday living. Attitudes, motives, drives, or impulses, if properly established, will result in the individual's seeking out scientific knowledge and utilizing it as a guide to living. This interest, drive, or motivation must be dynamic to the point where it results in behavior changes.

School and college health programs must be directed at developing those attitudes that will result in optimal health. Students should have an interest in, and be motivated toward, possessing a state of buoyant health, being well rested and well fed, feeling emotionally secure, and possessing the physical ability to perform life's routine tasks. They should have the right attitudes toward health knowledge, healthful school living, and health services. If such interests as these exist within the individual, proper health practices will be followed. Health should not be an end in itself except in cases of severe illness. Health is a means to an end, a medium that aids in achieving a state of well-being and contributes to enriched living.

Another factor that motivates individuals to good health is the desire to avoid the pain and disturbances that accompany ill health. People do not like toothaches, headaches, or indigestion because of the pain or distraction involved. However, developing health attitudes in a negative manner, through fear of pain or other disagreeable conditions, is a questionable approach.

A strong argument for developing proper attitudes or interests should center around the goals one is trying to achieve in life and the manner in which optimal health is an aid in achieving such goals. This is the strongest incentive or interest that can be developed in the

---

*See also Chapter 12.

individual. If one wishes to become a great artist, an outstanding businessman, or a famous dancer, it is greatly beneficial if he or she has good health. This is important so that the study, training, hard work, trials, and obstacles that one encounters can be met successfully. Optimal health will aid in the accomplishment of such goals. As Jennings, the biologist, has pointed out, the body can attend to only one thing at a time. If its attention is focused on a toothache, a headache, or an ulcer, it cannot be focused satisfactorily on some essential work that has to be done. Centering health attitudes or interests on life goals is dynamic because these attitudes represent an aid to accomplishment, achievement, and enjoyable living.

Development of desirable health practices. Desirable health practices represent the application of those habits that are most beneficial, according to the most qualified thinking in the field, to one's routine of living. The health practices that an individual adopts will determine in great measure the health of that person. If practices or habits harmful to optimal health are engaged in, such as failure to obtain proper rest or exercise,

overeating, overdrinking, smoking, and the use of harmful drugs and failure to observe certain precautions against contracting diseases, then poor health is likely to follow.

Knowledge does not necessarily ensure good health practices. An individual may have at his or her command all the statistics concerning the results of speeding at 70 miles per hour and the need for seat belts, but unless this information is applied it is useless. The health of an individual can be affected only by applying that which is known. At the same time, knowledge will not usually be applied unless an incentive, interest, or attitude exists that impels its application. It can be seen, therefore, that in order to have a good school health program, it is important to recognize the close relationship that exists among health knowledge, health attitudes, and health practices.

State and professional associations promote objectives

A significant advance at the state level was developed in New York State. As a result of the increased awareness of health problems,

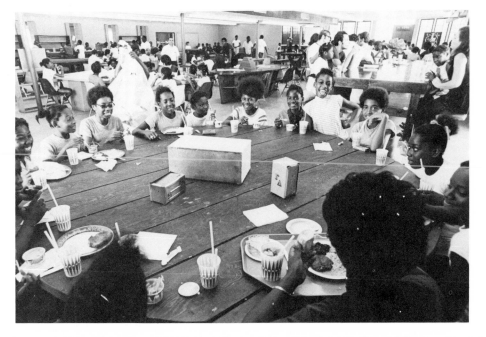

Young boys and girls participating at Miami-Dade Junior College North in the National Summer Youth Sports Program enjoy one of the well balanced free lunches they received each day. (Courtesy President's Council on Physical Fitness and Sports, which helped to sponsor this program.)

including the widespread use of drugs and narcotics, tobacco, and alcohol, the Speno-Brydges Bill was passed in May, 1967. This law required the teaching of health in all grades throughout the state of New York. A new health curriculum was developed and the program introduced in 1970. As a result of this legislation and the increased interest in health on the part of the citizens of this state, schoolchildren are receiving instruction in the critical health areas of tobacco, drugs, alcohol, and family living and also in such areas as nutrition, mental and emotional health, disease prevention and control, and accident prevention.

In 1971, The American Alliance for Health, Physical Education, and Recreation (AAHPER) drafted a position statement concerning recommendations for a comprehensive program of health instruction that provided a unified approach to the teaching of health. The recommendations included the following:

1. A program of health education should be unified and organized in such a manner that there is scope and sequence from Kindergarten through grade twelve.
2. A program of curriculum development should be undertaken that will stress (a) the identification of specific courses with content, learning activities, and evaluation requirements, and (b) coordination and integration with other subject areas.
3. The health curriculum should be jointly developed by school personnel, curriculum specialists, individuals from public and voluntary health agencies, and national and state consultants.
4. Health teachers should be specialists in health education and have a genuine interest in this field.

The AAHPER statement is increasingly reflected in health curriculums that have been recently established. A sequential and unified curriculum taught by health specialists is definitely what one will find in the future of health education.

OBJECTIVES OF SCHOOL AND COLLEGE PHYSICAL EDUCATION PROGRAMS*

A study of the individual reveals four general directions or phases in which growth and development take place—physical development, motor development, cognitive development,

---

*Bucher, C. A.: Foundations of physical education, ed. 7, St. Louis, 1975, The C.V. Mosby Co.

and social development. Physical education plays an important part in contributing to each of these phases of human growth and development.

The physical development objective. The physical development objective deals with the program of activities that builds physical power in an individual through the development of the various organ systems of the body. It results in the ability to sustain adaptive effort, the ability to recover, and the ability to resist fatigue. The value of this objective is based on the fact that an individual will be more active, have better performance, and be healthier if the organ systems of the body are adequately developed and functioning properly.

Muscular activity plays a major role in the development of the organ systems of the body. The *organ systems* include the digestive, circulatory, excretory, heat regulatory, respiratory, and other systems of the human body. These systems are stimulated and developed through such activities as hanging, climbing, running, throwing, leaping, carrying, and jumping. Health is also related to muscular activity; therefore, activities that bring into play all of the fundamental big muscle groups in the body should be engaged in regularly. Furthermore, the activity should be of a vigorous nature so that the various organ systems are sufficiently stimulated.

Through vigorous muscular activity several beneficial results take place. The developed heart provides better nourishment to the entire body. It beats slower and pumps more blood per stroke, with the result that more food is delivered to the cells and there is more efficient removal of waste products. During exercise the developed heart's speed increases more slowly and has a longer rest period between beats. After exercise it returns to normal much more rapidly. The end result of this state is that the individual who exercizes regularly is able to perform work for a longer period of time, with less expenditure of energy and much more efficiency, than the individual who exercizes little or not at all. This trained condition is necessary for a vigorous and abundant life. From the time an individual rises in the morning until he goes to bed at night, he or she is con-

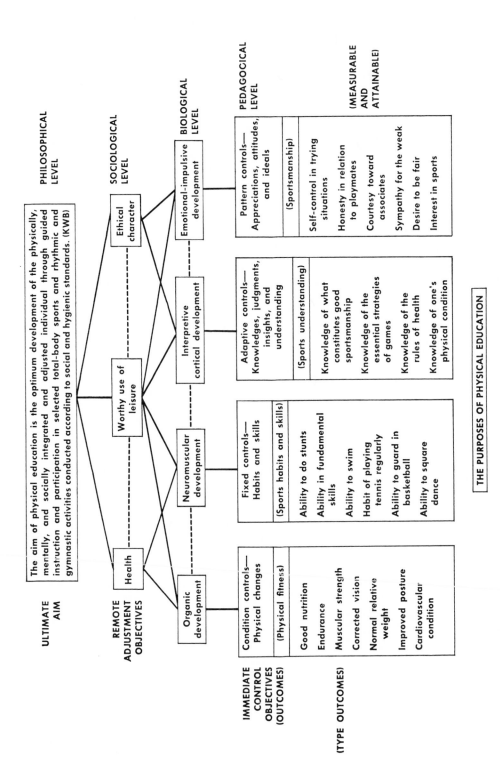

THE PURPOSES OF PHYSICAL EDUCATION

Objectives of physical education. (From Bookwalter, K. W.: Physical education in the secondary schools, Washington, D. C., 1964, The Center for Applied Research in Education, Inc.)

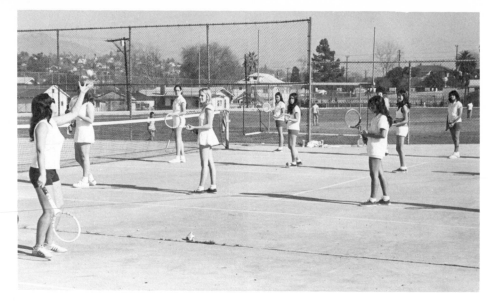

Girls at Franklin High School in Los Angeles developing skill in tennis. Los Angeles Unified School District, Student Auxiliary Services Branch. (Courtesy Gwen R. Waters.)

tinually in need of vitality, strength, endurance, and stamina to perform routine tasks, be prepared for emergencies, and lead a vigorous life. Therefore, physical education aids in the development of the trained individual so that he or she will be better able to perform routine tasks and live a healthy, interesting, and happy existence.

The motor development objective. The motor development objective is concerned with performing physical movement with as little expenditure of energy as possible and in a proficient, graceful, and esthetic manner. This has implications for one's work, play, and anything else that requires physical movement. The name *motor* is derived from relationship to a nerve or nerve fiber that connects the central nervous system, or a ganglion, with a muscle. Movement results, as a consequence of the impulse it transmits. The impulse it delivers is known as the motor impulse.

Effective motor movement is dependent upon a harmonious working together of the muscular and nervous systems. It results in greater distance between fatigue and peak performance; it is found in activities involving running, hanging, jumping, dodging, leaping, kicking, bending, twisting, carrying, and throwing; and

it will enable one to perform his or her daily work much more efficiently and without reaching the point of exhaustion so quickly.

In physical education activities, the function of efficient body movement, or neuromuscular skill as it is often called, is to provide the individual with the ability to perform with a degree of proficiency. This will result in greater enjoyment of participation. Most individuals enjoy doing those particular activities in which they have acquired a degree of mastery or skill. For example, if a child has mastered the ability to throw a ball consistently to a designated spot and has developed batting and fielding power, he or she will like to play baseball or softball. If he or she can swim 25 or 50 yards without tiring and can perform several dives, he or she will enjoy being in the water. If an adult can consistently serve tennis "aces," he or she will like tennis; if one can drive a ball 250 yards straight down the fairway, one will like golf; and if one can throw ringers, one will like horseshoes. A person enjoys doing those things in which he or she excels. Few individuals enjoy participating in activities in which they have little skill. Therefore, it is the objective of physical education to develop in each individual as many physical skills as possible so that interests will be wide and varied. This will not only result in more enjoyment for the participant, but at the same time will allow for better adjustment to group situations.

Physical skills are not developed in one lesson. It takes years to acquire coordination, and the most important period for development is during the formative years of a child's growth. The building of coordination starts in childhood, when an individual attempts to synchronize the muscular and nervous systems for such movements as creeping, walking, running, and jumping. A study of kinesiology shows that many muscles of the body are used in even the most simple of coordinated movements. Therefore, in order to obtain efficient motor movement or skill in many activities, it is necessary to start training early in life and to continue into adulthood. Furthermore, a child does not object to the continual trial-and-error process of achieving success in the performance of physical acts. He or she does not object to being observed as an awkward, uncoordinated beginner during the learning period. Most adults, however, are self-conscious when going through the period of learning a physical skill. They do not like to perform if they cannot perform in a creditable manner. The skills they do not acquire in their youth are many times never acquired. Therefore, the physical education profession should try to see that this skill learning takes place at a time when a person is young and willing and is laying the foundation for adult years.

The motor development objective also has important implications for the health and recreational phases of the program. The skills that children acquire will determine to a great extent how their leisure time will be spent. One enjoys participating in those activities in which one excels. Therefore, if a child excels in swimming, a great deal of his or her leisure time is going to be spent at a pool, lake, or beach. If he or she excels in tennis, he or she will be found on the courts on Saturdays, Sundays, and after dinner at night. There is believed to be a correlation between juvenile delinquency and lack of constructive leisure-time activity. If we want children to spend their leisure moments in a physically wholesome way, we should see that skills are gained in physical education activities.

The cognitive development objective. The cognitive development objective is concerned with the accumulation of a body of knowledge and the ability to think and interpret this knowledge.

Physical activities must be learned; hence, there is a need for thinking on the part of the intellectual mechanism, with a resulting acquisition of knowledge. The coordination involved in various movements must be mastered and adapted to the environment in which the individual lives, whether it be in walking, running, or wielding a tennis racquet. In all these movements the child must think and coordinate muscular and nervous systems. Furthermore, this type of knowledge is acquired through trial and error. Then, as a result of experience, there is a changed meaning in the situation. Coordination is learned, with the result that an act once difficult and awkward to perform becomes easy to execute.

The individual should not only learn coordination but should also acquire a knowledge of rules, techniques, and strategies involved in physical activities. Basketball can be used as an example. In this sport a person should know the rules, the strategy in offense and defense, the various types of passes, the difference between screening and blocking, and finally the values that are derived from playing in this sport. Techniques that are learned through experience result in knowledge that is also acquired. For example, a ball travels faster and more accurately if one steps with a pass, and time is saved when the pass is made from the same position in which it is received. Furthermore, a knowledge of leadership, courage, self-reliance, assistance to others, safety, and adaptation to group patterns is very important.

Knowledge concerning health should play an important part in the program. All individuals should know about their bodies, the importance of sanitation, factors in disease prevention, the importance of exercise, the need for a well-balanced diet, values of good health attitudes and habits, and the community and school agencies that provide health services. This knowledge will contribute greatly to physical prowess as well as to general health. Through the accumulation of a knowledge of these facts, activities will take on a new meaning and health practices will be associated with definite purposes. This will help each individual to live a healthier and more purposeful life.

In physical education activities one also gains insight into human nature. The various forms of activity in physical education are social experiences that enable a participant to learn about human nature. For all children and youth this is one of the main sources of such knowledge. Such knowledge contributes to social efficiency and good human relations.

The social development objective. The social objective is concerned with helping an individual make personal adjustments, group adjustments, and adjustments as a member of society. Activities in the physical education program offer one of the best opportunities for making these adjustments, if there is proper leadership.

Social action is a result of certain hereditary traits and learned behavior. There are interests, hungers, desires, ideals, attitudes, and emotional drives that are involved in everything we do. A child wants to play because of the drive for physical activity. A man will steal food because of the hunger drive. The responses to all these desires, drives, and hungers, may be either social or antisocial in nature. The value of physical education reveals itself when we realize that play activities are one of the oldest and most fundamental drives in human nature. Therefore, by providing the child with a satisfying experience in activities in which he or she has a natural desire to engage, the opportunity is presented to develop desirable social traits. The key is qualified leadership.

All human beings should experience success. This factor can be realized through play.

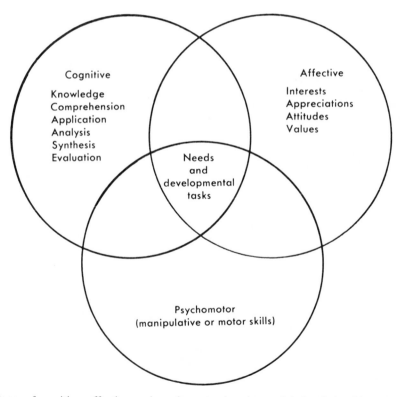

Interdependence of cognitive, affective, and psychomotor domains, and their relationship to needs and developmental tasks. (From Tanner, D.: Using behavioral objectives in the classroom, New York, 1972, The Macmillan Co.)

Through successful experience in play activities, a child develops self-confidence and finds happiness in his achievements. Physical education can provide for this successful experience by offering a variety of activities and developing the skills necessary for successful achievement.

In a democratic society all individuals should develop a sense of group consciousness and cooperative living. This should be one of the most important objectives of the physical education program. Whether or not a child will grow up to be a good citizen and contribute to the welfare of society will depend to a great extent upon the training he or she receives during youth. Therefore, in various play activities, the following factors should be stressed: aid for the less-skilled and weaker players, respect for the rights of others, subordination of one's desires to the will of the group, and realization that cooperative living is essential to the success of society. The individual should be made to feel that he or she belongs to the group and has the responsibility of directing his or her actions in its behalf. The rules of sportsmanship should be developed and practiced in all activities that are offered in the program. Courtesy, sympathy, truthfulness, fairness, honesty, respect for authority, and abiding by the rules will help a great deal in the promotion of social efficiency. The necessity for good leadership and the ability to follow should also be stressed as important to the interests of society.

A MODERN CONCEPT OF INSTRUCTIONAL OBJECTIVES

Behavioral or instructional objectives are being more widely used in order to better assess learning outcomes of students and teacher performance or accountability. Bloom, Krathwohl, and their associates* developed a threefold division of instructional objectives that included the following areas: (1) cognitive: recognition of knowledge and development of intellectual ability; (2) affective: changes in interest, attitudes, and values; and (3) psychomotor: development of manipulative or motor skills.

*Tanner, D.: Using behavioral objectives in the classroom, New York, 1972, The Macmillan Co.

These three areas or domains are interdependent, as shown in the figure on p. 44, but may also be examined independently in relation to general or specific curriculum objectives. Any instructional objective, whether it is learning how to swim or how to play a musical instrument, should take these three domains into consideration in establishing the learning process.

THE ROLE OF ADMINISTRATION IN ACHIEVING OBJECTIVES

Good administration is an essential in the fields of school and college health education and physical education if the goals that have been set for these professions are to be realized. Harmony must be encouraged among the various members of the staff, adequate facilities provided, the program planned and continually reevaluated, a public relations plan established, leadership provided, and many other essentials and details attended to with dispatch if the objectives are to be achieved.

The administrator is a key person; he or she sets the pace and provides the leadership. If this individual does not assume the responsibilities that go with such a position, there will be apathy and indifference throughout the organization or department, and consequently the aims for which the profession exists will not be realized. Administrators must continually keep in mind the goals toward which they are working. With these in mind they should gear their staff relationships, programs, and other factors in a way that will be most efficient and productive from the standpoint of realizing such goals.

Administrators frequently have the areas of both health and physical education within their administrative division. This affords the opportunity to promote the kind of cooperation that is needed to achieve the aims of each. One cannot be promoted at the expense of the other. One cannot be recognized as being more important than the other. If such is the practice, progress will be obstructed. Administrators must recognize the important place that each area has in the total picture. All administrative policies must preserve this balance.

If the administrators have only one of these

specialized areas within their division, this should not limit their relationship with the other. Both areas are closely allied and it is very important that they work closely together. Administrators will determine in large measure whether or not this becomes a reality.

PROFESSIONAL ORGANIZATIONS

Administrators should be familiar with the role of professional organizations in their work. They should realize that these associations help in the achievement of objectives, promote professional ethics, scholarship, leadership, and high educational standards.

Some of the organizations with which the health educator and physical educator should be familiar are listed below.*

National Education Association
American Alliance for Health, Physical Education, and Recreation
National Recreation and Park Association
American Academy of Physical Education
American School Health Association
National College Physical Education Association for Men
National Association of Physical Education for College Women
National Junior College Athletic Association
American Physical Therapy Association
Society of State Directors of Health, Physical Education, and Recreation
American Youth Hostels, Inc.
Young Women's Christian Association
Physical Education Society of the Young Men's Christian Associations of North America
Boy's Clubs of America
National Collegiate Athletic Association
National Association of Intercollegiate Athletics
Canadian Physical Education Association
Delta Psi Kappa
Phi Delta Pi
Phi Epsilon Kappa
American College of Sports Medicine

Questions and exercises

1. Survey ten schools or colleges in your area to determine the administrative relationship of health and physical education.
2. Why is it important for health and physical educators to work closely together?
3. Prepare a research paper on the reasons why health

*For a detailed discussion of these organizations, refer to Chapter 20 in Bucher, C.A.: Foundations of physical education, ed. 7, St. Louis, 1975, The C.V. Mosby Co.

and physical education were incorporated in the national association.

4. Why are both health and physical education specialists needed in the schools?
5. Define health and physical education.
6. List and discuss the objectives of both school and college health and physical education.
7. Interview or correspond with five health educators and five physical educators on the main problems confronting their professions.
8. To what extent are the objectives of school and college health and physical education being achieved today?
9. Define the term *school health program* Discuss the various aspects of the program.
10. Why are health attitudes so important?
11. What are the goals of physical education in addition to developing an individual physically?
12. What are some of the benefits to an individual that come from physical activity?
13. What is meant by a modern concept of instructional objective?
14. Why must there be cooperation to achieve the objectives in health and physical education? What part does the administrator play?

Reading assignment in *Administrative Dimensions of Health and Physical Education Programs, Including Athletics:* Chapter 2, Selections 5 to 10.

Selected references

American Association for Health, Physical Education, and Recreation: Health concepts—guides for health instruction, Washington, D. C., 1966, The Association.
American Association for Health, Physical Education, and Recreation: Knowledge and understanding in physical education, Washington, D. C., 1969, The Association.
American Association for Health, Physical Education, and Recreation: Physical education for college men and women, Washington, D. C., 1965, The Association.
Bauer, W. W.: Teach health, not disease, Journal of Health and Physical Education **12:**296, 1941.
Bookwalter, K. W.: Physical education in the secondary schools, New York, 1964, The Center for Applied Research in Education, Inc. (The Library of Education).
Braza, G. F.: The status and administration of required health courses—a resume, The Journal of School Health **41:**142, 1971.
Bucher, C. A.: Foundations of physical education, ed. 7, St. Louis, 1975, The C.V. Mosby Co.
Bucher, C. A.: Physical education for life, St. Louis, 1969, McGraw-Hill Book Co. (A textbook for high school courses in physical education.)
Bucher, C. A., and Dupee, R. K., Jr.: Athletics in schools and colleges, New York, 1965, The Center for Applied Research in Education, Inc. (The Library of Education).
Bucher, C. A., and Koenig, C.: Methods and materials for secondary school physical education, ed. 4, St. Louis, 1974, The C.V. Mosby Co.
Bucher, C. A., Olsen, E. A., and Willgoose, C. E.: The

foundations of health, New York, 1967, Appleton-Century-Crofts.

Bucher, C. A., and Reade, E. M.: Physical education and health in the elementary school, ed. 2, New York, 1971, The Macmillan Co.

Byrd, O. E.: School health administration, Philadelphia, 1964, W. B. Saunders Co.

Hicks, D. A.: Professional preparation of health educators in the 70's, The Journal of School Health **42:**243, 1972.

Irwin, L. W., and Mayshark, C.: Health education in secondary schools, St. Louis, 1968, The C.V. Mosby Co.

Joint Committee on Health Problems in Education of National Education Association and American Medical Association: Healthful school living, Washington, D. C., 1969, National Education Association.

Joint Committee on Health Problems in Education of National Education Association and American Medical Association: Health education, Washington, D. C., 1961, National Education Association.

Joint Committee on Health Problems in Education of National Education Association and American Medical Association: School health services, Washington, D. C., 1964, National Education Association.

Moore, C. A.: Changes: relevance or responsibility, Journal of Health, Physical Education and Recreation **44:**27, 1973.

National Committee on School Health Policies of the National Conference for Cooperation in Health Education: Suggested school health policies, ed. 3, Washington, D. C., 1966, National Education Association.

Neff, F. C.: Philosophy and American education, New York, 1966, The Center for Applied Research in Education, Inc. (The Library of Education).

Oberteuffer, D., and Beyrer, M. K.: School health education, ed. 4, New York, 1966, Harper & Row, Publishers.

Randall, H. B.: School health in the seventies, The Journal of School Health **41:**125, 1971.

Smolensky, J., and Bonvechio, L. R.: Principles of school health, Boston, 1966, D. C. Heath & Co.

Tanner, D.: Using behavioral objectives in the classroom, New York, 1972, The Macmillan Co.

A unified approach to health teaching—AAHPER position statement: The Journal of School Health **41:**171, 1971.

Willgoose, C. E.: Health education in the elementary school, ed. 2, Philadelphia, 1964, W. B. Saunders Co.

The administrative setting

Educational administration has changed with the increased complexity of the settings and services administered. As a result, the educational administrator today is a highly qualified, well-educated individual who must bring diverse abilities to his or her position. He or she must possess the traits of a teacher, philosopher, business executive, social worker, psychologist, public relations expert, architect, speaker, as well as many other desirable characteristics.

The educational administrator must approach his or her position with a desire to serve the students, teachers, and other school employees, parents, and the community at large. He or she must be involved in decisions that affect the entire school and community. Effective administration is dependent on the close cooperation of the administrator and his or her subordinates.

PRINCIPLES THAT ACT AS GUIDELINES FOR THE ADMINISTRATIVE STRUCTURE OF AN ORGANIZATION

Experts in many areas have compiled principles to aid in effective administration of an organization. Some of the most meaningful principles are given here.

1. *The administrative structure of an organization should clarify the delegation of authority and responsibility.* In order that the goals of the organization be efficiently and successfully met, the administration must delegate some of its powers to responsible agents. These powers should be clearly defined to avoid overlapping authority.
2. *Successful administration is dependent upon communication.* Communication is essential in avoiding duplication and waste and in aiding cooperation among departments.
3. *Coordination and cooperation among various departments in an organization are essential to effective administration.* Coordination of departments keeps them well-informed and working together in a complementary manner.
4. *The administrator must be an effective leader.* An effective leader is one who appreciates both the goals of the organization and the personnel working for the organization. Both are of extreme importance.
5. *Staff specialization aids effective administration.* In order to obtain their objectives, organizations must perform many different tasks requiring the abilities of various area specialists.
6. *Authority must be commensurate with responsibilities and lines of authority must be clearly drawn.* An organization chart is the best way to illustrate the chain of command. It is essential that the lines of authority be unambiguous.

ADMINISTRATIVE CHANGES IN SCHOOL ORGANIZATION
School districts

The school administration carries out its duties in a larger school district than was formerly the case, as a result of reorganization,

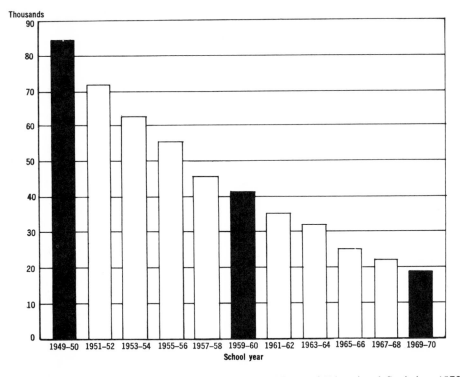

The number of school districts continues to decline. (From Digest of Educational Statistics, 1972 edition, National Center for Educational Statistics, U. S. Department of Health, Education and Welfare, Washington, D. C.)

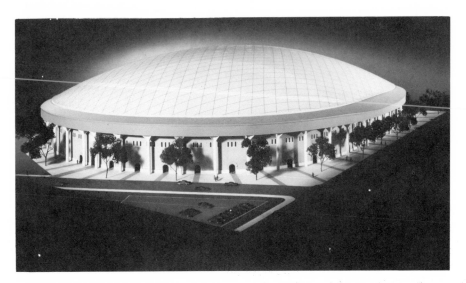

The proposed future administrative setting for athletics at the University of Minnesota. (Courtesy Gassner Nathan Browne, Architects Planners Inc., Memphis, Tenn.; Otto Baitz, Photography of Architecture, Cliffwood, N. J.)

centralization, and consolidation. The number of districts employing only a few teachers is declining rapidly. Enlargement of school districts has been necessary because of (1) the growth of student population, (2) small district financial problems, and (3) inadequate curricula.

The school district is the basic administrative unit for the operation of local elementary and secondary schools and is a quasimunicipal corporation established by the state. This basic educational unit ranges through the United States from a one-teacher rural system to a large metropolitan system serving thousands of pupils. A system may be an independent governmental unit or part of a state government, county, or other local administrative unit. The governing body of the system is the school board. The chief administrative officer is the superintendent of schools. The number of basic administrative units reported in 1931 and 1932 was 127,531. Today, there are less than 20,000 administrative units.

State and federal control

Traditionally, local communities have exercised almost complete control over local education, and the state has not interfered with local operations of school programs. Today, however, local communities have transferred some of their influence over education to state and federal governmental units. The control has advanced proportionately as the amount of state and federal financial aid to schools has increased. If school systems do not have quality educational programs as outlined by the state, fail to follow state and federal laws in such matters as civil rights, or fail to meet certain stipulations as attached to the use of governmental funds, such financial help can be withheld. This threat of withholding monies is proving to be a strong means of bringing local school districts into line with what is desired by state and federal authorities.

Patterns of school organization

The pattern of school organization at the elementary and secondary levels is in a period of transition. Some of the present patterns of school organization are as follows:

1. The traditional high school or 8-4 system—Under this type of organization the 4-year high school is preceded by the 8-year elementary school.
2. The combined junior and senior high school or 6-6 or 7-5 plan—Under this type of organization the junior and senior high schools are combined under one principal.
3. The emphasis upon junior high school or 6-3-3 system—Under this plan the junior high schools are grouped separately under one principal. Although the junior high school usually includes grades seven through nine, there are exceptions to this type of organization.
4. The 4-year high school or 6-2-4 system—Under this plan the 4-year high school is similar to the traditional high school in organization, and the junior high school consists of two grades.
5. The middle school or 4-4-4 plan—This type of organization retains the old high school idea but usually groups the early elementary grades together and the fifth to eighth (or other) grades in one unit.

There are many arguments that can be set forth for each plan of school organization or such other plans as the 6-3-3-2 or the 8-4-2, which includes 2 years of community college. The physical, psychologic, and sociologic aspects of the school setting and of child growth and development, the need for effective communication between schools, the range of subjects, the facilities provided, and the preparation of teachers are all pertinent to the type of administrative organization selected.

SCHOOL AND COLLEGE STRUCTURE

In this section the roles of the board of trustees, board of education, president of a college, superintendent of schools, principal and other administrative personnel, and lay groups will be discussed, as well as the place of physical education and health education within the educational framework. Much of this information applies directly to the school structure where most health education and physical education personnel are employed.

The college and university structure is analogous in some ways to the structure of the school system. For example, many of the administrative functions of a board of trustees of a college are similar in scope to those of a board of education, and the president of a college has duties similar in some respects to a superintendent of schools. The director of physical education or the director of health education

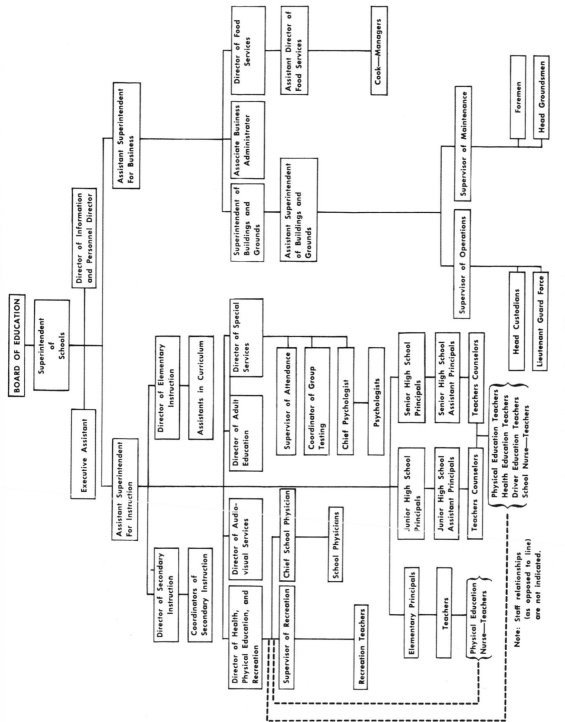

An organization chart for a public school system.

must perform many of the same duties in a college as the director does in a school system. A brief discussion of the college and university structure is included here to show the aspects of the structure that are especially unique to higher education.

A college or university is characterized by a governing board, usually known as a board of trustees, which is granted extensive powers of control by legislative enactment or by its charter. The governing board of a college usually delegates many of its powers to the administration and faculty of the institution. The administrative officers, usually headed by a president, are commonly organized into such principal areas of administration as academic, student personnel services, business, and public relations. The members of the faculty are usually organized into colleges, schools, divisions, and departments of instruction and research. In large institutions one frequently finds a university senate that is the voice of the faculty and that serves as a liaison between faculty and administration. The areas of health and physical education can have school, division, or department status. The duties of a dean, director, or chairman correspond in many ways

to those of a director of health or physical education in a school system.

Board of education, school committee, or board of directors*

The board of education is the legal administrative authority created by the state legislature for each school district. The responsibility of the board is to act on behalf of the residents of the district it represents. It has the duty of appraising and planning the educational program on a local basis. It selects executive personnel and performs duties essential to the successful operation of the schools within the district. The board develops policies that are legal and in the interest of the people it serves. It devises financial means within the legal framework to support the cost of the educational plan. It keeps its constituents informed of the effectiveness and needs of the total program.

Some of the more specific powers of boards

---

*The term *board of education* is used in this discussion although *school committee, community–school boards,* and *board of directors* are used in some sections of the country.

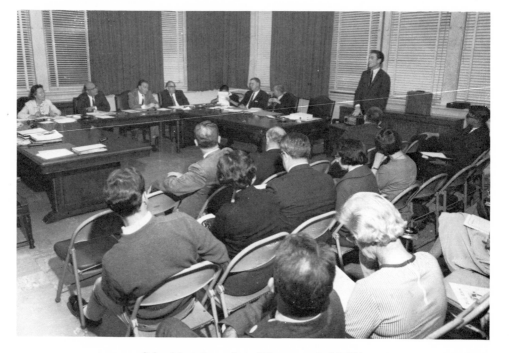

School board meeting. (Mamaroneck, N. Y.)

of education include purchasing property, planning school buildings, determining the educational program, securing personnel, levying taxes for school purposes, approving courses of study, determining the school calendar, and providing for the school census. The powers of boards of education are fixed by state statutory enactment.

The qualifications for board members are very few. There are usually general requirements that specify citizenship, age, residence, and sometimes ownership of property. In many communities women are playing very prominent roles on school boards. According to surveys that have been conducted, boards of education usually include individuals who are past middle age, have been successful in their community, and are conservative in nature. There has been an improvement in recent years in the organization and composition of boards of education. The addition of women and individuals who are nonpartisan in their outlook, the organization of smaller and less cumbersome boards, and provisions for longer terms of office are resulting in a more stable educational policy.

Boards of education vary in size. There is the usual three-member board in the common-school district that represents the independent one- or two-room school setup. Township boards of education range from five to nine members, county boards from three to fifteen, and city boards from three to sixteen. The trend is toward small boards of education. Board of education members are appointed in some cases, and in others they are elected.

The National School Boards Association has indicated the following characteristics of school boards in forty-two cities throughout the nation having more than 300,000 population.

Most school boards have seven, five, or nine members, in that order. Three cities have boards with fifteen members. The composition of school board members (3% women and 13% black) is broken down as follows: businessmen, 103; lawyers, 66; housewives, 51; physicians, 22; ministers, 11; and college professors, 8.

Most of the 137,000 members of the nation's 25,000 school boards are elected. Among the large cities, only Philadelphia, Pittsburgh, and Washington, D. C., choose boards through a committee of court judges. In Boston, Detroit, Los Angeles, and St. Louis, school boards are elected.

There is a growing feeling among professional and lay leaders alike for the need of reform in respect to school board operations. Reforms have been advocated by such an important group as the New York Committee on Educational Leadership and are receiving support in some of the more progressive sections of the country. These reforms include (1) the transfer of all administrative functions that encumber school board operations to the superintendent of schools, (2) better procedures for screening school board members so that the office seeks the person rather than the person seeks the office, (3) elimination of the annual public vote on the school budget where required and substituting budget hearings in its place, and (4) improved procedures for selecting superintendents of schools.

General administrative personnel

The administrative personnel that will be discussed include the superintendent of schools, assistant superintendent, clerk of the board, principal, supervisor, director, and lay groups.

Superintendent of schools. Within a large school system where many schools are involved there is a superintendent who has overall charge of the school program. Associate or assistant superintendents are in charge of technical detail, management, or various phases of the program, such as secondary education. There is also a superintendent's position associated with smaller schools. These officers are known as district superintendents. They are responsible for many schools extending over a wide geographic area.

The superintendent's job is to carry out the educational policies of the state and the board of education. He or she acts as the leader in educational matters in the community and also provides the board of education with the professional advice it needs as a lay organization. From an executive standpoint, the superintendent appraises the entire educational program over which he or she has control, working closely with the board of education to eliminate weaknesses and to establish a strong system of education. Any large organization needs leadership; so too does the educational system of any community.

The qualifications for the position of superintendent vary in different communities. In some villages and cities the individual must be a resident and in others this is not necessary. The educational requirement varies greatly from community to community. Some communities require a doctorate and others require a minimum of professional training. There is a trend, however, in the direction of increased education. Most superintendents of schools have their bachelor and master's degrees and an increasing number have taken work beyond the master's. Many have their doctorates. Both teaching and administrative experience are frequently listed as requirements.

Assistant superintendent for business services or school business administrator. The business administrator serves as director of business affairs and of buildings and grounds. In a college or university there is also one administrative officer who carries out similar duties. The business administrator usually has direct supervision of the business office staff, the building service and maintenance staff, and general supervision of the custodial staff. He or she has responsibility for supervising the operation and maintenance of all buildings and grounds. He or she may perform the duties of the superintendent as directed in the superintendent's absence. (Chapter 4 is devoted to a detailed discussion of the school business administrator.)

Assistant superintendent or director of instructional services. The director of instruction has under his or her direct supervision the divisions of elementary education, secondary education, adult education, health and physical education, music education, vocational and practical arts, summer school education, and inservice training of teachers. He or she gives major consideration to the development of curriculum materials, to organization, and to the supervision of instruction and teaching. The director of instruction may perform the duties of the superintendent of schools as di-

rected in the superintendent's absence. In a college or university the administrative officer in charge of the academic program could be a vice-president, dean, provost, or other officer.

Assistant superintendent or director of personnel services. The director of personnel supervises both professional and nonprofessional employees. He or she recruits and interviews candidates for positions. He or she is usually responsible for all pupil personnel services, guidance and psychologic services, handicapped children and special services, as well as attendance and adjustment, including pupil accounting. This administrator may supervise and coordinate the medical services, including medical, dental, and nurse-teacher services. This director may coordinate and direct the publications and information services and carry on testing and research activities. He or she may perform the duties of the superintendent as directed in the superintendent's absence. In a college or university many of these responsibilities are carried out by a dean of men or a dean of women.

Clerk of the board. The clerk of the board of education is usually under the direction of the superintendent of schools. He or she has custody of the seal of the board, notifies members of the board of regular and special meetings, and has charge of files and records of the board. The clerk sees that all files and records are properly maintained, presents a periodic financial statement, and supervises accounting for tuition pupils. He or she preaudits and certifies all bills, examines and certifies all payrolls, and keeps an active insurance register. The clerk usually conducts the annual school election and keeps the bond and coupon register of the board and public library, together with necessary reports of bonds and interest due.

Principal. The position of principal is very similar to that of the superintendent. It differs mainly in respect to the extent or scope of responsibility. Whereas the superintendent is usually in charge of all the schools within a particular community, the principal is in charge of one particular school. The duties of the principal include responsibility for executing educational policy as outlined by the superintendent, appraising the educational offering,

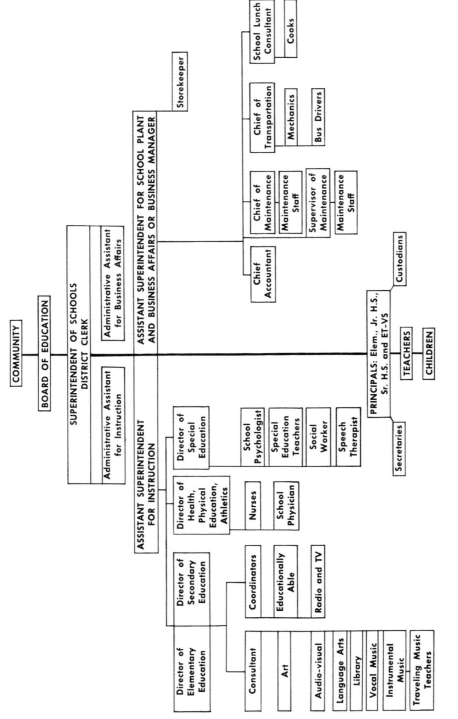

The operational organization chart clarifies channels of communication for the employees of the school district. The superintendent administers school district policies through the assistant superintendents, and they in turn utilize intermediate staff members in the process.

making periodic reports on various aspects of the program, directing the instructional program, promoting good relationships between the community and the school, and supervising the maintenance of the physical plant.

In many school situations, principals teach in addition to their administrative responsibilities. Some conduct extracurricular activites such as leading the band or coaching a varsity athletic team. Some principals have responsibilities on only one school level, but where various levels are combined in one structural unit, this responsibility may extend from the high school level down through the junior high school and even to the elementary school.

The qualifications for the position of principal vary. There is in evidence a trend toward increased academic qualifications for such positions. Some communities feel that the principal should have more academic preparation than the teachers.

Boards of education must select school administrators from the individuals available. The prestige, salary, security, and other factors that the positions offer play an important part in determining the quality of individual who can be secured.

Supervisor. This position usually implies a responsibility associated with the improvement of instruction. In some cases the assignment might be much broader in scope and in corporate responsibility for the entire elementary or secondary instructional program. In most cases, however, it usually applies to specific subject matter areas.

Director. The role of the director involves responsibility for functions of specific subject matter area or a particular educational level. The responsibilities have administrative as well as supervisory implications.

Director of health, physical education, and recreation. A common position to be found in educational systems is that of director of health, physical education, and recreation. In some cases a special certificate is granted for a director of health, physical education, and recreation after a stated program of studies has been accomplished, a stated amount of experience has been had, and other requirements met. Other communities and states have directors of health and physical education. Some have directors of physical education, directors of health, and directors of recreation where the fields of specialization are completely separated.

In a college or university there may be a director who heads up the entire physical education program and a director in charge of the health program, or the two fields may be combined into the same administrative unit, whether it be a college, school, division, or department.

A director's position exists to provide leadership, programs, facilities, and other essentials in these special areas. Specific areas of responsibility for a director of health, physical education, and recreation in general include the following:

General duties
1. Implement standards established by the state Department of Education and the local board of education. (In a college this would be the university administration.)
2. Interview possible candidates for positions in the special areas and make recommendations for these positions.
3. Work closely with the assistant superintendent in charge of business affairs, assistant superintendent in charge of instruction, and subject matter and classroom teachers.
4. Coordinate areas of health, physical education, and recreation.
5. Supervise all inside and outside facilities, equipment, and supplies concerned with special areas—this responsibility includes maintenance, safety, and replacement operations.
6. Maintain liaison with community groups—this responsibility includes such duties as holding educational meetings with doctors and dentists to interpret and improve the school health program, scheduling school facilities for community groups, and serving on various community committees for youth needs.
7. Prepare periodic reports regarding areas of activity.
8. Coordinate school civil defense activities in some school systems.
9. Serve on the school health council.

Health
1. Health services—in some cases include the supervision of school nurse teachers and dental hygiene teachers and coordination of the work of school physicians. Other responsibilities include preparation of guides and policies for the program of health services, organization of health projects, and obtaining proper equipment and supplies.
2. Health science instruction—includes supervision of health education programs throughout the school

system, preparation of curriculum guides and research studies, and upgrading the program in general.

3. Healthful school living—includes general supervision of school plant, psychologic aspects of school program, and formation of recommendations for improvement.

Physical education

1. Supervise total physical education program (class, adapted, intramurals, extramurals, and varsity interscholastic or intercollegiate athletics).
2. Administer schedules, practice and game facilities, insurance, and equipment.
3. Maintain liaison with county, district, and state professional groups.
4. Upgrade program in general.

Recreation

1. Supervise various aspects of the recreation program that, in addition to school program, may include summer and vacation playgrounds, teen centers, and so on.
2. Obtain, where necessary, facilities, equipment, personnel, and supplies.
3. Plan and administer program.

Women in administration

The inequities that women suffer in being excluded from leadership positions in education are enormous. Recent surveys indicate that although women still constitute 67% of the total teaching force, 97% of secondary school principals and more than 99% of superintendents are men. Men dominate the majority of educational leadership positions on all levels including the federal and state departments of education.

There are also disparities in salary among those women who do achieve administrative positions. Census data reveal that the average salary among 80,000 male school administrators in 1970 was $13,625. The average salary for 18,000 female school administrators was about $5,000 less. It was also found that women administrators do not progress as quickly as their male counterparts. Women are usually older than men in similar administrative positions.

Many studies have been conducted that establish that women do indeed make excellent administrators. Women frequently show greater ability to work with people and are more knowledgeable concerning teaching methods and techniques.

With all the data supporting female administrators, why are men chosen over women for leadership positions? Some of the reasons that have been given are:

1. Men usually dominate in school boards, teacher associations, research organizations, and professional groups.
2. Men usually dominate in education policy-making groups.
3. Men hold many leadership positions in the National Education Association and the American Federation of Teachers.

What is being done to change the pattern of discrimination against women in education? Professional groups have given their support for the passage of the Equal Rights Amendment to the U. S. Constitution. Conferences on the status of women have been held to educate people about the position of women in education. However, there is still much to accomplish. Discrimination of any type, including sex discrimination, has no place in our schools.

Lay groups

The general public is participating more and more in the work of schools and colleges. Parent-teacher associations, citizens' councils, alumni groups, and study groups are a few of the organizations that express the lay opinion of the community in regard to educational matters. This interest on the part of the public should be encouraged and helped in every way possible. There are more than 10 million members of parent-teacher associations throughout the country. The public school program should reflect what the public wants and thinks is best for their children. This can be accomplished only through active "lay" participation. Administrators and other school personnel should make sure that the citizens of the community are adequately informed in respect to educational matters so that the best type of program may be developed.

HEALTH WITHIN THE SCHOOL AND COLLEGE STRUCTURE*

The superintendent and principal or president and dean have the main responsibility for school and college health programs. The attitude they have toward health and the degree to which

---

*See also Chapters 12, 13, and 14.

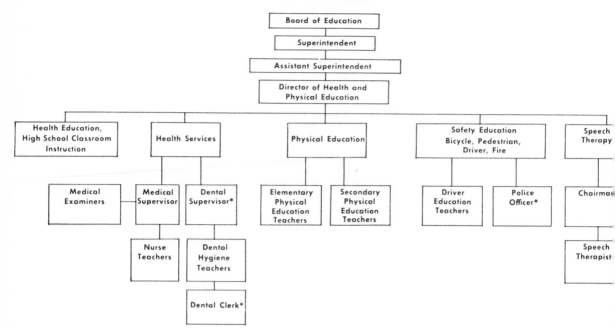

The director of health and physical education in the school structure.

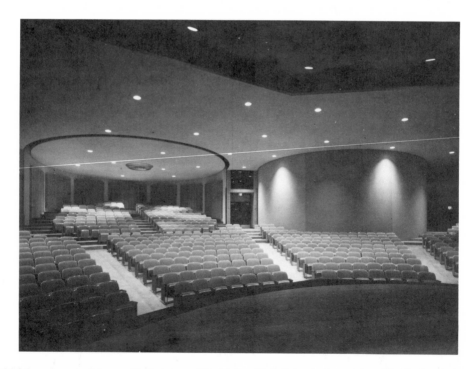

A healthful environment is provided at Agua Fria Union High School, Avondale, Ariz. Pods can be opened or shut as space is needed. (Photograph by Koppes.)

they recognize the importance of achieving professional objectives will determine the success of the school health program.

Administrators must recognize certain important principles in regard to health so that it may have an important place in the total school and college program. The following are basic concepts: Health should be an important and integral part of the overall educational program. All teachers and other personnel should understand and appreciate the importance of promoting health and the contributions they can make through their own work toward realizing such a goal. There should be individuals on the staff who have had special training in this field so that they may take the leadership in developing and promoting an adequate program. There should be coordination of the various instructional aspects of the educational program to ensure adequate coverage of health information and to avoid unnecessary overlapping. There should be provision for concentrated health teaching. Adequate facilities, time, money, and personnel should be provided to carry on this special work properly. A close working arrangement with the community should be recognized as an essential to a well-developed program. There should be a statement of policies in regard to health that is clear and understood by all.

Terminology for the school and college health program. The following definitions were drawn up by the Committee on Terminology that represented the American Association for Health, Physical Education, and Recreation, the Society of Public Health Educators, and the American Public Health Association. It is presented here for the reader's information.*

Cumulative school health record—A form used to note pertinent consecutive information about a student's health.

Dental examination—A procedure conducted by a dentist to determine all oral conditions including the normal as well as disease. It may include the use of x-rays.

Dental inspection—Observation and a limited evaluation of the oral structures to determine the presence of obvious

defects to be followed by referral to a dentist. The dental inspection provides an educational opportunity to encourage good oral practices including periodic visits to a dentist.

Health appraisal—The evaluation of the health status of the individual through the utilization of varied organized and systematic procedures such as medical and dental examinations, laboratory test, health history, teacher observation, etc.

Health counseling—A method of interpreting to students or their parents the findings of health appraisals and encouraging and assisting them to take such action as needed to realize their fullest potential.

Health environment—The promotion, maintenance, and utilization of safe and wholesome surroundings, organization of day-by-day experiences, and planned learning procedures to favorably influence emotional, physical, and social health.

Health instruction—The process of providing a sequence of planned and spontaneously originated learning opportunities comprising the organized aspects of health education in the school community.

Health observation—The estimation of an individual's well-being by noting the nature of his appearance and behavior.

Medical examination—The evaluation by a physician of the medical status of an individual.

Safety education—The process of providing or utilizing experiences for favorably influencing understandings, attitudes, and practices relating to safe living.

School health coordination—A process designed to bring about a harmonious working relationship among the various personnel and groups in the school and community that have interest, concern, and responsibility for development and conduct of the school health program.

School health education—That health education process associated with health activities planned and conducted under the supervision of school personnel with involvement of appropriate community health personnel and utilization of appropriate community resources.

School health program—The composite of procedures and activities designed to protect and promote the well-being of students and school personnel. The procedures and activities include those organized in: school health services, providing a healthful environment, and health education.

School health services—That part of the school health program provided by physicians, nurses, dentists, health educators, other allied health personnel, social workers, teachers, and others to appraise, protect, and promote the health of students and school personnel. Such procedures are designed to: (1) appraise the health status of pupils and school personnel, (2) counsel pupils, teachers, parents, and others for the purpose of helping pupils obtain health care and for arranging school programs in keeping with their needs, (3) help prevent and control communicable diseases, (4) provide emergency care for injury or sudden illness, (5) promote and provide optimal sanitary conditions and safe facilities, (6) protect and

*Report of the Joint Committee on Health Education Terminology, Journal of Health, Physical Education, and Recreation **33**:27, 1962, and the Report of the Joint Committee on Health Education Terminology, School Health Review **4**:25, 1973.

promote the health of school personnel, and (7) provide concurrent learning opportunities that are conducive to the maintenance and promotion of individual and community health.

Screening test—A medically and educationally acceptable procedure for identifying individuals who need to be referred for further study or diagnostic examination.

Essential aspects of the school and college health program. Health within the educational structure will be discussed under three headings: health instruction, health services, and healthful school and college living.

*Health instruction.** In the area of health science instruction, scientific knowledge is imparted and experiences are provided so that students may better understand the importance of developing good attitudes and health practices. Information concerning such subjects as nutrition, communicable disease, health quackery, rest, exercise, sanitation, drugs, alcohol, tobacco, environmental pollution, human sexuality, first aid, and safety is presented.

On the elementary level the responsibility for such health education rests primarily with the classroom teacher, although in some school systems trained specialists are provided as resource persons. On the secondary and college levels, it is recommended that individuals who have had special training in heath education be responsible for concentrated health instruction. This is not always the case. Sometimes, in the absence of a trained health specialist, the teacher of physical education, home economics, or science is given the responsibility. This procedure, however, is not always desirable because of the lack of necessary qualifications by persons other than specialists.

A concentrated course in health education should be required of all students for at least 1 and preferably 2 years at the secondary level. Some states are now requiring health in every grade. At the college level there should be at least a one-semester health course for all students. Health educators should teach such courses, and these subjects should be given the same credit and time allotments as other important causes.

The possibilities for health education should also be recognized in the various experiences the child has in school. When the school physician gives the medical examination, the dental hygienist examines the child's teeth, an emergency concerned with health exists in the community, or the curiosity of the child is aroused, "teachable moments" for imparting health information are presented. This type of health education often leaves a greater impression upon young minds than the more formal classroom teaching.

*Health services.** The health services phase of school and college health programs includes health appraisal, health counseling, correction of defects, provision for the exceptional child, prevention and control of communicable disease, and emergency care of injuries.

In this phase of the health program it is important to recognize concern for mental, emotional, social, and physical health. In providing health services that include all these phases of health, several persons in addition to the health educator play prominent roles.

The classroom teacher has an important responsibility in health services. He or she is probably closer to the child than any other person on the staff and therefore can detect deviations from the normal. The teacher is also in a position to give good advice, provide first aid when necessary, administer certain screening tests, and oversee the general welfare of the child.

The nurse plays a prominent role in the administration of the health program. Through counseling, acting as a resource person for other staff members, developing close relationships with parents, helping physicians, and other responsibilities peculiar to her profession, the nurse is a key person.

The physician has the potential for playing a very important part in school and college programs. Through medical examinations, health guidance, protection of students from communicable diseases, development of health policies, and consultations with parents, it is possible for the physician to exercise a great force for good in the health of the students and parents with whom he comes in contact. It has been the observation of many educators, how-

---

*See also Chapter 12.

*See also Chapter 13.

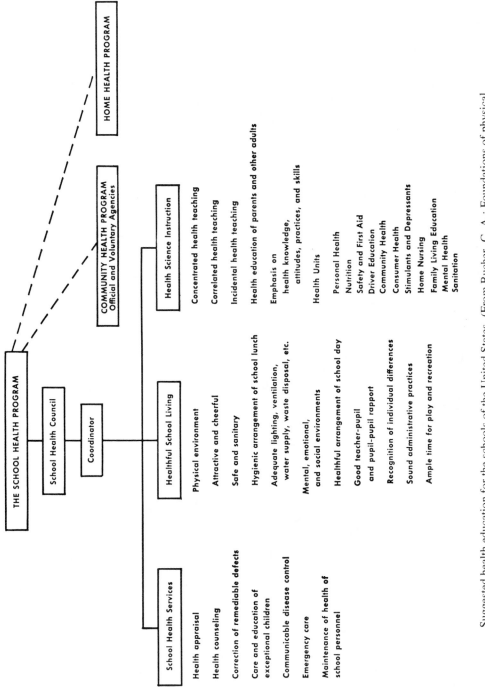

Suggested health education for the schools of the United States. (From Bucher, C. A.: Foundations of physical education, ed. 7, St. Louis, 1975, The C. V. Mosby Co.)

ever, that the physician often does not realize the educationsl implications of his role in the health program. As a result, he does not take advantage of teachable moments that occur whenever a student is being given a medical examination or when conferences are held with parents.

Dentists and dental hygienists play an important role wherever their services are provided. These specialists appraise the dental needs of students. Here again there is an unlimited opportunity to educate the student and the parent on the importance of proper oral hygiene.

Psychologists, psychiatrists, social workers, guidance counselors, speech therapists, and others are increasingly being brought into school and college health services programs. All have an important part to play and contribution to make to the total health of young people who attend schools and colleges in this country.

*Healthful school and college living.** Healthful living is also an important part of the total health program. In addition to a healthful physical environment, a wholesome emotional environment must also be provided. Both are important to the health of the student.

The physical environment should provide an attractive, safe, and wholesome place for students to congregate. This implies that such important considerations as lighting, ventilation, heating, location, sanitary facilities, play space, equipment, and other essentials are adequately provided for in the buildings and areas that are used for educational purposes. It also means there is proper maintenance by the custodial staff and includes any other factors that influence the physical arrangements of the school or college plant.

The emotional environment is just as important to the student's health as the physical one. To ensure a wholesome emotional environment, proper rapport must exist between the teacher and pupils and among the pupils themselves; educational practices pertinent to such matters as grades, promotions, assignments, schedules, play periods, attendance, class conduct, and discipline must be sound; and the teachers themselves must be emotionally well adjusted.

---

*See also Chapter 14.

Other phases of health administration. There are two other aspects of the health program that need special attention—the health council and the health coordinator.

The health council. Every school and every school system should have health councils or committees to help ensure a desirable and adequate health program. This means that there should be a health council for each school and one central health council for all the schools in a particular school system. The number of members comprising such councils may vary from three or four persons in a small school to fifteen or sixteen in a larger school. Potential members of such councils are the school principal, health coordinator, nurse, psychologist, guidance counselor, custodian, dental hygienist, speech therapist, physician, dentist, physical education teacher, science teacher, home economics teacher, classroom teacher, teacher of handicapped persons, nutritionist, students, parents, public health officer, mayor, clergymen, and any other individual who is particularly related to the health of the school or community and has something to contribute.

Health councils are responsible for coordinating the entire health program of the school. This would include determining subject matter to be taught, resources to be utilized, and experiences to be provided; securing a healthful environment for the school; arranging inservice training in health related areas; encouraging closer school-parent relationships in respect to such important health procedures as medical examinations; promoting sanitary conditions; providing for the safety of children; and distributing health literature.

Representatives from various community and school groups that are interested in health can accomplish much when sitting around a conference table discussing their problems. A spirit of cooperation and "oneness" will aid in developing procedures and taking action that will promote better health for all.

Health coordinator. Health affects many subject matter areas, the school plant, educational practices, and practically every aspect of school life. It is important therefore to have coordination. This means that responsibility must be fixed in one person. By having someone responsible it is possible to integrate health

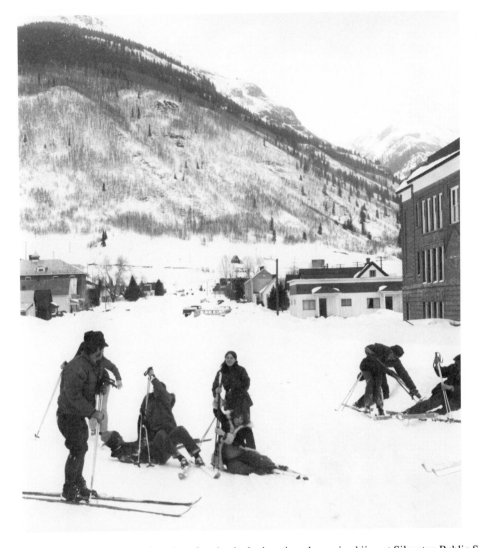

The out-of-doors provides an attractive place for physical education classes in skiing at Silverton Public Schools in Silverton, Colo. (Courtesy George Pastor.)

into the total education program and the total community health program.

As a result of the need for coordination of the various phases of health, many schools have appointed health coordinators. In some places this individual is known by another title such as health consultant or health educator. This person, in most cases, is appointed by the administration and has particular qualifications for the job.

The responsibilities of the health coordinator include such duties as integrating and correlat-

ing the various phases of health education in the subject matter areas, channeling health information to staff members, keeping records, preparing reports periodically on pertinent health matters, providing leadership for health councils, seeing that established health policies are carried out, appraising and evaluating the total health program, arranging special health examinations when needed, counseling students on health problems, aiding the physician in the performance of his duties, helping in the maintenance of a healthful environment, organizing safety and other programs that promote health, and helping in furthering school-home relationships.

PHYSICAL EDUCATION WITHIN THE SCHOOL AND COLLEGE STRUCTURE

Physical education is increasingly occupying a more important role in the school and college curriculum. During its early history, physical education was regarded by general school administrators as a fad, an appendage to the educational program, or a necessary evil to be tolerated. In recent years, however, it has been viewed by an increasing number of educators as an integral part of the total educational offering with many potentialities for contributing to enriched living.

Terminology in physical education. Components of the physical education program are characterized by many and varied terms. Since there has been no committee established to work out descriptive terms for the various phases of the program, as in the case of the health program, there is lack of uniformity within the profession. The suggestion is made that the four components of the physical education program, into which it logically divides itself, be called (1) the required class or basic instruction program, (2) the adapted program, (3) the intramural and extramural athletics program, and (4) the varsity interschool or intercollegiate athletics program.

The *required class* or *basic instruction program* is the provision of physical education for all students and is characterized by instruction in such matters as the rules, strategies, and skills in the various activities that comprise the program.

The *adapted program* refers to that phase of physical education that meets the needs of the individual who, because of some physical inadequacy, functional defect capable of being improved through exercise, or other deficiency, is temporarily or permanently unable to take part in the regular physical education program.

The *intramural and extramural athletics program* is voluntary physical education for all students within one or a few schools or colleges. It is characterized by such events as

competitive leagues and tournaments and play and sports days and acts as a laboratory period for the required class program. In the intramural program activities are conducted for students of only one school or college, while in the extramural program students from more than one school or college participate.

The *varsity interschool or intercollegiate athletics program* is designed for the skilled individuals in one school or college who compete with skilled individuals from another school or college in selected physical education activities.

Departments. The various departments of physical education throughout the country have many different plans of organization. A few years ago it was quite common to see such titles as Department of Physical Culture or Hygiene. The term *physical training* was also used as a descriptive term for the work performed in this special area.

Today, one also sees a variety of titles associated with physical education, such as the "Physical Education Department," "Department of Ergonomics and Physical Education," the "Department of Biokinetics," "Health and Physical Education Department," and the "Health, Physical Education, and Recreation Division." Camping and safety may also be included.

The titles that are given also show to some degree the particular work that is performed within these phases of the total program. In some schools and colleges physical education is organized into a separate unit with the various physical activities—intramural, extramural, and interschool or intercollegiate athletics—comprising this division. In other schools and colleges, health and physical education are combined in one administrative unit. In some cases, although the word *health* is used, there is little evidence of the particular specialized type of health work as it is known today. This is also true where the word *recreation* is used in the title. In the discussion to follow, the term *physical education* will be used.

There is usually a person designated as head or chairperson of the physical education department. The title of director of physical education is also used. In smaller schools, it is quite com-

SCHOOL AND COLLEGE PHYSICAL EDUCATION PROGRAM			
Chairman of Department			
The Basic Instructional Class Program	**Adapted Program**	**Intramural and Extramural Athletics Program**	**Varsity Interscholastic or Intercollegiate Athletics Program**
Instructional in nature	For special students including those with:	Competitive leagues and tournaments, play and sports days, etc.	For skilled boys, girls, men, and women
Required of all students	Faulty body mechanics	Voluntary in nature	Voluntary in nature
Daily period	Nutritional disturbances (over- and underweight)	For all students	Conducted during out-of-school hours
Credit given	Heart and lung disturbances	Conducted during out-of-class hours	Organized and administered with needs of participant in mind
Variety of activities	Postoperative and convalescent cases	Laboratory period for required class program	Rec.: For high school and college students only
Movement education	Hernias, weak and flat feet, menstrual disorders, etc.	Wide variety of activities based on needs and interests of students	Wide variety of activities based on needs and interests of students
Team games	Nervous instability		
Dual and individual games	Poor physical fitness	Rec.: Intramural athletics— fourth grade through college	
Rhythms and dances	Crippling conditions (infantile paralysis, etc.)	Rec.: Extramural athletics— seventh grade through college	
Games of low organization	Cultural deprivation Mental retardation Emotional disturbance Poor coordination		
Gymnastics	Provision for physical, mental, emotional, and social welfare of student		
Aquatics	Provision for program during regular class and special classes		
	Restricted and remedial physical activity		
	Utilization of special conditioning exercises, aquatics, and recreational sports		
	Harmonious working relationships with medical and nursing personnel		

mon to have only one man and one woman on the physical education staff, each acting as the head of his or her separate division.

The duties of the head of a physical education department include coordinating the activities within the particular administrative unit, requisitioning supplies and equipment, preparing schedules, making budgets, holding departmental meetings, teaching classes, coaching, hiring and dismissing personnel, developing community relations, supervising the intramural, extramural, and interscholastic programs, evaluating and appraising the required class program, representing the department at meetings, reporting to the principal, and having overall responsibility for the activities carried on.

The required class or basic instruction program.* In some states this phase of the program is required by state law, and in others it is governed by a local regulation. In a few schools and colleges participation is not required but voluntary. Classes are scheduled in much the same way as other subjects. Students, however, are too often assigned on the basis of administrative convenience rather than on the basis of homogeneity. Physical education people have advocated assigning students to

---

*See also Chapter 7.

classes in a way that would result in their realizing the greatest physical, social, and other benefits pertinent to this field of work. However, too few schools and colleges have followed these recommendations. The emphasis in the class program is instructional, and various games and activities are offered at different levels in the school program. On the elementary level, movement education, rhythmic activities, and simple games are stressed, whereas on the secondary level there is a change to more highly organized games and sports.

A survey of the country will show many inferior programs of physical education if they are compared to the standards that have been set for the profession. In many communities the required class program, although serving the entire student body, is hampered by lack of time, facilities, and leadership. Stress on varsity sports and lack of administrative support have also been influential factors. Furthermore, women have consistently been neglected in school physical education programs. This neglect has compounded the inferiority of many programs. This will be discussed in detail later in this chapter. The leadership that is found in some physical education programs is not resourceful, dynamic, and capable of promoting a sound program.

Where excellent required class or basic instruction programs of physical education exist, they have been developed on the basis of the physical, social, mental, and emotional needs of the students. A broad and varied program of activities, both outdoor and indoor, progressively arranged and adapted to the capacities and abilities of each student, is offered.

The adapted program. * One of the weakest phases of modern physical education programs is the lack of an effective adapted program at all educational levels. Since pupils should be required to take physical education each day they are in school, regardless of their physical condition or how they feel, the program must be adapted to their needs. The boy or girl should not be made to fit the physical education program. Instead, the physical education program should fit the individual. The child with a his-

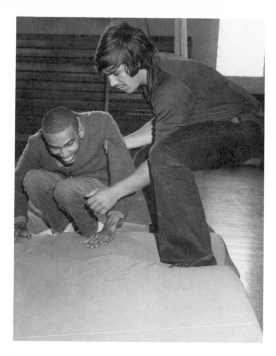

Boy being helped in adapted physical education program at the University of Bridgeport. (Courtesy Arnold College Division, University of Bridgeport, Conn. Parents and Friends Association of Mentally Retarded Children.) (Photograph by John Tasker.)

tory of rheumatic fever, the boy who has just returned from having an operation to remove his appendix, the girl who suffers menstrual difficulties, culturally disadvantaged students, and pupils with other health problems can all receive benefits from the physical education program, provided it is geared to their individual differences.

Special physical education programs must also meet the needs of the mentally retarded, physically handicapped, emotionally disturbed, and neurologically impaired children. To ensure the cooperation of parents, administrators, and others and to work out the best possible program, there should be a close working relationship between the nursing, medical, and other health professions. This procedure will also help to ensure that the prescription recommended properly fits the student's needs. Another consideration that cannot be overlooked is having qualified teachers assigned to the adapted program. The effectiveness of

---

*See also Chapter 8.

such a program will depend to a great extent upon the type of leadership that is provided.

The intramural and extramural athletics program. * The goal of the intramural and extramural program is to provide competition in games, sports, and other physical activities. This program is in addition to the required class or basic instruction program. Whereas the required class or basic instruction program is designed to be largely instructional in nature so that basic fundamentals for playing various activities can be learned, the intramural and extramural program is designed to provide an opportunity for students to utilize these learned skills in actual competitive situations.

There is a place in the intramural and extramural program for all students, regardless of degree of skill, strength, age, or field of specialization. It offers an opportunity for friendly competition between groups from the same school or college. Sometimes "sports" and "play" days are also included. These special events involve students from one or many schools who are invited to participate. Teams are composed of students from the same school and college and from many different schools and colleges.

As many as 90% or 95% of the students participate in the intramural and extramural programs where there is an active interest. Since these programs are conducted on a voluntary basis, this indicates the amount of enthusiasm and interest that can be generated through a well-organized program. High attendance in such a program usually reflects a broad offering of activities, with leagues or some other unit of competition, organized in a manner that appeals to the interest and needs of the students.

In small schools and colleges, intramural and extramural programs are usually conducted by one or two persons who are also in charge of the required class or basic instruction program. This places an additional workload on such individuals and consequently some fail to develop the type of program that could be offered if more personnel were available. In larger schools and colleges it is quite common to have a director of intramural athletics. This places the responsibility on one person and usually results in a better-organized and more effective program.

Close coordination should exist between the required class and intramural and extramural programs. Furthermore, department members, student managers, and interested faculty members should be encouraged to help in the conduct of the program. For the best administration of intramural and extramural programs, most schools also give careful consideration to units of competition; a program of fall, winter, and spring activities; eligibility requirements; provisions for medical examination; preliminary training periods; scheduling; variation in types of tournaments; coaching; and awards.

The varsity interschool and intercollegiate athletics program. * The varsity interschool program in athletics is designed for the individuals most highly skilled in sports. It is one of the most interesting and receives more publicity than the other two phases of physical education in the school setup. The reason for this is not that it is more important or renders a greater contribution; instead, it is largely the result of its popular appeal. The fact that sports writers and others discuss it in glowing terms and that it involves competition that pits one school or college against another school or college also increases its public appeal. A spirit of rivalry develops. This seems to be characteristic of the American culture.

The varsity interschool and intercollegiate athletics program has probably had more difficulties attached to it than any of the other phases of the physical education program. The desire to win and to increase gate receipts has resulted in some very unfortunate practices such as unethical recruitment policies, admission of students who are frequently academically unqualified, and extensive public relations programs. Large stadiums and sports palaces have been constructed that require large financial outlays for their upkeep.

Sex discrimination in physical education programs, especially in interschool and intercollegiate athletic programs, has been blatant. Many schools and colleges have no female

*See also Chapter 9.

*See also Chapter 10.

representation involved in interschool competition. Women have long been baton twirlers and cheerleaders but rarely seen as athletes.

When women's teams are represented, they often play preliminary games that serve as time-fillers prior to the male varsity team games. Their budgets are much less than that of the male teams, and their transportation is frequently restricted because of budgetary demands. In addition, they frequently have no uniform allowance (they wear their class gymsuits), no trainers, assistant coaches, scorekeepers, and water boys, and even their facilities and equipment are inferior.

Some solutions to these inequities are as follows:

1. Attitudes concerning women in athletics must be changed.
2. Activities should not be designated by sex but rather by interest and ability.
3. The fact that physical activity is not harmful to female reproductive organs must be stressed.
4. Facilities must be made available on an equal basis for boys and girls.
5. Court action should be considered when sex discrimination is pervasive and apparent.
6. People must be treated as individuals and not stereotyped by sex.

In some schools and colleges the interschool phase of the program comes under a director of athletics. It is his or her responsibility to arrange the schedules, make the necessary arrangements for athletic events, such as securing officials, and to care for the numerous details essential to a well-organized program. For many schools and colleges smaller in size, the individual or individuals who administer the required class and intramural and extramural programs also administer the interschool phase of the total physical education program. Since all are closely related, utilize the same personnel in most cases, share the same facilities, and are interested in achieving the same objectives, it is important that they all come under the jurisdiction of the same department. Such an organization makes it possible for all to accomplish their purposes under the leadership of an individual who recognizes the value and place of each in a well-rounded program.

In connection with financing athletic programs, many schools have what is called a general organization, which is in charge of the finances not only for the athletic program but also for other school activities, such as dramatics and music. This has been used with success in some schools and takes the financial responsibility out of the physical education department and places it in an impartial organization.

Other items of particular importance that should be arranged for in the administration of athletics are provision for medical supervision and an accident plan. Both should be carefully considered by any school desiring to have a sound athletics program.

The organization of physical education in colleges and universities

Physical education is organized as one administrative unit for men and women in a majority of colleges and universities in the United States. The administrative unit may be either a college, school, division, or department; the administrator in charge of the physical education program may be called a dean, director, supervisor, or chairman. In many institutions of higher learning this administrator is responsible directly to the president or to a dean, but in a few instances, he is responsible to the director of athletics. (In a majority of colleges, athletics are included as part of the same administrative setup with the rest of the physical education program.) In many cases the duties of the athletic director and the administrator of the physical education program are assigned to the same person. Many colleges and universities have intramural athletic directors, since in most of these institutions intramural athletics are a part of the physical education program.

Professional programs in physical education are a part of the physical education program at both the undergraduate and the graduate levels. Physical education and health *education* are frequently combined into the same administrative unit, but health *services,* as a general rule, are not organized as part of the physical education unit. Physical education is commonly responsible for the administration of recreation programs for both students and faculty.

State College Board of Trustees

President of the College

Vice President

or

Dean of the College

Associate Dean or Head ———— Executive Committee: All Department Chairmen

School of Physical Education, Health, and Recreation

Chairman, Department of Physical Education, Men	Chairman, Department of Physical Education, Women	Chairman, Department of Health Education	Chairman, Department of Recreation	Chairman, Department of Intercollegiate Athletics, Men (Director of Athletics)
Advisory Committee	Advisory Committee	Advisory Committee	Advisory Committee	Advisory Committee
Basic Instruction for Men	Basic Instruction for Women	Undergraduate Professional Curriculum	Undergraduate Professional Curriculum	Administration of Intercollegiate Athletics
Undergraduate Professional Curriculum	Undergraduate Professional Curriculum	Service Courses in First Aid	Service Courses, General Elementary Teachers	Coordination of Athletic Coaching Courses
Graduate Professional Curriculum	Graduate Professional Curriculum	State Field Service	Campus Recreation	Coordination of Intercollegiate Athletic Schedules
Intramural Sports	Intramural Sports	Coordination With Community Health Services	State Field Service	Coordination of Teaching Services of Coaches
Supervision of Sports Facilities	Extramural Sports	Health Education Institutes and Workshops	Administration of Outdoor Education Center	Coordination of Maintenance and Use of Athletic Facilities
Supervision of Aquatics	Dance Productions	Public and Private School Consultations	Recreation Institutes and Workshops	Coordination of Conference Affiliation, National Collegiate Athletic Association, American Amateur Athletic Union, etc.
Faculty-Staff and Community Instructional Services	Faculty-Staff and Community Instructional Services		Coordination with Community Recreation Services	
Research Laboratory	Research Laboratory		Public, Private, and Commercial Recreation Consultations	

Organization chart for a school of physical education, health, and recreation. (Developed by Don Adee.)

THE TWO-YEAR COLLEGE

The junior college, or community college as it is sometimes called, deserves special mention because this type of institution is expanding at such a rapid rate and will continue to do so as the number of college-bound students rise. This means that more and more high school boys and girls upon graduation will find their educational opportunities in this kind of college.

Though there are exceptions, most junior colleges (and by this term the community college is included) have the following three functions:

1. To give 2 years of preprofessional training or general education. A student may graduate with an associate degree in the arts or sciences after 2 years or transfer to a 4-year institution for a bachelor's degree. This transfer program is sometimes called the university parallel curriculum. Most 4-year colleges and universities will accept transfer students from accredited

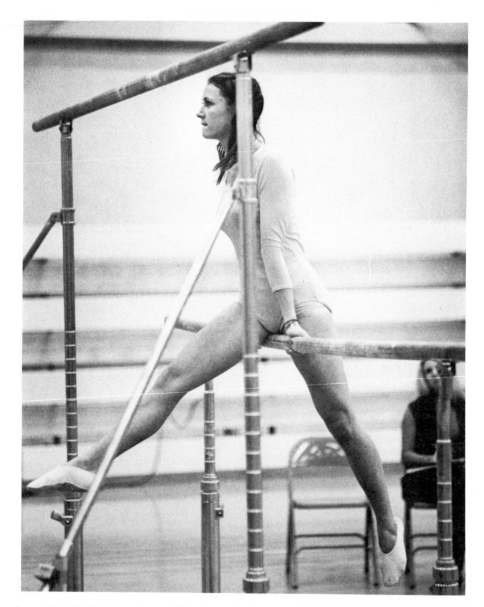

Women's varsity athletics has a large following at College of DuPage, Glen Ellyn, Ill. The college offers women opportunities in volleyball, football, swimming, tennis, softball, basketball, and gymnastics.

junior colleges if the academic achievement of the student is high and if the subjects studied are comparable to the curriculum of the higher institution.

2. To provide a complete program in a semiprofessional field such as secretarial work, home economics, medical laboratory techniques, drafting, and business education.

3. To provide classes for adults who want more education to help them in their jobs or who simply want to study subjects they never had a chance to study before.

The type of curricula offered by junior colleges is usually controlled by the needs and interests of the students they serve. Some junior college curricula are planned almost entirely for students who want a general education and who plan to transfer to a 4-year institution. Other junior colleges enroll the majority of students in semiprofessional courses.

A junior college in an agricultural area may feature agricultural courses, whereas another junior college in an industrial community may specialize in courses that prepare young people for jobs in nearby factories.

In respect to physical education and health education in the 2-year college, surveys conducted indicate that the pattern of 2 hours weekly for ½ unit credit is the most frequent procedure for physical education. Objectives in most cases stress the students' competence in maintaining good health and balanced personal adjustment. Some colleges are seriously attempting to meet these objectives, but others have not yet developed their programs sufficiently to accomplish this task. Athletics appear to be an especially strong point of physical education at the junior college level because of the great student and public interest. Some colleges provide broad programs of team com-

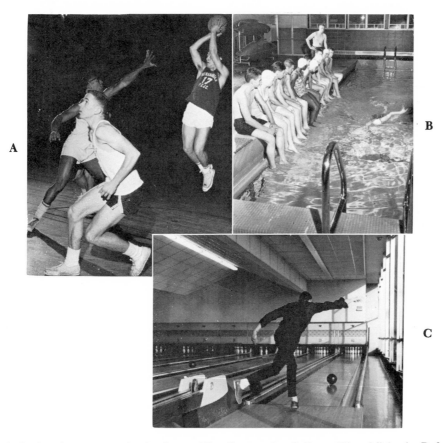

The physical education program in the 2-year Flint Community College, Flint, Mich. **A,** Defense is not stressed by all teams in the intramural league. **B,** All swimming classes are coeducational. Classes for beginning swimmers through water safety instructor courses are offered. **C,** Commercial alleys are used for bowling classes.

petition in many sports, whereas others are very limited.

Many 2-year colleges are offering a certificate in the field of parks and recreation. It is estimated that by 1980 more than 100 such institutions will offer this type of certificate. The person holding this type of associate degree can be involved in planning, organizing, and conducting recreational activities in such settings as hospitals, military bases, industrial organizations, and local agencies. However, unless these persons continue their education, their administrative and supervisory responsibilities will be minimal.

Most 2-year colleges have a health service program for their students, but instruction in personal and community hygiene or health is less usual than instruction in physical education. Where a health course is offered, it is usually a one-semester course for 2 credits.

Interviews with deans of instruction, faculty, and students of 2-year colleges indicate that they prefer to have one department chairperson in charge of both the health and physical education programs. The department chairperson usually is responsible to the dean of students or dean of instruction.

COMMUNITY ORGANIZATION FOR HEALTH

It is important to understand not only the structure of the school and college but also that of the larger community of which it is a part. If programs of health and physical education are to render the most valuable service at the community level, their leaders must clearly understand its structural organization. This important level of government touches human lives to a great degree.

Public health organization at the local level

Health department. There are few, if any, local departments with more important functions than the health department. In spite of this, the amount of money set aside and the emphasis placed on this phase of government are usually less than that spent on many other areas, such as for police or fire protection.

The department of health also works more closely with other branches of local government than most other departments. For example, it is closely related to bureaus having control of water supply and purification, garbage collection and disposal, sewerage system and street cleaning, and police department enforcement of the sanitary code. It also works with officers in charge of education, especially in regard to medical and dental examination of school children. Such essential relationships make it imperative to have a local health department that functions efficiently.

In some cities governed by a commission, health is combined with police and fire administration to form a department of public safety. However, in most cities, especially the larger ones, there is a separate department of health. At the head of the health department in these larger cities there is usually a board of health or a commission, headed by a health commissioner. In a few cities the health activities are guided by a single commissioner, who is appointed by the mayor or city council.

In many cases small or medium-sized cities and villages do not employ full-time health officers, and the public health activities are cared for by a physician who devotes only part time to this work. Under such conditions, a health department in the full sense of the term does not exist and the public health activities are bound to be limited.

On some occasions, two or three small communities have felt the need for full-time health personnel and consequently have pooled their efforts and resources and have combined to develop a joint health administration with a full-time health officer. This has resulted in advantages to all communities concerned. It is hoped that this policy will be used to a greater extent by small villages, towns, and cities located within a short enough radius to make such a system practical.

The recognized, successful health departments in larger cities have boards of health presided over by a commissioner of health. These boards enact the sanitary code of the city, issue emergency health orders, and have been given broad powers in all health matters. In some emergency situations such a group has been given the power to imprison persons, destroy property, forbid traffic, and perform similar duties to prevent the spread of disease.

The health department in larger communities is usually divided into certain specialized divisions, each having control over various health aspects of the community. Some of these divisions are as follows:

The *bureau of administration,* which coordinates all the various activities performed and serves as a central communication point with other city functions.

The *division of records,* which collects, preserves, and publishes vital statistics, issues burial permits, registers physicians, assists in enforcing child labor and school attendance laws, and performs statistical work for the department.

The *sanitary division* or *bureau,* which has jurisdiction over sanitary conditions and looks into such matters as reported nuisances and the sanitation of slaughter-houses and stables.

The *bureau of preventable diseases,* which is concerned with preventing and controlling communicable disease, holding tuberculosis and other clinics, disinfecting premises and goods, and supervising a staff of field nurses.

The *division of child hygiene,* which is concerned with child and infant care, eye and dental clinics, supervision of day nurseries, and placement and care of dependent children.

The *food and drug bureau,* which has control over the food and drug supply in the city and inspects premises where foods are stored, handled, sold, or prepared. It also is especially concerned with the persons who prepare or serve food in public eating places.

The *bureau of laboratories,* which carries on research work, maintains supply stations for diphtheria antitoxin and vaccine, and makes scientific studies of various diseases and combats them whenever possible.

The *bureau of hospitals,* which supervises the various hospitals that in large cities are maintained by the department for the care of individuals who have communicable diseases.

Last, but not least, there is the *bureau of public health education.* This bureau is gradually being added to more and more departments of health because it is becoming increasingly evident that individuals are not going to develop good health practices without an educational program. This bureau sends out various types of information concerning health matters, promotes cooperation between department officials and the public, publishes health literature for professional and lay persons, gives health lectures, and organizes exhibitions and other media for publicizing the importance of certain health practices.

The health department, as can be seen from the preceding description, provides many essential and important functions for a community. Unfortunately, many of the activities listed are not carried on by all cities. An analysis of the functions performed indicates a change of emphasis from that of merely eliminating nuisances and fighting epidemics to one of prevention and providing information and services essential for good health.

Health councils. One of the best ways to ensure that all the health resources in a community are being utilized effectively for the benefit of most people is to have a community health council.

A community contains many groups and individuals who are interested in health. With so many interested in such an endeavor, there is need for coordination and a clearinghouse for the solution of health problems. A council or committee that is composed of representatives of various community groups can serve a very useful purpose. Much progress can be made if representatives from such groups as voluntary and professional health agencies, schools, industry, merchants, and others interested in health meet to discuss health problems. Group discussion can take place, problems can be aired, plans can be made, and work can be done that would never be possible without some type of cooperative effort. The health council is a comparatively new organization but has been found to be most helpful in promoting health in the community. As an agency through which many groups may cooperate to promote health, it has great possibilities for mobilizing public support for necessary health measures.

Voluntary health agencies. Some voluntary health agencies usually exist in communities of any size. These are organizations concerned with health that receive their support from public drives for funds, gifts, membership fees, and donations. Some examples of these are the American Cancer Society, National Tuberculosis Association, National Committee for Mental Hygiene, and the American Red Cross. Voluntary agencies in the field of health take the leadership for solving particular health problems that affect great numbers of American people. Through voluntary contributions and work, these agencies attempt to meet the problems.

Many voluntary health agencies exist now and new ones are being formed periodically. The greatest need at the present time is to coordinate the work that all the various agencies for health—whether they be official, voluntary, or private—are doing. There is considerable confusion in the public's mind because of the numerous agencies that are asking for financial help and support. If the work were better coordinated and organized, the public would have a clearer picture of what is needed and consequently would lend greater support.

Relationship between public health and school health programs

The health of the school child is a major consideration of our educational systems. In 1918 it was placed first on the list of "Cardinal Principles for Education." In 1938 it was reemphasized by the Educational Policies Commission. Conferences have been held, legislation passed, personnel appointed, and programs planned for the express purpose of promoting the health of the youth in our schools. This great emphasis focused on the health of the child and the happiness and fitness of future citizens of the United States means that every effort must be made to accomplish this objective in the most efficient and best way possible. Therefore, all the personnel and resources that are available in the community must be mobilized for this purpose. This is not a one-agency job. Instead, it requires the help and assistance of all organizations affecting the health of the child. Voluntary and official agencies, hospitals, boards of education, and other interested individuals and organizations must pool their resources, facilities, equipment, and knowledge in order that the health of the child may receive utmost consideration.

On the other hand, the solution of community health problems outside the school needs the concerted effort of every agency. Public health programs are to a great degree based upon an enlightened public that understands the health problems of the community and gives its support to the solving of these problems. The school can play a major part in helping to educate the citizens of the community so that health progress may be realized. The school health program should fit into the total community health program in a well-coordinated manner so as to render utmost service to all concerned.

In discussing interrelationships between school and public health programs, it is important to consider the controversy between community health groups and the schools as to who is responsible for administering the various phases of the school health program.

There are primarily three points of view concerning where the responsibility lies. One group feels that the board of education should be responsible, another that public health officials should assume the responsibility, and a third group thinks that school health is a joint responsibility of both the board of education and public health officials. It is advisable to consider briefly some of the arguments in favor of each point of view.

Those individuals who advocate board of education control for the school health program set forth many pertinent arguments in their behalf. These arguments can be summed up in the following statements. Board of education supporters point to the fact that the Tenth Amendment to the Constitution of the United States places the authority for education in the hands of the states. The states delegate this authority to the local communities, which in turn vest the authority in the board of education. The board of education, in the absence of legislation to the contrary, is responsible for all education, and health education, therefore, falls logically under their jurisdiction. They point to the fact that teachers, as a result of their training in such areas as psychology and methodology, are much better prepared to instruct children in health matters than are public health officials. They are better prepared to make health services meaningful educational experiences for all pupils. As another argument, they maintain that if public health officials were responsible for the school health program, the teachers would have two bosses, thus making for inefficient administration.

Those individuals who advocate that the school health program should be controlled by public health officials also list many pertinent arguments in their favor. Public health supporters say that health is logically a province of the medical profession and should therefore be under supervision of medical personnel, such as those found in most public health departments. They point to the fact that the school is part of the total community, and therefore such an important matter as health is a responsibility of community health officials. Furthermore, the pupil is in school only 5 days of each week and 180 or so days per year. The rest of the time he is in the larger community outside the school environment. They argue that public health nurses, as a result of their training and experience, are the best qualified to develop and administer a health services program, especially in respect to home-school-community relationships. They maintain that according to law the control of communicable diseases is a prerogative of public health officials and that they can do the job much more efficiently than can the board of education.

Finally, there is a group of persons who maintains that the school health program should be controlled jointly by both the board of education and public health officials. These point out that there will be better utilization of personnel, facilities, and community resources and that, consequently, greater health progress can be made if there is joint control with both working together for the good of all.

There does not seem to be a simple solution to this controversy about where the responsibility for school health lies. Probably the answer to this problem will vary according to the community. The solution would seem to depend upon how each community can best meet the health needs of the people who inhabit its particular geographic limits. The type of administrative setup that most fully meets the health needs and makes for greatest progress should be the one that is adopted. Vested interests should not be considered, and the health

interests of the consumer should be the primary concern. *Health is everybody's business,* and everyone should strive for the best health program possible in his community, state, nation, and world.

COMMUNITY ORGANIZATION FOR PHYSICAL EDUCATION

Physical education within the larger community outside of the school is usually incorporated in the programs sponsored by recreation people or by voluntary and private agencies such as the Boys' Club, YMCA, churches, and camps. Since these organizations and programs are considered in detail in the last two chapters of this book, they will not be discussed here.

Questions and exercises

1. Discuss some of the principles that serve as guidelines for the administrative structure of an organization. What other principles can you suggest that may also function as guidelines?
2. Draw a structural organization chart for your school or college showing the various administrative divisions. Discuss the responsibilities of each of the divisions. Give special attention to the health and physical education divisions.
3. In regard to the board of education of the community in which you live, list the composition of the board, powers of the board, and qualifications of board members.
4. Discuss the role of the superintendent of schools, principal, and college administrators in a selected community.
5. Discuss some of the inequities suffered by women in administrative positions. Give some of the reasons why these inequities exist.
6. Define each of the following: (a) school health program, (b) school health services, (c) health appraisal, (d) health counseling, (e) health environment, (f) health instruction, and (g) school health coordination.
7. Describe in detail the three main divisions of the total school physical education program.
8. Discuss the relationship of local government to school health. What administrative provisions have been made for these important considerations?
9. Discuss the women's physical education programs in your school or a school you are familiar with. Try to ascertain whether sex discrimination exists, and if so, in what ways.
10. Discuss in detail the organization and administration of a program of physical education in a junior college of your choice.

Reading assignment in *Administrative Dimensions of Health and Physical Education Programs, Including Athletics:* Chapter 3, Selections 12 to 15.

Selected references

Blackwell, T. E.: College and university administration, New York, 1966, The Center for Applied Research in Education, Inc. (The Library of Education).

Bookwalter, K. W.: Physical education in the secondary schools, Washington, D. C., 1964, The Center for Applied Research in Education, Inc. (The Library of Education).

Bucher, C. A.: Foundations of physical education, ed. 7, St. Louis, 1975, The C. V. Mosby Co.

Bucher, C. A.: Physical education for life, St. Louis, 1969, McGraw-Hill Book Co.

Bucher, C. A., and Dupee, R. K., Jr.: Athletics in schools and colleges, Washington, D. C., 1965, The Center for Applied Research in Education, Inc. (The Library of Education).

Bucher, C. A., and Koenig, C.: Methods and materials for secondary school physical education, ed. 4, St. Louis, 1974, The C. V. Mosby Co.

Bucher, C. A., Olsen, E., and Willgoose, C.: The foundations of health, New York, 1967, Appleton-Century-Crofts.

Bucher, C. A., and Reade, E. M.: Physical education and health in the elementary school, ed. 2, New York, 1971, The Macmillan Co.

Educational Policies Commission: School athletics—problems and policies, Washington, D. C., 1954, National Education Association.

Eichhorn, D. H.: The middle school, New York, 1966, The Center for Applied Research in Education, Inc. (The Library of Education).

Gauerke, W. E.: School law, New York, 1965, The Center for Applied Research in Education, Inc. (The Library of Education).

Goldhammer, K.: The school board, New York, 1964, The Center for Applied Research in Education, Inc. (The Library of Education).

Hillson, M.: Change and innovation in elementary school organization, New York, 1965, Holt, Rinehart and Winston, Inc.

Hillson, M., and Hyman, R. T.: Change and innovation in elementary and secondary organization, New York, 1971, Holt, Rinehart and Winston, Inc.

Jarvis, O. T., editor: Elementary school administration: Readings, Dubuque, Iowa, 1969, William C. Brown Co., Publishers.

Jenson, T. H., and Clark, D. L.: Educational administration, New York, 1964, The Center for Applied Research in Education, Inc. (The Library of Education).

Joint Committee on Health Education Terminology, School Health Review 4:25, 1973.

Joint Committee on Health Problems in Education of National Education Association and American Medical Association: School health services, Washington, D. C., 1964, National Education Association.

Joint Committee on Health Problems in Education of National Education Association and American Medical Association: Healthful school living, Washington, D. C., 1969, National Education Association.

Joint Committee on Health Problems in Education of National Education Association and American Medical Association: Health education, Washington, D. C., 1961, National Education Association.

Miller, B. F. and Burt, J. J.: Good health, personal and community, Philadelphia, 1972, W. B. Saunders Co.

Morphet, E. L., Johns, R. L., and Reller, T. L.: Educational administration, Englewood Cliffs, N. J., 1967, Prentice-Hall, Inc.

Reynolds, J. W.: The junior college, New York, 1965, The Center for Applied Research in Education, Inc. (The Library of Education).

Singer, R. N., and others: Physical education—an interdisciplinary approach, New York, 1972, The Macmillan Co.

Taylor, S.: Educational leadership: a male domain? Phi Delta Kappan, 55:124, 1973.

Ulrich, C.: She can play as good as any boy, Phi Delta Kappan 55:113, 1973.

U. S. Department of Health, Education, and Welfare, Office of Education: How teachers make a difference, Washington, D. C., 1972, U. S. Government Printing Office.

Unruh, G. and Alexander, W. M.: Innovations in secondary education, New York, 1970, Holt, Rinehart and Winston, Inc.

Van Til, W.: Education: a beginning, Boston, 1971, Houghton Mifflin Co.

Van Til, W., editor: Curriculum: quest for relevance, Boston, 1971, Houghton Mifflin Co.

Willgoose, C. E.: Health education in the elementary school, ed. 3, Philadelphia, 1969, W. B. Saunders Co.

Willgoose, Carl E.: Health Teaching in secondary schools, Philadelphia, 1972, W. B. Saunders Co.

Wynn, R. D.: Organization of public schools, New York, 1964, The Center for Applied Research in Education, Inc. (The Library of Education).

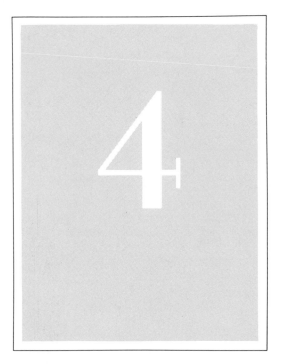

The business administrator*

Schools and colleges today are in the "business" of education. The size of the physical plant, increased enrollment, and greater expenditures than ever before require the talents of a qualified business administrator. The school or college business administrator is an integral part of the entire administrative team and ideally should have experience in both business administration and education. He or she is primarily responsible for the efficient and economic management of business matters concerning the educational institution.

It is important that health educators and physical educators understand and appreciate the vital role of the business administrator. Many administrative functions of health and physical educators fall within the responsibility of the business administrator. These functions include transportation, insurance, purchasing of supplies and equipment, and fiscal management. The business administrator is a specialist in these and other areas, and educators should work closely with this individual in reference to all business-related matters.

The American Association of School Administrators and the Association of School Business Officials of the United States and Canada have now jointly agreed that school business administrators may be defined as follows:

> The school business administrator shall be that employee member of the school staff who has been designated by the Board of Education and/or the Superintendent to have general responsibility for the administration of the business affairs of a school district. In any type of administrative organization, he shall be responsible for carrying out the general administration of the district and such other duties as may be assigned to him. Unless otherwise provided by local law or customs (as in dual control areas), he shall report to the Board of Education through the Superintendent of Schools.†

The school or college business administrator is an important member of the administrative team who has a significant contribution to make in the decisionmaking process as well as in executing business functions. He or she is well versed in education matters as well as in business management, and teaching experience is highly desirable. He or she is in a position to participate under the superintendent's or president's leadership and in making educational decisions as well as doing an efficient job of serving the district or college by providing educational activities for the staff and pupils.

---

*Thanks are due Mr. H. J. Stevens, Assistant Superintendent of Business Affairs, Nanuet, New York Public Schools, for his help in writing this chapter.
†Association of School Business Officials: The school business administrator (Bulletin 21), Evanston, Ill., 1960, The Association.

Since health educators and physical educators must work closely with school business administrators, special consideration is given to this key school or college administrator and the role he or she plays in the administration of school and college programs in general and in school and college health and physical education programs in particular.

THE COLLEGE BUSINESS MANAGER

The college business manager, or the vice president for business affairs as he or she is sometimes called, is responsible for budget preparation and fiscal accounting, investment of endowment and other monies, planning and construction of buildings, data processing, management of research and other contracts, business aspects of student loans, and intercollegiate activities.

Most key business officers have earned a master's or a doctor's degree, usually in business administration. However, some are certified public accountants and some have taken courses in management institutes. Most college business managers are recruited outside the academic world.

For the purposes of this chapter, the term *business administrator* is used, and the duties of such an educational officer are discussed in terms of schools and the school district. However, the functions that are outlined for the business administrator, the problems discussed, and the working relationship with health and physical education personnel are similar to or have implications for college as well as for school health educators and physical educators.

RESPONSIBILITIES OF THE BUSINESS ADMINISTRATOR

The business administrator's responsibilities are varied. He or she is as familiar with employee health insurance problems as with state and federal allocations for education. In the smaller school district, the business responsibilities are incorporated into the duties of the chief school administrator. As districts enlarge, there is a need to hire a person to oversee all the nonteaching areas of the district so that the chief school administrator is free to devote more time to the educational program of the district. No

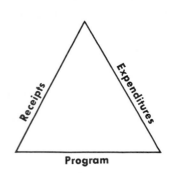

The Business Administrator's Isosceles Triangle.

two districts are alike in the handling of business responsibilities.

Following are some of the administrator's duties as listed by Frederick W. Hill,* past president of the Association of School Business Officials:

1. Budget and financial planning—This is an area in which the business official has to be sensitive to the needs of the staff in order to carry out a program. One also must have a sixth sense to understand how much the community can expend on the program. This can be related to the accompanying isosceles triangle. There has to be a direct relationship among all the components that make up the three sides of the triangle.

PPBS (Planning, Programming, Budgeting System) is being used by greater numbers of educators each year. This management tool allows for planning programs, budgeting available resources, evaluating performance, examining alternatives, and describing accomplishments to the public. By 1972 more than 1,500 school districts across the nation had phased in PPBS procedures. This management technique will be discussed in detail in Chapter 16—Budget Making and Financial Accounting.

2. Purchasing and supply management—The business official must utilize the best purchasing techniques to obtain maximum value for every dollar spent. After purchases are made and goods received, he or she is responsible for warehousing, storage, and inventory control. An article offered at the cheapest price is not always the most economical to purchase.

3. Plans—The business official works with

---

*Hill, F. W.: The rightful role of the school business official, School Business Affairs **29:**63, 1963.

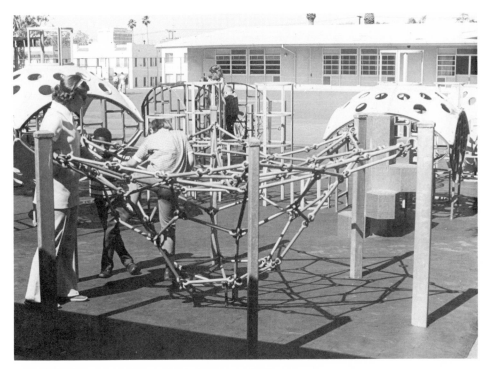

The business administrator has the responsibility of purchasing playground equipment. Special equipment utilized on playground in Los Angeles City Schools. (Courtesy Playground Corporation of America.)

administrators, teachers, architects, attorneys, and citizens of the community in developing plans for expansion of building facilities.

4. Personnel—The business official's duties vary in relation to the size of the district. In a small district he or she may be in charge of the nonteaching personnel, and in a large district he or she may be in charge of all personnel. In this capacity this official has to maintain records, pay schedules, retirement reports, and other personnel records.

5. Staff improvement—The business official is always interested in upgrading the people under his or her jurisdiction by providing workshops and inservice courses concerning latest developments in the field.

6. Community relations—Without community support the school would not operate. Some administrators tend to forget this when they become too far removed from the community. There is always a need to interpret the business area to the public.

7. Transportation—It has often been said that boards of education find themselves spend-ing too much time on the three B's—buses, buildings, and bonds. When this occurs, it is time to look into the hiring of a business official.

8. Food services—The business official is responsible for the efficient management of the lunchroom.

9. Accounting and reporting—The business official establishes and supervises the financial records and accounting procedures.

10. Debt service—The business official is involved with various capital developments and financial planning through short-term and long-term programs. Part of the financial rating of a school or a college district is judged on the way its debt service is handled.

11. Insurance—The business official must be familiar with a large schedule of insurance provisions ranging from fire and liability to health insurance. He or she has to maintain records for proof in case of loss.

12. Legal matters—The business official has to be familiar with education law and he or she has to know when to consult with attorneys.

13. System analysis—The business official must constantly question existing systems to see if they can be changed so that the job can be done more efficiently. New methods are being introduced utilizing data processing that will be a challenge as well as an aid to the business official.

14. Money raising—The business administrator is frequently called on to lead money-raising drives for colleges and universities.

15. Grants and financial aid—The business official must be aware of money available for programs through private, state, and federal grants and money available for scholarship candidates from private and public sources.

FUNCTION OF BUSINESS MANAGEMENT IN THE EDUCATIONAL PROGRAM

The business administrator is in a position to serve the educational program. His or her function is strictly limited by the size of the educational triangle—program, receipts, expenditures. The greater the perimeter of the triangle, the larger will be the sphere of operations. This applies to all departments in the system. Likewise, in times of inflation, the expenditures and receipts may increase, the program side will also increase, but the actual program could remain the same. Hence, it is obvious that the business administrator must project both expenditures and receipts if a constant program is going to be maintained.

The business office represents a means to an end, and it can be evaluated in terms of how well it contributes to the realization of the objectives of education.

OBJECTIVES OF BUSINESS MANAGEMENT

In serving schools and colleges, the business administrator constantly has the goal of helping them obtain the greatest educational service possible from each tax or aid dollar spent. He or she should take a democratic approach on decisions affecting others. A decision will then be reached that will be for the best, with the assurance that the educational benefits are worth the cost.

The business administrator is part of the team of administrators—along with presidents, principals, superintendents, and board members—who may be expected to look into the years ahead and have some ideas in regard to the future plans of the school or college.

The business administrator spends large sums of money for educational purposes. Total expenditures for education as a percentage of the gross national product: United States, 1929-30 to 1971-72. (From National Center for Educational Statistics, U. S. Department of Health, Education and Welfare, Digest of Educational Statistics, 1972 edition.)

GUIDELINES FOR HEALTH AND PHYSICAL EDUCATORS

Some of the guidelines for health and physical educators to follow as viewed by business administrators are as follows:

1. Business matters concerning health and physical education programs in the buildings of the district should be approved by the building principal before going to the school business administrator.

2. The school business administrator should keep the central administration informed of any budget changes for the athletic programs since the curriculum will also be affected.

3. Supplies that are requested to be purchased should be accompanied by a complete specification, including model, catalogue size, and so on. Health and physical educators should make themselves available to the business administrator to evaluate bids submitted.

4. Requisitions should be submitted only after a careful study of the needs of the health and physical education department.

5. The director of the health and physical education program should meet with the business administrator to determine the financial philosophy of the school or college toward the educational program.

6. The director of the health and physical education programs should keep the business administrator informed of new materials and ideas in his field.

7. All requests for special trips should be in writing on forms provided by the business office.

8. A monthly calendar should be submitted by the director of health and physical education, listing all athletic events and all pertinent transportation details.

9. The director of health and physical education should cooperate with the insurance program by submitting lists of students participating in sports, reporting accidents, and following through with physical examinations.

10. All personnel should be instructed in regard to administrative policies for dealing with accidents.

RELATIONSHIP WITH HEALTH AND PHYSICAL EDUCATION DEPARTMENTS

The business administrator has a very close working relationship with physical educators and health educators.

Director of health and physical education

In a large school district the business administrator works directly with the director of the department on budgetary and financial mat-

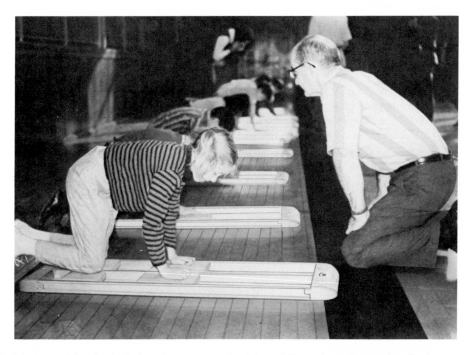

The administrator of the physical education program should carefully evaluate the merchandise he recommends to the business administration for purchasing. This illustrates an Exer-cor, an instrument developed by Health and Education Services Corporation, Bensenville, Ill., for persons to get needed exercise.

ters. It is important that all matters concerning physical education programs in the various buildings of the school district be approved by the building principal before they go to the central office. This is especially true in the secondary school because the physical education program is one part of the total curriculum. After the programs have been approved by the principal, they should be presented by the principal to the central office. If any program is to be modified, the principal is notified accordingly. Purchasing of materials is done on a bid basis, and when substitutes are offered for specified items, the business administrator should consult with the director of the department. The director then acts as a consultant in determining the quality of the items being purchased. One of the most serious mistakes that can be made when working with the business administrator is to "pad" the budget request for supplies and materials. The old expression "murder will out" comes to the fore at this point. The physical education person may decide that he needs twenty-four basketballs for next year, but he decides to list thirty-six on his budget request—hoping for the twenty-four—and if he receives thirty-six, he will have that many extra in the storage closet. Likewise, the business administrator should not make blind deletions in the requisitions without a consultation. There has to be a feeling of rapport between the two areas—so when the physical educator requests twenty-four basketballs, he will know he will receive twenty-four, unless a mutual budget change has been made.

A teacher in the physical education department should analyze the community and school philosophy to determine how much emphasis is to be placed on the program. This will have a direct bearing on the expenditures. In some school districts the academic program is a runner-up to the athletic program. A teacher new to a school system soon finds out how liberal or conservative the district is when he or she commences to submit purchase requisitions. An early meeting with the business administrator would be very helpful in determining the financial philosophy of the school district toward health and physical education programs.

The health educator and health coordinator

The health educator plays a significant role in the school and college curriculum today. Educational growth is most effective when the students are progressing healthfully as well as intellectually. It has been found that one of the reasons for the lack of educational attainment has been the physical inability to cope with the school or college program. Many items come to the business office that can be passed on to the health educator such as teaching aids for the health program.

Health coordinators or persons in charge of school health programs need to work closely with the business administrator in at least three ways. First, they should work together to provide a healthful school environment, which includes good lighting, seating, sanitary conditions, and ventilation. They should also contribute to the faculty and staff by interpreting and providing retirement and other financial benefits and being available for consultation on other matters that pertain to their academic positions. Second, there should be provision for adequate supplies and equipment to make the health instruction program most effective. Third, the health services program should be staffed with adequate personnel, facilities, and budget to assure an effective program.

The dental hygienist

The dental hygienist is a relatively new addition to the health education team. Until recent years most school districts have utilized the services of the local dentists to make an annual dental inspection. In some districts the dentists were paid for this service. In other districts the dentists served on a volunteer basis. In the latter school districts it is more difficult to initiate the idea of hiring an individual to make dental inspections. A dental hygienist should be utilized in the classroom as a consultant, similar to the school nurse-teacher. At the time the dental hygienist's schedule is prepared, consideration should be made for classroom visitations to discuss dental hygiene with the students. It is the responsibility of the school business administrator to provide the means for the dental hygienist to obtain materials and equipment to carry out his or her function in the school district.

OTHER AUXILIARY SERVICES

The business administrator renders many additional services that have a direct bearing on health and physical education programs.

Team transportation

The business administrator is usually responsible for the transportation program. A good business administrator, with an educational background, will be cognizant of the importance of exercise of not only the mind but also of the body. He or she will, therefore, make a provision in the transportation program for buses to carry athletic teams to sport contests so that they will arrive safely on time at their destinations. The director of athletics must be informed of the type of facilities that will be available so that he or she can plan accordingly. This involves a direct relationship between the director of athletics and the transportation supervisor. All requests for special athletic trips should be in writing and acknowledged by the secondary school principal or college administrator where he or she is involved. This is necessary since the principal or college administrator will be aware of any conflicts with other

parts of his or her program. The business administrator finds it very difficult to schedule special athletic trips on a moment's notice, although it is understandable when games are canceled for reason of weather or other unforeseen events. The director of athletics should submit a monthly calendar of athletic events, listing the date, time and place of departure, event, destination, number of participants, time of pickup, and remarks (see sample on p. 84).

The events scheduled on April 8 are routine, and the transportation supervisor can request a bus accordingly. The events on April 9 are a little more complex, and the director of athletics can state a preference for a station wagon. It is much more economical for a school district or college to furnish a station wagon rather than a sixty-passenger bus to transport five students. The events on April 10 are more complex, and the remarks indicate that one bus can be utilized for both teams. It is necessary to list the number of participants so that the proper size bus, or buses, can be assigned. This calendar should be submitted in triplicate (carbons) to the business administrator. After the transportation department has scheduled the trips, the business administrator initials all three copies and returns two copies to the athletic director. The director keeps one copy, and the

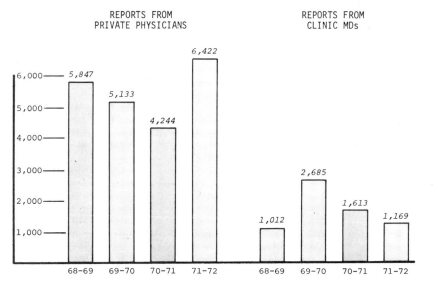

The health coordinator works closely with the business administrator in providing for the health needs of students. Medical evaluations of children and youth in Denver Public Schools. (From Forty-Seventh Annual Report 1971-72, Department of Health service, Denver Public Schools, Denver, Colo.)

Month of April

April 8

Depart: 3:00 P.M.
From: Senior High School
Team: Junior Varsity Baseball
To: Jones High School
Students: 35
Pickup: 5:30 P.M.
Remarks:

April 9

Depart: 3:00 P.M.
From: Junior High School
Team: Varsity Tennis
To: Albany High School
Students: 5
Pickup: 5:00 P.M.
Remarks: Station wagon requested;
        Coach Lewis will drive.

April 10

Depart: 3:00 P.M.
From: Senior High School
Team: Varsity Baseball and
      Varsity Tennis
To: Baseball to Jones High School
    Tennis to Albany High School
Students: 40
Pickup: Baseball—5:00 P.M.
      Tennis—5:30 P.M.
Remarks: One bus for both teams—
      drop off baseball first.

---

other copy is sent to the principal or college administrator. The procedure for submitting transportation requests could vary in different schools. The administrator might receive the schedule for approval before the business office.

Facilities, equipment, and supplies

The business administrator has a responsibility to provide adequate indoor and outdoor facilities and sufficient equipment and supplies for the health and physical education department, and the latter has the responsibility to keep these items in the best condition possible.

There are three phases related to facilities, equipment, and supplies.

The first phase is to secure needed items in order to provide a program. The size of the health suite and gymnasium, the field acreage, and the quantity and quality of the equipment are all related to money. The health educator and physical educator can present to the business administrator alternate programs with price tags for the business administrator to transfer into tax rates for the board of education or board of trustees. This is usually done prior to a building program.

The second phase is in regard to a maintenance program. The director of health and physical education is usually the custodian of all the equipment and supplies. He or she has an obligation to the district to see that health supplies, uniforms, bats, balls, and other equipment are not unnecessarily damaged. He or she should delegate responsibility to the various teachers and coaches to supervise all participants at all times. Locker room damage can be extensive after a game if the players are not under continual supervision. Damaged uniforms can be repaired if the physical education personnel are aware of deteriorating conditions. Usually it is much more economical to repair them rather than to replace them.

The use of the grounds requires cooperation between the physical educator and the superintendent of buildings and grounds. There must be a direct line of communication between these two positions. The former is primarily interested in a first-rate physical education program, and the latter is primarily interested in first-rate facilities. Neither can be first rate without cooperation between the two individuals involved and a mutual understanding of each other's problems.

The third phase of the utilization of facilities, equipment, and supplies relates to replacement of existing units. Equipment does wear out, and the life of the equipment does depend somewhat on the second phase. The business administrator, in the capacity as the director of the budget, prefers to replace items over a period of years—not all at once. It is a budget hardship to replace all football uniforms, for example, in 1 year, whereas the budget can absorb the cost if a few uniforms are replaced annually.*

---

*See also Chapter 17.

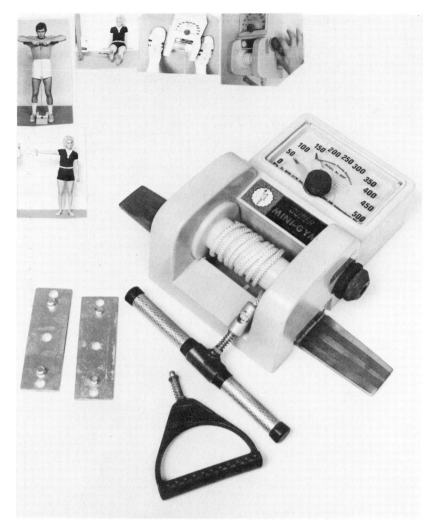

The business administrator needs to secure needed equipment and supply items for the physical education program. A super Mini-Gym Model no. 180, used in Skylab Mission, provides isokinetic exercise. (Courtesy Mini-Gym, Independence, Mo.)

At times there are some large replacement expenses that cannot be avoided, for example, replacing bleachers. The business administrator is in a position to include this in the budget as a capital expense or perhaps add it to a bond issue. But such a large budget item does merit special consideration from the business administrator. Too many special considerations added to the budget from the department will soon give people the impression that the program receives greater emphasis than the other phases of the instructional program. One of the ways to obtain economical and efficient use of the facilities, equipment, and supplies is for the business administrator and health and physical educators to reside as taxpayers in the community where they are employed.

Insurance*

The business administrator has to maintain a constant vigil on developments in the health and physical education insurance programs. Athletics represent one of the most important areas of coverage. Some schools and colleges

---

*Insurance is also discussed in Chapter 18.

do not provide an athletic insurance program. If a student is injured in an athletic event, the family would then be responsible for all medical expenditures. There would be no provision for the school or college to reimburse the family for its expense. Of course, the school or college is always open to a lawsuit by the parents in an effort to reclaim expenses. This is expensive for the school or college, for if the claim is settled in favor of the parents, the school's or college's insurance premiums for the next few years are increased. If the lawsuit is settled in favor of the school or college, the insurance company has already placed a sum of money in reserve until the final decision is reached. This is also costly because the premium is increased during the time the money is in reserve. An intangible effect is the damage to the school's or college's public relations.

An alternative is to provide an opportunity for the students to purchase athletic insurance or, better yet, for the school or college to purchase a policy for students participating in sports. Of course, the latter is the best method because all students are covered, regardless of their wealth, and the students' liability policy is not subject to suit. Most parents are only interested in recovering monies actually spent, and they are satisfied accordingly. Usually a blanket policy purchased by the school or college can be obtained at a lesser unit cost than a policy purchased by individuals. The athletic insurance program can be administered by a local or regional broker, relieving the school or college of going into the insurance business.

It is the responsibility of the director of physical education to supply accurate lists of participating students to the business office prior to the beginning of sports seasons. It is imperative for the various coaches to become aware of the insurance coverage so that when accidents do happen, they can inform the athletes of the proper procedure to follow in filing reports and claims. Usually the business office will supply policies for every participant in a covered athletic team. The coach should not only be knowledgeable, but he or she should also show concern for accident victims. This is not only a form of good public relations, but it may also make the difference in the parents' minds

concerning a lawsuit. The coaches then must be instructed in the proper attitude to take when such mishaps occur.

Medical examinations

The business administrator has a responsibility to the department to ascertain that there are enough physicians appointed by the board of education and that the health services are adequate to serve the needs of the school district or college. Every student participating in physical education should have a medical examination before he or she enters into activities. In athletics there should be a medical examination before each sport season. This means that if a student is participating in football, basketball, and baseball, he or she would have three medical examinations.

PROBLEMS BUSINESS ADMINISTRATORS ENCOUNTER

Some of the pitfalls and problems encountered by business administrators in working with health and physical educators, as seen through the eyes of business administrators, are as follows:

1. Overestimation of budget requests with the idea of expecting a reduction in the request
2. Not being able to justify budget requests as they relate to the total educational program
3. Deadlines not met in submitting requests for transportation, supplies, and other needs
4. Lack of awareness of the school district or college philosophy in regard to the place of the athletic program in the curriculum; hence, budget complications
5. Lack of cooperative planning in regard to the transportation equipment that is available and the scheduling of special athletic events away from school or college necessitating the use of buses
6. Late notification to the business administrator's office when a special athletic event is cancelled that requires cancellation of a prearranged bus
7. Negligence in filing accident reports on students injured in sports or classes, no matter how insignificant an accident may seem at the time
8. Incomplete records on students participating in sports—especially in regard to the requirement that all students receive a physical examination *before* trying out for the sport
9. Lack of concern for accident victims
10. Lack of knowledge of an injured student's rights and privileges under the student accident policy
11. Failure to realize that the educational goals repre-

sented in the philosophy of the school or college take priority over selfish, petty, and political interests

12. Lack of respect for the "chain of command"—a health and physical education teacher should not bypass the director of the department when communicating with the business office

13. Lack of interest in the facilities at his or her disposal, causing breakdowns and extra added expense

Questions and exercises

1. Interview a business administrator to obtain the following information: (a) the relations he or she has with health educators or physical educators, (b) how the business aspects of health education or physical education programs can be most effectively carried out, and (c) what a new teacher of health education or physical education should know about business administrators.

2. Why is a person who is a specialist in business management needed in school or college systems today?

3. Read one book or one article in a school or college administration magazine of your choice that concerns itself with the role of the business administrator in schools or colleges. Give a report to the class.

4. How is business management of health education and/or physical education carried on at the college level?

Reading assignment in *Administrative Dimensions of Health and Physical Education Programs, Including Athletics:* Chapter 3, Selection 11.

Selected references

Avedisian, C. T.: PPBS: Planning, programming, budgeting systems, Journal of Health, Physical Education, Recreation **43:**37, 1972.

Casey, L. M.: School business administration, New York, 1964, The Center for Applied Research in Education, Inc. (The Library of Education).

Green, M.: Prestige and finance, Physical Education **29:** 127, 1972.

Hill, F. W.: The school business administrator, Evanston, Ill., 1960, American Association of Business Officials of the United States and Canada.

Hill, F. W.: The rightful role of the school business official, School Business Affairs **29:**63, 1963.

Hill, F. W., and Colmey, J. W.: School business administration in the smaller community, Minneapolis, 1964, T. S. Denison & Co., Inc.

Knezevich, S. J., and Fowlkes, J. G.: Business management of local school systems, New York, 1960, Harper & Row, Publishers.

Linn, H. H.: School business administration, New York, 1956, The Ronald Press Co.

Malone, W. C.: Team concept in school administration, Clearing House **47:**259, 1973.

Naughton, J. J.: Profile of the chief school business administrator, Connecticut Teacher **34:**16, April, 1967.

Roe, W. H.: School business management, New York, 1961, McGraw-Hill Book Co.

Stevens, H. J.: Are you issuing blank checks? School Management **9:**80, 1965.

Whaling, T.: Managing the school system: a performance improvement approach, Education Digest **38:**18, 1973.

Personnel administration for health and physical education programs

The very nature of personnel administration is rapidly changing. On both high school and college campuses, students and faculty are participating more in the administrative process. Administrators are consulting with faculty, students, and general staff prior to making final decisions on such aspects of academic life as curriculum, scheduling, and working conditions. In addition, administrators are being required to negotiate with unions in collective bargaining sessions. Administration is no longer a unilateral prerogative of a few executives but is increasingly becoming a cooperative endeavor involving students, faculty, staff, and community members.

For all these reasons, the administration of personnel is perhaps the most challenging responsibility of an effective leader. A leader who does not have the cooperation of his or her personnel will have great difficulty in implementing any decision or policy. Some principles essential to effective personnel administration are discussed in the following sections.

PRINCIPLES OF PERSONNEL ADMINISTRATION
Cooperation

To achieve cooperation implies that the specialties and unique abilities of individuals must be noted and utilized in situations where their services will be rendered under optimal conditions. The permanency of cooperation will depend upon the degree to which the purposes of the organization are achieved and individual motives are satisfied. The function of administration is to see that these essentials are accomplished.

The individual as a member of an organization

Administration should seek to imbue the organization with the idea that every individual has a stake in the enterprise. The undertakings can be successful only as all persons contribute to the maximum of their potentials, and with success will then come increased satisfaction to each individual. Above all, it must be recognized that submergence of self is necessary for the achievement of the organization's goals.

The fallacy of final authority

The authority that does exist belongs to the job and not to the person. The administrator should never feel powerful and all-important. Authority does not reside in one human being but in the best thinking, judgment, and imagination that the organization can command. Every individual has the authority that goes with his or her position and only that much. In turn, this authority is conditioned by other members whose work is closely allied to achieving the objectives for which the organization exists. Authority comes from those who perform the more technical aspects of the organization's work as well as from those who, because of their positions, are responsible for the ultimate decisions. Department heads, foremen, and staff consultants issue reports interpreting the facts. Their judgments, conclusions, and recommendations contribute to the formulation of the final decisions that are the responsibility of the administrator. If these interpretations, judgments, conclusions, and recommendations are not accepted, the organization may fail. Its best thinking has been ignored. Furthermore, individuals cannot be induced to contribute their efforts in an organization that has little respect for their thinking. Authority is not resident in one person. Instead, it permeates the entire organization from top to bottom.

Staff morale

There are certain conditions that are known to contribute to staff morale. Some of the more important of these will be discussed. The administration should continually strive to create such conditions in their organizations. The degree to which high staff morale exists will be in direct proportion to the degree to which such conditions are satisfied.

Leadership. The quality of the leader will determine staff morale to a great degree. From the top down, there should be careful selection of all individuals who act in leadership capacities. Other things being equal, individuals will contribute better service, produce more, have an overall better morale, and have more respect for individuals who are leaders in the true sense of the word.

Physical and social environment. A healthful physical and social environment is essential to good staff morale. The physical health of the worker must be provided for. There must also be provisions for mental health that include proper supervision, opportunity for advance-

ment, plans for any emergency that may arise, and avenues for intellectual improvement.

The social environment is also an important consideration. The individuals with whom one works and the activities in which one engages can strengthen or dampen the human spirit. An individual is the product of his interactions with others. Therefore, in order to improve oneself it is very important to associate with those who can contribute to this improvement. Since the working day represents, to a great degree, the majority of an individual's social relationships, it is important that these relationships be wholesome and conducive to individual improvement.

Advancement. Human beings like to feel that they are "getting ahead in the world." This is an important consideration in developing and continuing a high degree of staff morale. This consideration necessitates informing each member of an organization concerning what is essential for progress and promotion. Opportunities should be provided for self-improvement in learning new skills, gaining new knowledge, and having new experiences. In addition, encouragement should be given those who are anxious to improve and are willing to devote extra time and effort for such a purpose.

Recognition of meritorious service. Another requirement, similar to advancement, which is requisite for staff morale, is recognition for outstanding contributions to the organization. As has been previously pointed out, all human beings need to be recognized. Those who make outstanding contributions to the organization should be so honored. This is very important to further greater achievements.

Individual differences. An important principle of personnel management is the recognition of individual differences and different types of work. Individuals differ in many ways —abilities, skills, training, and physical, mental, and social qualities. There are also various types of work that require different skills, abilities, and training.

These differences in individuals and types of work must be recognized by the administrator. One of his or her main duties in respect to personnel should be to make sure that the right person is in the right niche. An individual who is a "round peg in a square hole" does not contribute to his or her own or the organization's welfare. To be placed in a position that should be held by a person with lesser qualifications or vice versa is unjust and devastating in its results.

It is important for the administrator to recognize in some formal way individual differences that exist in the organization. A system of status must exist for purposes of communication and orderly procedure. Such systems of status must be readily understood, authoritative, and authentic. These systems of status not only make for better communication but also provide the basis for personnel improvement and ad-

vancement within the organization. Furthermore, they help to develop a sense of responsibility in the individual. The status that is granted any one person should be in line with capacities and importance of the function he or she performs. Many disruptive features can develop in status systems if there is no recognition of individual abilities, if the system is allowed to become an end rather than a means to an end, and if proper incentives are not provided at each level.

Differentiated staffing. Just as administrations must recognize individual differences, they must also recognize a teacher's interests, talents, and general suitability to teach different phases of the curriculum. This is where the con-

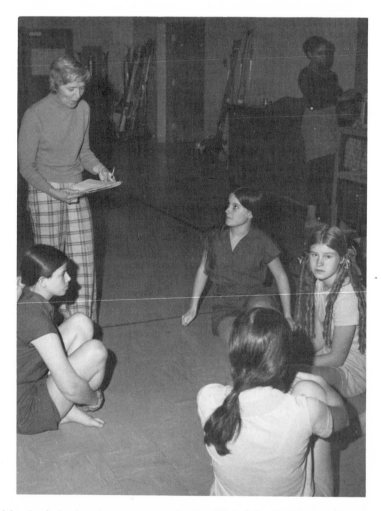

Paraprofessional in physical education program at Regina High School, Minneapolis, takes attendance and keeps all records for program. (Photograph by Rollie Baird, Dellarson Studios.)

cept of differentiated staffing comes into play. Teachers should be assigned activities where they demonstrate particular skills, so that one teacher does not assume the same educational role or teach the same class in every activity. In addition, schools are also employing staff members such as paraprofessionals, activity specialists, teacher-interns, and teacher-aides, as well as clerks, custodians, and equipment and facility managers. Differentiated staffing will be discussed in greater detail in Chapter 7.

QUALIFICATIONS OF THE ADMINISTRATOR

Although the qualities of a good administrator need to be considered in relation to the qualities of the persons in the organization he or she is attempting to lead, nevertheless it is helpful to recognize certain leadership characteristics that appear to be necessary if an administrator is to be successful on the job. The identification of these qualities is essential to help determine whether or not one should go into this important field if the occasion arises. This identification will also help in evaluating the type of administration one is experiencing in his or her own organization, whether he or she is an administrator or holds another position.

The qualifications of an administrator are many. Some (administrative mind, integrity, ability to instill good human relations, ability to make decisions, health and fitness for the job, willingness to accept responsibility, understanding of work, command of administrative technique, and intellectual capacity) are discussed in the following sections. There has been no attempt to list these in order of importance, although in the discussion of each, one may be able to discern the most essential and important qualifications.

Administrative mind

A research project that involved a self-analysis of nearly 1000 executives, all of whom were presidents of industrial organizations, pointed up the following important considerations for the person who wants to be a good administrator. Using time effectively, ability to get other people to do things, building a

team, setting the direction, finding expert advice, making crisis decisions, negotiating, and effective self-improvement were considered important. Personal improvement, especially directed along lines involving public speaking, planning work, memory skills, conference leadership, writing, producing better ideas, and reading, were also considered necessary.

Some individuals have qualities that, perhaps, have been developed through training and experience and that peculiarly adapts them to administrative work. These individuals are able to analyze situations objectively, have the ability to clarify generalizations, and possess the quality of administering in a constructive manner rather than in an exploitative way. Such persons are sensitive to human relations and the important part they play in the successful functioning of any organization. These individuals think in imaginative terms. They are able to see into the future and plan a course of action with an open mind. They recognize problems in order of importance, are able to analyze a situation, develop various plans of action, and reach logical conclusions. They have the ability to organize.

Integrity

One of the most important qualifications of any administrator is integrity. Whether or not a leader can inspire the staff, have their cooperation, and achieve the purposes of the organization will depend to a great degree upon his or her integrity. Everyone likes to feel that an administrator is honest and sincere, keeps promises, can be trusted with confidential information, and is an individual in whom one has faith. Such confidence cannot emanate from administrators unless they have integrity. Failure to fulfill this one qualification will result in low morale and an inefficient organization.

Ability to instill good human relations

Ray O. Duncan, former president of the American Alliance for Health, Physical Education, and Recreation (AAHPER), suggested the following as considerations for administrators: be friendly and considerate, be alert to the opinions of others, be careful what you say and how you say it, be honest and fair, be wise enough to weigh and decide, be able to tolerate human failings and inefficiency, be able to acquire humility, and plan well for staff meetings.

The ability to get along with associates in work is an essential qualification for an administrator. Only through cooperative effort is it possible for an organization to achieve its goals. This cooperative effort is greatest when the individuals responsible for the coordination of human efforts have the welfare of the various members of the organization at heart. This means that an administrator must be able to convert the abilities of many individuals into coordinated effort. This is done in many ways. Some of these methods include setting a good example, inspiring confidence, selecting proper incentives, possessing poise, making the right decisions in tense moments, having an impersonal attitude, cooperating and helping others when necessary, and developing and practicing ethical standards. The administrator must be adept at the art of persuasion, which takes into consideration such important items as the points of view, interests, and other factors characterizing those to be persuaded.

There is very little associated effort without leadership. The administrator must be a leader and possess the attributes and qualities that people expect if they are to achieve the purposes for which the organization has been established.

Ability to make decisions

The administrator must be able to make decisions when the situation necessitates such action. This presumes an understanding of what constitutes the important and the unimportant in the particular situation that is in question, the ability to foresee future developments and the results of a decision, and a knowledge of what is reasonable and what is unreasonable. It also assumes knowledge of what is in the best interests of the organization and what is not, and what has the best chance for success and what has the least chance.

Decision is essential in order to accomplish objectives at the most opportune time. The administrator should have the capacity and be willing to make a decision. Many times if a decision is not forthcoming lethargy, suspense,

and poor morale are created. The administrator who procrastinates, is afraid of making the wrong decision, thinks only of his or her own security, and is oblivious to the organization's needs should never hold an administrative position.

Health and fitness for the job

Good health and physical fitness are essentials for the administrator. They often have a bearing on making the right decisions. Socrates once said that people in a state of bad health often made the wrong decisions in regard to affairs of state. Jennings, the famous biologist, pointed out that the body can attend to only one thing at a time. Therefore, if attention is focused on a pain in the chest, a stomach ailment, or a nervous condition, it is difficult to focus it on the functions that an administrator must perform. Poor physical or mental health may cause poor administration.

Vitality and endurance are essential to the administrator. They affect one's manner, personality, attractiveness, and disposition. Administrative duties often require long hours of tedious work under the most trying conditions. Failure to have the necessary strength and endurance under such conditions could mean the inability to perform tasks that are essential to the welfare of the organization. Members of an organization have confidence in those administrators who watch over their interests at all times. It is possible for an administrator to retain this confidence continuously only if he or she is in good health and physically fit to perform arduous duties.

Willingness to accept responsibility

Every administrator must be willing to accept responsibility. There are duties to be performed that greatly influence the welfare of many individuals. Plans have to be fulfilled if the purposes of the organization are to be accomplished. Action is required to ensure production and render services. The person who accepts an administrative job is morally bound to assume the responsibility that is part and parcel of that position. A good administrator will experience a feeling of dissatisfaction whenever he or she fails to meet responsibilities.

Understanding of work

The administrator will benefit from having a thorough understanding of the specialized work in which the organization is engaged. If it concerns a particular industry, it will be an advantage to know the production process from the ground up. If it is government, knowledge of related legislative, executive, and judicial aspects will help. If it is education, familiarity with that particular field will be an asset. If it is a specialized field within education or other area, it is necessary to have a knowledge of the particular specialty and also the part it plays in the total educational process. It is difficult to guide purposefully unless the individual knows his or her particular educational specialty and how it relates to other subject-matter areas. One often reads about the Congressman who was once a page in the Senate, the railroad executive who was a yard worker, the bank president who started as a bookkeeper, and the superintendent of schools who many years before started as a teacher. The technical knowledge and understanding of the total functioning of an organization are best gained through first-hand experience. An administrator will find that detailed knowledge of an organization's work is of great help in successfully guiding its operations.

Command of administrative technique

Administrative technique in many ways is similar to the first qualification listed—administrative mind. There is one essential difference. Administrative mind refers more to the "know how" and temperament of the individual, whereas *administrative technique* refers to the application of this knowledge and ability. An individual who possesses this quality can plan and budget his or her time and effort and also the time and work of others, in the most effective way possible. Time is not spent on details when more important work should be done. Tasks are performed in a relaxed, efficient, calm, and logical manner. Work is accomplished in conformance with established standards. Duties are effectively executed, including those that involve strong pressure and great amounts of time. Resources for performing the job are utilized.

It has been said there are three conditions that burn out an administrator in a short length of time: performing his or her own duties in a tense, highly emotional manner, performing too many details, and being part of an organization that is not considerate of its administrators.

Intellectual capacity

Intellectual capacity in itself will not guarantee a good administrator. In fact, the so-called intellectual often makes a very poor administrator. Such traits as absent-mindedness and tardiness are often not compatible with acceptance of responsibility. Intellectuals sometimes cannot make decisions because they visualize so many sides of an issue. Furthermore, such an individual is often not interested in people but in books, figures, or other data. This makes a poor leader since lack of interest in human beings results in poor followership.

However, one should not gain from this discussion that intellectual capacity should be disregarded. To be a good administrator one must be intellectually competent. One should be able to think and reason logically, to apply knowledge effectively, to communicate efficiently, and to possess other factors that are closely allied to the intellectual process. There have been many so-called "brains" who failed miserably as administrators, whereas most good administrators can be classified as at least average in respect to their intellectual capacities.

Space has not permitted a discussion of all the qualifications of the administrator. Others, such as courage and initiative, are also important. There is in addition the ability to be an ambassador for the organization. Liaison work with higher echelon groups in the organization and also with outside groups is important. It is necessary at times to stand up and fight for one's own department or division. To a great degree this will determine whether it is respected and has equal status with other administrative divisions.

ADMINISTRATIVE STYLES

An administrative style may be defined as the method used by the leader in carrying out duties. Leadership styles are usually recognized as autocratic, democratic, or laissez-faire. These styles of leadership are discussed in the following sections.

The autocratic leader

The autocratic leader determines all policy by himself or herself. He or she approaches each part of a decision one step at a time; the future is never quite clear. The responsibilities of subordinates are assigned and thoroughly defined. The leader may make personal remarks to individual faculty or staff members but remains apart from group participation.

Some advantages of autocratic leadership are: (1) subordinates are given a definite pattern to follow, (2) less secure members of the faculty or staff are free from decision making, (3) dependency is encouraged, and (4) decision making is expeditious.

Disadvantages of autocratic leadership include: (1) individuality is suppressed, (2) hostility and aggressive tendencies increase, and (3) discontent is created. Many faculty and staff members have both a need and desire to contribute to policy making decisions. To be denied this participation is extremely frustrating and may lead to apathetic behavior.

The democratic leader

The democratic leader encourages group participation and discussion and provides alternative solutions to problems. Division of responsibilities is decided by faculty and staff who participate in the choice of whom they wish to work with. The democratic leader is objective in evaluating faculty and staff and is an active participant in group meetings.

Advantages of such leadership include: (1) greater group productivity, (2) lessened hostility and discontent, and (3) encouragement of creativity and individuality. Faculty and staff members who are very involved in decision making tend to be more at ease and contribute more freely to their departments.

The disadvantages of a democratic leader include: (1) divided opinions in open discussions, (2) apathy and ignorance present in meetings, (3) authority that is not clearly defined, and (4) delay in reaching decisions. However, these problems can be reduced by sufficient planning on the part of the leader.

The laissez-faire leader

The laissez-faire leader believes in complete freedom for group or individual decision making, with a minimum of interference from the leader. He or she supplies resource materials and will only become more involved when asked to participate. He or she avoids determining responsibilities and coworker assignments.

The advantages of a laissez-faire leader include: (1) encouragement of individuality and creativity and (2) less apparent faculty and staff discontent. Creative persons, especially, seem to thrive under laissez-faire leadership. However, the disdvantages seem to overpower the advantages in this case. Studies of laissez-faire situations have found them to be loosely structured, disorganized, apathetic, and even chaotic. A poorer quality of work and diminished accomplishment is also noted.

THE ADMINISTRATOR AS A LEADER

In the last 30 years research findings have indicated that some beliefs, such as certain qualities per se indicate who the leaders are, that leaders are born and not made, and that some people will lead and others will follow, are not exactly true. Instead, in recent years research seems to indicate that personal characteristics must be related to the characteristics of the followers, because of the interaction of the two that takes place. The identification of qualities of certain individuals as leaders without relating these qualities to the persons they are going to try to lead has little meaning.

Stogdill* studied the relationship of personality factors to leadership and found that the leader of a group exceeds the average of the group in respect to such characteristics as intelligence, scholarship, acceptance of responsibility, participation, and socioeconomic status.

Berelson and Steiner† surveyed the scientific findings in the behaviorial sciences and formulated some propositions and hypotheses relating

---

*Stogdill, R. M.: Personal factors associated with leadership, a survey of the literature, Journal of Psychology **25:**63, 1948.
†Berelson, B., and Steiner, G. A.: Human behavior: an inventory of scientific findings, New York, 1964, Harcourt, Brace & World, Inc., pp. 341-344.

to leadership. In essence some of these are as follows:

1. The closer an individual conforms to the accepted norms of the group, the better liked he will be; the better liked he is, the closer he conforms; the less he conforms, the more disliked he will be.
2. The higher the rank of the member within the group, the more central he will be in the group's interaction and the more influential he will be.
3. In general, the "style" of the leader is determined more by the expectations of the membership and the requirements of the situation than by the personal traits of the leader himself.
4. The leadership of the group tends to be vested in the member who most closely conforms to the standards of the group of the matter in question or who has the most information and skill related to the activities of the group.
5. When groups have established norms, it is extremely difficult for a new leader, however capable, to shift the group's activities.
6. The longer the life of the leadership, the less open and free the communication within the group and probably the less efficient the group in the solution of new problems.
7. The leader will be followed more faithfully the more he makes it possible for the members to achieve their private goals along with the group goals.
8. Active leadership is characteristic of groups that determine their own activities, passive leadership of groups whose activities are externally imposed.
9. In a small group, authoritarian leadership is less effective than democratic leadership in holding the group together and getting its work done.

Other studies that provide pertinent information on leadership include those of Myers,* Hemphill,† Homans,‡ and Halpin.§

The physical educator or health educator who desires to exercise a leadership role in his or her organization should study the administrative theory reflected in the research studies available on this subject. This will help to better assure success as a leader in any particular situation.

---

*Myers, R. B.: The development and implications of a conception for leadership education, Unpublished doctoral dissertation, University of Florida, 1954.
†Hemphill, J. K.: Administration as problem solving. In Halpin, A. W., editor: Administrative theory in education, Chicago, 1958, Midwest Administration Center, University of Chicago.
‡Homans, G. C.: The human group, New York, 1950, Harcourt, Brace and World, Inc.
§Halpin, A. W.: A paradigm for the study of administrative research in education. In Campbell, N. R., and Gregg, R. T., editors: Administrative behavior in education, New York, 1957, Harper & Row, Publishers.

MAJOR ADMINISTRATIVE DUTIES

Gulick and Urwick* have utilized the word POSDCORB to outline the functions of an administrator. This is based on Henri Fayol's work, *Industrial and General Administration*. An organization of duties under these major headings is apropos to the section under discussion although the semantics of the subject in some cases is not appropriate to modern administration. POSDCORB refers to the functional elements of (1) planning, (2) organizing, (3) staffing, (4) directing, (5) coordinating, (6) reporting, and (7) budgeting.

Planning

Planning is the process of outlining the work that is to be performed, in a logical and purposeful manner, together with the methods that are to be utilized in the performance of this work. The total plan will result in the accomplishment of the purposes for which the organization is established. Of course this implies a clear conception of the aims of the organization.

In order to accomplish this planning, the administrator must have vision to look into the future and to prepare for what is seen. He or she must see the influences that will affect the organization and the requirements that will have to be met.

Organizing

Organizing refers to the development of the formal structure of the organization, whereby the various administrative coordinating centers and subdivisions of work are arranged in an integrated manner, with clearly defined lines of authority. The purpose behind this structure is the effective accomplishment of established objectives. Organizational charts aid in clarifying such organization.

This formal structure should be set up in a manner that avoids red tape and provides for the clear assignment of every necessary duty to some responsible individual. Whenever possible, standards should be established for acceptable performance for each duty assignment.

---

*Gulick, L., and Urwick, L., editors: Papers on the science of administration, New York, 1937, Institute of Public Administration.

The coordinating centers of authority are developed and organized chiefly on the basis of the work to be done by the organization, services performed, individuals available in the light of incentives offered, and efficiency of operation. A single administrator cannot perform all the functions necessary, except in the smallest organizations. Hence, responsibility must be assigned to others in a logical manner. These individuals occupy positions along the line, each position being broken down in terms of its own area of specialization. The higher up the line one goes, the more general is the responsibility; the lower down the line one goes, the more specific is the responsibility.

Staffing

The administrative duty of staffing refers to the entire personnel function of selection, assignment, training, and providing and maintaining favorable working conditions for all members of the organization. The administrator must have a thorough knowledge of the staff. He or she must select with care and ensure that each subdivision in the organization has a competent leader and that each employee is assigned to the job where he can be of greatest service. Personnel should possess energy, initiative, and loyalty. The duties of each position must be clearly outlined. All members of the organization must be encouraged to utilize their own initiative. They should be rewarded fairly for their services. The mistakes and blunders of employees must be brought to their attention and dealt with accordingly. Vested interests of individual employees must not be allowed to endanger the general interests of all. The conditions of work should be made as pleasant and as nearly ideal as possible. Both physical and social factors should be provided for. Services rendered by the individual increase as the conditions under which he or she works improve.

Directing

Directing (leading is a more appropriate term) is a responsibility that falls to the administrator as the leader. He or she must direct the operations of the organization. This means

distinct and precise decisions must be made and embodied in instructions that will ensure their completion. The administrator must direct the work in and impersonal manner, avoid becoming involved in too many details, and see that the organization's purpose is fulfilled according to established principles. Executives have a duty to see that the quantity and quality of performance of each employee are maintained.

The administrator is a leader. His or her success is determined by the ability to guide others successfully toward established goals. Individuals of weak responsibility and limited capability cannot perform this function successfully. The good administrator must be superior in determination, persistence, endurance, and courage. He or she must clearly understand the organization's purposes and keep them in mind as he or she guides and leads the way. Through direction, it is essential that faith be created in the cooperative enterprise, in success, in achievement of personal ambitions, in the integrity of the leadership provided, and in the superiority of associated efforts.

Coordinating

Coordinating means interrelating all the various phases of work within an organization. This means that the organization's structure must clearly provide for close relationships and competent leadership in the coordinating centers of activity. The administrator must meet regularly with chief assistants. Here arrangements can be made for unity of effort, reports can be submitted on progress, and obstacles to coordinated work can be eliminated. Good coordination also means that all factors must be considered in their proper perspective.

This duty requires the development of a faith that runs throughout the organization. Coordination can be effective only if there is faith in the enterprise and in the need for coordinated effort. Faith is the motivating factor that stimulates human beings to continue rendering service so that goals may be accomplished.

There should also be coordination with administrative units outside the organization where such responsibilities are necessary.

Reporting

Reporting is the administrative duty of supplying information to administrators or executives higher up on the line of authority or to other groups to which one is responsible. It also means that subordinates must be kept informed through regular reports, research, and continual observation. In this respect the administrator is a point of intercommunication. In addition to accepting the responsibility for reporting to higher authority, he or she must continually know what is going on in the area under his or her jurisdiction. Members of the organization must be informed on many topics of general interest, such as goals to be achieved, progress being made, strong and weak points, and new areas proposed for development. This information will come from various members of the organization.

Budgeting

As the word implies, budgeting refers to financial planning and accounting. It is the duty of the administrator to allocate to various subdivisions the general funds allotted to the organization. This must be done in a manner that is equitable and just. In carrying out this function, he or she must keep the organization's purposes in mind and apportion the available money to those areas or projects that will help most in achieving these purposes. It also means that controls must be established to ensure that certain limits will be observed, so-called budget padding will be kept to a minimum, and complete integrity in the handling of all the budgetary aspects of the organization will be maintained. PPBS (Planning, Programming, Budgeting System), discussed in Chapter 3, is being implemented increasingly in school systems throughout the country. This management technique will be discussed in detail in Chapter 16.

QUALIFICATIONS OF HEALTH AND PHYSICAL EDUCATORS

The most important consideration in administration is personnel. The members of an organization determine whether it will succeed or fail. Administration must take into account the qualifications of health and physical educators,

factors that promote cooperation, principles of good human relations, the fallacy of final authority, the importance of decisiveness, the need for good staff morale, and other principles to be observed in personnel management.

Qualifications for health educators

The qualifications of health educators may be discussed in reference to health education, school health services, and healthful school living.

Health education. The qualified health educator should be knowledgeable in what constitutes well-balanced and well-functioned health teaching and its implications for different students at different levels. He or she should also be very familiar with health curriculums and materials. In addition, he or she should show skills in detecting student health interests and needs and motivating students to achieve and maintain an optimal level of personal health. He or she should also be skilled in using health resources and in acting as a health counselor.

School health services. The qualified health educator should be knowledgeable concerning available health care personnel and should be skilled in establishing school health policies for various health services, using health screening techniques, encouraging correction of health problems, and working with parents and community in promoting healthful living.

Healthful school living. The qualified health educator should be aware of opportunities in and about the school that promote healthful living and be interested in improving both the physical environment and psychologic setting so that healthy living is encouraged.

The personality of the health educator is of particular concern. The individual must be well adjusted and well integrated emotionally, mentally, and physically if he or she is to do a good job in developing these characteristics in others. Such a person must also be interested in human beings and possess skill and understanding in human relations so that health objectives may be realized.

It is very important that the health educator have a mastery of certain scientific knowledge and specialized skills and have proper attitudes.

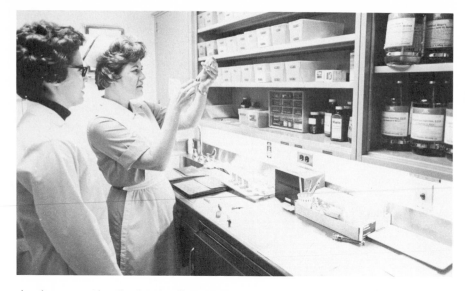

The nurse is a key person in school and college health services. The nursing program at College of DuPage, Glen Ellyn, Ill., has provided the Chicago area with qualified nurses since 1971.

Such knowledge, skills, and attitudes will help the health educator identify the health needs and interests of individuals with whom he or she comes in contact, provide a health program that will meet these needs and interests, and promote the profession so that human lives may be enriched. This means that many experiences should be included in the training of persons entering this specialized field. These experiences can be divided into general education, professional education, and specialized education.

General education experiences should provide knowledge and skill in the communicative arts, understanding in sociologic principles, an appreciation of the history of various peoples with their social, racial, and cultural characteristics, and the fine and practical arts that afford a means of expression, a means of releasing the emotions, a medium for richer understanding of life, and a medium for promoting mental health. The behavioral sciences are especially important for the health educator. The science area is also very important to the health educator and should include anatomy and kinesiology, physiology, bacteriology, biology, zoology, chemistry, physics, and also such behavioral sciences as child and adolescent psychology, human growth and development, general psychology, mental hygiene, and sociology.

In professional education it is important for the health educator to have a mastery of the philosophies, techniques, principles, and evaluative procedures that are characteristic of the most advanced and best thinking in education.

The qualifications for teachers of health to be certified in New Jersey are listed on p. 99.

Qualifications for physical educators

The following are some special qualifications of the physical educator.

The physical educator should be a graduate of an approved teacher training institution that prepares teachers for physical education. The college or university should be selected with care.

Since physical education is based upon the foundational sciences of anatomy, physiology, biology, kinesiology, sociology, and psychology, and research, the leader in this field should be well versed in these areas.

The general education of physical educators is under continuous scrutiny and criticism. Speech, knowledge of world affairs, mastery of the arts, and other aspects of this area are important in the preparation of the physical educator. Since his or her position requires frequent

HEALTH EDUCATION

AUTHORIZATION. This certificate is required for teaching health education in the elementary and secondary schools.

REQUIREMENTS

I. A bachelor's degree based upon a four-year curriculum in an accredited college

II. Successful completion of *one* of the following:

    A. A college curriculum approved by the New Jersey State Department of Education as the basis for issuing this certificate

OR

    B. A program of college studies including:

general background

1. A total of thirty semester-hour credits in *general background* courses distributed in at least three of the following fields: English, social studies, science, fine arts, mathematics, and foreign languages. Six semester-hour credits in English and six in social studies will be required.

2. A minimum of eighteen semester-hour credits in *professional education* courses distributed over four or more of the following groups including at least one course in each starred area. A maximum of three semester-hour credits will be accepted in health education. These eighteen credits do not include student teaching.

    * Methods of teaching health education

professional education

    * Educational psychology. This group includes such courses as psychology of learning, human growth and development, adolescent psychology, educational measurements, and mental hygiene.

    * Health education. A maximum of three semester-hour credits will be accepted in this area. This group includes such courses as personal health problems, school health problems, nutrition, health administration, and biology.

    Curriculum. This group includes such courses as principles of curriculum construction, the high school curriculum, a study of the curriculum in the specific field, and extracurricular activities.

    Foundations of education. This group includes such courses as history of education, principles of education, philosophy of education, comparative education, and educational sociology.

    Guidance. This group includes such courses as principles of guidance, counseling, vocational guidance, educational guidance, research in guidance, and student personnel problems.

3. A minimum of forty semester-hour credits in the *field of specialization* distributed among the following four areas, and covering both the elementary and secondary fields, with major emphasis on health education.

    Bacteriology, biology, and chemistry

    Psychology and sociology, including mental hygiene, adolescent psychology, sociology, and educational sociology

specialized field

    Health education, including anatomy, physiology, child growth and development, personal and community health, foods and nutrition, health aspects of home and family life, health counseling, safety and first aid, and organization, administration, and supervision of school health programs

    Methods of teaching, including a study of the public school health education curriculum

student teaching

4. One hundred and fifty clock hours of *approved student teaching*. At least ninety clock hours must be devoted to responsible classroom teaching; sixty clock hours may be employed in observation and participation. This requirement is in addition to the eighteen credits in professional education.

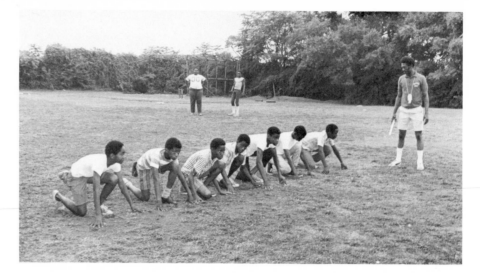

The physical educator should have a sincere interest in the teaching of physical activities. An instructor at Morehouse College in Atlanta works with some youngsters in track. (Courtesy President's Council on Physical Fitness and Sports.)

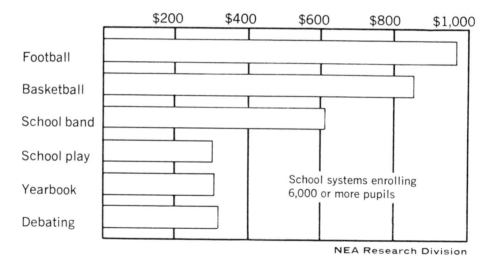

Average maximum annual salary supplements 1967-1968 for the physical educator qualified to coach selected pupil-participating activities. (From NEA Research Bulletin **46**:79, 1968.)

appearances in public, adequate knowledge and skill in the art of communication are essential.

Physical education work is strenuous and therefore demands that members of the profession be in a state of buoyant, robust health in order that they may carry out their duties with efficiency and regularity. It should also be remembered that physical educators are supposed to build healthy bodies. Therefore, they should be a good testimonial for their preachments.

Many moral and spiritual values are developed through participation in games and other physical education activities. It is essential, therefore, that the teacher of physical education have a proper background and possess such qualities that he or she will stress fair play, good sportsmanship, and a sound standard of values. The nature of his or her leadership should be such that the highest standards of moral and spiritual values are developed.

PHYSICAL EDUCATION

AUTHORIZATION. This certificate is required for teaching physical education in elementary and secondary schools. (Health education shall be included in this authorization if the curriculum contains at least eighteen semester-hour credits in this field.)

REQUIREMENTS

I. A bachelor's degree based upon a four-year curriculum in an accredited college

II. Successful completion of *one* of the following:

A. A college curriculum approved by the New Jersey State Department of Education as the basis for issuing this certificate

OR

B. A program of college studies including:

general background

1. A minimum of thirty semester-hour credits in *general background* courses distributed in at least three of the following fields: English, social studies, science, fine arts, mathematics, and foreign languages. Six semester-hour credits in English and six in social studies are required.

professional education

2. A minimum of eighteen semester-hour credits in *professional education* courses distributed over four or more of the following groups, including at least one course in each starred area. A maximum of three semester-hour credits will be accepted in health education. These eighteen credits do not include student teaching.

   * Methods of teaching physical education in elementary and secondary schools

   * Educational psychology. This groups includes such courses as psychology of learning, human growth and development, adolescent psychology, educational measurements, and mental hygiene.

   * Health education. A maximum of three semester-hour credits will be accepted in this area. This group includes such courses as personal health problems, school health problems, nutrition, health administration, and biology.

   Curriculum. This group includes such courses as principles of curriculum construction, the high school curriculum, a study of the curriculum in the field of specialization, and extra-curricular activities.

   Foundations of education. This group includes such courses as history of education, principles of education, philosophy of education, comparative education, and educational sociology.

   Guidance. This group includes such courses as principles of guidance, counseling, vocational guidance, educational guidance, research in guidance, and student personnel problems.

student teaching

3. One hundred and fifty clock hours of *approved student teaching*. At least ninety clock hours must be devoted to responsible classroom teaching; sixty clock hours may be employed in observation and participation. This requirement is in addition to the eighteen credits in professional education.

4. A minimum of forty semester-hour credits in the *field of specialization*, distributed among the following areas and covering both the elementary and secondary fields:

   Anatomy, physiology, kinesiology

   Coaching, development of personal skills, nature and function of play

   History, principles, and organization and administration of physical education

specialized field

   Materials and methods in physical education for the elementary grades and materials and methods in physical education for the high school

   Health education including personal and community hygiene, first aid, and safety

The physical educator should have a sincere interest in the teaching of physical education. Unless the individual has a firm belief in the value of his or her work and a desire to help extend the benefits of such an endeavor to others, he or she will not be an asset to the profession. A sincere interest in the teaching of physical education means that one enjoys teaching individuals, participating in the gamut of activities incorporated in such programs, helping others to realize the happiness and thrilling experiences of participation that he or she enjoys, and helping to develop citizenship traits conducive to democratic living.

The physical educator should possess an acceptable standard of motor ability. Physical skills are basic to the profession. To be able to teach various games and activities to others, it is necessary to have skill in many of them. The physical educator must enjoy working with people, since there is continuous association in an informal atmosphere when teaching physical education activities. The values of such a program will be greatly increased if the physical educator teaches in a manner conducive to happiness, cooperation, and a spirit of friendship. The qualifications for teachers of physical education to be certified in New Jersey are listed on p. 101.

ATHLETIC TRAINERS

A relatively new concept in high school and college physical education programs is the certified athletic trainer. These men and women complete a 4-year college curriculum that emphasizes the biologic and physical sciences, psychology, coaching techniques, first aid and safety, nutrition, and other courses in physical and health education.

Specific responsibilities are outlined by each school involved; however, the major duties of the athletic trainer are prevention, emergency treatment, and rehabilitation of athletes who incur injuries. The athletic trainer works closely with administrators, coaches, physicians, the school nurse, students, and parents in a cooperative effort to provide the best possible health care for all athletes under his or her authority.

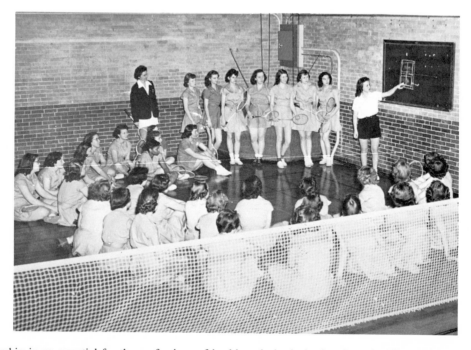

Leadership is an essential for the professions of health and physical education. An Illinois State University senior gives a demonstration lesson on badminton to a group of high school girls. Observing in the background is the supervising staff member.

Table 5-1. Teacher strikes, work stoppages, and interruptions of service, by type of organization, month, and state, 1972-73 school year*

Type of organization, month, and state	Number of strikes, work stoppages, and interruptions of service	Estimated number of personnel involved	Estimated number of man-days involved †
Type of organization			
Professional association	120	48,230	416,927
Teacher union	23	66,278	1,136,296
Month			
August	26	7,341	65,009
September	60	38,391	426,411
October	12	4,912	35,192
November	2	550	2,850
January	10	43,278	852,574
February	10	2,424	22,032
March	8	3,711	9,980
April	6	10,058	121,548
May	9	3,843	17,627
State			
California	2	1,350	1,850
Colorado	2	611	1,222
Connecticut	2	1,361	4,022
Delaware	3	859	3,568
District of Columbia	1	6,200	74,400
Hawaii	1	9,000	117,000
Illinois	16	31,067	321,573
Indiana	2	2,595	21,055
Kansas	1	81	1,944
Massachusetts	2	970	8,700
Michigan	16	5,404	29,522
Missouri	2	4,082	64,164
Montana	1	130	910
New Hampshire	2	205	1,570
New Jersey	6	1,056	8,440
New York	10	3,225	25,868
Ohio	13	3,275	11,168
Oregon	1	210	1,890
Rhode Island	10	5,327	23,339
Pennsylvania	35	32,158	784,225
Tennessee	1	80	1,360
Washington	3	1,477	6,047
Wisconsin	11	3,785	39,386
Total	143	114,508	1,553,223

*Compiled from published and unpublished information collected by the Bureau of Labor Statistics, U. S. Department of Labor, and NEA Research.

†Based on instruction days of full-time teachers during regular school year. Teacher report-in days, holidays, week-ends, and vacation days are excluded.

From National Education Association Research Information Service, Washington, D. C., 1973, National Education Association.

He or she is also responsible for development and supervision of a student athletic training staff.

The University of Arizona recently instituted a graduate internship in athletic training in cooperation with the Tucson Public Schools. This internship is a one-year course of study leading to a master's degree in physical education or health education. The intern is a part-time, paid member of a high school athletic staff and works approximately 25 hours a week in addition to classroom studies.

There is a definite need for more women as well as men to become involved in athletic training. In many undergraduate physical education programs, women have not received adequate preparation in athletic training courses. Most athletic training in women's competitive sports is performed by men who cannot best handle the physical and emotional trauma suffered by female athletes. In addition, a female athlete may be reluctant to seek the services of a male athletic trainer. Women are more likely to be open about personal problems to other women. Athletic training is important in all sports, male as well as female. Injuries and other related problems occur regularly in women's sports, and women should be adequately trained to meet these situations.

QUALITIES THAT MAKE FOR SUCCESSFUL TEACHING

Several persons were interviewed as to the qualities and characteristics they thought existed in the best teachers to whom they were exposed. A list of those qualities that were mentioned most frequently are as follows:

1. Teacher knew the subject matter well.
2. Teacher took a personal interest in each student.
3. Teacher was well respected and respected the students.
4. Teacher stimulated the students to think.
5. Teacher was interesting and made the subject matter come to life.
6. Teacher was an original thinker and creative in his or her methods.
7. Teacher was a fine speaker, presented a neat appearance and was generally well groomed.
8. Teacher had a good sense of humor.

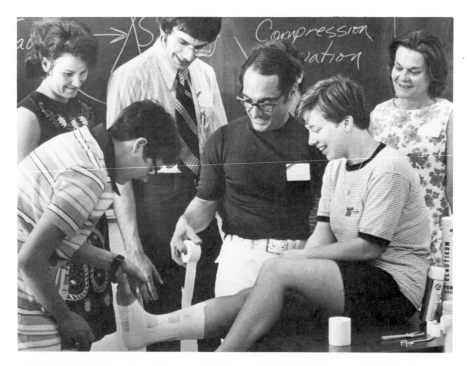

College of DuPage, Glen Ellyn, Ill., held a special 2-day athletic team trainer seminar showing techniques and methods to current and prospective team trainers.

9. Teacher was fair and honest in dealings with his students.

10. Teacher was understanding and kind.

PROBLEMS OF BEGINNING TEACHERS

Beginning teachers need considerable encouragement and help. The administration should be aware of this need and work to ensure that it is met. As a guide to some of the problems of beginning teachers, a survey of fifty teachers indicated the following:

1. Difficulties arising as a result of the lack of facilities

2. Large size of classes, making it difficult to teach effectively

3. Teaching assignments in addition to the primary responsibility of teaching health education or physical education

4. Discipline problems with students

5. Conflicting methodology between what the beginning teacher was taught in professional preparing institution and established patterns of experienced teachers

6. Clerical work—difficulty in keeping records up to date

7. Problems encountered in obtaining books and supplies

8. Problems encountered in obtaining cooperative attitude from other teachers

9. Lack of departmental meetings to discuss common problems

10. Failure to find time for personal recreation

WORKING EFFECTIVELY WITH GENERAL SCHOOL AND COLLEGE ADMINISTRATORS

School and college health and physical education programs are part of general education. Consequently, such items as the budgets allocated, facilities provided, and personnel appointed are subject to the thinking and decisions of general educators. Presidents of colleges, deans, superintendents of schools, principals, and administrators of instructional and business services, through their decisions and actions, affect these special programs in elementary and secondary schools and in colleges and universities of the nation. It is therefore important to get the thinking of these general administrators in respect to programs of school health, physical education, and recreation. The information that follows was taken from a review of general administration books and interviews with general administrators for the purpose of determining what constitutes effective working relationships between general school administrators and health and physical educators.

What constitutes effective working relations between general school administrators and health and physical educators?

Effective working relationships between general administrators and health and physical educators may be discussed under the headings of (1) responsibilities of general administrators, (2) responsibilities of health and physical educators, (3) common points of conflict, and (4) checklist for effective working relationships.

Some responsibilities of general administrators. There are many responsibilities of general administrators that have an impact upon good working relationships. A few of the more important are listed in the following paragraphs:

1. Administrators should possess a sound understanding of human nature in order to work effectively with people. General administrators should not look upon the administrative process

Table 5-2. Major problems of teachers*

	Urban	Suburban	Rural
Large class size	40.4%	33.4%	30.6%
Classroom management and discipline	23.3	10.8	12.1
Inadequate assistance from specialized teachers	22.5	21.0	30.3
Inadequate salary	34.9	24.5	30.3
Inadequate fringe benefits	27.7	22.3	31.3
Ineffective grouping of students into classes	24.3	18.2	24.2
Lack of public support for schools	27.8	17.4	23.7
Ineffective testing and guidance program	21.1	14.2	20.8

*From NEA Research Bulletin **46:**116, 1968.

in an impersonal manner but, instead, should always keep in mind the human dimensions. As such, human problems should be given high priority.

2. Administrators should understand their own administrative behavior. They should see conflicts where they exist and not fabricate them where they do not exist. They should given an accurate account of group expectations although they may not be in agreement with them. They should recognize the differences and rationale between their own views and those of other people.

3. Administrators should exercise wisely the authority vested in the administrative position. The authority goes with the office and not with the person. Administrators should recognize that the administrative position exists to further the goals of the school system and the education of children and youth. It should never be used as a personal vendetta.

4. Administrators should establish effective means of communication among members of the school system. Opportunities should be readily available for a discussion of personal and professional problems, new ideas, and ways of improving the effective functioning of the organization.

5. Administrators should provide maximum opportunity for personal self-fulfillment. Each person has a basic psychologic need of being recognized, having self-respect, and possessing a feeling of belonging. Within organization requirements, general administrators should make this possible for each teacher on the job and every member of the school organization, regardless of subject area or job role.

6. Administrators should provide leadership. General administrators speak for their schools. They are the acknowledged leaders both in the internal and external functioning of the educational program. Such responsibility implies leadership qualities that will bring out the best individual effort on the part of each member of the staff and a total coordinated endeavor working toward common goals.

7. Administrators should provide clear-cut policies and procedures. Policies and procedures are essential to efficient functioning of the school organization; therefore, they should

be carefully developed, thoroughly discussed with members who are concerned, put in written form in clear concise language, and then followed.

8. Administrators should plan meaningful faculty meetings. Meetings of the staff should be carefully planned and efficiently conducted. Meetings should not, as a regular rule, be called on impulse and dominated by the general administrator. Plans and procedures agreed upon should be carried out.

9. Administrators should make promotions on the basis of merit with an absence of politics and favoritism. Promotions should be arrived at through a careful evaluation of each faculty member's qualifications and objective criteria.

10. Administrators should protect and enhance the mental and physical health of the faculty and staff. In carrying out this responsibility the general administrator should eliminate petty annoyances and worries that can weigh heavily upon staff members, attempt to increase the satisfactions that each person derives from the organization, promote friendly relationships, develop an esprit de corps, improve respect for and social status of staff members in the community, and establish a climate of understanding that promotes goodwill.

Some responsibilities of health and physical educators. All the responsibilities of health educators and physical educators cannot be discussed in the limited space available for this subject. A few of the more important responsibilities that affect good working relationships with general administrators are listed:

1. Health and physical educators should lend thought and energy to supporting the total educational program. Each staff member must see his or her responsibility to the total educational program. This means serving on committees, attending faculty meetings, contributing ideas, and giving support to worthy new developments regardless of the phase of the total program to which it belongs. Also, the staff member should view his or her own field of specialization in proper perspective with the total educational endeavor.

2. Health and physical educators should take an interest in the administrative process. Such interest can be tangibly shown by participating in policy making and decision making, doing some role playing as to the problems and pressures faced by the general administrator in his or her job, and contributing ideas that will help cut down on administrative red tape and thus streamline the educational process.

3. *Health and physical educators should carry out their individual responsibilities with dispatch and efficiency.* Each teacher or staff member has a job to do. If each job is performed effectively, the total school organization will function more efficiently. Only as each person assumes the responsibility for doing his or her own job in a responsible manner can the educational effort be accomplished effectively.

4. *Health and physical educators should get their reports in on time.* Purchase requisitions, attendance, excuse, accident, and the multitude of other forms and reports that have to be completed and then collated in the general administrator's office must be done on time. Punctuality on the part of all staff members makes the general administrator's job much easier.

5. *Health and physical educators should be loyal to the administration.* Each staff member has the responsibility to be loyal to the administrators of his or her school organization. There can be differences of opinion and disagreement on the administrative process and the way it is conducted, but loyalty to the leaders is essential.

6. *Health and physical educators should observe proper administrative protocol.* Administrators do not appreciate a teacher going over their heads to a higher authority without their knowing about it. There are lines of authority that must be recognized and followed in every organization. Schools are no exception to the rule.

7. *Health and physical educators should be professional.* In relationships with colleagues, general administrators, or the public in general, a staff member should recognize that there is a professional way of behaving. Confidences are not betrayed, professional problems are ironed out with the people concerned, and personality conflicts are discussed with discretion.

Common points of conflict between general administrators and health and physical educators. Although there are many implications

for conflict in the listing of responsibilities for general administrators and for health and physical educators, some additional areas where poor working relationships occur are listed as follows:

1. The failure on the part of general administrators to recognize health and physical educators as vital subjects of the academic and educational process
2. A failure on the part of general administrators to see health education and physical education as two distinct and separate fields
3. The existence of an authoritarian and undemocratic administration with the general administrator ruling with an iron hand
4. The failure to outline clearly goals and responsibilities for the organization and for each member of the organization
5. The existence of some teachers' unions and organizations that obstruct rather than further the democratization of administration
6. The failure of general administrators to provide dynamic leadership
7. The failure of the administrator to provide clearly defined policies
8. The practice of administrators encroaching upon classes and schedules without good reason or adequate previous announcement
9. The assignment of unreasonable teaching loads and extra class assignments
10. The failure of teachers to read bulletins that contain important administrative announcements
11. The failure of teachers to conscientiously assume the duties and responsibilities associated with administrative routine, such as the checking of attendance
12. The failure of teachers to handle disciplinary cases properly
13. The existence of unsatisfactory plant, buildings, and working conditions
14. The lack of adequate teacher materials and equipment
15. Overemphasis upon athletics

What administrative groups worry about

The professional magazine, *Nation's Schools,* * conducted an opinion poll to determine what school administrators and board members worry most about. A 4% sampling was done of 16,000 school administrators in 50 states, which brought a 54% response. An 8% sampling was done of 8,000 school board members, which brought a 22% response. Pre-

---

*Schoolmen worry most about teacher, money shortages, Nation's Schools **81:**81, 1968.

CHECKLIST FOR EFFECTIVE WORKING RELATIONSHIPS BETWEEN GENERAL ADMINISTRATORS AND HEALTH AND PHYSICAL EDUCATORS

	Yes	No
1. Job descriptions of all school personnel are formulated, written, and disseminated to each individual involved.		
2. Policies are cooperatively formulated.		
3. Teachers are encouraged to participate in the determination of policies. Administration utilizes committees of faculty to develop policies.		
4. Policies cover priorities in the use of physical education facilities.		
5. Policies have been developed and are in writing for the major areas of the educational enterprise as well as specifically for the fields of health education and physical education.		
6. Departmental policies and procedures are up to date and complete.		
7. Board of education establishes and approves policies and programs.		
8. Health and physical educators know the policies for their school system and work within this framework.		
9. Open channels of communication are maintained between administrator and teacher.		
10. Inservice education is provided teachers.		
11. Teachers are encouraged to participate in the activities of professional organizations.		
12. Supervisors act in an advisory and not an administrative capacity.		
13. The teaching load of all teachers is equitable in that the following factors are considered: work hours per week, number of students per week, and number of after-school activities scheduled.		
14. Athletics are open to all students and conducted according to sound educational principles.		
15. Policies are in writing and disseminated and cover the organization and administration of varsity interscholastic athletics.		
16. Coaches are certified in physical education.		
17. The group process is effectively used in faculty and committee meetings.		
18. There is a strong belief in and a willingness to have a democratic administration.		
19. Faculty meetings are well organized.		
20. New staff members are oriented in respect to responsibilities, school policies, and other items essential to their effective functioning in the school system.		
21. Departmental budgets and other reports are submitted on time and in proper form.		
22. Staff members attend faculty meetings regularly.		
23. Staff members participate in curriculum studies.		
24. Classroom interruptions are kept to an absolute minimum.		
25. Proper administrative channels are followed.		
26. Relationships with colleagues are based on mutual integrity, understanding, and respect.		
27. The administration is interested in the human problems of the school organization.		
28. Maximum opportunity is provided for personal self-fulfillment consistent with organization requirements.		
29. Department heads are selected on the basis of qualifications rather than seniority.		
30. Staff members are enthusiastic about their work.		
31. All personnel are provided opportunities to contribute to the improved functioning of the school system.		
32. The school board's executive officer executes policy.		
33. Faculty and staff assignments are educationally sound.		
34. The administration works continually to improve the working conditions of school personnel.		
35. Out-of-class responsibilities are equitably distributed.		
35. The administration provides recreational and social outlets for the staff.		
37. The administration recognizes and records quality work.		
38. Health and physical educators seek to improve themselves professionally.		
39. Health and physical educators view with proper perspective their special fields in the total educational enterprise.		

CHECKLIST FOR EFFECTIVE WORKING RELATIONSHIPS BETWEEN GENERAL ADMINISTRATORS AND HEALTH AND PHYSICAL EDUCATORS—cont'd

	Yes	No
40. Health and physical educators organize and plan their programs so as to best meet the needs and interests of their students.	_____	_____
41. Health and physical educators continually evaluate themselves and the professional job they are doing in the school system.	_____	_____
42. Budgetary allocations are equitably made among departments.	_____	_____
43. The administration is sensitive to the specific abilities and interests of teachers and staff.	_____	_____
44. Health and physical educators take an active role in school planning.	_____	_____
45. Health and physical education objectives are consistent with general education objectives.	_____	_____
46. The administration recognizes and gives respect and prestige to each area of specialization in the school system.	_____	_____
47. Health and physical educators are consulted when new facilities are planned in their areas of specialization.	_____	_____
48. Funds are available for professional libraries, professional travel, and other essentials for a good inservice program.	_____	_____
49. Health and physical educators carefully consider constructive criticism when given by the administration.	_____	_____
50. The administration is skilled in the organization and administration of a school system.	_____	_____

sented here in adapted form are some of the main worries of school officials.

Superintendents of schools

Shortages of teachers
Inadequate funds
Militant teachers
Overcrowded conditions
Relations with school board
Transportation problems
Student problems of dress
Desegregation
New curricula
Community pressures
Use of drugs

School board members

Inadequate funds
Shortages of teachers
Militant teachers
Overcrowded conditions
Transportation problems
Relations with school administrators
Desegregation
Vandalism
Community pressures
New curricula
Student problems of dress
Use of drugs

Questions and exercises

1. Draw up a list of competencies that you consider essential for all teachers.
2. Draw up a list of competencies that in your opinion are essential for teachers of health and physical education.
3. Define the term *administration* in your own words and give illustrations to point out the various facets of your definition.
4. Discuss the qualifications of a good administrator, giving concrete examples to support the importance of each qualification listed.
5. Prepare an organization chart for some department, school, or agency with which you are associated. Discuss significant aspects of the administrative setup of this organization.
6. Explain the concept of differentiated staffing. Briefly discuss your opinion of this concept.
7. Prepare a rating sheet that could be utilized by students to determine the extent of their qualifications for the field of administration.
8. From your own experience, prepare a list of principles that you feel are essential to good personnel relations.
9. What is meant by the term *fallacy of final authority?* Cite two illustrations to support the idea involved.
10. Interview five general administrators and summarize their feelings about health education and physical education.
11. Discuss administrative styles. Which administrative style would you prefer a leader to follow? Explain.

12. Explain the responsibilities of athletic trainers. Why is it important that women be trained in this area?
13. What do you feel are the responsibilities of health educators and physical educators in the total educational program?
14. If you were a general administrator, what kind of a health educator or physical educator would you hire for your school or college system? Outline the type of person you would want working for you.

Reading assignment in *Administrative Dimensions of Health and Physical Education Programs, Including Athletics:* Chapter 4, Selections 16 to 20.

Selected references

American Association of School Administrators: Profiles of the administrative team, Washington, D. C., 1971, The Association.

Bucher, C. A.: Foundations of physical education, ed. 7, St. Louis, 1975, The C. V. Mosby Co.

Byrd, O. E.: School health administration, Philadelphia, 1964, W. B. Saunders Co.

Castetter, W. B.: The personnel function in educational administration, New York, 1971, The Macmillan Co.

Committee on Organizational Pattern: Organizational patterns for instruction in physical education, Washington, D. C., 1971, American Association for Health, Physical Education, and Recreation.

Delforge, G., and Klein, R.: High school athletic trainers internship, Journal of Health, Physical Education, Recreation **44:**42, March, 1973.

Hutton, L., and Silkin, J.: Needed: women athletic trainers, Journal of Health, Physical Education and Recreation **43:**77, January, 1972.

Jenson, T. J., and Clark, D. L.: Educational administration, New York, 1964, The Center for Applied Research in Education, Inc. (The Library of Education).

Moore, H. E.: The administration of public school personnel, New York, 1966, The Center for Applied Research in Education, Inc. (The Library of Education).

Ridini, Leonard: An experimental design for the training of paraprofessionals in physical education, Journal of Health, Physical Education, and Recreation **41:**23, October, 1970.

Schwank, W., and Miller, S.: New dimension for the athletic training profession, Journal of Health, Physical Education, Recreation **42:**41, September, 1971.

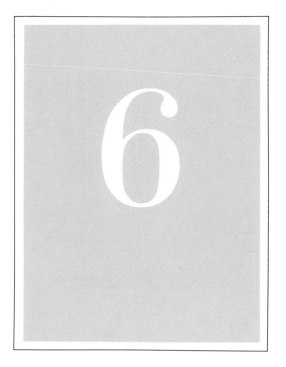

Student involvement and leadership in physical education

One of the most significant trends in education today is the involvement of students in charting their own educational careers. Students today are actively involved in curriculum planning, school board meetings, decision making, and in matters of administrative and teacher accountability.

Traditionally, there have been student leaders who have performed responsible tasks in many different areas of school and college life. These student leaders have more of a performance orientation than a decision making responsibility. However, both types of students are leaders in the sense that they are taking responsibility upon themselves; they are trying to improve human relations among students, faculty, and community, and they are acting in a law-abiding manner following established guidelines. Change is usually beneficial, but it must take place according to democratic principles.

In this chapter, the role of the involved student and the traditional student leader will be explored. It is important to note here that very frequently the involved student and the traditional leader are one and the same person. In recent years many leaders' groups have been involved in the planning and evaluating of their own programs and their participation in the programs.

WHY DO STUDENTS BOTH NEED AND WANT TO BE INVOLVED?

Today's students are different from students in the years prior to the late 1960s. Students of today have been brought up in an involved society where groups have spoken openly about such matters as war, segregation, poverty, crime, abortion, drug use, and political campaigns. Students wish to become part of the involved society for many reasons. Some of these reasons are cited here for consideration:

Students feel that they are not understood as individuals by their teachers and administrators.

They think they should be involved in the decisions that directly affect their lives in school.

They think many courses they are required to study are not relevant to their present or future life and find these offerings dull and defeating.

Students also feel that their school curriculum has not kept pace with the rapidly changing society all around them.

Young people of today have many diverse concerns, as illustrated by a recent survey of 200 college-bound men and women. Many of these concerns become apparent in a survey of their personal attitudes. Some of these attitudes are listed here.

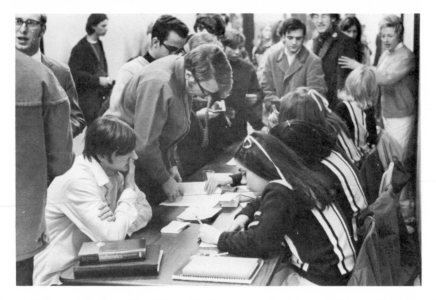

Cheerleaders at College of DuPage, Glen Ellyn, Ill., become involved by registering students for a blood drive to help local residents.

Students favor a more liberalized curriculum.

Approximately one-third of the students felt that women should be free to choose their own life style.

More than one-half of the students felt that conscientious objectors should be excused from military service during wartime.

Most students expressed an antiwar sentiment.

Students were very concerned with poverty and showed a general disturbance with the growing preoccupation with material possessions.

Most students expressed politically liberal or very liberal ideas.

It is hoped that these attitudes will provide some insight into today's young people and an understanding of why so many seek total involvement in their schools and the larger society.

WHAT CAN BE DONE TO INVOLVE STUDENTS?

There are many ways in which administrators can involve students in physical education programs. Teachers and administrators alike should stress communication with their students and create situations where open dialogue can oc-cur. Students should be included on advisory committees that discuss school athletic programs, scheduling, new activities, and the need for additional facilities or equipment. In addition, students should be encouraged to form sports clubs, participate in community sponsored athletic activities, and to work on independent study programs in physical education areas. Students should participate in evaluation programs designed to ascertain student as well as teacher performance. Evaluation should also include student appraisal of curriculum and suggestions for change.

STUDENT RIGHTS AND RESPONSIBILITIES

In a recent study of 68 colleges, conducted by Fairleigh Dickenson University, the extent to which these colleges have followed the principles of the *Joint Statement on the Rights and Freedoms of Students* was ascertained. This *Statement* was sponsored by such organizations as the American Association for University Professors (AAUP) and the United States National Student Association (USNSA), and it set the minimum standards for student rights in institutions of higher learning. Some of the results of the survey show that:

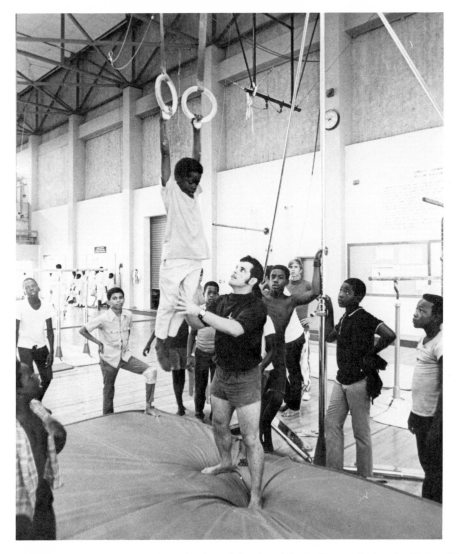

A student leader instructs disadvantaged youths from Miami and Dade County during the National Summer Youth Sports Program conducted by Miami-Dade Junior College North. (Courtesy President's Council on Physical Fitness and Sports.)

1. Students are included in decision making meetings concerning student affairs in 87% of the responding colleges.
2. Students are voting members of decision making groups on student affairs in 25% of the responding colleges. A higher percentage (approximately 50%) exists at small private colleges.
3. Students are frequently involved in policy making groups concerned with curriculum, physical planning, and financial aid.
4. Hearings for students who have com-

mitted on-campus crimes are provided by 86% of the responding schools. Hearing committee representation is comprised of both faculty and students in 33% of the responding colleges and all students in 29% of the responses.

In the physical education area, the American Alliance for Health, Physical Education, and Recreation (AAHPER) has recently formed The Student Action Council (SAC). Student members of SAC elect officers and have become an active voice in the profession. A recent project of the Student Action Council (Looking Into Free Environment) is related to the Energy Crisis. Another project, LIFE, provides for active participation of students in many issues confronting society including environmental pollution, political issues, world peace problems, and provisions for recreation development in inner-city areas.

AREAS OF STUDENT INVOLVEMENT

In past years many schools have been more concerned with the subject matter they were teaching than in the students that were being taught. In recent years, students have been demanding greater involvement in the educational process, and in most cases, this increased involvement has been satisfactory to both students and administrators. Some of these areas of involvement are briefly discussed here.

General planning

Students should be involved in planning meetings that discuss schedule changes, curriculum innovations, physical plant changes and new construction, and recent changes in educational methodology. Students should be invited to attend school board meetings, parent association meetings, and should also accompany teachers and administrators to other schools

where certain innovations may be directly observed. Some schools and colleges have instituted student advisory boards that meet with staff members to discuss problems, changes, and future planning ideas.

The sports club program at the University of Tennessee is an excellent example of a program for students and planned by students. The purposes of this program are:

1. To offer activities in sport areas to all interested students.
2. To develop skills in special sports.
3. To provide opportunities for extramural competition.

All students, regardless of the skill in a particular sport, are welcome to join. Instruction is provided for learners in every club. The sports club program is financed through support from the Sport Club Office, dues, games, and contributions. Coaches are usually drawn from faculty or community members, and all coaching is on a voluntary basis. These clubs are student-organized but under the supervision of the assistant director for sports clubs.

Another interesting example of a student designed program is the elective physical education program at Silverton High School, Silverton, Colorado. This course is available to eleventh and twelfth grade students, and its

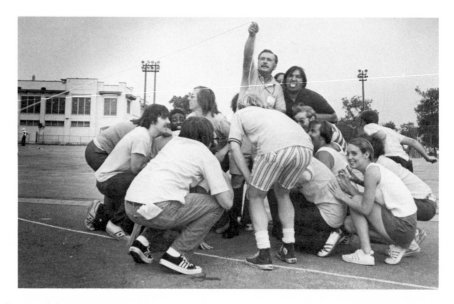

Play leaders receiving leadership training in Milwaukee. (Division of Municipal Recreation and Adult Education, Milwaukee Public Schools.)

primary objective is to give students a voice in curriculum construction. The course planned by the students allows for participation in such sport areas as alpine and Nordick skiing, backpacking, mountaineering, fly fishing, and weekend camping trips. The course has met with active student participation from all school departments. The home economics department aided in keeping food costs down, and the shop class made hunting bows. The community also participated in giving discounts on certain pieces of sports equipment. This student-designed elective course has been successful in expanding the classroom to include the out-of-doors.

Curriculum planning

Through the use of student surveys one can ascertain the extent of curriculum changes desired by the student body. Administrators, teachers, and students should carefully weigh this information in the light of the current literature in the field, research studies, and actual curriculum changes in other schools and colleges. Student participation and feedback is essential; however, students do have limited experience in educational matters, and this must also be taken into consideration. Frequently, the use of experimental programs on a limited basis can test the change before implementing it on a larger scale.

Many schools and colleges have recently instituted independent study programs where students receive credit for individual projects conducted under staff guidance. Some schools, colleges and universities have eliminated certain requirements for graduation and major field study. In addition, college grades have been replaced in some cases by pass/fail ratings. Many of these innovations were initiated by student groups.

In Framingham North High School, Framingham, Massachusetts, students take an active role in curriculum planning. Students plan what they are going to learn and how they would like to learn the gymnastics unit of the physical education class. Several days were set aside for students to set goals, plan the steps needed to reach a specific goal, and make a commitment to learning and improvement. The students put their goals in writing and then set about to achieve them. Instruction was provided and grading was a cooperative venture between students and teachers. An evaluation sheet completed near the end of the program indicated that the students had very positive feelings about gymnastics and the concept of goal-centered learning.

Leadership training programs

Leadership training programs in physical education are a constructive answer to the often heard criticism that students are not given opportunities to assume independent responsibility. A pilot program entitled Recreation Leadership was initiated and coordinated by the chairman of the Girls Physical Education Department at Concord High School, Concord, California. Twenty junior and senior boys and girls were selected to participate in the Recreational Leadership class. Criteria used for the selection include: maturity, enthusiasm, interest and ability in working with children, and ability to accept responsibility. There were five phases of the program that continued through the entire semester. The phases included: (1) preparatory and objective phase, (2) first aid course, (3) camp-counseling training and eventual use in helping to counsel sixth grade students in a camping situation, (4) physical fitness testing, and (5) elementary school teaching where they aided in teaching physical education classes. The culminating activity for the semester was a presentation to the parents of the elementary school children depicting through films and tapes the activities participated in by the student leaders and children.

Another innovative student leadership program is the Physical Education Leadership Training Program (PELT) sponsored by the Department of Health, Physical Education, and Safety of the Norfolk City School System. As part of an elective course in the physiology of exercise, juniors and seniors can relate their learning experiences to leadership experiences in elementary schools.

The PELT program has as its primary objectives: (1) assistance in instruction, particularly when the physical education teacher is absent; (2) to provide in-depth study of health and phys-

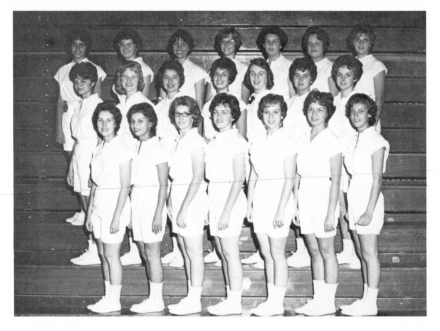

Student leaders. (Rich Township High School, Park Forest, Ill.)

ical education for students who want to teach as a career; (3) to provide students with leadership opportunities; and (4) to provide individualized instruction. The content and leadership experiences are developed and coordinated by the eleventh and twelfth grade classes. Supervision of the program is provided by the elementary physical education teacher, elementary classroom teacher, senior high school physical education teacher, head of the senior high school physical education department, and supervisor of physical education.

The four phases of the PELT program are: (1) in-service training, (2) observation, (3) teaching, and (4) teaching without supervision. This program is valuable to both teachers and students and helps the elementary grade teachers to provide individualized help for each student.

THE VALUE OF
STUDENT LEADERSHIP

Physical educators have the ability to develop leadership qualities in the students who participate in their programs. Many opportunities exist in curricular and extracurricular physical education programs to enable students to as-

sume leadership responsibilities under the direction and guidance of experienced physical educators. Under qualified supervision students can develop such attributes as cooperation, self-control, and good human relations and become imbued with the desire to serve other people. In addition, students can become involved with such responsibilities as planning and evaluating the programs in which they participate. To achieve the best results, however, the climate in which they participate should be friendly and permissive, be a place where initiative and creativity are encouraged, and provide frequent opportunities to discuss problems with their classmates and teachers and to understand clearly the meaning of good leadership. Finally, certain principles must be recognized if successful student leadership is to be developed. These principles include a clear delineation of student and staff responsibilities and a leadership program where individual development and self-direction are encouraged.

When a program of student leadership is established with such principles and conditions in mind, it will not only help each student to grow and develop but it will also be of value to the fields of physical education and health.

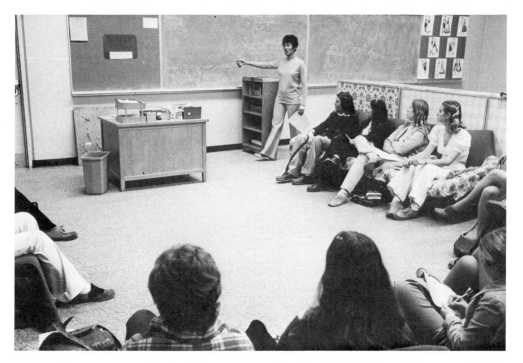

Student Leadership Program at El Camino Real High School in Los Angeles. (Los Angeles Unified School District, Student Auxiliary Services Branch. Courtesy Gwen R. Waters.)

Students frequently become more interested in these specialized fields and often decide to pursue a career in them as a result of seeing firsthand the opportunities they provide. Student leadership also renders a valuable service to the department by making it possible for more students to receive individualized instruction from their better skilled classmates; by providing better safety conditions under which activity participation can take place, since more spotters and other staff members are available; and by providing for the maximum utilization of class time as a result of a larger and more effective instructional staff. Many times student leadership also enables the teacher to spend more of his or her time in teaching rather than having to give attention to small clerical details such as attendance taking and equipment and supply management. Furthermore, it helps to enrich the program by providing expanded leadership for such extras as exhibitions, demonstrations, and intramural and interscholastic athletics.

ADVANTAGES AND DISADVANTAGES FOR THE STUDENT LEADER

Many students have been spoken to who have engaged in student leadership responsibilities in their respective physical education programs. As seen through their eyes, there are many advantages and disadvantages to serving in a student leadership capacity. An analysis of their evaluations of such a responsibility indicates that many of the disadvantages, however, can be eliminated if the program is conducted in a sound educational manner.

Students who have taken on student leadership responsibilities find that they are recognized by classmates and faculty as leaders who have special skills and personal attributes that qualify them for such a role. They also mention some of the more tangible material rewards that go with such a responsibility, for example, special uniforms, lockers, award dinners, assembly programs, and other forms of recognition. Those students who are interested in physical education or health as a possible career point out that they are provided an opportunity to learn more about the field and to get experience as a leader in this area of specialization. Furthermore, they point out that leadership qualities are developed with such experience, such as the ability to think, analyze problems, and make judgments concerning how a class should be conducted. The social experiences, such as associating with other leaders within their own school as well as student leaders in other schools, are also rewarding.

Student leaders feel that they gain a sense of duty and responsibility from their experience. They learn to abide by a code of ethics that has been established so that their responsibilities as a leader can be carried out as effectively as possible. They enjoy the responsibilities that are given to them and find that the additional duties help to further develop their minds and bodies.

Student leaders have also commented on the disadvantages that accrue from taking on such responsibilities. Some students indicate that they are asked to take on duties in order that the teacher may get an additional free period. Others say they are requested to assume duties for which they are not qualified, for example, teaching certain skills in which they are not proficient. Some students have found that the leadership program is poorly organized and administered and as a result they are not motivated to develop leadership qualities. In addition, they point out that some of the jobs assigned are menial in nature and not related to the development of leadership traits. In addition to pointing out disadvantages that evolve from the teacher's actions, they also point the finger at certain students who are autocratic and undemocratic in the execution of their responsibilities, thus preventing the achievement of desirable educational goals.

An interesting observation of some student leaders is that at times they feel that only a few select students are given the opportunity to have leadership experiences and, as a result, many potential leaders are overlooked. Students feel that more persons should be provided with the opportunities to develop leadership traits through such an experience. A last observation of students is that the actual leaders who have gone through the training programs are sometimes combined with the leaders-in-training in many of the experiences, social and curricular, that are provided. The students who make this observation indicate that they do not feel this procedure is the best one to follow since there is much duplication in the program provided.

QUALIFICATIONS OF THE STUDENT LEADER

The student leader obviously must have certain qualifications if he or she is to achieve the goals for which a leadership program is established. Since the student leader will have an impact on all the students with whom he or she works, it is important that such exposure yield sound educational results. Therefore, it is important to have established standards by which student leaders are selected. There are five qualifications that should be used as guides in the selection of student leaders.

Personality. The personality of the student leader should be conducive to interaction with the other students and faculty in a harmonious and desirable manner. A student leader should be cheerful and friendly, possess a sense of humor, and be able to smile at himself or herself. He or she should be enthusiastic about and enjoy the work, but at the same time must command the respect of his or her classmates and be viewed as the leader who must guide and make decisions for the welfare of the entire class.

Intelligence and scholarship. Intelligence and the application of this intelligence as demonstrated by getting passing grades in all subjects should be a requirement of the student leader. Intelligence and sound judgment are needed as a basis for making wise decisions, solving problems, and gaining the respect of one's classmates.

Interest in other people. Leadership cannot be exercised by a person unless he or she has a sincere interest in other people. The student leader should have an understanding of the needs of human beings and possess a desire to serve them. In addition, he or she should have a sympathetic attitude toward classmates with less skill who are awkward and uncoordinated in physical movement. Also, he or she should demonstrate qualities of good sportsmanship at all times.

Health and a love of physical activity. The student leader in physical education should exemplify the qualities that he or she is trying to develop in other students. Good health and sport skills and general motor ability are important considerations for the student leader in this field of specialization. In addition to providing a desirable image of the physical education leader, these qualities are prerequisites to the energy and productivity that are needed to carry out the responsibilities associated with the job of student leader.

Leadership qualities. In addition to the qualities that have been discussed as essential to a student's leadership role, other qualities are also necessary. These qualifications include the need to recognize the importance of the democratic process in teaching, the ability to efficiently organize classes and groups for activities, and other attributes such as dependability, desire, resourcefulness, initiative, industriousness, and patience.

METHODS OF SELECTING THE STUDENT LEADER

There are several methods utilized by physical educators to select student leaders. Some physical educators advocate the appointment of temporary leaders during the first few sessions of a class until the students become better known to their classmates and instructor. Some of the methods by which student leaders are selected are discussed in the following paragraphs.

Volunteers. Students are asked to volunteer to become a student leader. It may happen that the least qualified persons are the ones who volunteer. If this method is used, it should probably be used with the understanding that the student leader will serve for only a relatively short period of time. Also, there can be a rotation of student leaders with this method so that all volunteers may have such an experience.

Appointment by the teacher. The physical education instructor may appoint the student leader, utilizing his or her experience and judgment as a basis for the selection, based upon the qualities that are needed for such a position.

One of the limitations of this procedure is that it is not democratic since it does not involve the students who are going to be exposed to the student leader. However, if the teacher has the objective of letting each student in the class have a student leadership experience, this limitation can be overcome.

Election by the class. Another method of selecting student leaders is to have the students in the physical education class vote and elect the person or persons they would like to have serve in this capacity. A limitation of this method is that the person selected is often the most popular student as a result of participation in sports, student government, or some other school activity. Being the most popular student does not mean that he or she is qualified to be a leader. This is a democratic procedure, however, and if the guidelines for selection of a leader are established and if the proper climate prevails, it can be an effective method.

Selection based on test results. A battery of tests is sometimes used by physical educators as a means of selecting student leaders. Tests of physical fitness, motor ability, sports skills, other instruments that indicate leadership and personality characteristics yield useful information. They provide tangible evidence that a person has some of the desirable qualifications that are needed by a student leader in a physical education class. In addition, if the physical educator desires to have the entire class participate in the student leadership program, the test results may also be of value to the teacher in helping each student to identify weaknesses that need to be overcome during the training period.

Selection by Leaders' Club. Physical educators sometimes organize Leaders' Clubs as a means of providing a continuing process for the selection of student leaders. The students who are members of the Leaders' Club, under the supervision of a faculty advisor, select new students to participate as leaders-in-training. Then, after a period of training, these students in turn become full-fledged student leaders. This method, with its advantages and disadvantages, is discussed at greater length in the paragraphs to follow.

TRAINING THE STUDENT LEADER

One method of selecting and training student leaders is through a Leaders' Club. These clubs commonly have their own constitution, governing body, faculty advisor, and training sessions.

The written constitution of a Leaders' Club usually states the purpose of the club, requirements for membership, qualifications and duties of officers, financial stipulations, procedures for giving awards and honors, and other rules governing the organization.

The governing body of the Leaders' Club may consist of a president, vice-president, treasurer, and secretary all of whom are elected by the members of the club.

The faculty advisor is a teacher who works closely with the leaders to ensure that the objectives of the Leaders' Club are accomplished. The faculty advisor exercises close supervision over the affairs of the club and, in addition, provides inspiration and motivation to the leaders, encouraging creativity, and helping the students to achieve their goals.

The Leaders' Club usually has regular meetings on a weekly, biweekly, or monthly basis.

The Leaders' Club involvement in the selection and training of student leaders

In some schools, the students who are interested in becoming student leaders apply for membership in the Leaders' Club. Certain requirements are usually established as a means of judging whether or not a student is eligible for membership in the Club. In one school these requirements are listed as follows:

1. Grade of 80% or above in physical education
2. Scholastic average of at least 70% in major subjects
3. Passing grades in all subjects
4. Satisfactory health record
5. Membership in school's general organization
6. Recommendation of the physical education teacher concerning personality, character, and quality of work
7. All-around physical performance
8. Good rating on physical fitness tests

When a student's application to membership in a Leaders' Club is accepted, a period of training for one semester usually follows. During this period students learn the requirements and responsibilities of a student leader, practice demonstrating and leading as an assistant in physical education classes, and become familiar with the rules of games, the techniques of officiating, and other responsibilities that go with the role of student leader.

After the training period has ended, the qualifications of the trainees are again reviewed by the Leaders' Club. Such items as scholastic average, health and medical record, character, recommendations of physical education teachers, performance on skill tests, scores on written tests of rules, ability to officiate, and skill proficiency are examined. The next step may be the personal interview or a visit before the entire governing body of the Leaders' Club. Here the candidate's record is reviewed, pertinent questions are asked, and action is taken. The faculty advisor, however, usually makes the final judgment.

Some physical educators feel that the Leaders' Club involvement in the selection and training of student leaders is quite formal and not in the best interests of the goals of the leadership program. These critics especially question the personal interview at the end of the training period and action being taken by a student's peers in determining whether or not a student should become a member of the Leaders' Club. Furthermore, some physical educators object to clubs and societies in general as being contrary to the democratic ideals that should guide any leadership program.

Methods of guiding the student leader

There are several methods that have proved effective in guiding student leaders, either during their training period or while they are actually serving as fullfledged student leaders. These methods include movies, guest lecturers, leaders' physical education period, and meetings. *Movies* can be shown on such subjects as strategies involved in sports or how to play a game or sport. *Guest lecturers,* such as visiting physical education teachers, sports personalities, and educational specialists in such areas as motor learning and teaching techniques, can be utilized advantageously. A *leaders' physical education period,* where the student leaders themselves comprise the class and the faculty advisor covers various duties that the student leader must assume, can be helpful. *Meetings* in which the faculty advisor offers advice and instruction, problems are discussed, and other matters involving the student leader are covered are also an excellent medium of guiding student leaders.

HOW THE STUDENT LEADER MAY BE UTILIZED

Student leaders may be used in the physical education program in several capacities.

Class leaders. There are many opportunities in the basic physical education instructional class period where student leaders can be utilized to advantage. These include:

1. Acting as squad leader, where the student takes charge of a small number of students for an activity
2. Being a leader for warm-up exercises at the beginning of the class period
3. Demonstrating how activities—skills, games, strategies—are to be performed
4. Taking attendance
5. Supervising the locker room
6. Providing safety measures for class participation, such as acting as a spotter, checking equipment and play areas, and providing supervision
7. Assuming measurement and evaluation responsibilities, such as helping in the testing program, measuring performance in track and field, and timing with a stop watch

Officials, captains, and other positions. Student leaders can gain valuable experience by serving as officials within the class and intramural program, being captain of an all-star or other team, coaching an intramural or club team, and acting as scorers and timekeepers.

Committee members. Many committee assignments should be filled by student leaders so that they gain valuable experience. These include being a member of a *rules committee,* where rules are established and interpreted for games and sports; serving on an *equipment and grounds committee,* where standards are established for the storage, maintenance, and use of these facilities and equipment, and participating on a *committee for planning special days or events* in the physical education program, such as play, sports, or field days.

Supply and equipment manager. Supplies and special equipment are needed in the physical education program when the various activities are being taught. This includes such equipment as basketballs, archery, golf, and hockey equipment, and audiovisual aids. The equipment must be taken from the storage areas, transferred to the place where the activity will be conducted, and then returned to the storage area. The student leader can help immeasurably in this process and profit from such an experience.

Program planner. Various aspects of the physical education program need to be planned,

---

STUDENT LEADERSHIP SURVEY OF NINE NEW YORK STATE SCHOOLS

Questions

1. Do you use any kind of student leadership in your physical education classes?
2. If yes, do you use boys or girls or both?
3. What are their duties?
   Squad leaders, demonstrators, etc.
4. Do you use student leaders during athletic events at your school?
5. Do your student leaders in any way help formulate curriculum through suggestions to the teacher?
6. Do you use your athletic captains in a leadership role during practice or game situations? How?
7. Do you find the work of student leaders beneficial to the overall implementation of the program?
8. How do you select your leaders—teacher-appointed, class-elected, squad-elected classes, athletics?
9. How long do they serve?
10. Do you feel that the system of student leadership you have now is adequate, should be enlarged or changed, or done away with? Why?

Utilization of student leaders. Survey conducted by Norman Peck. See answers on p. 122.

Questions*	Rye	Rye Neck	Mamaroneck	New Rochelle	Valhalla	Hastings	Port Chester	Scarsdale	Bronxville
1	Yes	Yes	Yes	Yes	Yes	Yes	Yes—senior high only	Yes	Yes
2	Yes	Girls only	Yes	Yes	Yes	Yes	Yes	Yes	—
3	Squad leaders Demonstrators	Squad leaders Demonstrators	Squad leaders Demonstrators Spotters Instructors	Squad leaders	Squad leaders to set up equipment	Squad leaders Demonstrators	Squad leaders	Leaders in various physical education activities	—
4	Yes—varsity club members	Yes—varsity club members	Yes—"M" club members	Yes—varsity club members	Yes—varsity club members	Yes—varsity club members	No	Yes—varsity club members	Yes—leaders club (girls) and varsity club (boys)
5	No	No	Yes—through suggestion to teacher	No	No	Yes—through G.O. council	No	To very limited extent—not important part of program	No
6	Yes	No	Yes	Yes—strategy	Yes—sportsmanship and training	Yes—strategy	Yes	Yes	Yes
7	Yes	Yes—in school service functions	Yes—in all areas and functions	Yes—very much	Yes—in most cases	Yes—in all cases	Doubtful—sometimes good and sometimes poor	Yes	Yes—very much
8	Class—teacher appointed Athletics—appointed by teacher	Class—teacher appointed Athletics—elected by team	Class—high school teacher appointed Athletics—elected by team	Class—teacher appointed Athletics—elected by team	Class—teacher appointed Athletics—elected by team	Class—teacher appointed Athletics—elected by team	Class—teacher appointed Athletics—elected by team	Class varies with age groups and instructors Athletics—elected by lettermen	Leaders club Teachers selected Varsity club elected by team
9	Class—rotating basis Captain—elected for season	Class—rotating—equal chance for all Captain—elected for season	Class—usually for unit of instruction Captain—elected for season	Class—rotating basis, day—week unit Captain—elected for season	Class—one period all must serve Captain—elected for season	Class—unit Captain—elected for season	Class—rotating basis Captain—elected for season	Class varies—depends on ability and athletics—elected for season	Leaders club Varsity club for all year Captain—elected for season
10	Increasing	Expand to include boys' physical education classes	Change in curriculum will allow for more student leadership	Enlarge program and include safety techniques	Adequate	Increasing	Increasing	Adequate	Needs improvement

*See p. 121.

and students should be involved. Student leaders, because of their special qualifications and interest, are logical choices to participate in such planning. Their knowledge and advice can be utilized to ensure that the program meets the needs and interests of the students who participate in the program. Any curriculum development program should involve such students.

Record keeper and office manager. Attendance records and inventories must be taken, filing and recording done, bulletin boards kept up to date, visitors met, and other responsibilities attended to. These necessary functions provide worthwhile experiences for the student leader and benefit the program.

Special events coordinator. There are always a multitude of details to attend to when play days, sports days, demonstrations, and exhibitions are planned and conducted. Student leaders should be involved in the planning of these events and also in their actual conduct.

EVALUATION OF THE PROGRAM

An evaluation of the student leadership program should take place periodically to determine the degree to which the program is achieving its stated goals. Students should be involved in this evaluation. Such questions as the following might be asked. "Are the experiences that are provided worth while?" "Are the students developing leadership qualities?" "Is the teacher providing the necessary leadership to make the program effective?" "Are any of the assigned tasks incompatible with the objectives sought?" "If a Leaders' Club exists, is it helping to make for a better leaders' program?"

Questions and exercises

1. Explain briefly why students both need and desire to be involved. Suggest some ways by which students can become involved in physical education programs.
2. What are some of the advantages of a student leadership training program? Discuss one of those mentioned in the text or one you are personally familiar with.
3. Write a brief essay expressing your thoughts on student involvement in general and specific student involvement in physical education programs.
4. Do a job analysis of a student leader in each of three different schools and evaluate the responsibilities assigned in terms of the development of leadership traits.
5. Interview three experienced physical educators who were student leaders during their high school days and draw up a list of guidelines for a student leadership program based on their experiences and their evaluations of their own experiences.

Selected references

Annand, V.: PELT-Physical education leadership training, Journal of Health, Physical Education, and Recreation **44**:50, October, 1973.

Bell, M. M.: Are we exploiting high school girl athletes? Journal of Health, Physical Education, and Recreation **41**:53, 1970.

Blaylock, M.: Student unrest from a middle group, Improving College and University Teaching 211, Summer, 1971.

Chaffee, L., and Nickel, K.: Students vs administrators. Does it have to be? Journal of Health, Physical Education, and Recreation **43**:258, April, 1972.

Heisler, B., and Park, R.: Total involvement, Journal of Health, Physical Education, and Recreation **42**:24, October, 1971.

Herr, E.: Student activism: perspectives and responses, High School Journal 219, February, 1972.

Kudela, R.: Facing student unrest, The Clearing House 547, May, 1970.

McKenna, B.: Student unrest: some causes and cures, National Association of Secondary School Principals Bulletin 54, February, 1971.

Pastor, G.: Student-designed, Journal of Health, Physical Education, and Recreation **42**:30, September, 1971.

Romine, S.: Seven uncomfortable thoughts about student unrest, American School Board Journal 10, April, 1971.

School Board Members: Share the power with students, The Education Digest 39, October, 1970.

Sliger, I.: Student aquatic center recreation complex, Journal of Health, Physical Education, and Recreation **41**:42, February, 1970.

Voege, R.: Innovating? Involve the student, The Clearing House 543, May, 1969.

Williamson, E. G.: Student unrest and the curriculum, Educational Technology 18, May, 1970.

PART TWO

Administration of physical education programs

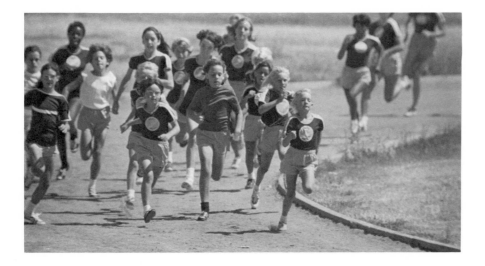

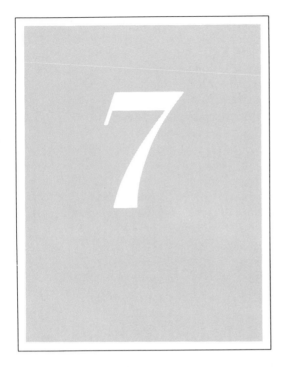

The basic instructional physical education program*

The physical skills that one has developed through the basic instructional physical education program are frequently carried over into adult life. A favorable attitude toward physical activity can often be traced back to favorable experiences in school instructional programs. Great satisfaction can be derived from physical education programs that teach the individual valuable skills and take advantage of the natural enjoyment inherent in physical activity.

The physical educator must see each boy and girl as an individual and work to develop that individual's interests and potentialities. From the earliest ages, children should experience a variety of activities that are not determined by sexual distinctions. Boys and girls can be taught to enjoy many of the same activities if they are given an opportunity to do so. Very often the quiet, unaggressive girl and the boisterous, active boy are only acting out roles that they have been taught or socialized into playing. Physical education programs can prevent this type of behavior by letting all children participate in some of the same activities regardless of sex.

ENCOURAGING NEW DEVELOPMENTS IN THE TEACHING OF PHYSICAL EDUCATION

Innovative methods of making physical education come alive for boys and girls are being researched and utilized increasingly in instructional programs. Students are being given greater freedom to select their own activities and to supplement these activities with community resources. Some examples of new physical education programs are discussed in the following section.

An experimental high school. John Dewey High School in Brooklyn, New York is an experimental high school that divides its 8-hour day into 22 computer scheduled modules. Classes may last for two or three modules (called mods) and vary in length on different days. There are also blocks of independent study time included in the daily schedule. Progress is evaluated in terms of achievement of

*School and college physical education programs will be discussed in the next four chapters. This chapter is concerned with the basic instructional physical educational class or service program. Chapter 8 concerns itself with the adapted physical education program. Chapter 9 deals with the intramural and extramural athletic programs, and Chapter 10 is concerned with interscholastic and intercollegiate varsity athletic programs.

designated behavioral objectives rather than by letter grades.

Each department maintains a resource center staffed by teachers and paraprofessionals. Available at the resource centers are Dewey Independent Study Kits (DISKs) that are prepared courses offered by each department for full credit. The physical education resource center is held in the gymnasium when regular classes are not scheduled. Activities offered at the resource center are the same as those taught in regular classes or are purely recreational in nature. Students may work independently in physical education with DISKs.

Opportunities for field work in physical edu-

cation also exist. Involvement as teachers' aides, participation in advanced college dance groups, and utilization of community recreational resources are only a few of the ways that John Dewey students become involved in outside field work.

Mini-courses. Thomas Carr Howe High School of Indianapolis, Indiana has introduced the idea of mini-courses into the activity program. Twice a month during the spring semester the students attend 60 different special interest activities selected from 170 offerings. Time for these activities is gained by shortening each regular period by 5 minutes. Activities include guidance, instructional, and rec-

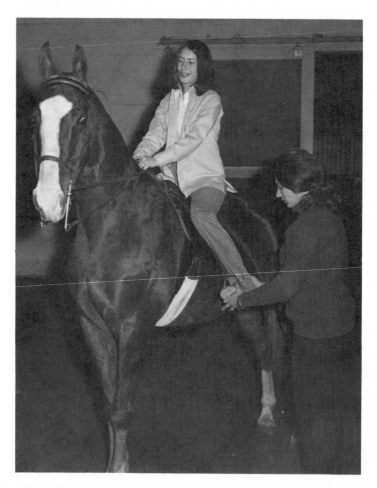

Paraprofessional teaching riding at Regina High School, Minneapolis. (Photograph by Rollie Baird, Dellarson Studios.)

reational offerings, and community resource people are utilized wherever possible. Table tennis, yoga, golf, riflery, sport fishing, and hunting are only a few of the recreational activities offered.

Computer monitored physical education. Simmons Junior High School, Aurora, Illinois offers daily coeducational activities where students progress at their own rate through a series of self-directed activities. A computer is used to keep track of each student's progress. Performance objectives are the basis of evaluation, and physical skills are supplemented by

cognitive concepts. Each student works at a particular activity with a learning unit planned for his level of achievement. Performance objectives are clearly outlined for each level, and final achievement is frequently the ability to demonstrate a skill to the teacher.

Mini-gyms. The concept of mini-gyms is that children should be encouraged toward physical expression beyond the scheduled gym period. Suggestions for accomplishing this include: (1) activity areas in every classroom, (2) chinning bars in the halls, (3) mats in the cafeteria, (4) carpeted areas for tumbling, (5)

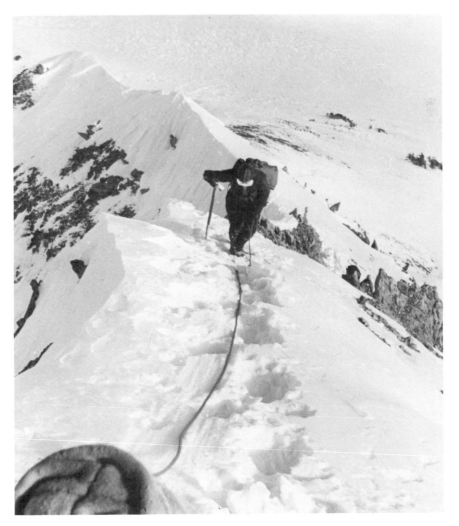

Silverton, Colo. High School utilizes community resources for its activities. Students in an eleventh and twelfth grade physical education class completing a unit in mountaineering with an assault on a local 13,600 foot peak.

stationary bicycles and rowing machines, (6) outdoor exploration areas, and (7) most importantly, a philosophy of education that encourages children to utilize these areas.

Using community resources. John Dickinson High School in Wilmington, Delaware has been able to add such activities as horseback riding, karate, fencing, and bowling to its physical education program by using community resources. Most of these elective activities are coeducational, and any fees are paid for by the students. Physical education for seniors is optional, and many include these courses in their schedules because of the outside activity offerings.

There have been several other developments that also augur well for the teaching of physical education. These are (1) getting at the "why" of physical activity, (2) movement education, (3) perceptual-motor programs, (4) the Broadfront Program, and (5) the Battle Creek Physical Education Project.

Getting at the "why" of physical activity

An encouraging new development in physical education is the progress being made toward in-

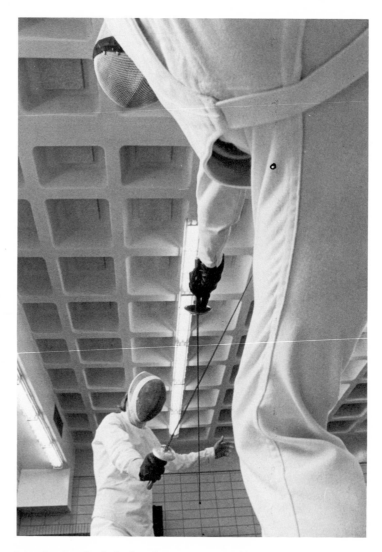

Fencing is one activity that the physical education program provides at Florissant Valley Community College in St. Louis. (Photograph by LeMoyne Coates.)

corporating the "why" of physical activity into physical education programs, particularly at the high school level. Traditionally, physical education has consisted entirely of physical activity with very little explanation being given to students as to *why* they should be active. Physical education appears to have operated under the assumption that participation in games, sports, and other activities alone will develop an understanding of the potential values of these activities, although it is widely accepted that students will function more positively if they know, understand, and appreciate the reasons for participating in various forms of physical activity. Today, it is being increasingly recognized that students need to understand basic concepts about health and fitness in order to be truly physically educated.

The American Alliance for Health, Physical Education, and Recreation has had a committee working for several years identifying the knowledge and understanding needed in physical education.* This report by an outstanding group of leaders is divided into an introduction and four parts: Introduction, Why Teach A Body of Knowledge in Physical Education?; Part I, Activity Performance (covers such items as basic sport skills, body mechanics, concepts fundamental to movement, skills in strategies and activity patterns, rules and procedures, and protective requirements); Part II, Effects of Activity, Immediate and Long Term; Part III, Factors Modifying Participation in Activities and the Effects of Participation; and Part IV, Standardized Tests.

In keeping with the trend toward getting at the "why" of physical activity, a few textbooks have been published that outline the material essential for boys and girls to know in order to be physically educated. A text has been written entitled *Physical Education for Life,*† which is specifically designed for this purpose and for the use of high school boys and girls. The

material included in this text, in both English and Spanish editions, is outlined here in order to give the reader some idea of what material might be included regarding the "why" of physical activity.

Physical Education for Life includes a full coverage of sports and activities appropriate for both sexes, for boys only, and for girls only. Part One concentrates on such topics as the organ systems of the body related to and affected by physical activity, the requirements for good body mechanics, exercises to correct some atypical posture conditions, how physical movement takes place and the laws of physics that apply to such movement, how skills are learned based on the latest scientific principles of motor learning, the requirements for and the ingredients of a personal regimen for achieving and maintaining physical fitness, and isometric and isotonic exercises for high school students. Furthermore, a chapter is devoted to safety guidelines and first aid procedures common to participation in physical education activities. Each chapter concludes with a series of questions and answers covering additional information pertinent to the subject of the chapter.

Part Two consists of twenty chapters. Each chapter presents a different physical education activity, ranging from archery, badminton, and basketball to dancing, gymnastics, and wrestling. Each chapter includes the history of the activity, terminology, rules of the game, and recommendations for attire, equipment, etiquette, and safety precautions. There is a progressive treatment of the basic skills involved in the beginning, intermediate, and advanced ability levels of each activity. Each chapter ends with a discussion of strategy and activities for improving skill.

Movement education

Movement education is a significant new approach to teaching physical education. It frees the individual student to work and progress at his or her own pace, while it offers opportunities for creative expression and exploration. It helps the student to better understand the physical laws that govern human movement. Physical skills are developed

*American Association for Health, Physical Education, and Recreation: Knowledge and understanding in physical education, Washington, D. C., 1969, The Association.
†Bucher, C. A.: physical education for life, St. Louis, 1969, Webster Division, McGraw-Hill Book Co. Bucher, C. A.: Tratadode Educacion Fisica y Deportes, Mexico, 1973, Compañia, Editorial Continental, S. A.

through an individualized problem-solving technique.

Movement education is being introduced into many elementary schools throughout the nation, and various aspects of movement education are taking root in secondary schools and colleges as well.

What is movement education? Experts do not agree on a single definition. They do agree, however, that movement education is dependent on physical factors in the environment and on the individual's ability to intellectually and physically react to these factors. Movement education attempts to help the student to become mentally as well as physically aware of his bodily movements. It is based on a conceptual approach to human movement. Through movement education, the individual develops his or her own techniques for dealing with the environmental factors of force, time, space, and flow as they relate to various movement problems.

Movement education employs the problem-solving approach. Each skill to be explored

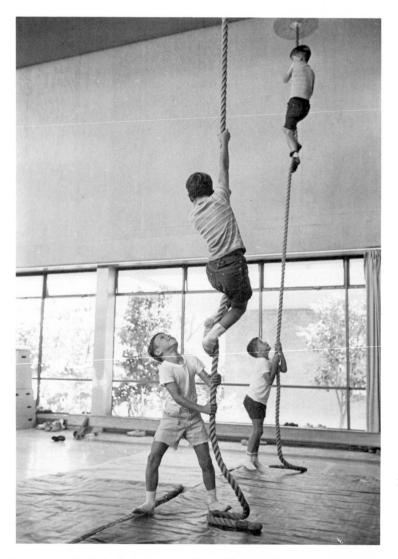

Students in an elementary school physical education class. (Courtesy President's Council on Physical Fitness and Sports.)

presents a challenge to the student. Learning results as the student accepts and solves increasingly more difficult problems. For this reason, the natural movements of childhood are considered to be the first challenges that should be presented to the student.

Traditional physical education emphasizes the learning of specific skills through demonstration, drill, and practice. Movement education emphasizes the learning of skill patterns through individual exploration of the body's movement potential. Traditional physical education stresses the teacher's standard of performance. Movement education stresses the individual child's standard of performance.

Perceptual-motor foundations

Another development in physical education that should be noted is the increased recognition of perceptual-motor foundations. For some time there has been an increased recognition of the importance of meaningful perceptual-motor programs for underachievers in the elementary schools. Research conducted by psychologists, physical educators, and others has shown that motor activity, when properly presented, can enhance perceptual development.

One of the most significant developments of this interest was the publication of the report of a task force of the AAHPER, which studied such subjects as the evolution of perceptual-motor behavior with implications for the teaching-learning process. It also explored interdisciplinary implications and identified areas for future study and research.* This study indicates there is a relationship between physical education and the development of perceptual-motor skills and that perceptual-motor skills are essential to learning and scholastic achievement. Therefore the conclusion is drawn that physical education, through the contribution that can be made in this area, has the potential for contributing to and facilitating the educational and academic achievement of certain children in our schools.

---

*American Association for Health, Physical Education, and Recreation: Perceptual-motor foundations: a multidisciplinary concern, Washington, D. C., 1969, The Association.

The Broadfront Program

Ellensburg, Washington, has developed a comprehensive program in physical education, health, recreation, which has been in existence for several years but still has many implications for professional fields. The project was started as a result of a Title III grant from the national government. It is designed to help each boy and girl in elementary, junior high, and senior high school develop physical skills, desirable attitudes, and knowledge about physical education, health, and recreation. It not only focuses attention on the normal boy and girl but also the handicapped and the retarded student. Furthermore, it is concerned with linking the school and community together in a program with both student and adult participation. Specifically, the Broadfront Program has five major aspects: (1) the acquisition of skills on the part of the student in individual sports, (2) health education, (3) a community-school program, (4) outdoor education and school camping, and (5) an adapted health and physical education program.

Broadfront is designed to accomplish such goals as ensuring that students develop skill competency in at least two lifetime sports, providing inservice education for classroom teachers both elementary and secondary, utilizing professors and major students from nearby colleges, instructing the adult population of Ellensburg, Washington, in lifetime sports, utilizing all facilities in both the school and community, and providing for the orientation of student teachers who are majors in physical education, as well as elementary school education majors, so that they will understand and appreciate the program.

The Battle Creek Physical Education Curriculum Project

The Battle Creek Curriculum Project represented an effort on the part of a public school system working with a university to develop and implement a model curriculum for physical education at both the elementary and secondary educational levels. The project team consisted of specialists in physical education, curriculum development, child growth and development, sociology, physiology, and educational measurement. The major objectives of the project were to first identify a body of knowledge that would form the framework for a curriculum model. This was accomplished by an intensive search of the literature to find out such things as the influence of physical activity on one's biologic, sociologic, and psychologic development and the relationship of one's various activity patterns to culture and environment. The second objective was to take the findings of this intensive search of the literature and organize it in terms of such things as a philosophy that would act as a guide for the curriculum model and also as a guide for general and behavioral objectives and outcomes. Finally, the development of a model program in physical education was derived from the previous two steps. The Battle Creek Project has national implications for physical education programs.

THE BASIC INSTRUCTIONAL PROGRAM

The basic instructional program of physical education is the place to teach, not a setting for free play and intramurals or an opportunity for the varsity team to practice. The entire period should be used to teach skills, strategies, understandings, and essential knowledge concerning the relation of physical activity to physical, mental, emotional, and social development.

Skills should be taught from a scientific approach so that the various kinesiologic factors that affect movement are understood clearly by the student. Utilization of demonstrations, super-8 films, loop films, models, slide films, videotapes, posters, and other visual aids and materials can help in clarifying instruction. Team teaching and differentiated staffing enable the master teacher of specific skills to be utilized more extensively than in the past.

The material presented throughout the school life of the child should be sequential in development and progressive in application. Just as a student advances in mathematics from simple arithmetic to algebra, geometry, and calculus, so in physical education the pupil should progress from basic skills and materials to more complex and involved skills and strategies.

Performance objectives should be established for individual student achievement. When boys and girls advance from one grade to another, they should have achieved certain objectives in various physical education activities, just as they master various levels of skills and understandings in subject matter areas of instruction.

The physical education class should involve more than physical activity itself. As the student understands more fully the importance of sports and activities in life, what happens to the body during exercise, the relation of physical activity to one's biologic, psychologic and sociologic development, the history of various activities, and the role of physical activity in the cultures of the world, the class takes on more intellectual respectability and meaning for the student and the profession in general.

Just as textbooks are used in other courses in the educational system, so should physical education use a textbook, with regular assignments given. Textbooks should contain not only material on physical skills but should also get at the subject matter with which physical education is concerned.

Records that follow a child from grade to grade should be kept throughout his or her school life. These records will indicate the degree to which the objectives have been achieved by the student, his or her physical status, skill achievement, knowledge about the field, social conduct, and other aspects that will help to interpret in a meaningful manner what physical education has done for the student and what still needs to be done.

There should also be homework in physical education. The subject matter needs to be mastered, the skills acquired, and standard of physical fitness achieved. Much of this information, skill, and various standards can be met at least partially through homework assignments.

Guidelines

The basic instructional physical education period cannot be conducted in a "hit-and-miss" fashion. It must be planned in accordance with the needs and interests of the individuals it serves.

Some of the initial considerations in planning and developing a physical education program are suggested by committees of the AAHPER Physical Education Division. These committees

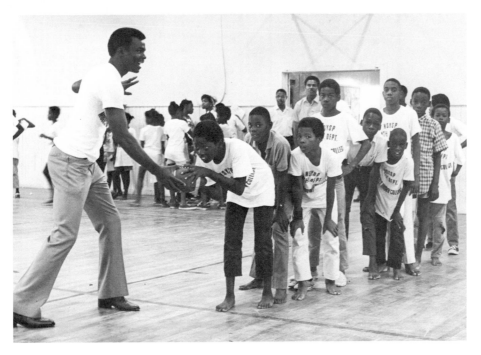

Secondary school students engaging in relay race at Morris Brown College in Atlanta. (Courtesy President's Council on Physical Fitness and Sports.)

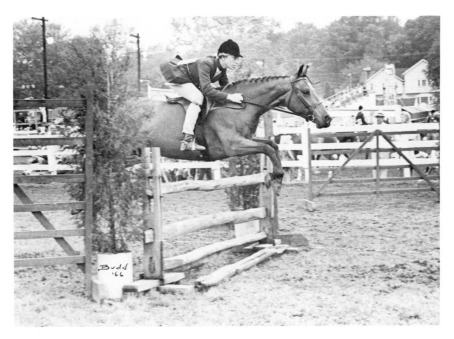

Student engaging in riding. (Courtesy Budd Studios, New York City.)

prepared three position papers: *Essentials of a Quality Elementary School Physical Education Program, Guidelines for Secondary School Physical Education,* and *Guide to Excellence for Physical Education in Colleges and Universities.* These papers have as their prime objective the delineation of essential elements for excellence in physical education programs. In this section the basic instructional guidelines are set forth in adapted format for each group discussed in the position papers.

Elementary school program. The instructional program for elementary students should have the following guidelines:

1. Program excellence should contribute to self-reliance and complete functioning of students.
2. A comprehensive physical education program must meet the needs of all children: gifted, slow-learners, handicapped, culturally deprived, and the average child.
3. Maximum involvement of each student in mental, motor, and emotional responses will result in positive changes in behavior.
4. A variety of learning experiences should result in

the development of concepts, values, and behavior of a physically educated person.
5. Curriculum content should be organized so that attitudes, learning, and skills take place in a sequential and developmental manner.
6. Teaching must be both teacher-directed and self-directed, and the instructional program should be designed to: (a) teach the whole child, (b) encourage development of physical fitness, (c) develop motor skills, (d) encourage creativity, (e) emphasize elements of safety, (f) motivate self-expression and realization of self-concept, and (g) stimulate social development.
7. Instruction should include use of audiovisual materials, small groups, and individualized instruction, as well as intramural and extramural activities.

Secondary school program. Many of the guidelines proposed by the elementary committee are also valid for secondary and college instructional programs. The conclusions of the secondary school position paper are given here in adapted format.

1. The instructional program must meet the differing needs of all students and be geared to the developmental needs of each pupil.
2. The program should be balanced between team and

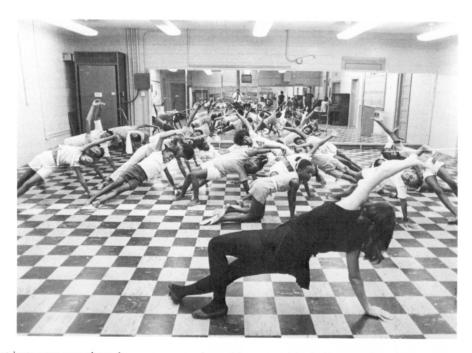

Student instructor goes through warm-up exercises with young girls during a modern dance class for participants in the National Summer Youth Sports Program conducted by Miami-Dade Junior College North. (Courtesy President's Council on Physical Fitness and Sports.)

individual sports, aquatics, gymnastics, self-testing activities, dance, and rhythms.

3. Progression should be sequential in specific skills and movement patterns.
4. Elective learning opportunities should be offered.
5. Knowledge of the human body and the principles of human movement are essential.
6. Creativity, self-direction, and vigorous activity, in addition to safety principles, should be encouraged.
7. Physical fitness and skills that can be employed in a comprehensive intramural, interscholastic and recreational program for all pupils should be emphasized.
8. The development of human relationships and the encouragement of pupils who have difficulty because of physical, social, and emotional problems is essential to an excellent program.

College and university program. The college position paper concluded that colleges and universities should provide instruction in physical education as part of the general education program. The instructional program should include the following considerations:

1. All students should have an opportunity to participate in physical education programs of their choice, and professional counsel should be made available to aid students in their choice of courses.
2. Programs should be innovative in meeting the needs of all students and should include independent and tutorial study.
3. Policies that pertain to advanced placement, credit by examination, requirements, and grading should reflect the institutional philosophy.
4. Participation in intramurals, extramurals, and intercollegiate athletics should not substitute for instructional classes in physical education.
5. Likewise, nonphysical education activities should not substitute for physical education requirements.
6. Research should be conducted to improve the quality of the physical education program.

The next step in considering the basic instructional program is to examine some of the administrative problems involved in its organization. These include scheduling, time allotment, daily physical education period, size of classes, teaching loads, and differentiated staffing and grouping; administrative policies concerned with having physical education on a required or elective basis, substitutions, credit allowances, class attendance, and excuses; separation of boys and girls in grades one to six; physical education specialist or classroom teacher and the question of self-defense courses; items of class management concerned with planning, dressing and showering, dress, roll taking, grading, and records; matters relating to activities, such as criteria for their selection, classification, and coeducational aspects; and program considerations at the elementary, junior high school, senior high school, and college levels.

SCHEDULING

The manner in which physical education classes are scheduled reflects the physical education leadership in the school or college and the attitude of the central administration. The physical education class will be more meaningful for students if it is scheduled in a manner that is linked to their interests, rather than in the interest of administrative convenience.

Scheduling should be done according to a definite plan. Physical education should not be inserted in the overall master scheduling plan whenever there is time left over after all the other subjects have been provided for. This important responsibility cannot be handled on a hit-and-miss basis, since that disregards the interests and needs of the students. Instead, at the secondary educational level, for example, physical education classes should be scheduled first on the master plan, along with such subjects as English and science that are required of all students most of the time they are in school. This allows for progression and for grouping according to the interests and needs of the individual participants. The three important items to take into consideration in scheduling classes are (1) the number of teachers available, (2) the number of teaching stations available, and (3) the number of students who must be scheduled. This is a formula that should be applied to most subjects in the school offering. Physical education will normally be scheduled correctly, as will other subjects, if this formula is followed.

All students should be scheduled. There should be no exceptions. If the student can go to school or college he or she should be enrolled in physical education. Special attention should be given, however, to the handicapped and gifted individual to ensure that he or she is placed in a program suited to individual needs. Also, special attention should be given to the weak student who needs extra help in the development of physical skills.

At the elementary and secondary levels, but especially at the elementary, scheduling should be done on 1-year basis. Special attention should be given to the needs and interests of students in respect to such items as the availability of facilities, equipment, and supplies and the weather. Planned units of work will usually become increasingly longer as the student progresses in grades, because of the longer interest span, greater maturity, and the increased complexity of the activities.

Every physical educator should make a point of presenting to the central administration his or her plans for scheduling physical education classes. The need for special consideration in this area should be discussed with the principal, scheduling committee, and others involved. Through persistent action, progress will be made. The logic and reasoning behind the formula of scheduling classes according to the number of teachers and teaching stations available and the number of students who must be scheduled cannot be denied. It must be planned in this way if there is to be progression in instruction and if a meaningful program is to result.

The introduction of flexible scheduling into school programs has implications for the administration of school physical education programs. Flexible scheduling assumes that the traditional system of having all subjects meet the same number of times each week for the same amount of time each period is passé. Flexible scheduling provides that class periods be of varying lengths, depending on the type of work being covered by the students, methods of instruction, and other factors pertinent to such a system. Whereas the master plan makes it difficult, if not impossible in many cases, to have flexible scheduling, the advent of the computer has made such an innovation practical and common.

Flexible scheduling also makes it possible to schedule activities for students of differing abilities in a different manner so that all are not required to have a similar schedule based on a standard format of the school day. Under the traditional system all students who were the slowest, for example, took as many courses as the brightest. Under flexible scheduling, some students may take as few as four courses and some as many as eight.

Modular scheduling is one type of flexible scheduling that breaks the school day into periods of time called modules. In Ridgewood High School in Norridge, Illinois, the school day is composed of 20-minute modules, and classes may vary from one to five modules, depending on the purpose of the course. The school is on a 6-day cycle and operates by day one, two, or three rather than the traditional days of the week. In physical education, each year level meets for three modules per day, four days per week. Each year level also has a two-module large group meeting once every cycle. In this meeting students hear guest speakers and lectures concerned with physical education concepts.

In other schools using modular scheduling, students frequently have unscheduled modules that can be used for swimming pool or gymnasium activities. In addition, intramurals, open lab sessions (free time to use facilities), sport clubs, and demonstrations provide incentive for students to use the skills they have learned.

Time allotment

Just as scheduling practices vary from school to school, college to college, and state to state, so does the time allotment. In some states there are mandatory laws that require that a certain amount of time each day or week be devoted to physical education, whereas in others permissive legislation exists. For grades one to twelve the requirement varies in different states from none, or very little, to a daily 1-hour program. Some require 20 minutes daily and others 30 minutes daily. Other states specify the time by the week, ranging from 50 minutes to 300 minutes. The college and university level does not usually require as much physical education as grades one to twelve. The usual practice in higher education is to require physical education two times a week for 2 years.

The general consensus among physical education leaders is that in order for physical education to be of value, it must be given with regularity. For most individuals this means daily

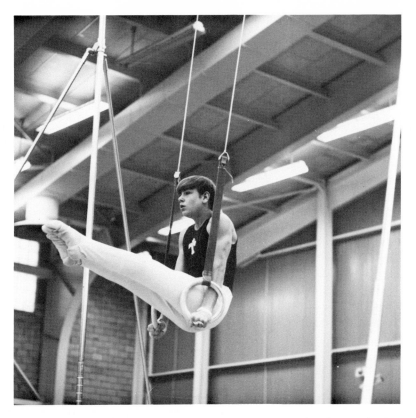

Student at Thornwood High School, South Holland, Ill., performing on the rings.

periods. There is also agreement among experts in the field of health that exercise is essential to everyone from the cradle to the grave. Smiley and Gould pointed out several years ago the exercise needs of individuals at various ages. These needs still exist today:

Ages 1 through 4. Free play during hours not occupied by sleeping

Ages 5 through 8. Four hours a day of free play (running, jumping, dancing, climbing, teetering, etc.) and of loosely organized group games (tag, nine pins, hoops, beanbags, etc.)

Ages 9 through 11. At least three hours a day of outdoor active play (hiking, swimming, gymnastsics, group games and relays, soccer, volleyball; broad-and-high jump, 25- and 50-yard dashes, folk dancing, etc.)

Ages 12 through 14. At least two hours a day of outdoor active play (hiking, swimming, gymnastics, group games, relays, soccer, volleyball, indoor baseball, basketball, baseball, tennis, 60-yard dash, the jumps, shot-put, low hurdles, short relays, folk and gymnastic dancing). Still no endurance contests

Ages 15 through 17. At least one and one-half hours a day of outdoor active play (hiking, swimming, apparatus work, group games and relays, soccer, volleyball, indoor baseball, basketball, baseball, tennis,

football, golf, ice hockey, 60-yard dash, the jumps, shot-put, low hurdles, short relays, folk and gymnastic dancing). Still no endurance contests

Ages 18 through 30. At least one hour a day of active outdoor exercise (all the types listed in the preceding paragraph and, if examined and found physically fit, in addition, cross-country running, crew, wrestling, boxing, fencing, and polo)

Ages 31 through 50. At least one hour a day of moderate outdoor exercise (golf, tennis, riding, swimming, handball, volleyball, etc.)

Ages 51 through 70. At least one hour a day of light outdoor exercise (golf, walking, bowling, gardening, fishing, croquet, etc.)*

Daily physical education period at elementary and secondary school levels

The time allotment recommendation usually considered adequate is a daily physical education period that can vary in length for each student. Some individuals feel that, especially in the elementary schools, a program cannot be

---

*Smiley, D. F., and Gould, A. G.: A college textbook of hygiene, New York, 1940, The Macmillan Co., pp. 346-347.

adapted to a fixed time schedule. However, as a standard, there seems to be agreement that a daily experience in such a program is needed. Such a recommendation is made and should always be justified on the basis of value and contribution to the student and his or her needs. There should be provision for regular, instructional class periods and, in addition, laboratory periods where the skills may be put to use.

On the secondary level especially, it is recommended that sufficient time be allotted for dressing and showering in addition to the time needed for participation in physical education acitivites. Some leaders in physical education have suggested a double period every other day rather than a single period each day. This might be feasible if the daily class periods are too short. However, the importance of daily periods should be recognized and achieved wherever possible. Administrators should work toward providing adequate staff and facilities to allow for a daily period.

One of the most intensive and enlightening public interpretation programs ever carried on in modern times in support of a daily program of physical education was conducted in California. The California Association for Health, Physical Education, and Recreation rendered an outstanding service to the profession in cataloguing, describing, and interpreting the values

inherent in the daily program of physical education in their state. They incorporated their scientific evidence and research findings in a special issue of the *Journal of the California Association for Health, Physical Education, and Recreation.* *

This special issue included supporting statements from such people and organizations as the President of the United States, citizens' committees, American Medical Association, California Heart Association, physiologists and psychologists, educators, and parent-teachers' associations. As a result of this intensive and aggressive campaign, the public became much better informed regarding the need for daily physical education.

The President's Council on Physical Fitness and Sports has made this statement in regard to the daily physical education period:

The unanimous support for recommendations of the President's Council on Physical Fitness by a national jury of eminent medical leaders accompanying similar support by the American Medical Association and its committee on Exercise and Physical Fitness, Medical Aspects of Sports, and the Joint Committee of the AMA and its National Education Association indicate the sound position the President's Council has taken in recommending daily

* Values inherent in the daily program of physical education: fitness for California children and youth, Journal of the California Association for Health, Physical Education, and Recreation, special issue, March, 1965.

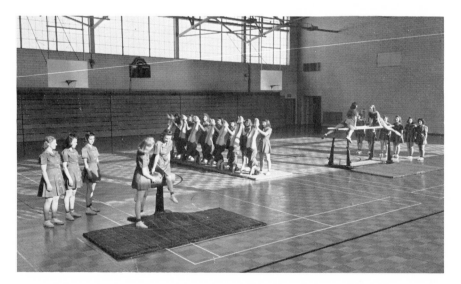

Girls' physical education. (East Stroudsburg State College, East Stroudsburg, Pa.)

physical education instruction involving vigorous exercise in grades 1 to 12.*

Size of classes

Some school and college administrators feel that physical education classes can accommodate more students than the so-called academic classes. This is a misconception that has developed over the years and is in need of correction. Physical educators themselves are in many cases at fault for such a practice. Some have failed to interpret their field of endeavor adequately to the central administration. Others have followed the practice of throwing a ball to a class and utilizing free play, with little or no organization. This has led some administrators to feel that the same type of teaching job would be done with a small class, and therefore they see no reason to incur the administrative problems and extra expense of more staff and smaller classes.

The problem of class size seems to be more pertinent at the secondary than at other educational levels. At the elementary levels, for example, the classroom situation represents a unit for activity and the size of this teaching unit is usually reasonable. However, there are some

schools that combine various classrooms for physical education, resulting in large classes that are not desirable.

Classes in physical education should be approximately the same size prevalent for the other subjects in the school or college offering. This is just as essential for effective teaching, individualized instruction, and progression in physical education as it is in other subjects. Physical education contributes to educational objectives on at least an equal basis with other subjects in the curriculum. Therefore, the size of the class should be comparable so that an effective teaching job can be accomplished and the objectives of education attained.

The standard established by LaPorte's committee* after considerable research which is still considered to be valid today, points up the acceptable size of physical education classes. It recommends not more than thirty-five students as the suitable size for activity classes. Normal classes should never exceed forty-five for one instructor. Of course, if there is a lecture or other activity scheduled, which is adaptable to greater numbers of students, it may be possible to have a larger number of students in the class. For remedial and corrective classes the

*President's Council on Physical Fitness, Washington, D. C., distributed in 1965 (mimeographed).

*LaPorte, W. R.: The physical education curriculum (a national program), ed. 6, Los Angeles, 1955, University of Southern California Press, pp. 50-51.

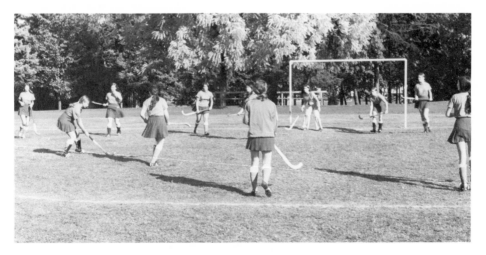

High school girls practice field hockey at Memorial South Park in Vancouver. (Courtesy Board of Parks and Public Recreation, Vancouver, B. C.)

suitable class size is from twenty to twenty-five and should never exceed thirty. With flexible scheduling, the size of classes can be varied to meet the needs of the teacher, facilities, and type of activity being offered.

The American Association for Health, Physical Education, and Recreation has recommended that class size should not exceed thirty-five.

TEACHING LOADS AND STAFFING

The load of the physical education teacher should be of prime concern to the administrator. In order to maintain a top level of enthusiasm, strength, and other essential characteristics, it is important that the teaching load be adjusted so that the physical educator is not overworked.

Years ago the New York State Physical Fitness Conference* recommended that one full-time physical education teacher should be provided for every 240 elementary pupils and one for every 190 secondary pupils enrolled. If such a requirement is implemented, it would aid considerably in providing adequate staff members in this field and avoid an overload for so many of the teachers.

LaPorte's national study† made recommendations in respect to teaching load at precollege educational levels that should be considered carefully by any teacher or administrator striving to meet acceptable standards. It recommended that class instruction per teacher not exceed 5 clock hours or the equivalent in class periods per day, or 1,500 minutes per week. It never should exceed 6 clock hours per day or 1,800 minutes a week. This maximum should include afterschool responsibilities. A daily load of 200 students per teacher is recommended and never more than 250. Finally, each teacher should have at least one free period daily for consultation and conferences with students.

It is generally agreed that the normal teaching load in colleges and universities should not exceed 15 hours per week.

*Report to the Commissioner of Education on the State Fitness Conference, Albany, N. Y., 1952, State Education Department, p. 7.
†La Porte, W. R., op. cit., p. 51.

Differentiated staffing

There are many innovations, such as differentiated staffing, that are directed toward aiding the teacher in the performance of his or her duties. The introduction of paraprofessionals, certified undergraduate interns, and student teachers provides Oak Grove Junior High School in Bloomington, Minnesota with valuable staff members. The major responsibilities of each of the assistants are:

Paraprofessionals. Responsibilities include: (1) supervised instructional assistance, (2) assistance in swimming pool, (3) clerical duties, (4) student conduct supervision, and (5) preparation of learning materials.

Certified undergraduate interns. Responsibilities include: (1) clerical assistance, (2) record keeping, (3) material preparation, (4) conduct supervision in noninstructional areas, (5) individual assistance, and (6) observation.

Student teachers. Their major areas of responsibility include: (1) observation, (2) supervised clerical teaching experience, (3) assisting supervising teachers, (4) preparation of learning materials, (5) individual assistance, and (6) extracurricular guidance.

Differentiated staffing relates to increased responsibilities or differentiation of functions among staff members. For example, in team teaching, higher salaries are given to team leaders or head teachers. Staff members who assume such roles as heads of departments or staff assistants are usually compensated accordingly. Outstanding, competent teachers with expertise in certain areas are assigned to special projects in some school systems and compensated accordingly. In other words, differentiated staffing means that the skills and contributions of staff members are different, and therefore, they play different roles in the educational process and are compensated accordingly.

The benefits derived from differentiated staffing are obvious from the responsibilities given to various staff members. The teacher is able to devote more time to help students, and he or she can also be free to work with small groups in different skills. Differentiated staffing allows the teacher to be free to teach and not be directly involved in clerical and physical responsibilities.

GROUPING OF STUDENTS

Homogeneous grouping in physical education classes is very desirable. To render the most valuable contribution to students, factors influencing performance must be taken into consideration in organizing groups for physical education instructional work or competition. The lack of scientific knowledge and measuring techniques to obtain such information and the administrative problems of scheduling have handicapped the achievement of this goal in most schools and colleges.

The reasons for grouping are sound. Placing individuals with similar capacities and characteristics in the same class will make it possible to better meet the needs of each individual. Grouping individuals with similar skill, ability, and other factors aids in equalizing competition. This helps the student to realize more satisfaction and benefit from playing. Grouping makes for more effective teaching. Instruction can be better organized and adapted to the level of the student. Grouping facilitates progression and continuity in the program. Furthermore, grouping makes for a better learning situation for the student. Being in a group with persons of similar physical characteristics and skills ensures some success, a chance to excel, recognition, a feeling of belonging, and security. Consequently, this helps the social and personality development of the individual. Finally, homogeneous grouping helps protect the child. It ensures his or her participation with individuals who are similar in physical characteristics. This protects the child physically, emotionally, and socially.

The problem of grouping is not as pertinent in the elementary school, especially in the lower grades, as it is in the junior high school and upper levels. At the lower levels the grade classification appears to serve the needs of most children. As children grow older, the complexity of the program increases, social growth becomes more diversified, competition becomes more intense, and consequently, there is a greater need for having similar individuals in the same group.

At the present time students are homogeneously classified on such bases as grade, sex, health, physical fitness, multiples of age-height-weight, ability, physical capacity, motor ability, interests, educability, speed, skill, and previous experience. Such techniques as health examinations; tests of motor ability, physical capacity, achievement, and social efficiency; conferences with students; and determination of physiologic age are utilized to obtain such information.

The suggestions of the American Alliance for Health, Physical Education, and Recreation* are appropriate when considering recommendations for grouping:

1. The need for grouping students homogeneously for instruction and competition has long been recognized, but the inability to scientifically measure such important factors as ability, maturity, interest, and capacity has served as a deterrent from accomplishing this goal.

2. The most common procedure for grouping today is by grade or class.

3. The ideal grouping organization would take into consideration all factors that affect performance—intelligence, capacity, interest, knowledge, age, height, weight, and so on. To utilize all these factors, however, is not administratively feasible at the present time.

4. Some form of grouping is essential to provide the type of program that will promote educational objectives and protect the student.

5. On the secondary and college levels, the most feasible procedure appears to be to organize subgroups within the regular physical education class proper.

6. Classification within the physical education class should be based on such factors as age, height, and weight statistics and other factors, such as interest and skill, that are developed as a result of observation of the activity.

7. For those individuals who desire greater refinement in respect to grouping, utilization of motor capacity, motor ability, attitude, appreciation, and sports-skills tests may be used.

Some physical education departments have adopted a nongraded curriculum that places students in learning situations according to

*American Association for Health, Physical Education, and Recreation: Administrative problems in health education, physical education, and recreation, Washington, D. C., revised 1969, The Association.

present levels of skill achievement and physical maturity. A child's chronologic age or grade level attainment is not a factor in the nongraded physical education curriculum. This allows for individual student differences and interests. Athens High School, Athens, Ohio, has introduced the nongraded approach to physical education. This school combines the nongraded curriculum with modular flexible scheduling to achieve an interesting, innovative program.

ADMINISTRATIVE POLICIES

The administrator of any physical education program is perennially confronted with such questions as: Should physical education be required or elective? How much credit should be given? Is it possible to substitute some other activity for physical education? What should be the policy on class attendance? How should one deal with excuses? What provision should be made for sex differences? Should there be courses in self-defense? These and other questions are answered in the following discussion.

Should physical education be required or elective?

There is general agreement that physical education should be required at the elementary level. However, there are many advocates on both sides of the question of whether it should be required or elective on the secondary and college levels. Both groups are sincere and feel that their beliefs represent what is best for the student. Probably most specialists feel that the program should be required. Some school administrators feel it should be elective. Following are some of the arguments presented by each.

Required

1. Physical education represents a basic need of every student.

2. The student is compelled to take so many required courses that the choice of electives is limited, if not entirely eliminated, in some cases.

3. The student looks upon those subjects that are required as being the most important and the most necessary for success.

4. Various subjects in the curriculum would not be provided for unless they were required. This is probably true of physical education.

Until state legislatures passed laws requiring physical education, this subject was ignored by many school administrators. If physical education were on an elective basis, the course of some administrative action would be obvious. Either the subject would not be offered at all or the administrative philosophy would so dampen its value that it would have to be eliminated because of low enrollment.

5. Even under a required program, physical education is not fulfilling its potentialities for meeting the physical, social, and cognitive needs of students. If an elective program were instituted, deficiencies and shortages would increase, thus further handicapping the attempt to meet the needs of the student.

Elective

1. Physical education "carries its own drive." If a good basic program is developed in the elementary school, with students acquiring the necessary skills and attitudes, the drive for such activity will carry through in the secondary school and college. There will be no need to require such a course, because students will want to take it voluntarily.

2. Objectives of physical education are focused on developing skills and learning activities that have carryover value, living a healthful life, and recognizing the importance of developing and maintaining one's body in its best possible condition. These are goals that cannot be legislated. They must become a part of each individual's attitudes and desires if they are to be realized.

3. Many children and young adults do not like physical education. This is indicated in their manner, attitude, and desire to get excused from the program and to substitute something else for the course. Under such circumstances the values that accrue to these individuals are not great. Therefore, it would be best to place physical education on an elective basis where only those students participate who actually desire to do so.

Should substitutions be allowed for physical education?

A practice exists in some school and college systems that allows students to substitute some other activity for their physical education requirement. This practice should be scrutinized and resisted aggressively by every administrator.

Some of the activities that are used as substitutions for physical education are athletic participation, Reserve Officers' Training Corps and band.

There is no substitute for a good program of physical education. In addition to healthful physical activity, it is concerned also with developing an individual socially, emotionally, and mentally. It develops in the individual many skills that can be utilized throughout life for worthy use of leisure time. These essentials are lost if a student is permitted to take some other activity in place of physical education. Professional persons who condone substitutions for their physical education classes are not clear about the goals of their profession.

Should credit be given for physical education?

Whether or not credit should be given for physical education is another controversial problem with which the profession is continu-

ally confronted. Here again can be found advocates on both sides. There are those who feel the joy of the activity and the values derived from participation are sufficient in themselves without giving credit. On the other hand, there are those who feel that physical education is the same as any other subject in the curriculum and should also be granted credit.

The general consensus among physical education leaders is that if physical education is required for graduation and if it contributes to educational outcomes, credit should be given, just as in other subjects.

What policy should be established on class attendance?

It is important for every department of physical education to have a definite policy on class attendance that covers absenteeism and tardiness. Since it is felt that students should attend school and college regularly, it follows that they should also attend physical education classes on a regular basis. However, time for independent study should be allowed for in the schedule.

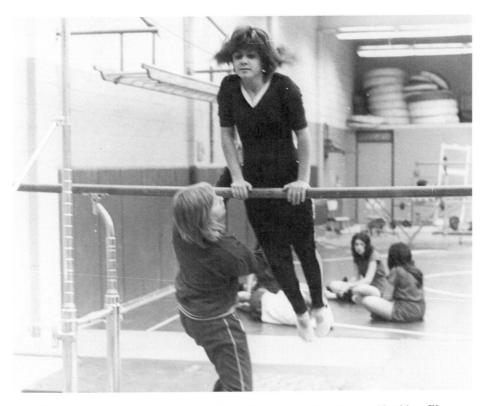

High school girl performing on the bar at Ridgewood High School, Norridge, Ill.

Regular attendance in physical education is important in order to derive the values and outcomes that accrue from participation. Since attendance is necessary in order to achieve such outcomes, every physical education department should have a clear-cut policy on attendance regulations. These regulations should be few in number and clearly stated in writing so that they are recognized, understood, and strictly enforced by teachers and students. They should allow for a reasonable number of absences and tardinesses, which can always occur in emergency situations over which the student has no control. Perfect attendance at school or college should not be stressed. Many harmful results can develop if students feel obligated to attend classes when they are ill and should be at home. There should probably be some provision for makeup work when important experiences are missed. However, makeup work should be planned and conducted so that the student derives essential values from such participation,

rather than enduring it as a disciplinary measure. There should also be provision for the readmission of students who have been ill. A procedure should be established so that the program is adapted to these individuals.

A final point to remember is the importance of keeping accurate, up-to-date attendance records. Unless meaningful records are kept, administrative problems will increase.

What about excuses?

The principal, nurse, or physical educator frequently receives a note from a parent or family physician asking that a student be excused from physical education. Many abuses develop if all such requests are granted. Many times for minor reasons the student does not want to participate and obtains the parent's or family physician's support.

Tom Peiffer, a physical educator in the New York State public schools, conducted a survey to determine both the extent of required physical

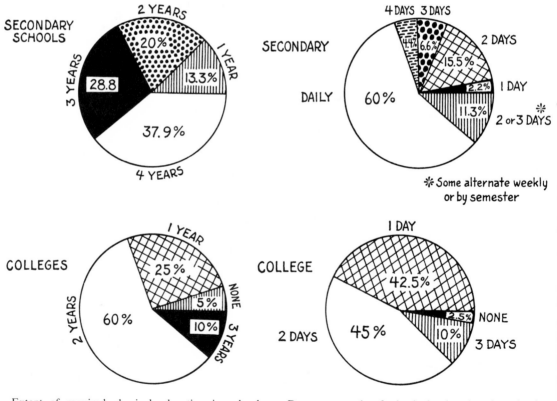

Extent of required physical education in schools surveyed.

Days per week of physical education in schools surveyed.

education and practices in regard to physical education excuses in secondary schools, colleges, and universities. The questionaire used in the survey was sent to schools selected at random from fifteen states situated in various sections of the United States. The questionnaire was sent to the high school in the largest city, to a suburban school of that city, to one city in the state with a population of 20,000 to 25,000, to one city in the state with a population of 10,000 to 15,000, and to one community with a population of 3,000 to 5,000. On the college level, questionnaires were sent to one state university, one private institution, and one teacher training institution. Questionnaires were sent to seventy-five secondary schools and sixty-seven colleges and universities. Replies were received from forty-five secondary schools and forty colleges and universities. Among the secondary schools, 37.9% required 4 years of physical education, 28.8% required 3 years, 20% required 2 years, and 13.3% required 1 year. In higher education, 60% of the colleges required 2 years, 25% required 1 year, 10% required 3 years, and 5% did not have a requirement. The number of days per week devoted to physical education is also shown in the diagram on p. 146.

Peiffer's survey showed that high schools permitted a student to be excused on the basis of a parental note, a memorandum from the family physician, or the discretion of the physical education teacher. While some schools would accept the recommendation of any of these three persons, other schools would accept only an excuse from the school physician. At the college level most programs accept the college physician's excuse or permit the instructor of each class to use his or her own discretion in granting excuses to students.

The reasons listed concerning why excuses in physical education were granted were an interesting part of the preceding survey. Secondary schools grant most of their excuses for participation in athletics and for being in the school band. Some schools permit their athletes to be excused only on the day of the game, while others grant a blanket excuse for the entire sports season. Other reasons for excuses on the secondary level, in addition to athletics, included makeup tests, driver training, counseling, a too-heavy extracurricular load, and medical reasons. At the college level, excuses were granted to athletes, veterans, students who could pass physical fitness tests, honor students, older students, for medical reasons, in "hardship cases," and so on.

Another part of the questionnaire on excuses attempted to discover what was done with the students who were excused. Students in secondary schools were sent to study halls; required to score, officiate, or help around the physical education department; write reports; remain on the sidelines; or report after school. At the college level most colleges did nothing except follow a pattern of failing a student in some cases if he or she exceeded the legal number of excused absences per semester. A few either required the student to observe the class, substitute a health class, or study in the gymnasium or left it up to the instructor's discretion.

Some school systems have exercised control over the indiscriminate granting of requests for excuses from physical education. Policies have been established, sometimes through conferences and rulings of the board of education, requiring that all excuses must be reviewed and approved by the school physician before they will be granted. Furthermore, family physicians have been asked to state specific reasons for requesting excuses from physical education. This procedure has worked out very satisfactorily in some communities. In other places physical educators have taken particular pains to work very closely with medical doctors. They have established a physical education program in collaboration with the school physician so that the needs of each individual are met, regardless of his or her physical condition. They have met with the local medical society in an attempt to clear up misunderstandings in regard to the purpose and conduct of the program. Family physicians have been brought into the planning. As a result of such planning, problems in regard to excuses from physical education have been considerably reduced.

There may be a correlation between the respect, prestige, and degree to which physical education is understood in any community and the number of excuses that are requested.

Furthermore, respect, prestige, and understanding are reflected in the type of leadership that exists. It has been found that in those communities where parents, family physicians, and the lay public in general understand physical education, the number of requests for excuses is relatively small. In such communities, the values that can be derived from participation in the program are clearly recognized, and since most parents and physicians want children to have worthwhile experiences, they encourage rather than attempt to limit such participation. The leadership of any program can eliminate many of the administrative problems in regard to excuses, provided physical education is properly interpreted to the public at large.

A few years ago, a conference concerned with close cooperation between physical education and medical doctors drew up a list of statements in respect to the problem under discussion. These are as follows:

1. Orient the student, parent, and physician at an early date in regard to the objectives of the physical education program.
2. Route all requests for excuse through the school physician. In the absence of the physician the school nurse should have this responsibility. The sympathetic and informed nurse can be a real asset to the physical education program.
3. Discard permanent and blanket excuses. The school physician should share in planning certain areas of the individual physical education program. Instead of being categorically excused, boys and girls can be given an activity in keeping with their special needs.
4. Students involved in the excuse request should have a periodic recheck on the need for excuse (this tends to reduce requests up to 50%).
5. Conferences between the school physicians and the head of the physical education department on the local level need to be emphasized.
6. The problem of excuse from physical education should be tied up with the total guidance program of the school. It helps also if the administrator and classroom teachers are familiar with the general physical education aims.

Should boys and girls be separated for physical education in grades one to six?

There is disagreement concerning whether or not boys and girls should be separated for physical education classes in the elementary school.

Those persons who advocate keeping the pupils together list such reasons as the following to support their position:

1. Separation hinders the social objective.
2. Separation causes unnecessary curiosity on the part of both boys and girls.
3. Schools cannot provide the resources and teachers needed to conduct separate programs.
4. Interests of both boys and girls prior to the adolescent period are much the same.
5. Playing together can carry over to later years, resulting in a happy, shared recreational life.

Those persons who advocate separating the sexes, at least during some of the elementary school years, list such reasons as the following to support their position:

1. Boys are interested in feats requiring strength, endurance, and skill, whereas girls are primarily interested in grace and moderate amounts of skill.
2. Girls and boys shy away from each other and want to be separated in physical activities.
3. Physical activities that the boys like, placing heavy demands on organic vitality, are not appropriate for girls.
4. A segregated program can do more to accomplish the separate objectives of both boys and girls.
5. A program that brings boys and girls together results in boys taking over key positions. Also, boys are more demanding, resulting in less time for girls to practice skills and have fun.

An analysis of the characteristics of boys and girls at the various grade levels shows that in the first and second grades the boys and girls have no preference as to sex, and, at the third grade, boys and girls are just beginning to become conscious of the distinctions between them. Interests and abilities of boys and girls during the first three grades are not significant. Therefore, it is recommended that through the third grade, boys and girls might well take their physical education classes together.

At the fourth-, fifth-, and sixth-grade levels there are some significant distinctions that suggest that certain physical education activities be conducted separately. Girls are nearing puberty and are more physically and emotionally mature than boys of the same age. Interest patterns may vary between the sexes in relation to their maturity differences and socialization. It is important for the physical educator to understand that girls may be as interested in certain activities as boys, but their socialization has worked against them in realizing this potential. For example, boys can derive great satisfaction from dance activities, and girls can derive the same satisfaction from touch football. Physical education programs should be geared toward developing all of the interests of both sexes by providing a well-rounded program that does not limit participation because of sex.

Should the physical education specialist or the classroom teacher conduct the physical education class in the elementary school?

This question has been continually discussed for many years. There are educators who advocate the classroom teacher handling physical education classes and also many supporters who want a specialist to take over this responsibility. The issue is quite involved, and limited space does not permit covering in depth each side of the issue. These facts, however, should be pointed out. The classroom teacher has limited professional education in physical education. Some classroom teachers are not interested in teaching physical education. Furthermore, there is increased interest in physical education today, which implies that qualified and interested persons should handle these classes. There is a trend toward more emphasis on movement education, perceptual motor development, physical fitness, skills, and other aspects of education with which physical education is concerned. There is a need for more research on physical education programs as they relate to the learning and growth of children. There is an increased emphasis upon looking to the specialist in physical education for help and advice in planning and conducting the elementary school program. These developments have implications for a sound inservice program to help the classroom teacher do a better job in physical education.

In light of the present status of physical education in the elementary schools of this country, such recommendations as the following should be very carefully considered. Each elementary school should be staffed with a man or woman specialist in physical education. The classroom teacher may find his or her best contribution to physical education programs in kindergarten to grade three, but to do the best job he or she needs preparation in this special field and the advice and help of a physical education specialist. Although the classroom teacher can contribute much to the physical education program in grades four to six, factors such as the growth changes and interests taking place in boys and girls and the more specialized program that exists at this level make it imperative to seek the help of a specialist. A specialist possesses the ability, experience, and training required to meet the needs of growing boys and girls as well as gain their respect and interest. The specialist and the classroom teacher should pool and share their experiences so that the most desirable learning experience may be provided children in the physical education program. Each teacher has much to contribute and should be encouraged to do so.

What about self-defense courses?

There are many arguments pro and con concerning self-defense courses for both men and women. On the affirmative side, the arguments include the need to be prepared in case of attack from a robber, assailant, rapist, and molester. The advocates further stress that knowing the various tricks of dirty fighting and self-defense will enable one to defend herself or himself in various kinds of emergency situations.

Those persons who oppose self-defense courses argue that a little knowledge is a bad thing; a criminal always has the advantage with weapons carried, the surprise of the attack, and greater strength and experience. Those opposed also indicate that the tricks learned in such courses may be used to the detriment of friends and associates in playful situations. They also stress that the number of instances of attack do not warrant devoting time to such a course. Furthermore, some persons stress that such courses are entirely opposed to the values that physical education stresses, namely, social effectiveness and sportsmanship. Finally, some educators indicate that the majority of the students exposed to such courses would find such instruction ineffective in warding off assailants.

CLASS MANAGEMENT

Good class management requires planning. Forethought is needed in order to have a group

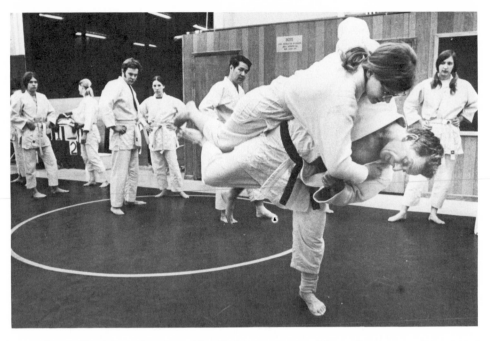

Judo is sometimes offered in conjunction with self-defense courses. Men and women participate in the judo program in physical education at College of DuPage, Glen Ellyn, Ill.

of students act in an orderly manner, accomplish the tasks that have been established, and have an enjoyable, satisfying, and worthwhile experience. The leader who is in charge of a class where these optimal conditions exist has spent considerable time in planning the details of the class from start to finish. Good class management does not just happen. It requires considerable thought, good judgment, and the making of many plans before the class begins.

There are many reasons for good organization. These should be recognized by every teacher and administrator. Some of these are listed below:

1. It gives meaning and purpose to instruction and to the activities.

2. It results in efficiency, the right emphasis, and the best use of the time available.

3. It more fully ensures that the needs and interests of the students will be satisfied.

4. It more fully ensures progression and continuity in the program.

5. It provides for measurement and progress toward objectives.

6. It ensures provision for child health and safety.

7. It encourages program adaptations to each individual's needs and interests.

8. It reduces errors and omissions to a minimum.

9. It helps to conserve the instructor's time and strength and aids in giving her or him a sense of accomplishment.

Some guides with which the teacher and administrator should concern themselves are as follows:

1. There should be long-term planning—for the semester and the year, as well as daily, weekly, and seasonal.

2. A definite time schedule should be planned for each period, taking into consideration time to be devoted to showering and dressing, taking roll, class activity, and other essentials.

3. The activity should be carefully planned so that it proceeds with precision and dispatch, with a minimum amount of standing around and a maximum amount of activity for each student.

4. The physical education class period should be regarded primarily as an instructional period. It is not one for free play. However, in order to have sustained interest and as much

satisfaction and joy result from the class as possible, there should be provision for using the instruction received in actual activity.

5. There should be a definite system established for such essentials as taking roll, keeping records, grading, adhering to policy on uniforms, and dressing and showering.

6. Attention should be given to the preparation of materials to be used in class. The teacher should know beforehand the materials to be used, and they should be ready when the class begins.

7. The setting for the class should be safe and healthful. The equipment should be safe and line markings, arrangements for activities, and other essential details attended to.

8. Procedures to be followed in locker room should be established, to provide for traffic, valuables, clothes, and dressing and showering.

9. A procedure should be established for falling in, taking attendance, organizing for activity, and dismissal.

10. The instructor should always use proper English and explain things in a simple, clear, and informative manner. During explanations the class should be attentive.

11. The instructor should always be prompt and punctual for class meetings.

12. The instructor should be tactful and considerate of every pupil. Pupils should not be condemned for making mistakes. It should be remembered that an educational situation is a normal and natural setting for mistakes.

13. Pupils should be encouraged and motivated to do their best.

14. All pupils should be treated in the same manner. There should be no favorites.

15. A planned program of measurement and evaluation should be provided to determine progress being made by pupils and the effectiveness of teaching.

16. The instructor and the class should wear suitable dress.

17. There should be as few rules of behavior as possible, making sure that those that are established are adhered to. Pupils should participate in the establishment of such rules.

18. The instructor should circulate among the entire class, giving help to those who are in need of it. Individual differences should be adequately provided for.

19. The instructor should have a good command of the subject. The values of demonstrations, visual aids, and other techniques to promote learning should be recognized and used.

20. Desirable attitudes and understandings toward physical fitness, skill learning, good sportsmanship, and other concepts inherent in physical education should be stressed at all times.

21. Standards of achievement and specific goals that are attainable should be established. Pupils' progress should be recorded so that they know how they are advancing toward these goals.

Some of the factors concerned with class management that deserve special attention are dressing and showering, taking roll, grading, and records. Each of these will be discussed in more detail.

Dressing and showering

Such factors as the age of the student, time allowed, grade participating, and type of activity should be considered in a discussion of dressing and showering for physical education classes.

The problem of showering and dressing is not so pertinent at the lower elementary level where the age of the participants and type of activities as a general rule do not require special dress and showering. Also the time allotted is too short in many cases. In the upper elementary and at the junior and senior high school and college levels, however, it is a problem.

Physical education, by its very nature, embodies activities that result in considerable movement. Participation also frequently results in perspiration. In the interests of comfort and good hygiene practices, provisions should be made for special clothing and showering. The unpleasant features of a student's returning to class after participating in physical education activity, with clothes dripping from perspiration and with the accompanying odors, are not in conformance with establishing good habits of personal cleanliness and grooming. Therefore, all schools should make special provisions for places to dress in comfortable uniforms and for showering. Such places should be convenient to the physical education areas, be comfortable, and afford privacy. Although boys and girls are increasingly becoming accustomed to using a group shower, there are still many who prefer the private showers. In the interests of these individuals, such facilities should be provided. There should also be some type of towel service. In many schools there are facilities for laundering towels that have worked out very satisfactorily.

Dress

There are many reasons for the use of special uniforms in physical education classes above the elementary level:

1. It makes for better appearance if an individual is dressed in clothing that is appropriate to the activity in which is or she is engaging.
2. It provides for more comfort and safety and allows for freedom of movement.
3. It is more economical, since it saves on street clothes. If uniforms are purchased in lots by the school, there can be a considerable saving to the student. Those students who cannot afford uniforms should have them provided free of charge.
4. If all students have the same uniform, it aids morale and promotes equality.

Dress does not have to be elaborate. For girls simple, washable shorts and blouses or one-piece suits are suitable. For boys white cotton jerseys and trunks will suffice. Of course, appropriate footwear should also be worn. An important consideration is to keep the uniform clean. The instructor should establish a policy on clean uniforms and work diligently toward seeing that hygienic standards are met by all.

Taking roll

There are many methods of taking roll. If a method satisfies the following three criteria, it is usually satisfactory. (1) It is efficient—roll taking should not consume too much time. (2) It is accurate—it is important to know accurately after the class has been held who was present and who was not. This means taking into consideration those who might come to class late or leave early. (3) It should be uncomplicated—any system that is used should be very simple and easy to administer.

Some of the methods for roll taking that may be used are as follows:

1. *Having numbers on the floor*—each member of the class is assigned a number that he or she must stand on at the time the signal for "fall in" is given. The person taking attendance records the numbers that are not covered.

2. *Reciting numbers orally*—each member of the class is assigned a number that he or she must say out loud at the time the signal for "fall in" is given. The person taking attendance then records the numbers that are not given.

3. *Tag board*—each member of the class has a number that is recorded on a cardboard or metal tag that hangs on a peg on a board in a central place. Each member of the class who is present removes his or her tag from the board and places it in a box. The person taking attendance records the absentees from the board.

4. *Delaney system*—a special system developed by Delaney involves using a folder with cards that are turned over when a person is absent. It is a cumulative system that records the attendance of pupils over a period of time. There are adaptations of this system that are used elsewhere.

5. *Squad system*—the class is divided into squads and the squad leader takes the roll for his squad and in turn reports to the instructor.

6. *Issuing towels and equipment*—the roll is taken when a towel is issued to each student or when it is turned in, or when a basket with uniform is issued or returned.

7. *Signing a book or register*—students are required to write their names in a book or register at the beginning of the class. Some systems require the writing of a name at the beginning of a period and crossing it out at the end of a period. The person taking attendance records the names not entered.

Records

Records are essential in keeping valuable information in regard to pupils' welfare. They also are essential to efficient program planning and administration. They should, however, be kept to a minimum and should be practical and functional. They should not be maintained just as busy work and for the sake of filling the files. Instead they should have use and a place in the program.

Some of the records should be concerned

directly with the welfare of the pupil and others with certain administrative factors.

Those records that concern the welfare of the student are the health records, the cumulative physical education form, anecdotal accounts, attendance reports, grades, and accident reports.

Health records are essential. They contain information on the health examination and other appraisal techniques, health counseling, and any other data pertaining to the student's health.

The cumulative physical education record should start when the student first attends school and contain information about activities engaged in, afterschool play, test, anecdotal accounts, interests, needs, and any other pertinent information that should be known in respect to the student and his participation in the physical education programs.

There should be special records for attendance and grades and any special occurrences that have a bearing on the child and that are not recorded in other records.

If a student is involved in an accident, a full account of the circumstances surrounding the accident should be recorded. Usually special forms are provided for such purposes. *

The records dealing with administrative factors are concerned with general administrative information and equipment records. These would include a list of the year's events: activities; records of teams; play days, sports days, intramurals; events of special interest; techniques utilized that have been helpful; budget information; and any other data that would be helpful in planning for succeeding years. Memory often fails over a period of time, with the result that many good ideas are lost and many activities and techniques of special value not utilized because they are forgotten.

There should be records in regard to equipment, facilities, and supplies. Such records should show the material needing repair, new materials needed, and also the location of various materials, so that they can easily be found.

There is also a need for records in regard to such items as locker or basket assignments and any other pertinent information that is essential to the efficient running of a physical education program.

PHYSICAL EDUCATION ACTIVITIES

Physical education activities represent the heart of the program. They are the means for accomplishing objectives. They represent the media that attract the attention of the student and through participation aid him or her in the achievement of life's goals. Because they are so important to the physical education profession, they must be selected with considerable care.

Criteria for selection

1. Activities should be selected in terms of the values they have in achieving the objectives of physical education. This means they would not only possess potentialities for developing body awareness, movement fundamentals, and physical fitness but also would have implications for developing the cognitive, affective, and social makeup of the individual.

2. Activities should be interesting and challenging. They should appeal to the students and present them with problem-solving activities and situations that challenge their skill and ability. For example, golf always presents the challenge of getting a lower score.

3. They should be adaptable to the growth and developmental needs and interests of children and youth. The needs of individuals vary from age to age. Consequently, movement activities and the pattern of organization must also change if these needs are to be met. The activity must be suited to the child, not the child to the

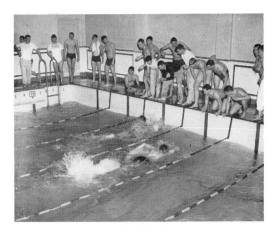

---

* See Chapters 10 and 14 for more information on accidents.

Washington State College, Pullman, Wash.

activity. Wherever possible, students should be allowed some choice in the activities in which they participate.

4. Activities should be modifications of fundamental movements such as running, jumping, throwing, walking, and climbing.

5. Activities, of course, must be selected in the light of the facilities, supplies, equipment, and other resources available in the school, college, or community. One cannot plan an extensive tennis program if only one court is available.

6. Activities should be selected not only with a view to their present value while the child is in school but also with a view to postschool and adult living. Skills learned during school and college days have potentialities for use throughout life, thus contributing in great measure to enriched living. Patterns for many skills utilized in adult leisure hours are developed while the individual is in the formative years of childhood.

7. Activities must be selected for health and safety values. Such an activity as boxing has been questioned as to its effect on the health and the safety of individuals

8. The local education philosophy, policies, and school or college organization must be taken into consideration.

9. School activities should provide situations that are similar to those children experience in natural play situations outside the school environment.

10. Activities should provide the student with opportunities for creative self-expression.

11. Activities should be selected which have potentialities to elicit the correct social and moral responses through high-quality leadership.

12. Activities should reflect the democratic way of life.

Classification

One survey* produced a list of physical education activities offered throughout the country, here classified into various categories. These do not necessarily meet criteria that have

*Bucher, C. A.: Foundations of physical education, ed. 6, St. Louis, 1975, The C. V. Mosby Co.

been listed. They merely indicate current offerings in physical education programs in the United States:

Team games
Baseball — Soccer
Basketball — Softball
Code ball — Speedball
Field hockey — Touch football
Flag football — Volleyball
Football

Outdoor winter sports
Ice hockey — Snow games
Roller skating — Snowshoeing
Skating — Tobogganing
Skiing

Other activities
Camping and outdoor activities — Correctives
Mountaineering — Fly-tying
Yoga — Games of low organization
Jogging — Movement education
Kayaking — Relays
Orienteering — Self-testing activities
Combatives (judo, karate)

Rhythms and dancing
Folk dancing — Square dancing
Gymnastic dancing — Social dancing
Modern dancing — Tap dancing
Rhythms

Formal activities
Calisthenics — Marching

Water activities
Canoeing — Lifesaving
Surfing — Rowing
Water skiing — Swimming
Scuba diving — Sailing
Diving — Water games

Gymnastics
Acrobatics — Rope climbing
Apparatus — Stunts
Obstacle course — Trampoline
Pyramid building — Tumbling

Dual and individual sports
Achery — Handball
Badminton — Horseback riding
Bait and fly casting — Horseshoes
Skeet shooting — Paddle tennis
Trap shooting — Rifle
Horseback riding — Rope skipping
Cycling — Shuffleboard
Bowling — Skish
Checkers — Table tennis
Darts — Tennis
Deck tennis — Tether ball
Fencing — Track and field
Fishing — Wrestling
Golf

The state of California lists the following types of activities:

1. Aquatics, where facilities are available
2. Gymnastics and tumbling
3. Individual and dual sports
4. Mechanics of body movement and health aspects of physical activity
5. Rhythms and dance
6. Team sports
7. Combatives for boys*

Coeducational activities

The need for more coeducational activity is being recognized. History shows that activities for boys and girls have been combined at the lower elementary levels but at the upper elementary, secondary, and college levels they have been separated. A common sight on college campuses and even at the secondary level is separate sets of facilities for the men and women or boys and girls. In the light of education objectives, this does not seem to be in the interests of what the profession is striving to attain in the schools.

Men and women are continually together in work, home, social, and other situations throughout life. If they are to adjust properly in such situations, it is essential that attention be given to this matter in their childhood and youth

*California State Department of Education, Bureau of Health Education, Physical Education, and Recreation. Letter dated August 14, 1964, from C. Carson Conrad, Chief, Bureau of Health Education, Physical Education, and Recreation, Sacramento, Calif.

years. This country is faced with the problems of increased divorce rates and disintegration of family life. Individuals who have not had the opportunity to play, work, and socialize with the opposite sex in childhood and youth often find it difficult to adjust satisfactorily when they become adults. Furthermore, if family life is to be a happy experience, the various members of the families should be attuned to such items as the others' interests, temperaments, likes, dislikes, and habits. Such adjustment is obtained only through constant association in a variety of situations. The physical education program should encourage and provide for such associations rather than be indifferent or oppose such a natural phenomenon. The contributions this specialized field can make to such an objective are very great and should be utilized to the fullest.

PROGRAMS

Many aspects of the elementary, junior high, senior high, and college physical education basic instructional programs have already been discussed. This information will not be repeated. Instead, certain administrative guides are suggested for each level to aid the administrator, teacher, or other interested person in the conduct of a physical education program.

Program for kindergarten through grade six

The various aspects of the physical education program for elementary school, including char-

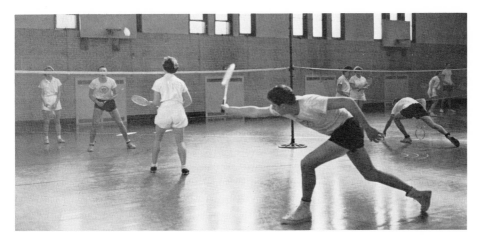

There is need for coeducational activity. (Wisconsin State College, La Crosse, Wis.)

acteristics of children at various ages, opportunities they need, and activities that meet these needs and characteristics, were developed by a group of experts at the National Conference on Physical Education for Children of Elementary School Age. The following information has been taken from their report and updated in part by the author because of its value to all persons interested in elementary school physical education. *Of course, the discussion of movement education recorded earlier in this chapter indicates a vital and important emphasis for elementary school physical education programs.*

PROGRAM*

Growth is a continuous process—an emerging—an unfolding. At no time does a child abruptly complete a particular stage of development and begin the next. Neither is there a time when all children in a group are at exactly the same stage of growth.

Any classification into groups along the route of growth is artificial. The following charts [Tables 7-1 to 7-3 on pp. 157-160] are merely devices to help give a picture of activities that seem to suit the changing needs of children. The subdivision and classifications used serve as convenient labels for periods of growth through which children gradually move, each child holding to a path that is his alone.

Program for grades seven and eight

Facilities, time, pupils, and teacher load are some of the factors that will determine the basic physical education instructional program for grades seven and eight. The absence or presence of a swimming pool, for example, would influence the type of program offered.

Boys and girls in grades seven and eight are in a period of rapid physical growth with awkwardness and lack of coordination frequently in evidence. Muscles, bones, heart, and lungs are experiencing the growth spurt. Some boys surpass some girls in strength and speed, and interests in different types of physical activities are common. There is keen interest in competitive activities, and this motivating factor may create the desire to want to continue participating beyond fatigue to exhaustion. The enjoyment of organized sports is common. The students develop loyalty to groups, have a desire for peer-group approval, and a strong desire for recognition. Emotions are easily aroused.

Boys and girls in the seventh and eighth grades need to have opportunities to participate in activities in which they can experience success—activities that do not emphasize their frequent awkwardness, that provide vigorous activity, that provide for group participation, and that challenge their interest and physical capabilities.

A description of children's characteristics and needs at the seventh and eighth grade levels together with physical education activities suited to these needs is taken from the report of the National Conference on Physical Education (Table 7-3).

Program for grades nine through twelve

A discussion of characteristics and the physical education program for youth 14 through 17 years of age, or grades nine through twelve, is included here.

During this period students display distinct characteristics in regard to physical growth and development. In respect to skeletal growth, the girls are about 2 years ahead of the boys. Some girls reach adult height at about 14 years, whereas others continue to grow for several years beyond this age. In the case of boys, some attain adult height at about 16 years and others continue their growth to 20 years or later.

In regard to muscular development, the "awkward age" is ending and there is a definite improvement in coordination. Posture is improving and control and grace are in evidence, especially by those who have participated in rhythmic activities such as dancing, swimming, and sports.

In respect to organic development, the heart increases in size, with a question being raised about strenuous competitive sports, since the heart and arteries may be disproportionate in size. The puberty cycle is completed in the majority of cases. There may be a period of glandular instability with fluctuations in respect to energy level. Some characteristic ailments at

---

*Report of National Conference of Physical Education for Children of Elementary School Age: Physical education for children of elementary school age, Chicago, 1951, The Athletic Institute, Inc. Updated by author 1974.

Table 7-1. Early childhood—5 to 8 years of age—kindergarten through third grade *

What they are like	What they need OPPORTUNITIES	What to do
Their large muscles (trunk, legs, and arms) are more developed than the smaller muscles (hands and feet)	To experience many kinds of vigorous activities that involve many parts of the body To engage in many developmental activities for small muscles	Activities such as hanging, running, jumping, climbing, dodging, or throwing at an object. Beanbag Toss, Jacks, Bouncing Balls, Hopscotch, O'Leary Movement activities involving space, time, flow, tempo Activities to explore various body movements Rhythm activities
They have a short attention span	To engage in many activities of short duration To develop body awareness To develop a favorable self-concept To develop fundamental movement activities	Choice of activity where a child can change frequently, and activities that can be started quickly, such as Magic Carpet, Pincho, Hill Dill, and stunts
They are individualistic and possessive	To play alone and with small groups To play as an individual in larger groups	Individual activities, such as throwing, catching, bouncing, kicking, climbing, stunts, running, hopping, skipping, building blocks, jumping. Dance activities that allow for expression of self, such as clowns, aviators, firemen, tops, airplanes. Sport skills and activities Swimming and water safety, apparatus, stunts and tumbling Creative rhythms, movement exploration
They are dramatic, imaginative, and imitative	To create and explore To identify themselves with people and things	Invent dance and game activities, such as Cowboys, Circus, Christmas toys; work activities such as pounding, sawing, raking, and hauling. Other play activities: farmers, postmen, grocers, elevators, bicycles, leaves, scarecrows
They are active, energetic, and responsive to rhythmic sounds	To respond to rhythmic sounds such as drums, rattles, voice and nursery rhythms, songs, and music	Running, skipping, walking, jumping galloping, dodging, swimming. Singing and folk games such as Oats, Peas, Beans, and Barley Grow; Farmer in the Dell; Dixie Polka
They are curious and want to find out things	To explore and handle materials with many types of play	Using materials such as balls, ropes, stilts, beanbags, bars, ladders, trees, blocks. Games and activities such as hiking, Run-Sheep-Run, Huckle-Buckle, Bean-stalk
They want chances to act on their own and are annoyed at conformity	To make choices, to help make rules, to share and evaluate group experiences	Variety of activities with minimum of rules, such as Center Base, Exchange, Midnight, and Red Light. Make-up activities, dances, and games
They are continuing to broaden social contacts and relationships	To cooperate in play and dance, to organize many of their own groups	Group games, such as simple forms of Dodge Ball, Kickball. Dance and rhythmic activities, such as Gustaf's Skoal, Dance of Greeting, Bow Balinda
They seem to be in perpetual motion	To play many types of vigorous activities	Running, jumping, skipping, galloping, rolling, fitness routines and activities

*From Report of National Conference on Physical Education for Children of Elementary School Age: Physical education for children of elementary school age, Chicago, 1951, The Athletic Institute, Inc. Adapted and updated by author, 1974.

Table 7-2. Middle childhood—9 to 11 years of age—fourth through sixth grades *

What they are like	What they need OPPORTUNITIES	What to do
They grow steadily in muscles, bone, heart, and lungs	To engage in strenuous activity that regularly taxes these organs to the limits of healthy fatigue	Running, jumping, climbing, and hard play. Movement experiences and body mechanics. Fitness routines. Tumbling, apparatus and stunts
They enjoy rough and tumble activities	To participate in activities that use the elements of roughness	Bumping, pushing, contact activities such as King of the Ring, Poison Pen, Indian Wrestle, Hand Wrestle, Beater Goes 'Round
Sex differences begin to appear with girls taller and more mature than boys. Sex antagonisms may appear	To enjoy their roles as boys and girls, to have wholesome boy-girl relationships in activities	Activities such as folk dances, mixers, squares. Swimming and water safety, relays, sport skills and activities. Group games such as Volleyball type games, Newcomb or Fist Ball, Softball. Others may be enjoyed separately or together
They respond differently in varying situations	To participate in wide range of activities and organizations using many kinds of materials	Individual, dual, or small and large group activities such as swimming, tumbling, stilts, track, catch, handball, relays, folk dances, mixers, and simple square dances such as Csebogar, Captain Jinks, Life on the Ocean Wave
They have a strong sense of rivalry and crave recognition	To succeed in activities that stress cooperative play along with activities that give individual satisfaction	Self-testing activities such as track events, stunts, chinning, sit-ups, push-ups, ball-throwing, for distance and accuracy. Group and team play such as Newcomb, Kickball, Circle or Square Soccer, End Ball, Club Snatch, Progressive Dodge Ball
They may show increasing independence and desire to help	To plan, lead, and check progress. To be involved in planning their own program	Assist with officiating, serve as squad leaders, act as scorers, help with equipment, elect captains, help with younger children and each other
They want to be liked by their own classmates, to belong. They have a strong loyalty to teams, groups, or "gangs"	To belong to groups, to be on many kinds of teams. To engage in a wide range of activities	Group games such as Bounce Volleyball, Line Soccer, Keep Away, Hit Pin Kickball, Net Ball. Partner play such as Deck Tennis (Ring Toss), Tennis, Aerial Darts, Horseshoes
They want approval, but not at the expense of their group relationships	To gain respect and approval of others	Participate in activities in which they achieve in the eyes of their group

*From Report of National Conference on Physical Education for Children of Elementary School Age. Physical education for children of elementary school age, Chicago, 1951, The Athletic Institute, Inc. Adapted and updated by author, 1974.

Table 7-3. Later childhood—early adolescence—12 to 13 years of age—seventh and eighth grades *

What they are like	What they need OPPORTUNITIES	What to do
This is a period of rapid physical growth that is frequently uneven in various parts of the body. Awkwardness and inability to coordinate sometimes occur	To develop skill and coordination and to take part in activities that do not call attention to their awkwardness or put them in embarrassing situations To develop a favorable body image	Movement experiences and body mechanics Skills in various activities such as batting, throwing, catching kicking, dribbling, and serving, as used in—Softball, Soccer, Volleyball, Basketball. Skills in body controls as—how to walk, to run, to stand, to sit, to relax. Individual activities as—rope jumping, horseshoes, target throw, jumping, skating, hiking, skiing, and swimming
Muscles, heart, lungs, and bones share liberally in the growth sput	Vigorous activity to stimulate each of these organs to attain its fullest development	Activities conducted as vigorously as possible with respect for individual reaction. Fitness routines and activities.
Boys and girls are showing differences in interests and in abilities. Boys may tend to surpass girls in strength and speed; girls may be more interested in dance forms than boys	To participate in some activities in separate groups and some together based largely on individual choice	Activities recommended in groupings as follows: 　Group sports 　　Soccer 　　Touch football 　　Softball 　　Basketball 　　Volleyball 　Individual, dual, and group sports 　　Track 　　Badminton 　　Tennis 　　Swimming 　　Outing activities 　Formal dancing 　　Square 　　Social 　　Creative 　　Folk
Interest in members of one's own sex broadens to include an interest in members of the opposite sex	To have coeducational activities in small and large groups	Activities such as Square, Social, and Creative Dance, Tennis, Swimming, and Outing Activities, Volleyball, Table Tennis, Badminton
Great loyalty to groups as clubs, gangs, and teams, and group acceptance	To belong to various teams and to plan and develop their own groups	Many teams in all team games such as class teams, homerooms, and clubs
Strong desire for individual recognition and the urge to be free of adult restrictions	To take part in activities of their own choosing, to be leaders and captains of groups, to create and modify games, and to evaluate progress To develop a favorable body image To be involved in planning program To be able to choose some activities	Squad-leader directed activities as: 　a. Testing skills—sit up, push-up 　b. Officiating in games 　c. Assigning positions on teams

Continued.

*From Report of National Conference on Physical Education for Children of Elementary School Age: Physical education for children of elementary school age, Chicago, 1951, The Athletic Institute, Inc. Adapted and updated by author, 1974.

Table 7-3. Later childhood—early adolescence—12 to 13 years of age—seventh and eighth grades—cont'd

What they are like	What they need OPPORTUNITIES	What to do
Emotions are easily aroused and swayed	To be frequently in situations requiring practice of fair play, when winning or losing. To participate in policy decisions affecting their physical education program	Wide variety of activities requiring individual decisions and scoring as in: a. High and broad jumps (boys only) b. Ball-throwing events c. Running against time d. Stunts and tumbling, as jump stick, Indian wrestle, pull-up, sit-up Independent study Officiating at games as umpiring in Softball, timing in races and relays
The interest span lengthens. They may want to continue in activities beyond fatigue to exhaustion	To participate in activities that are modified to overcome fatiguing factors as time, speed, distance, and pressures to win. To learn when to stop	Games that involve skills of major sports as: Line Soccer (Soccer), Keep Away (Basketball), End Ball (Basketball), Touch Football (Football), Newcomb (Volleyball), Long Base (Softball) Modifications of standard games involve changing fatiguing factors, as: a. Shortening playing periods in vigorous sports: shorter halves in soccer, shorter quarters in basketball b. Frequent time-outs c. Restricting space: Three-Court Soccer, Six-Court Basketball, One-Basket Basketball
There is a keen interest in competitive activities	To compete in a variety of activities that involve a wide range of skills and organization	Self-testing types with competition against self as tumbling, track events. Skill tests as throwing for baskets, pitching at a target. Games not highly organized as Bombardment, End Ball, Ten Trips, Kick Over, Fist Ball
The enjoyment of organized team sports is keen	To give every boy and girl an opportunity to be a participating member on the types of teams that challenge his interest and ability	Wide variety of team sports such as Soccer, Volleyball, Softball, Basektball, Field Ball. Many teams in each sport organized on such bases as skill and ability, age-height-weight, squads

this age would include headache, nosebleed, nervousness, palpitation, and acne.

The characteristics of the secondary school students are many. The boy or girl of 14 through 17 may have reached physiologic adulthood but needs many new experiences for fuller social and emotional development. He or she is emotional and is seeking a feeling of belonging in the life around himself or herself. This attempt to adjust may result in some emotional instability. The desire to conform to the standards of the group with whom he or she is closely associated is often greater than the desire to conform to adult standards. However, there are cases of "hero worship," and in such cases adults have considerable influence on youth. This age group is capable of competing in more highly organized games. Groups and "cliques" evolve in accordance with interests and physical maturation. In both sexes there is interest and an attempt to be physically attractive. As a result, good grooming increases. Appetite is good at this age. Various sexual manifestations during this age may cause undue self-consciousness. Since girls mature before boys, girls are, as a rule, more interested in boys than boys are in girls.

The needs of youth at these ages are many.

There is a need for adult guidance, which should allow for considerable freedom and choice on the part of youth. Family life is important and plays a steadying influence on the child at a time when life is becoming more and more complex. There is a need for wholesome activity and experiences where excess emotions and energy can be properly channeled. Certain physical education activities require separate participation on the part of boys and girls. However, there is a need for many experiences where boys and girls play together. Coeducational activities should be adapted to both sexes so that no physiologic or physical harm results. Social dancing is very important at this level. Also, at this age students are interested and receive much satisfaction from sports. Although individual differences determine the amount of sleep needed, most can profit from 8 to 10 hours. There is need for a planned afterschool program that is adapted to the needs of youth and that includes active recreation as well as the manipulative or contemplative activities.

The types of activities that will best meet the needs of the secondary school student should be wide and varied. Team games of high organization occupy an increasingly important place at the junior high and even more at the senior high school level. The junior high and early senior high school programs should be mainly exploratory in nature, offering a wide variety of activities with the team games modified in nature and presented in the form of leadup activities. Toward the end of the senior high school period there should be opportunity to select and specialize in certain activities that will have a carryover value after formal education ceases. Furthermore, many of the team games and other activities are offered in a more intensive manner and in larger blocks of time as one approaches the terminal point of the secondary school. This allows for greater acquisition of skill in selected activities.

As a general rule, boys and girls at the secondary level, including both junior and senior high, can profit greatly from rhythmic activities such as square, folk, and social dancing; team sports such as soccer, field hockey, softball, baseball,

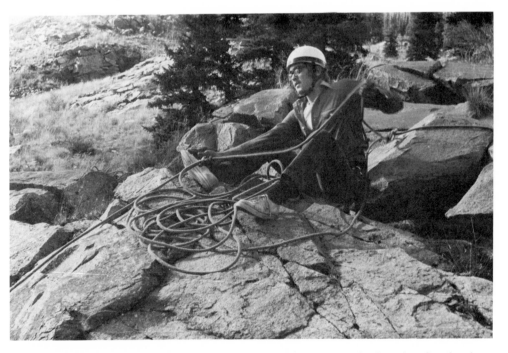

The manual management of a rope requires the concentration of a gymnast, the dexterity of a tuba player, and the confidence of a fighter pilot. Activity in physical education program in Silverton, Colo. public schools. (Courtesy George Pastor.)

touch football, volleyball, and speedball; individual activities such as track and field, tennis, paddle tennis, badminton, hiking, handball, bowling, archery, and fly casting; many forms of gymnastics such as tumbling, stunts, and apparatus activities; and various forms of games and relays. These activities will comprise the major portion of the program at the secondary level. Of course the activities would be adapted to boys and to girls as they are played separately or on a coeducational basis.

Program for colleges and universities

Oxendine * conducted a recent survey on the status of required physical education in 788 colleges and universities in the United States. His survey indicated that 74% of these institutions require physical education for all students, with another 8% having a requirement for students in certain departments or schools. The majority of the institutions that require physical education indicate that the requirement is for a 2-year period. The survey indicated a 10 to 15% decrease in institutions requiring physical education since 1968. Oxendine's survey also indicated that programs of physical education are on a sounder academic basis in large institutions than in small ones, in public compared to private institutions, and in coeducational as compared to noncoeducational institutions. Finally, Oxendine's survey indicated the trends toward more emphasis on "recreation" and "fitness" activities and on coeducational classes. There is less emphasis on team sports and all-male or all-female classes.

The college and university physical education program is the terminal point for formal physical education in the lives of many students. The age range of individuals in colleges and universities is very wide, incorporating those as young as 16 and as old as 60. However, most college students are in their late teens or early twenties. These individuals have matured in many ways. They are entering the period of greatest physical efficiency. They have devel-

oped the various organ systems of the body. They possess a high degree of strength, stamina, and coordination. In this respect the program does not have to be restricted for the average college population. College and university students have many interests. They want to prepare themselves adequately for certain vocations. They desire to be successful in their chosen fields of work. Such an objective offers potentialities for the physical education teacher who can show how the outcomes derived from the physical education program can contribute to success in their work. College students are interested in the opposite sex. They want to develop socially. This has implications for a broad coeducational program. They are interested in developing skills that they can use throughout life and from which they will obtain a great deal of enjoyment.

In formulating a program at the college and university level one needs to remember that many students enter with limited activity backgrounds. Therefore, the program should be broad and varied at the start, with opportunities to elect activities later. There should be considerable opportunity for instruction and practice in those activities in which a student desires to specialize. As much individual attention as possible should be given to ensure the necessary development of skill.

Most colleges offer physical education twice a week for 2 years. There are others, however, where the requirement is for 1, 3, or 4 years' duration. It would seem that the longer the requirement, the greater would be the assurance that the individual would leave school with the necessary skills. Some colleges and universities require only that the allotted time be put in, whereas others state that certain standards of achievement must be met. Both requirements are important if the objectives of physical education are to be realized.

The program of activities should be based on the interests and needs of students and the facilities and staff available. Some colleges have introduced "Foundations" courses getting at the subject-matter of physical education. There is an important place for coeducation at the college level in such activities as tennis, dancing, swimming, badminton, volleyball, and golf.

---

*Oxendine, J. B.: Status of general instructional programs of physical education in four-year colleges and universities: 1971-72, Journal of Health, Physical Education, and Recreation **43:**26, 1972.

Some of the experiences that might be included in the women's program are as follows: team activities—field hockey, soccer, speedball, basketball, softball, and fieldball; aquatics in all forms; dancing—folk, square, social, and modern; individual activities—bowling, table tennis, skating, badminton, archery, tennis, deck tennis, horseback riding, mountaineering, orienteering, platform tennis, snow skiing, skydiving, judo, karate, and hiking; formal activities—tumbling and stunts; and camping activities. Some of the activities that have been popular in men's programs are team activites—basketball, touch football, softball, volleyball, soccer, and speedball; aquatics in all forms; dancing—folk, square, and social; individual activities—skating, fishing, squash, badminton, tennis, golf, bowling, archery, hiking, horseshoes, handball, fencing, and wrestling; formal activities—tumbling and apparatus work; and camping activities.

A publication of the President's Council on Physical Fitness and Sports entitled *Fitness for Leadership** contains many suggestions for col-

lege and university programs in physical education.

Some of the pertinent suggestions for physical education programs in this report include the recommendation that physical achievement tests should be utilized to assess student needs and assure progress. Special help and prescribed programs should be offered to help physically underdeveloped students. Another suggestion is to institute a requirement that would make it necessary for all students to demonstrate and develop proficiency in swimming, conditioning exercises, and several other physical activities.

Special considerations for junior college physical education programs

The growth of the 2-year college in recent years has been phenomenal. Approximately one and one-half million students are enrolled in about 900 junior colleges from coast to coast. In many respects the activities for the 2-year college are the same as those for the 4-year institution. However, since approximately 70% of community colleges students will terminate their education after 2 years of study, there is

---

*President's Council on Physical Fitness and Sports: Fitness for leadership, Washington, D. C., 1964, U. S. Government Printing Office.

Table 7-4. Coeducational carryover physical activities offered in California junior colleges *

Activity	Number of schools in which taught	Rank	Offered	Rank
Aquatics	16	4	109	3
Archery	20	2	87	4
Badminton	15	5-6-7	74	5
Bowling	10	8	38	8
Fencing	4	12	10	12
Folk and square dance	9	9-10	17	10
Golf	21	1	132	2
Ice skating	1	13-14	6	13
Modern dance	8	11	15	11
Sailing	1	13-14	3	14
Social dance	15	5-6-7	44	7
Tennis	18	3	157	1
Tumbling, gymnastics, and trampoline	9	9-10	22	9
Volleyball	15	5-6-7	73	6

*Eiland, H. J.: Emphasis in junior college physical education programs should be on carryover physical recreation activities, Journal of Health, Physical Education, and Recreation **36:**35, 1965.

a need to provide skills and interests to enrich their leisure and stimulate a desire to keep themselves fit throughout their lifetimes.

Most of the 2-year colleges require students to take physical education both years. Most of the programs require 2 hours each week and stress the successful completion of the service program as a requirement for graduation. A 1971 study of 448 junior colleges found that 90% required physical education.

The California 2-year colleges take into consideration their responsibility for a wide variety of coeducational carryover physical activities. Table 7-4 shows information accumulated from the spring schedules of twenty-two junior colleges and California.

INTERRELATIONSHIPS OF ELEMENTARY, SECONDARY, AND COLLEGE AND UNIVERSITY PROGRAMS

Provision should be made for close interrelationships of the physical education programs at the elementary, secondary, and college levels. Continuity and progression should mark the program from the time the student enters school until he or she graduates. Overall planning is essential to guarantee that duplication of effort, waste of time, omissions, and shortages do not occur in respect to the goal of ensuring that each student become physically educated.

Continuity and progress do not exist today in many of the school systems of the United States. To a great degree each institutional level is autonomous, setting up its own program irrespective of the other levels and with little regard as to what has preceded and what will follow. Many are concerned only with their own little niche and not with the overall program. If the focus of attention is on the student—the consumer of the product—then it would seem that program planning would provide the student with a continuous program, developed in the light of his or her needs and interests, from the time he or she starts school until graduation. There should also be consideration given to adult years. Directors of physical education for the entire community should shoulder this responsibility and ensure that such a program

exists. Some communities like Great Neck, Long Island, and Long Beach, California, have directors over all the school and community physical education and recreation programs. This offers many possibilities for ensuring a continuous program for community residents.

PROVIDING FOR THE HEALTH OF THE STUDENT

Every effort must be put forth by the physical education staff to safeguard the health of all individuals in the program. To accomplish this objective satisfactorily, there must be a close working relationship with staff members in the school health program. Every child should have periodic health examinations with the results of these examinations scrutinized by the physical educator. Frequent conferences should be held with the school physician. A physical education program must be adapted to the needs and interests of each student. The physical educator must assume responsibility for health guidance and health supervision in the activities over which he or she is responsible. The school physician should be consulted when students return after periods of illness, when accidents occur, when students want excuses from the program, and at any other time that qualified advice is needed.

Special precautions must be taken to make activity safe for the student. The desire to win in sports competition must not be used to exploit a student's health. If a disagreement arises, the physician's decision should be final. These and many other phases of the physical education department's interrelationship with the school health program must be carefully attended to.

CRITERIA FOR EVALUATING PHYSICAL EDUCATION ACTIVITY CLASSES

Piscopo has developed the accompanying checklist for evaluating physical education activity classes. It should help in better understanding the essentials of this phase of the physical education program.

CRITERIA FOR EVALUATING PHYSICAL EDUCATION ACTIVITY CLASSES *

	Poor (1)	Fair (2)	Good (3)	Very good (4)	Excellent (5)
Meeting physical education objectives					
1. Does the class actively contribute to the development of physical fitness?	☐	☐	☐	☐	☐
2. Does the class activity foster the growth of ethical character, desirable emotional and social characteristics?	☐	☐	☐	☐	☐
3. Does the class activity contain recreational value?	☐	☐	☐	☐	☐
4. Does the class activity contain carryover value for later life?	☐	☐	☐	☐	☐
5. Is the class activity accepted as a regular part of the school curriculum?	☐	☐	☐	☐	☐
6. Does the class activity meet the needs of *all* students in the group?	☐	☐	☐	☐	☐
7. Does the class activity encourage the development of leadership among students?	☐	☐	☐	☐	☐
8. Does the class activity fulfill the safety objective in physical education?	☐	☐	☐	☐	☐
9. Does the class activity and conduct foster a better understanding of democratic living?	☐	☐	☐	☐	☐
10. Does the class activity and conduct cultivate a better understanding and appreciation for exercise and sports?	☐	☐	☐	☐	☐

Perfect score: 50 *Actual score:* _____

	Poor (1)	Fair (2)	Good (3)	Very good (4)	Excellent (5)
Leadership (teacher conduct)					
1. Is the teacher appropriately and neatly dressed for the class activity?	☐	☐	☐	☐	☐
2. Does the teacher know the activity thoroughly?	☐	☐	☐	☐	☐
3. Does the teacher possess an audible and pleasing voice?	☐	☐	☐	☐	☐
4. Does the teacher project an enthusiastic and dynamic attitude in class presentation?	☐	☐	☐	☐	☐
5. Does the teacher maintain discipline?	☐	☐	☐	☐	☐
6. Does the teacher identify, analyze, and correct faulty performance in guiding pupils?	☐	☐	☐	☐	☐
7. Does the teacher present a sound, logical method of teaching motor skills, for example, explanation, demonstration, participation, and testing?	☐	☐	☐	☐	☐
8. Does the teacher avoid the use of destructive criticism, sarcasm, and ridicule with students?	☐	☐	☐	☐	☐
9. Does the teacher maintain emotional stability and poise?	☐	☐	☐	☐	☐
10. Does the teacher possess high standards and ideals of work?	☐	☐	☐	☐	☐

Perfect score: 50 *Actual score:* _____

	Poor (1)	Fair (2)	Good (3)	Very good (4)	Excellent (5)
General class procedures, methods, and techniques					
1. Does class conduct yield evidence of preplanning?	☐	☐	☐	☐	☐
2. Does the organization of the class allow for individual differences?	☐	☐	☐	☐	☐

*From Piscopoe, J.: Quality instruction: first priority, The Physical Educator **21:**162, 1964.

Continued.

CRITERIA FOR EVALUATING PHYSICAL EDUCATION ACTIVITY CLASSES—cont'd

	Poor (1)	Fair (2)	Good (3)	Very good (4)	Excellent (5)
General class procedures, methods, and techniques–cont'd					
3. Does the class exhibit maximum pupil activity and minimum teacher participation? e.g., overemphasis on explanation and/or demonstration?	☐	☐	☐	☐	☐
4. Are adequate motivational devices such as teaching aids and audiovisual techniques effectively utilized?	☐	☐	☐	☐	☐
5. Are student or squad leaders effectively employed where appropriate?	☐	☐	☐	☐	☐
6. Does the class start promptly at the scheduled time?	☐	☐	☐	☐	☐
7. Are students with medical excuses from the regular class supervised and channelled into appropriate activities?	☐	☐	☐	☐	☐
8. Is the class roll taken quickly and accurately?	☐	☐	☐	☐	☐
9. Are accurate records of pupil progress and achievements maintained?	☐	☐	☐	☐	☐
10. Are supplies and equipment quickly issued and stored?	☐	☐	☐	☐	☐

Perfect score: 50   *Actual score:* _____

	Poor (1)	Fair (2)	Good (3)	Very good (4)	Excellent (5)
Pupil conduct					
1. Are the objectives of the activity or sport clearly known to the learner?	☐	☐	☐	☐	☐
2. Are the students interested in the class activities?	☐	☐	☐	☐	☐
3. Do the students really enjoy their physical education class?	☐	☐	☐	☐	☐
4. Are the students thoroughly familiar with routine regulations of class roll, excuses, and dismissals?	☐	☐	☐	☐	☐
5. Are the students appropriately uniformed for the class activity?	☐	☐	☐	☐	☐
6. Does the class exhibit a spirit of friendly rivalry in learning new skills?	☐	☐	☐	☐	☐
7. Do students avoid mischief or "horseplay"?	☐	☐	☐	☐	☐
8. Do students take showers where facilities and nature of activity permit?	☐	☐	☐	☐	☐
9. Do slow learners participate as much as fast learners?	☐	☐	☐	☐	☐
10. Do students show respect for the teacher?	☐	☐	☐	☐	☐

Perfect score: 50   *Actual score:* _____

	Poor (1)	Fair (2)	Good (3)	Very good (4)	Excellent (5)
Safe and healthful environment					
1. Is the area large enough for the activity and number of students in the class?	☐	☐	☐	☐	☐
2. Does the class possess adequate equipment and/or supplies?	☐	☐	☐	☐	☐
3. Are adequate shower and locker facilities available and readily accessible?	☐	☐	☐	☐	☐
4. Is the equipment and/or apparatus clean and in good working order?	☐	☐	☐	☐	☐
5. Does the activity area contain good lighting and ventilation?	☐	☐	☐	☐	☐

CRITERIA FOR EVALUATING PHYSICAL EDUCATION ACTIVITY CLASSES—cont'd

	Poor (1)	Fair (2)	Good (3)	Very good (4)	Excellent (5)
6. Are all safety hazards eliminated or reduced where possible?	☐	☐	☐	☐	☐
7. Is first aid and safety equipment readily accessible?	☐	☐	☐	☐	☐
8. Is the storage area adequate for supplies and equipment?	☐	☐	☐	☐	☐
9. Does the activity area contain a properly equipped rest room for use in injury, illness, or rest periods?	☐	☐	☐	☐	☐
10. Does the activity area contain adequate toilet facilities?	☐	☐	☐	☐	☐

Perfect score: 50   Actual score: _____

Criteria	Perfect score	Actual score
Meeting physical education objectives	50	_____
Leadership (teacher conduct)	50	_____
General class procedures, methods, and techniques	50	_____
Pupil conduct	50	_____
Safe and healthful environment	50	_____
Total points	250	_____

Questions and exercises

1. Write a 300-word essay on the total physical education program, bringing out the three main components and the contributions that each phase makes to the education of the individual.
2. Outline a physical education program for one of the educational levels. Show how the experiences that you include in your program contribute to the goals of physical education.
3. Discuss some innovative methods of teaching physical education. Visit a high school or junior high school and briefly describe any innovative methods in current use.
4. What are some initial considerations that must be brought about before a program can be planned?
5. Develop a set of standards that could be used to evaluate a physical education program.
6. Develop a list of principles that would serve as guides in the scheduling of physical education activities.
7. What part does each of the following play in scheduling: (a) time allotment, (b) size of classes, (c) teaching stations, (d) teaching loads, (e) grouping, and (f) administrative philosophy?
8. Have a class discussion on each of the following:
   (a) Physical education should be elective in school.
   (b) The Reserve Officer's Training Corp is not a substitute for physical education.
   (c) Credit should be given for physical education.
   (d) Attendance should be voluntary in physical education.
   (e) All excuses should be accepted in physical education.
9. What are some essential points to keep in mind in regard to good class management?
10. Discuss the objectives of differential staffing and the responsibilities of each staff member in the Oak Grove Junior High School. What is your own viewpoint concerning differential staffing?
11. Prepare a list of principles to guide the selection of activities in physical education.
12. What place do coeducational activities have in the physical education program? Justify your stand.
13. Develop a plan to ensure continuity in physical education from the elementary through the college level.
14. How can physical education and health education work together to help promote the health of each individual?
15. Why is an adapted program needed in physical education?

Reading assignment in *Administrative Dimensions of Health and Physical Education Programs, Including Athletics:* Chapter 5, Selections 21 to 27.

Selected references

American Association for Health, Physical Education, and Recreation: Broadfront, Journal of Health, Physical Education, and Recreation **38:**10, 1967.

American Association for Health, Physical Education, and Recreation: Knowledge and understanding in physical education, Washington, D. C., 1969, The Association.

American Association for Health, Physical Education, and Recreation: Perceptual-motor foundations: a multi-disciplinary concern, Washington, D. C., 1969, The Association.

Association for Childhood Education International: Physical education for children's healthful living, Washington, D. C., 1968, The Association.

Battle Creek Physical Education Curriculum Project Team: Battle Creek Physical Education Curriculum Project, Journal of Health, Physical Education, and Recreation **40:**25, 1969.

Bookwalter, K. W.: Physical education in the secondary schools, New York, 1964, The Center for Applied Research in Education, Inc. (The Library of Education).

Bucher, C. A., editor: Methods and materials in physical education and recreation, St. Louis, 1954, The C. V. Mosby Co.

Bucher, C. A.: Foundations of physical education, ed. 7, St. Louis, 1975, The C. V. Mosby Co.

Bucher, C. A.: Physical education for life, St. Louis, 1969, McGraw-Hill Book Co. (A textbook in physical education for high school boys and girls.)

Bucher, C. A., and Koenig, C.: Methods and materials for secondary school physical education, ed. 4, St. Louis, 1974, The C. V. Mosby Co.

Bucher, C. A., and Reade, E. M.: Health and physical education in the modern elementary school, New York, 1971, The Macmillan Co.

Bureau of Health Education, Physical Education, Athletics, and Recreation, California State Department of Education: Evaluation of the effects of flexible scheduling on physical education, Sacramento, California, 1972.

Corbin, C. B.: A textbook of motor development, Dubuque, Iowa, 1973, William C. Brown Co.

Dowell, L. J.: Conceptual foundations of physical education, health and recreation, Dubuque, Iowa, 1973, William C. Brown Co.

Elementary School Physical Education Commission of the American Assocation for Health, Physical Education, and Recreation Physical Education Division (1968-69): Essentials of a quality elementary school physical education program, Journal of Health, Physical Education, and Recreation **42:**42, 1971.

Espenschade, A. S.: Physical education in the elementary schools—what research says to the teacher, Washington, D. C., March, 1963, Department of Classroom Teachers, American Educational Research Association of the National Education Association.

Fitness for California Children and Youth: Values inherent in the daily program of physical education, Journal of the California Association for Health, Physical Education and Recreation, March, 1965 (special issue).

Hellison, D. R.: Humanistic physical education: a behavioral perspective, Englewood Cliffs, New Jersey, 1973, Prentice-Hall, Inc.

Insley, G. S.: Practical guidelines for the teaching of physical education, Reading, Massachusetts, 1973, Addison-Wesley.

LaPorte, W. R.: The physical education curriculum (a national program), ed. 6, Los Angeles, 1955, University of Southern California Press.

Oxendine, J. B.: Status of general instruction programs of physical education in 4-year colleges and universities: 1971-72, Journal of Health, Physical Education, and Recreation **43:**26, 1972.

Physical Education Division Committee: Guidelines for secondary school physical education, Journal of Health, Physical Education, and Recreation **42:**47, 1971.

Physical Education Division Committee: Guide to excellence for physical education in colleges and universities, Journal of Health, Physical Education, and Recreation **42:**51, 1971.

Physical education in the junior college, Journal of Health, Physical Education, and Recreation **36:**33, 1965.

President's Council on Physical Fitness: Fitness for leadership, Washington, D. C., 1964, Superintendent of Documents.

Reams, D., and Bleier, T. J.: Developing team teaching for ability grouping, Journal of Health, Physical Education, and Recreation **39:**50, 1968.

Stahly, D.: Care and feeding of a good activity program, The Clearing House **46:**3, 1972.

The now physical education, Journal of Health, Physical Education, Recreation **44:**23, 1973.

The University of the State of New York, The State Education Department, Bureau of Secondary Curriculum Development: Physical education in the secondary school, Curriculum Guide, Albany, 1964, State Department of Education.

U. S. Office of Education, U. S. Department of Health, Education, and Welfare: How teachers make a difference, Washington, D. C., 1971, Superintendent of Documents.

Von Bergen, E.: Flexible scheduling for physical education, Journal of Health, Physical Education, and Recreation **38:**29, 1967.

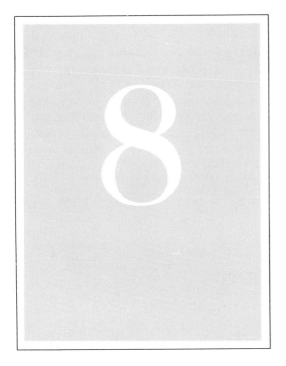

The adapted program*

A former Commissioner of Education, S. P. Marland, Jr., observed in his annual report to Congress that ". . . change is in the air . . ."* This is indeed true and is reflected in the innovative techniques utilized in school systems and universities. Change is also reflected in programs for the gifted, retarded, handicapped, and disadvantaged individual. All persons have the right to fulfill themselves to their highest potential, and that is the ultimate purpose of an adapted program in physical education.

The term *adapted* is used here, although many books and programs use other terms, such as *corrective, individual, modified, therapeutic, remedial, special, restricted,* and *atypical.* In fact, *physical education programs for the handicapped* is the term being used more and more frequently. The adapted program refers to that phase of physical education that meets the needs of the individual who, because of some physical inadequacy, functional defect capable of being improved through physical activity, or other deficiency, is temporarily or permanently unable to take part in the regular physical education program. It also refers to a significant segment of a school or college student population that does not fall into the classification "average" or "normal" for their age or grade. These students deviate from their peers in a physical, mental, emotional, or social characteristics or in a combination of these traits.

The principle of individual differences is being recognized increasingly by educators. The observance of this principle has resulted in special provisions in the schools for retarded as well as for gifted children, for those with heart abnormalities, defective sight, physical disabilities, and other deviations from the normal, and for those who are culturally deprived or emotionally disturbed.

The principle of individual differences that applies to education as a whole should also apply to physical education. Most administrators believe that as long as a student can come to school or college, he or she should be re-

*Marland, S. P., Jr.: A report on the condition of education, American Education **8**:3, 1972.

*A detailed discussion of the care and education of exceptional children is given in Chapter 13 on school health services. Much of this material is pertinent to the adapted program but will not be repeated here. However, the reader may wish to read that important section.

This chapter is designed to outline briefly the adapted program as a component of total school and college physical education programs.

quired to participate in physical education. If this tenet is adhered to, it means that programs must be adapted to individual needs. Many children and young adults who are recuperating from long illnesses or operations or who are suffering from other physical or emotional conditions require special consideration in their programs.

It cannot be assumed that all individuals in physical education classes are normal. Unfortunately, many programs are administered on this basis. One estimate has been made that one out of every eight students in our schools is handicapped to the extent that special provision should be made in the educational program.

Schools and colleges will always have students who, because of many factors such as heredity, environment, disease, accident, or other reason, will have physical or other impairment. Many of these students have difficulty in adjusting to the demands that society places upon them. It is the responsibility of physical

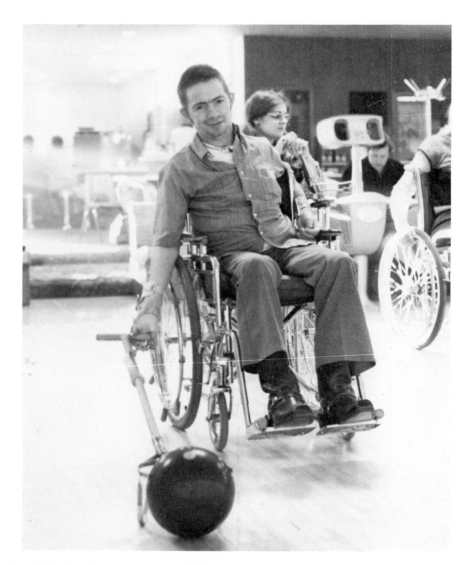

Adapted physical education can enable many handicapped individuals to realize the joy of sports. A patient participating in a bowling program, utilizing bowling device for quadriplegics. (Younker Memorial Rehabilitation Center, Iowa Methodist Hospital, Des Moines, Iowa.)

education programs to help each and every individual who comes into class. Even though a person may be atypical, this is not cause for neglect. In fact, it should represent an even greater challenge to see that he or she enjoys the benefits of participating in physical activities adapted to his needs. Provision for a sound adapted program has been a shortcoming of physical education throughout the nation because of a lack of properly trained teachers, the financial cost of remedial instruction, and the fact that many administrators and teachers are not aware of their responsibility and the contribution they can make in this phase of physical education. These obstacles should be overcome as the public becomes aware of the need of educating *all* individuals in *all* phases of the total education program.

Parker grasped the importance of providing for the exceptional person in these words:

The exceptional person needs an opportunity to become a responsible citizen; to become an economically efficient producer and consumer of goods, or services; to develop an understanding of human relationships of home, neighbor-

---

LOS ANGELES CITY SCHOOL DISTRICTS
Health Education and Health Services Branch—Auxiliary Services Division
Corrective Physical Education Section

CORRECTIVE PHYSICAL EDUCATION ACTIVITY GUIDE
A Guide for the Teacher and Physician
In Planning a Restricted Program of Physical Education

Pupil_____ Date_____

School_____ Corrective Phys. Ed. Teacher_____

I. TYPES OF MOVEMENTS	OMIT	*MILD	**MODERATE	UNLIMITED	REMARKS
Bending					
Climbing					
Hanging					
Jumping					
Kicking					
Lifting					
Pulling					
Pushing					
Running					
Stretching					
Throwing					
Twisting					

II. TYPES OF EXERCISES	OMIT	*MILD	**MODERATE	UNLIMITED	REMARKS
Abdominal					
Arm					
Breathing					
Foot					
Head					
Knee					
Leg					
Trunk					
Relaxation					

III. TYPES OF POSITIONS	LIMITED	UNLIMITED	IV. TYPES OF ACTIVITIES	YES	NO
Lying supine			Competitive sports		
Lying prone			Games——Sitting		
Sitting			Games requiring standing but no running or jumping		
Standing			Officiating		
			Swimming		
Recommended until_____ 196_			Coeducational activities		
			Social dancing		
Remarks:			Square dancing		
			Sports and games		

_____
Signature of Physician

*Very little activity.
**Half as much as the unlimited
program.

A guide for planning adapted physical education for students.

hood, and wider social groups; and to realize whatever personal potentialities the Creator has bestowed. For an exceptional child it means a well-planned curriculum of many rich experiences of the kinds he is capable of having, which brings to him some measure of ability to make and keep friends, to share with others some if not all of the common social experience, to care for himself personally and for his home, perhaps even to earn his living or a reasonable part of it, and to enjoy life as he must live it.*

Stone and Deyton framed the value of adapted physical education in these terms:

These children receive health and vocational guidance from interested teachers, who have discovered the value of rehabilitation through corrective physical education. Through these cooperative efforts, physically and psychologically atypical children are trained to face and accept their handicaps, to realize their limitations, and to adapt to them. The aims of the corrective programs for these children are to meet the physical and emotional needs of each one, to prove to each individually that there is a place for him which he alone can fill best, to help fit himself for that place, and within his handicap to allow him to "play, too."†

CLARIFICATION OF TERMS

The term "adapted" was defined at the beginning of this chapter and is used primarily throughout this text to identify the physical education program for students with certain disabilities. These disabilities are further defined by changing terminology. For example, in 1967 New York State amended its education law to redefine "handicapped child." The handicapped child under New York State law is one who ". . . because of mental, physical, or emotional reasons cannot be educated in regular classes but can benefit from special services. . . ."‡

The New York State Education department uses the term "exceptional child" to identify the pupil who ". . . differs from his peers to such an extent that he cannot profit fully from the regular prescribed curriculum and for whom

special provisions need to be made in order for him to realize his potential."*

The Office of Education of the United States Department of Health, Education and Welfare uses the term "disadvantaged" to designate a child who is economically deprived, racially and geographically isolated, untrained and unskilled, and handicapped and neglected.

The importance of understanding different uses of terminology is stressed because of federal legislation and funds available to educational programs and children who meet the requirements of the definition utilized by particular government and other agencies. Some of this legislation is discussed in the following section.

LEGISLATION FOR THE DISADVANTAGED

In order to stimulate the development of a national commitment to equal educational opportunities for every disadvantaged child, federal legislation in recent years has provided funds and grants to local school districts, public and private nonprofit institutions, and individual states.

The 1965 Elementary and Secondary Education Act played a leading role in providing assistance to adapted physical education programs. The provisions for assistance are best referred to by their titles.

1. Title I, Education of Disadvantaged Children (P.L. 89-750, as amended), is the largest program of federal aid to elementary and secondary education. The major purpose of Title I is to provide programs effectively designed to meet the educational needs of disadvantaged children.

2. Titles III and IV promote a strong liaison between school and community and encourage innovative programs. These titles are essential to implementing adapted programs.

3. Title VI, as amended in 1969, created a single Education of the Handicapped Act (P.L. 91-230). The Bureau for the Edu-

---

*Parker, R.: Physical education for the handicapped, Journal of Health and Physical Education **17:**254, 1946.
†Stone, E. B., and Deyton, J. W.: Corrective therapy for the handicapped child, New York, 1951, Prentice-Hall, Inc., pp. 1-2.
‡Blatt, B.: Public policy with the education of children with special needs, Exceptional Children **38:**7, 1972.

---

*University of the State of New York: Physical education for the exceptional child, Albany, New York, 1970, Curriculum Development Center, p. iii.

cation and Training of the Handicapped was created under the Office of Education to implement this law. Part D of this law authorizes grants for the training of personnel in the education of the handicapped. Part E authorizes research and demonstration projects in the areas of physical education and recreation for the handicapped.

4. Title VIII, the Education Professions Development Act, has broad implications for adapted programs. Its main purposes include the improvement of preservice and inservice teacher education, provisions for specialist training, training of prospective and experienced administrators, and provisions for better use of school personnel and instructional materials.

It is essential that school administrators be familiar with this legislation and all new legislation that is pertinent to the development of all educational programs, including the adapted program. Financial aid and grants that can help in training personnel and developing innovative programs are often overlooked by administrations.

EXTENT OF ATYPICAL CONDITIONS AMONG STUDENTS

Although records are insufficient, there have been several estimates of the number of children with handicapping conditions in the nation's schools. One estimate indicates that 8% to 10% of schoolage children are handicapped, emotionally disturbed, brain injured, auditorily impaired, or have chronic health problems. Statistics for 1971 cite that at least 7 million children in the United States between the ages of 4 and 19 years are physically handicapped. The great majority of these boys and girls are in the elementary schools.

Some specific figures in regard to handicapping conditions have been given. One source states that there are approximately 10,000 children who are totally blind and 58,000 children of school age who have partial sight. There are more than 500,000 in each of the following classifications: crippled, deaf, or hard of hearing. There are approximately 700,000 speech-

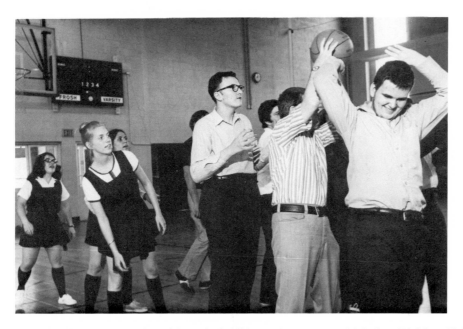

A physical education instructor working with atypical children. (Courtesy Arnold College Division, University of Bridgeport, Conn., Parents and Friends Association of Mentally Retarded Children.) (Photograph by John Tasker.)

handicapped children, and a similar number of children are considered socially maladjusted. Each year in the United States more than 126,000 babies are born with some degree of mental retardation. At present there are more than 7 million mentally retarded children and adults in the United States. According to the Director of Programs for the Handicapped of the AAHPER, 4 million children of school age in the United States have physical, mental, or emotional handicaps. In addition to the handicapped, there are those students with poor motor ability, low physical fitness, and weight problems who represent 20% to 25% of the total school population. The Ford Foundation indicates at least 50% of the children living in cities are culturally disadvantaged. There are also over 500,000 children with special health problems.

OBJECTIVES OF THE ADAPTED PROGRAM

Physical education can be of great value to the atypical individual in many ways. It can help in identifying deviations from the normal and in referring students to proper individuals or agencies, when necessary. It can help the atypical person to have a happy, wholesome play experience. It can help the student to achieve, within his or her limitations, physical skill and exercise. It can provide many opportunities for the learning of skills that are appropriate for the handicapped person to achieve success. Finally, physical education can help to contribute to a more productive life on the part of the handicapped individual by developing those physical qualities that are needed to meet the demands of day-to-day living.

Daniels and Davies developed a comprehensive list of objectives for the adapted physical education program, which represents a worthy guide for administrators everywhere. The list follows:

1. Accomplish needed therapy or correction for conditions which can be improved or removed (pertains particularly to temporary disabilities such as reduced dislocations and post appendectomies).
2. Aid in the adjustment and/or resocialization of the individual when the disability is permanent (permanent disabilities like amputation, cerebral palsy

can benefit greatly from adapted physical education programs).
3. Protect the condition from aggravation by acquainting the student with his limitations and capacities and arranging a program within his physiological work capacity or exercise tolerance.
4. Provide students with an opportunity for the development of organic power within the limits of the disability.
5. Provide students with an opportunity to develop skills in the recreational sports and games within the limits of the disability.
6. Provide students with an opportunity for normal social development through recreational sports and games appropriate to their age group and interests.
7. Contribute to security through improved function and increased ability to meet the physical demands of daily living. *

Arnheim and others† list objectives for the adapted physical education program. Their specific objectives are listed in the context of helping students with handicaps to achieve effective physical, mental, emotional, and social growth through the medium of a program of selected physical education and recreational activities. Their specific objectives to help students in achieving these goals are given here in adapted form:

To help students to correct conditions that are capable of being improved
To help students protect themselves from injuries and conditions that might occur as a result of participating in physical education activities
To provide opportunities for students to learn a variety of appropriate recreational activities
To help students to develop optimal organic power and physical condition in light of their physical resources
To help students to understand and appreciate their physical and mental limitations
To help students to develop socially and achieve a worthy self-image
To help students understand, appreciate, and develop good body mechanics
To help students understand and appreciate sports in which they will be spectators

An analysis of these objectives indicates that through their accomplishment the needs of every individual will be provided for, regardless

---

*Daniels, A. S., and Davies, E. A.: Adapted physical education, ed. 2, New York, 1965, Harper & Row, Publishers, pp. 82-88.
†Arnheim, D. D., and others: Principles and methods of adapted physical education, ed. 2, St. Louis, 1973, The C. V. Mosby Co.

of whether he or she has a temporary or a permanent disability, a need for organic, mental, emotional, or social adjustment, or a need for a broad or limited program. These are excellent goals for physical educators.

PLANNING THE ADAPTED PHYSICAL EDUCATION PROGRAM

To have an effective adapted physical education program requires considerable thought and planning. The Bureau of Health Education, Physical Education, and Recreation of the California State Department of Education has prepared a special publication for distribution to their schools and physical educators.* Among many outstanding features of this publication are suggestions for planning an adapted physical education program. These suggestions presented in adapted form include the following:

1. Instruction and practice in basic skills of locomotion and skills for physical recreation should be provided for all age groups.

2. The regular physical education program in the intermediate grades and secondary schools should provide for a minimum of two units in the mechanics of body movement.

3. Where there is a need for special help by students in overcoming poor body alignment, there should be special classes in those schools in which such classes are possible and by individual assignments in regular classes in other schools.

4. From kindergarten through high school, each teaching unit should be planned to teach motor skills for movement patterns that will, in turn, provide for a successful experience in those physical activities included in the program.

5. Where the pupil's ability is limited, he or she should either be permitted to participate in regular courses if the experience can be successful, or provision should be made for other units of instruction that will provide the special help needed.

6. If a student's condition is such that rest and relaxation are needed, these should be provided for.

7. Policies concerned with pupils who are absent from class should take into consideration the welfare of the student.

8. When assigning students with severe physically handicapping conditions to special classes or when following other procedures to provide special instruction for pupils, all experiences should be regarded and operated as integral parts of the total, regular physical education program.

9. A special program should be offered to those pupils who score below the twenty-fifth percentile of the California Physical Performance Tests or a similar battery of tests.

10. Both school and family physicians should understand the nature and scope of the adapted physical education program in order to intelligently recommend a student's participation in physical education.

CONTRIBUTION OF PHYSICAL EDUCATION TO VARIOUS TYPES OF ATYPICAL CONDITIONS

There is no one way to group students in the adapted program. As has been indicated, there are many different types of boys and girls in the program. It would be wise for the physical educator and health educator to sit down with the school physician, school psychologist, and nurse and include in their planning the various types of atypical students they have in their institution. The discussion in this section includes the following atypical conditions: (1) physically handicapped, (2) mentally retarded, (3) emotionally disturbed, (4) culturally disadvantaged, (5) poorly coordinated, and (6) physically gifted and creative students.

Physically handicapped students

Historically, various methods have been utilized to classify physically handicapped persons. Two types of classification that have been used are given here.

The University of the State of New York*

---

*Dexter, G.: Special physical education classes for physically handicapped minors. Sacramento, Calif., June, 1964, California State Department of Education, pp. 3-4.

*University of the State of New York: Physical education syllabus, book 4. Secondary schools (grades 7 to 12 inclusive), boys, Albany, 1944, University of State of New York Press.

lists the following specific deficiencies or growth abnormalities that require adapted physical education activities:

1. Heart and lung disturbances
2. Postoperative and convalescent patients
3. Faulty body mechanics, including posture
4. Underweight
5. Overweight
6. Nervous instability
7. Functional defects
8. General muscular weakness resulting from lack of exercise, or systemic deficiencies
9. Conditions, congenital or acquired, affecting bone or muscle mechanism
10. Certain eye conditions

LaPorte* points to the fact that corrective cases may be classified under the following headings:

1. Nutrition (overweight and underweight)
2. Poor posture
3. Weak and flat feet
4. Functional and organic heart conditions
5. Hernias
6. Infantile paralysis and other crippling conditions
7. Neurasthenia or nervous instability
8. Menstrual and endocrine disorders

Whatever the physical disability, a physical education program must be provided. Some handicapped students will be able to participate in a regular program of physical education with certain minor modifications. A separate adapted program must be provided for those students who cannot participate in the basic instructional program of the school. The physically handicapped student cannot be allowed to sit on the sidelines and become only a spectator. The handicapped student needs to have the opportunity to develop and maintain adequate skill abilities and fitness levels.

Physical handicaps, which may stem from congenital or hereditary causes or may develop later in life through environmental factors, such as malnutrition, disease, or accident, sometimes cause negative psychologic and social traits to develop because of the limitations imposed on the individual. A physically handicapped student is occasionally ignored or rebuffed by classmates who do not understand

the nature of the disability or who ostracize the student because the disability prevents him or her from participating fully in the activities of the school. These attitudes toward the handicapped force them to withdraw in order to avoid becoming hurt and result in their becoming further isolated from the remainder of the student body.

Some experts have noted that the limitations of the handicap often seem more severe to the observer than they are in fact to the handicapped individual. When this misconception occurs, the handicapped student must prove his or her abilities in order to gain acceptance and a chance to participate and compete on an equal basis with nonhandicapped classmates.

The blind or deaf student or the student with a severe speech impairment has a different set of problems from the orthopedically handicapped student. The partially sighted, the blind, the deaf, and the speech-impaired student cannot communicate with great facility. The orthopedically handicapped student is limited in the physical education class but not necessarily in the academic classroom. The student with vision, hearing, or speech problems may be limited in both physical education and the academic classroom.

Very often there is a tendency toward overprotection of handicapped children. Recent programs, however, have specifically included the visually handicapped child in the regular physical education program. Injuries and accidents among these children were proved to be negligible. The purposes of having these children participate in regular physical education programs are to provide activities with their peers and to aid them in developing skills in lifetime sport areas so they can enjoy these sports outside school and in later life.

Some innovative programs that include blind students in regular physical education classes are:

1. *Robert E. Lee School, Long Beach, California.* Here blind children participate in all activities including softball and track. Students are offered aid by classmates when necessary.

2. *Fargo Public Schools, Fargo, North Dakota.* The visually handicapped students participate with their peers at the elementary level.

*LaPorte, W. R.: The physical education curriculum (a national program), ed. 6, Los Angeles, 1955, University of Southern California Press, p. 59.

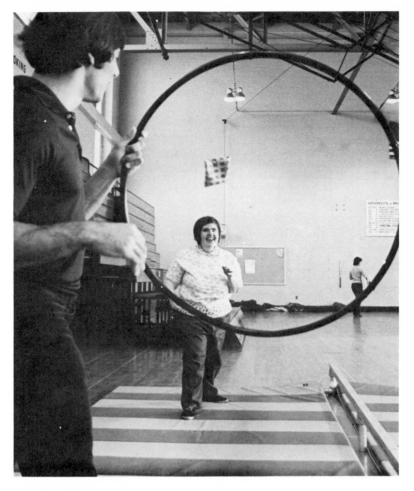

A physical education instructor involved with helping a handicapped student. (Courtesy Arnold College Division, University of Bridgeport, Conn., Parents and Friends Association of Mentally Retarded Children.) (Photograph by John Tasker.)

They are unrestricted in such areas as exercise, rope jumping, balance beam work, relays, tumbling, and ice skating.

3. *Wheeling High School, Wheeling, Illinois.* Blind students regularly play softball with their sighted classmates. The bases are roped off to guide the students, and a large soft ball is used. Signals to bat and throw are called by sighted team members.

There is a lack of physical educators who are especially trained to teach physically handicapped students. School systems find that the cost of providing special classes taught by specially trained physical educators is sometimes prohibitive. Where there are no special classes, the physical educator must provide, within the regular instructional program, those activities that will meet the needs of the handicapped student. Further, placing the physically handicapped student in a regular physical education class will help give him or her a feeling of belonging. This advantage is not always possible where separate adapted classes are provided.

Some handicapped students will be able to participate in almost all of the activities that nonhandicapped students enjoy. As previously mentioned, blind students have successfully engaged in team sports where they can receive oral cues from their sighted teammates. Some athletic equipment manufacturers have placed bells inside game balls; the blind student is then able to rely on this sound as well as the supplementary oral cues. Ropes or covered wires acting as hand guides also enable the blind student to participate in track and field events. Still other activities such as swimming, dance, calisthenics, and tumbling require little adaptation or none at all, except in regard to heightened safety precautions.

In general, deaf students will not be restricted in any way from participating in a full physical education program. Some deaf students experience difficulty in those activities requiring precise balance, such as balance-beam walking, and may require some remedial work in this area. The physical educator should be prepared to offer any extra help needed.

Other physically handicapped students will have a variety of limitations and a variety of skill abilities. Appropriate program adaptations and modifications must be made in order to meet this range of individual needs. The physician is the individual most knowledgeable about the history and limitations of a student's handicap. He or she is therefore in the best position to recommend a physical activity program for the student. The student's abilities and levels of fitness should be tested in those areas where medical permission for participation has been granted. This will ensure not only a proper program for the individual but will also help in placing the student in the proper class or section of a class. Careful records should be kept showing the student's test scores, activity recommendations, activities, and progress through the program.

Organized competition for the handicapped has been very successful and meaningful for its participants. An innovative competitive program in the form of an "activity day" has recently been introduced at Cypress Orthopedic School in California. This activity day serves as a climax to the learning of physical skills developed as a part of the vigorous physical education program. Such activities as a wheelchair beanbag race, balloon bounce, and crutch walking race demonstrate some of the activities these children can and do participate in.

The adapted and the regular physical education programs should be as similar as possible. Where the programs are totally divergent, the physically handicapped student is isolated from his or her classmates. When the programs are as similar as possible, the handicapped student can be made to feel a part of the larger group and will gain self-confidence and self-respect. Physically handicapped students need the challenge of a progressive program. They welcome the opportunity to test their abilities, and they should experience the fun of a challenge and the success of meeting it. The handicapped should be given an opportunity to seek extra help and extra practice after school hours. During this time they can benefit from more individualized instruction than is possible during the class period. The fitness level of each student, his or her ability, recreational needs, sex, age, and interest will help to determine the activities the student will engage in pleasurably. Safe facilities and safe equipment are essential. Intramural and club programs should be provided, but they should be of such a nature that physically handicapped students can enjoy them in a safe and controlled atmosphere that precludes the danger of injury.

Mentally retarded students

In some schools, special physical education classes are offered for mentally retarded students, while in still other schools the mentally retarded participate in the regularly scheduled physical education classes.

Mental retardation can be a result of hereditary abnormalities, birth injury, or an accident or illness that leads to impairment of brain function. There are degrees of mental retardation ranging from the severely mentally retarded, who require custodial care, to the educable mentally retarded, who function with only a moderate degree of impairment.

Many agencies are conducting research in the field of mental retardation in an attempt to discover the causes and nature of mental retardation and the methods through which retardation may be prevented. Some agencies are operating innovative training schools for the mentally retarded. The Joseph P. Kennedy, Jr., Foundation is spearheading much of the research concerned with mental retardation and is also a leader in providing camping and recreational programs for the mentally retarded. The

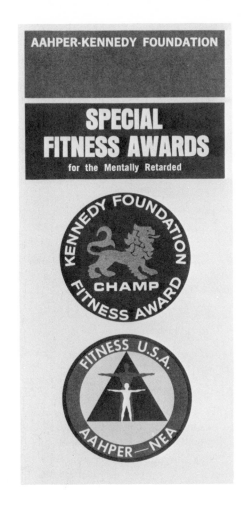

Special fitness awards for the mentally retarded, AAHPER–Kennedy Foundation.

Kennedy Foundation has also sponsored training programs for teachers of the mentally retarded. The United States government is sponsoring experimental physical education programs for mentally retarded persons staffed by special education teachers, specially trained physical educators, vocational rehabilitation technicians, and architectural engineers. Special programs and special equipment have been designed especially for use by the mentally retarded. Climbing devices, obstacle courses, and unique running areas, as well as a swimming pool, are part of the special facilities. The objectives of this program include social and personal adjustment and development of physical fitness, sports skills, and general motor ability.

Mentally retarded students show a wide range of intellectual and physical abilities. Experts seem to agree that a mentally retarded child is usually closer to the norm for chronologic age in physical development than in mental development. Some mentally retarded students are capable of participating in a regular physical education class, whereas others have been able to develop only minimal amounts of motor ability. In general, most mentally retarded students are 2 to 4 years behind their normal peers in motor development alone.

Despite a slower development of motor ability, mentally retarded students seem to reach physical maturity faster than do normal boys and girls of the same chronologic age. The mentally retarded tend to be overweight and to lack physical strength and endurance. Their posture is generally poor, and they lack adequate levels of physical fitness and motor coordination. Some of these physical problems develop because the mentally retarded have had little of the play and physical activity experiences of normal children. The problems of some mentally retarded youngsters are further multiplied by attendant physical handicaps and personality disturbances.

The mentally retarded require a physical educator with special training, special skills, and a special brand of patience. The mentally retarded lack confidence and pride and need a physical educator who will help them to change their negative self-image. The physical educator must be able to provide a program designed to give each student a chance for success. The physical educator must be ready to praise and reinforce each minor success. He or she must be capable of demonstrating each skill, give simple and concise directions, and be willing to participate in physical education activities with the students. Discipline must be enforced and standards adhered to, but the disciplinary approach must be a kind and gentle one.

The physical educator must be especially mindful of the individual characteristics of each mentally retarded student. Those students who need remedial work should be afforded this

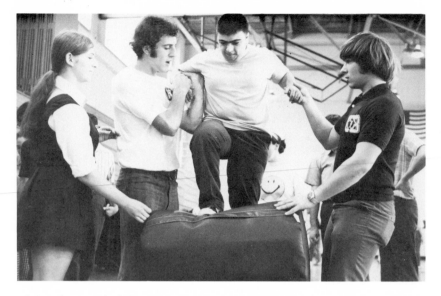

Mentally retarded students can be helped through physical education activities. (Courtesy Arnold College Division, University of Bridgeport, Conn., Parents and Friends Association of Mentally Retarded Children.) (Photograph by John Tasker.)

opportunity, while those students who can succeed in a regular physical education program should be placed in such a class or section.

Most mentally retarded students need to be taught how to play. They are frequently unfamiliar with even the simplest of childhood games, and they lack facility in the natural movements of childhood, such as skipping, hopping, and leaping. The mentally retarded are often seriously deficient in physical fitness and need work in postural improvement. Further, the mentally retarded find it difficult to understand and remember game strategy such as the importance of staying in the right position, and cannot relate well to the rules of sports and games.

The majority of mentally retarded students need a specially tailored physical education experience. For those who can participate in a regular physical education class, care must be taken so that these students are not placed in a situation where they will meet failure. In a special physical education class, the mentally retarded student can be exposed to a variety of physical education experiences. Physical fitness and posture improvement, along with self-testing activities and games organized and designed according to the ability and interests

of the group, will make up a vital part of the special program. In such a class, activities can be easily modified and new experiences introduced before interest wanes. Research has indicated that specially tailored physical education classes can help mentally retarded students to progress very rapidly in their physical skill development. Movement education is especially suited to the mentally retarded. These students have often not engaged in the natural play activities of childhood and need to develop their gross motor skill abilities in order to be able to find success in some of the more sophisticated motor skills.

There are many new and exciting innovations in physical education programs for mentally retarded youngsters. The AAHPER-Kennedy Foundation Special Fitness Awards program encourages retarded children and youths to engage in vigorous physical activities to compete in the Olympics for the retarded. In order to qualify for these Olympics, the child must first earn the "champ" award. The three awards given are silver, gold, and champ. Standards of performance are based on a national sample of educable retarded children. In order to achieve awards in this program, the child must meet the standards of seven test items and spend 30 hours of active sports participation within a 3-month period.

In July, 1968, the first International Special Olympics for mentally retarded boys and girls was held at Chicago's Soldier Field. More than 1,000 boys and girls participated. The second such Olympics was held in 1970 and featured more than two hundred events.

Olympics programs for children with all types of handicaps including retardation have also been held. The first Special Olympics was held in southwest Cooke County, Illinois, and involved the entire community in the program. Children were divided into nonphysically and physically handicapped groups and then into chronologic age, ability, and sex groupings.

Emotionally disturbed students

The emotionally disturbed student presents special problems for the physical educator, who must be concerned not only with teaching but also with the safety of the students in the class.

A single emotionally disturbed student can have a disastrous effect on a class and can affect the behavior of the rest of the students in that class. Effective teaching cannot take place when discipline deteriorates.

Emotionally unstable students have difficulty maintaining good relationships with their classmates and teachers. Some of their abnormal behavior patterns stem from a need and craving for attention. Sometimes the disruptive student exhibits gross patterns of aggressiveness and destructiveness. Other emotionally unstable students may be so withdrawn from the group that they refuse to participate in the activities of the class, even to the extent of refusing to report for class. In the case of physical education, the emotionally disturbed student may refuse to dress for the activity when he or she does report. These measures draw both student and teacher reaction and focus attention on the nonconforming student.

Emotionally unstable students are often restless and unable to pay attention. In a physical education class they may poke and prod other students, refuse to line up with the rest of the class, or insist on bouncing a game ball while a lesson is in progress. These are also ploys to

gain attention. The student behaves in the same manner in the academic classroom for the same reason.

Some emotionally disturbed students may have physical or mental handicaps that contribute to their behavior. Others may be concerned about what they consider to be poor personal appearance such as extremes of height or weight or physical maturity not in keeping with their chronologic age. Still other emotionally disturbed students may simply be in the process of growing up and are finding it difficult to handle their adolescence.

If negative student behavior stems from some aspect of a student's personality, then the physical educator must take positive steps to resolve the problem so that teaching can take place. The physical educator must deal with each behavior problem on an individual basis and seek help from those school personnel who are best equipped to give aid. The school psychologist and the student's guidance counselor will have information that will be of help to the physical educator. A conference with these individuals may reveal methods that have proved effective with the student in the past. Further, the observations made by the physical educator will be of value to the continuing study of the student.

The physical educator will find that not all emotionally disturbed students are continual and serious behavior problems. The physical educator should have a private conference with the student whose behavior suddenly becomes negative and try to understand why the student has reacted in a way unusual for him or her. Such a conference will lead to mutual understanding and often help to allay future problems with the same student.

Much of the physical educator's task is student guidance. In individual cases of disruptive behavior, the physical educator should exhaust all of his or her personal resources to alleviate the problem before enlisting aid from other sources. Any case of disruptive behavior demands immediate action on the part of the physical educator to prevent minor problems from becoming major ones.

The majority of school pupils enjoy physical activity and physical education. They look forward to the physical education class as one part of the school day in which they can express themselves and gain a release of tension in an atmosphere that encourages this. For this reason, the student who is disruptive in the classroom is often one of the best citizens in the physical education class.

Physical education is in a unique position to help the emotionally disturbed student. Most students profit from the activities of physical education, and through their actions in this phase of the school curriculum teaching personnel can gain many insights into understanding student behavior. Individual knowledge of each student is of utmost importance in physical education and in understanding individual behavior patterns. Recognizing a student's needs and problems early in the school year will help in offsetting future behavior problems.

While physical education classes are conducted in a less formal manner than are classroom subjects, this does not mean that lower standards of behavior are acceptable. Students should know what the standards are on the first day of class and should be expected to adhere to these standards in all future classes.

Respect for the individual student is a necessity. No student likes to be criticized or embarrassed in front of his or her peers. When a student is singled out from a group and used as a disciplinary example, the atmosphere in the class will deteriorate. Respect for the student means maintenance of respect for the teacher. If disciplinary matters are handled on a one-to-one basis, rapport is enhanced. If the disruptive student knows that the physical educator expects him or her to behave in a bizarre manner, he or she will react in just this way. Good behavior should be expected until the student acts otherwise. Constant failure only abets disruptive behavior. If a student is known to be hostile and disruptive, an attempt should be made to avoid placing that student in situations where he or she feels inadequate and shows this in his or her behavior. If, for example, a disruptive student does not run well, he or she may still make a superior goalie in soccer, a position that would not require running. If the emotionally disturbed student has a special skill talent, he or she might be asked to demonstrate for the class. This will give the recognition and atten- tion needed. Praise should be given for a skill that is well performed.

No student is going to participate in extra class activities unless he or she really wants to. Therefore, behavioral standards should be set for each activity, and it should be available to all students in the school who meet the standards. Acceptance into a club or participation on an intramural team may help the disruptive student gain self-respect and peer recognition and approval.

Culturally disadvantaged students

Recently, culturally disadvantaged students have become a real concern to various communities and to the schools serving these communities. It is a common error for the public to associate only the black child with cultural deprivation. Professional educators especially must realize that cultural deprivation crosses all color lines and ignores none of them. The culture of poverty is especially apparent in the large urban centers. Culturally disadvantaged persons may be found in Appalachia, suburbia, and isolated small towns and rural villages all across the United States.

The culturally disadvantaged student feels isolated from the mainstream of life. Home and neighborhood environments serve as negative influences, destroying confidence, robbing him or her of a chance for success, and defeating any aspirations he or she may have. A culturally disadvantaged student does not achieve success in school because the cultural standards of the school and the home environment are usually inconsistent. Even schools in ghetto or slum areas are staffed by teachers who represent the middle-class segment of society. Continual failure in the classroom negatively affects the school behavior of the culturally disadvantaged student. Short attention span, emotional instability, excitability, and restlessness often contribute to disruptive behavior patterns.

In physical education the culturally disadvantaged student can be given an opportunity to meet success. Physical activity has a strong appeal for these youngsters whether they are students in a school in their neighborhood or community or part of the student body in a school in an affluent area.

The physical educator is the most important single factor in a school physical education program for the disadvantaged. The physical educator should have a sincere interest in these students and must be willing to assume the responsibility for physically educating them. He or she should have an adequate background and special training in general education and physical education courses concerned with teaching the disadvantaged. These courses will help in attaining a fuller understanding of the culturally disadvantaged student and the educational problems he or she faces. The physical educator should have the ability to develop rapport with the culturally disadvantaged so that he or she can better respect, understand, and help these students. The physical educator should be able to provide an enriched program that will help to motivate the culturally disadvantaged student to make the best use of his or her physical, intellectual, and creative abilities.

Through physical education activities many general educational knowledges, skills, and abilities can be enhanced. Through folk dances, for example, it is possible to acquaint the student with the dress and customs of various cultures. This knowledge will help a class in history to become more interesting to the student and develop pride in his or her own culture. Through a sport such as baseball, mathematics can be brought to life. The students will be able to see the relationship between mathematics and its uses in determining baseball batting averages, computing team won-lost percentages, and the importance of understanding angles as applied to laying out a baseball diamond.

The school physical education program frequently is the only supervised physical activity program for the culturally disadvantaged student. These students usually do not have a neighborhood recreational facility available and must conduct their sports and games on unsupervised streets or in dangerously littered lots. The school physical education experience must be designed to afford this student the physical education and recreational activities that are denied elsewhere. There must be a wide choice of physical education activities offered so that these students can select not only those experiences they find pleasurable but also those in which they can find success.

The program should include activities that will help these students to increase their physical fitness and optimal skill levels. Lack of structured programs outside the school denies culturally disadvantaged students the opportunity to participate in a regular program of physical activity. This often prevents these students from maintaining even minimal fitness levels. Competitive sports and games must be a part of the class program, but time must also be alloted for the individual to compete with himself or herself to raise a physical fitness test score or to improve in a skill performance.

Innovative programs for the culturally disadvantaged have been gaining in recent years. One such program was recently sponsored by the Health and Physical Education Department at Trenton State College. A group of inner-city boys, classified as educationally disadvantaged and potential drop-outs were chosen to participate in a 6-week program that was part of a federally funded institute for preparing vocational and practical arts teachers in the teaching of disadvantaged youth.

The daily program for the youths was divided into three parts. The morning was spent in motivational concept learning, followed by an hour-and-a-half recreation period. The afternoon was spent in employment in a local industry. The recreation period activities were geared to the other learning activities of the program. There was a minimum of verbal explanation, and many different activities were made available to the boys. A change of activity was necessary, since these boys had a very short attention span.

Recreation activities were used to reinforce learning concepts in many ways. In trampoline activity, for example, the boys also learned about velocity, balance, air lift, and gravity. In wrestling, concepts of leverage, weight factors, and resistance were taught. Percentages and other mathematical concepts were enhanced by scoring basketball games. This close relationship between subject learning and recreation was very successful in motivating this group of disadvantaged youths.

Culturally disadvantaged students need to develop a background in the lifetime sports. Swimming, dancing and tennis, as well as other recreational activities such as bowling, should be included in the program. There should be records, a phonograph, and a variety of rhythm instruments. The culturally disadvantaged enjoy rhythmic activities and find that they are successful in such areas as dance, gymnastics, and tumbling, where they can demonstrate their creativity and express their individuality. Many warm-up activities, as well as many games, can be done to a musical accompaniment.

The culturally disadvantaged are especially conscious of their individuality, and the program must allow ample opportunity for self-expression and creativity. Teacher recognition and praise for the most minor accomplishment is of utmost importance to the continued success of these students. If possible, culturally disadvantaged students should not be in a large class because little teaching takes place and because the individual student becomes lost in the mass.

Poorly coordinated students

The student with low motor ability is often ignored by the physical educator. This person may be unpopular with classmates and be considered a detriment in a team sport. He or she may be undesirable as a partner in a dual sport and may wind up paired with an equally uncoordinated and awkward partner. Students with low motor ability need special attention so that they can improve physical skill performances, derive pleasure from success in physical activity, and gain a background in lifetime sports.

Poorly coordinated students are frequently placed in regular physical education classes when they have no mental or physical handicaps. The only concession made to their problem is through ability grouping in schools where facilities and personnel are adequate. Even then, ability grouping sometimes is used only to separate the "duds" from the "stars," thus increasing the poorly coordinated student's feelings of inadequacy. The poorly coordinated student may be held up to ridicule by fellow students as well as by physical education teachers, who use him or her as an example of how not to perform a physical skill.

The poorly coordinated student will resist learning new activities because the challenge this presents offers little chance for success. The challenge of a new skill or activity to be learned may create such tension within the student that he or she becomes physically ill. In other instances this tension may result in negative behavior.

Poor coordination may be the result of several factors. The student may not be physically fit, or may have poor reflexes, or may not have the ability to use mental imagery. For some reason such as a lengthy childhood illness, the poorly coordinated student may not have been normally physically active. Other poorly coordinated students may enter the secondary school physical education program from an elementary school that lacked a trained physical educator, had no facilities for physical education, or had a poor program of physical education.

In working with poorly coordinated students the physical educator must exercise the utmost patience. He or she must know why the student is poorly coordinated and be able to devise an individual program for each student that will help the person to move and perform more effectively. The physical educator must be sure that the student understands the need for special help and try to motivate him or her to succeed. When a skill is performed with even a modicum of improvement, the effort must be praised and the achievement reinforced.

With a large class and only one instructor, there can be relatively little time spent with each individual. Buddy systems—that is, pairing a poorly coordinated student with a well-coordinated partner—often enables both students to progress faster. The physical educator must be careful not to push the student beyond his or her limits. A too difficult challenge coupled with the fatigue that results from trying too hard may result in retardation, rather than acceleration, of improvement. Any goal set for the poorly coordinated student must be a reasonable one.

The objectives of the program for poorly coordinated students will not differ from the objectives of any physical education program.

Before a program is devised, the status of the

students will need to be known so that their individual abilities and needs can be identified. Physical fitness and motor ability testing should be ongoing phases of the program. Through the physical education program the students should come to realize that their special needs are being met because they are as important as the well-skilled students in the eyes of the physical educator.

Separating students into ability groups may cause poorly coordinated students to feel that they are being pushed out of the way. If ability grouping is used, the poorly coordinated must receive adequate instruction, a meaningful program, and have equal access to good equipment and facilities.

If a student has poor eye-hand or eye-foot coordination, he or she will not succeed in such activities as tennis or soccer. Activities should be chosen that suit the abilities of the students and at the same time help them to develop the needed coordinations. Work on improving fitness and self-testing activities should form only a part of the program. Appropriate games, rhythmics and dance, and such activites as swimming and archery will help to stimulate and maintain interest. Physical fitness clubs, swimming clubs, and other clubs open to all students will also benefit the poorly coordinated.

With carefully arranged teams and schedules in an intramural program, the poorly coordinated can be given a chance to compete with other students on their own level of ability. Preparation for intramural competition should be a part of the class program.

Dancing lends itself to coeducational instruction. When classes can be combined and coeducational instruction offered, the poorly coordinated will have an opportunity to develop social skills. Different groupings for different activities will stimulate interest and provide students with a variety of partners.

The student's progress should be evaluated periodically. When an adequate level of success has been attained in a particular activity, the student should be assigned to a faster moving and more highly skilled group. A selection of activities should be offered that will appeal to the poorly coordinated and guide their selections in relation to their abilities.

Physically gifted and creative students

Gifted and creative students in physical education also need a specially tailored physical education experience.

The physically gifted student has superior motor skill abilities in many activities and maintains a high level of physical fitness. This student may be a star athlete, but in general is simply a good all-around performer. In a game situation, he or she always seems to be in the right place at the right time. The physically gifted student learns quickly and requires a minimum of individual instruction. He or she is usually enthusiastic about physical activity and practices skills without being told to do so. Any individual instruction required is in the form of coaching rather than remedial correction. The physically gifted student has a strong sense of kinesthetic awareness and understands the principles of human movement. The student may not be able to articulate these latter two qualities, but observation by the physical educator will reveal that the student has discovered how to exploit his or her body as a tool for movement.

The creative student also has a well-developed sense of kinesthetic awareness and knows how to use his or her body properly. This student is the girl who dances with ease and grace or who is highly skilled in free exercise. It is the boy who is the lithe tumbler or gymnast. These students develop their own sophisticated routines in dance, tumbling, gymnastics, apparatus, and synchronized swimming. They may or may not be extraordinarily adept in other physical education activities, but they are as highly teachable as are the physically gifted.

The beginning physical educator may find it especially difficult to teach a student who possesses many more physical abilities than the teacher. However, there is no student in school who knows all there is to know about an activity. Many experiences will still be new to them.

The physically gifted and creative students may not have attempted a wide range of activities, but they may have experienced all the activities offered in the school physical education program. Both the physically gifted and the creative student as well as the average stu-

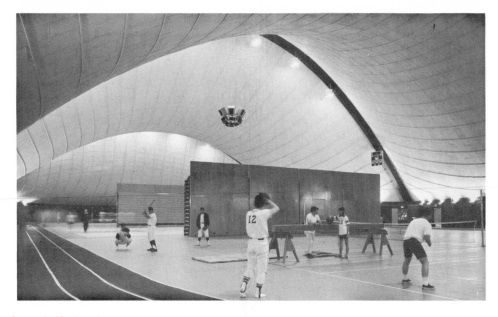

Creative and gifted students, such as these varsity baseball players playing in Graceland Fieldhouse, La Moni, Iowa, have developed a kinesthetic awareness. (Courtesy Shaver & Company, Salina, Kan.)

dent will be stimulated and challenged by the introduction of new activities. The creative student in dance may be introduced to a new kind of music, or the boy skilled on apparatus may enjoy adding new moves to his routines. The athlete may be a good performer, but perhaps needs to become a better team player. Or he or she may rely on superior skills rather than on a complete knowledge of the rules and strategies of sports and games.

A well-planned physical education program will be adaptable to the needs of all the students it serves. But before the program can be definitively developed, the specific needs, limitations, and abilities of the students in the program must be defined. The activities offered must be adapted to the needs of the students, since the students cannot be adapted to the program.

The exceptional student needs a structured program of physical activity, since this is a vital part of his or her mental, social, emotional, and physical development. Some schools have made it a policy to excuse athletes from the activity program when their varsity sport is in season. This is a disservice to the student, especially when the varsity sport and the unit

being taught in class are different. A student benefits from physical activity in a regular program. The physical educator can keep the interest of the exceptional student high by adopting some tested methods.

A leader's program has proved valuable in many schools. Leaders can assist the physical educator in innumerable ways, and they develop a sense of responsibility for the program because they are directly involved. Members of Leaders' Clubs have served as gymnastics and tumbling spotters in classes other than their own and can assist as officials in both the class program and during intramural contests. Members of Leaders' Clubs thus still participate in the activities of their own class, but at the same time receive the benefit of extra exposure to activities. Movies, film strips, loop films, and slides interest and benefit all students. The exceptional student can compare his or her performance with those of experts and can gain new insights into skills.

Textbooks in physical education are not in wide use in secondary school physical education programs. Students can benefit from the use of a textbook, special outside readings, assignments, and research problems, and these provide an additional challenge for the exceptional student.

Many highly skilled or creative students will be able to assist those students who have low motor skill abilities. By working on a one-to-one basis, the amount of individualized instruction will be increased. The student with low motor ability will receive the special assistance he or she needs, and the gifted student will be helped to realize that not all students possess high levels of ability.

The exceptional student can assist in the intramural program by acting as a coach on a day when his or her team is not playing. Coaching a team will help the student to become more cognizant of the importance of team play, sportsmanship, and the need for rules.

The gifted student can especially profit from independent study programs where he or she can choose a desired area of study and proceed at his or her own rate. Resource centers, field trips, and library research are all important parts of independent study programs. The gifted or creative student may also want to contribute to the physical education programs by suggesting and demonstrating innovative methods of learning an activity or by creating new activities. These students should be encouraged and their interest in physical education should be discussed as a possibility for a future career in this area.

SCHEDULING THE ADAPTED PROGRAM

Before scheduling a student in the adapted program, a thorough understanding should be gained of the boy's or girl's atypical condition and the type of procedure that will best meet his or her total development.

Because of the shortage of funds, space, and staff, many scheduling difficulties arise in respect to the adapted program. Many times equipment has to be improvised, special groups must be scheduled within the regular class period, and staff members have to devote out-of-school time to this important phase of the total physical education program. Unfortunately, some teachers solve the problem by sending the exceptional student to study hall or letting him or her observe from the bleachers,

thus failing to provide for a modified program.

There is a feeling among physical education leaders that scheduling atypical children and youth in separate groups is not always satisfactory. Many educators who have studied this problem feel that the atypical student should take his or her physical education along with the normal students and, to provide for the handicapped condition, the program should be modified and special methods of teaching used. In such cases, the administrator should make sure that the modification of the program for the student is physically and psychologically sound. Sometimes mental and emotional defects can be minimized if the teacher acquaints other students with the general problems of the handicapped person and encourages their cooperation in helping the student to make the right adjustment and maintain his or her self-esteem and social acceptance. There also seems to be a trend, at least in secondary schools, to follow an adapted sports program rather than to have a corrective type of program.

In the larger schools it sometimes has been possible to schedule special classes for students with some types of abnormalities. There also have been special schools established for the severely handicapped. These two types of procedures have not always proved satisfactory, however, because of the financial cost and the feeling that boys and girls should be scheduled with normal students for social and psychologic reasons.

In some smaller schools and colleges where there is a staff problem, those students needing an adapted program have been scheduled as a separate section within the regular physical education class period. In some cases group exercises have been devised together, with the practice of encouraging pupils to assist one another in the alleviation of their difficulties. These methods are not always satisfactory but, according to the schools and colleges concerned, are much better than not doing anything about the problem. In other schools and colleges, atypical pupils have been scheduled during special periods, where individual attention can be given to them.

The procedure that any particular school or college follows in scheduling students for the

ANNUAL PHYSICAL ACTIVITY FORM

Junior and Senior High School

Sponsored by Bureau of School Health Service, Division of Pupil Personnel Services, New York State Department of Education and New York State Heart Assembly, Inc.

Date _____

To Dr. _____

From Dr. _____ School Physician
_____ School

_____
Address

Re: _____ _____
Name of pupil Grade in school

All pupils registered in the schools of New York State are required by the education law to attend courses of instruction in physical education These courses are required to be adapted to meet individual needs. This means that a pupil who is unable to participate in the entire program should have his activities modified to meet and/or improve his condition. The physical education classes are approximately _____ minutes in length and are held __ times a week.

The final responsibility for the determination of a student participation rests with the school physician. Your recommendation will assist him in making a decision. If further clarification is needed, the school physician will arrange a conference with you.

This child may participate in all physical education class activities and in competitive sports, intramural and interscholastic. Yes_____ No_____

DIAGNOSIS: _____

If activity is limited, please check what he may do, in the following list:

PHYSICAL EDUCATION CLASS ACTIVITIES

( ) Basketball   ( ) Trampoline   ( ) Square dancing
( ) Baseball   ( ) Tumbling   ( ) Social dancing
( ) Football   ( ) Volleyball   ( ) Apparatus
( ) Soccer   ( ) Wrestling   ( ) Archery
( ) Softball   ( ) Track   ( ) Field hockey
                                        ( ) Swimming

INTRAMURAL AND INTERSCHOLASTIC SPORTS

( ) Basketball   ( ) Wrestling   ( ) Golf
( ) Baseball   ( ) Track and field ( ) Swimming
( ) Football   ( ) Cross country   ( ) Cheerleading
( ) Soccer   ( ) Bowling

1. Does this child require a rest period during school hours? Yes_____ No_____
2. Duration of restrictions: weeks_____ months_____ school year_____
3. Do you wish the patient to return to you for reevaluation? Yes_____ No ___Date___

_____ _____ M. D. _____
Date   Address
Prepared and pretested by: Nassau TB, Heart and Public Health Association, Inc.

Adapted physical education record. (Bureau of School Health Service, Division of Pupil Personnel Services, New York State Department of Education and New York State Heart Assembly, Inc.)

adapted program will depend upon its educational philosophy, finances, facilities and staff available, and the needs of the students.

SELECTING ACTIVITIES FOR ADAPTED PHYSICAL EDUCATION

The activities should be selected for the adapted physical education program with the needs of the atypical student in mind. It must usually be done on an individual basis after consultation with proper medical authorities. The activities should be selected in light of the objectives so that worthwhile skills are developed, a proper state of organic fitness is maintained, and the social and emotional needs of the student are considered. In no case should an activity ever aggravate an existing injury or atypical condition. Of course, all activities should be appropriate to the age level of the student and be ones in which he or she can find success. As far as possible and practical, activities should reflect the regular program of physical education offered at the school or college. The fewer changes made in the original activity, the more the atypical person feels that he or she is being successful and not different from the other students. Activities should contribute to the development of basic movements and skills. There should be as much group activity as possible since the socializing benefits of participation are important in providing students with a feeling of belonging and being a part of a group.

THE TEACHER IN THE ADAPTED PROGRAM

In the United States today there are several institutions offering specialization in adapted physical education programs. The specialist in adapted physical education is usually in a master's or doctoral program and is required to complete courses in special education, psychology, sociology, and other allied areas, as well as in adapted physical education.

It is also important that physical educators and classroom teachers be given the opportunity to take courses in adapted physical education so that they will be able to approach their students with greater understanding. Course work in adapted physical education on the undergradu-

ate level should also be made more available. Very few undergradute departments in physical education currently require a course in adapted physical education.

In discussing the qualifications of health and physical educators, much has been said about the training needed by physical education teachers. These qualifications are very important and necessary for the teacher in the adapted program. However, in addition to these qualifications, the teacher should understand the student with the atypical condition—the various atypical conditions, their causes, and treatment. The teacher should like to work with students who need special help and be able to establish a good rapport in order to instill confidence and faith in the work that needs to be done. The teacher should appreciate the various mental and emotional problems that confront an atypical person and the methods and procedures that can be followed to cope with these problems. The teacher must in some ways be a psychologist, creating interest and stimulating motivation toward physical activity for the purpose of hastening improvement. The teacher should be sympathetic to the advice of medical personnel. She or he should be willing to give corrective exercise under the guidance of physicians and to plan the program with their help. In addition, it is necessary to know the implications of medical and other findings for the adapted physical education program, to be familiar with the medical, psychologic, or other examinations of each student, and, with the help of the physician, psychologist, social worker, or other specialist, to work out a program that best meets the needs of the student.

THE ADAPTED PROGRAM IN SCHOOLS AND COLLEGES

The administrator of physical education should understand the components that make up a well-rounded adapted program and should strive toward including these essential phases in his or her particular school or college system.

One of the best descriptions that has been developed to point out the broad outlines of an adapted program primarily for the physically handicapped was published in the Yearbook of the American Association for Health, Physical

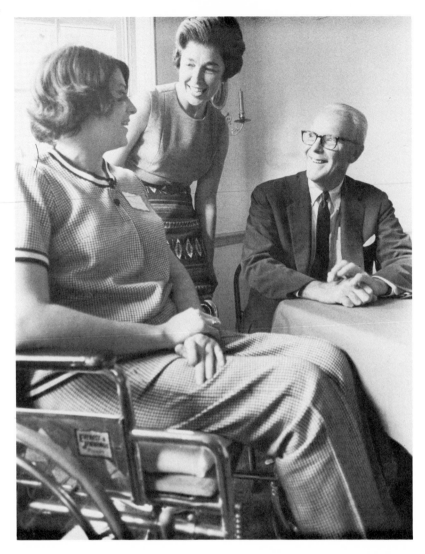

Honor student at College of DuPage, Glen Ellyn, Ill., and President of Rehabilitation Institute and hospitality chairwoman of the Institute talk with student about her plans to become a teacher and her trips to Europe with other wheelchair students.

Education, and Recreation entitled *Children in Focus.** It will be valuable for any administrator to have the main points of this program reproduced here in slightly adapted form:

1. *Health examinations.* A thorough examination should be given to all students by either the school or the family physician.

2. *Classification for physical education based on the*

*Daniels, A.: What provision for the handicapped? In American Association for Health, Physical Education, and Recreation: Children in focus, 1954 Yearbook, Washington, D. C., 1954, The Association.

examination. The results of the health examination will determine the type of handicap, if any, and whether the student should be in the regular or adapted program.

3. *Conference with students needing special consideration.* Conference can uncover student's needs, interests, limitations, and capabilities in the area of adapted physical education.

4. *Scheduling accomplished in accordance with school policy or size of school.* A suggested plan is as follows:

(a) Large schools—separate classes.

(b) Medium-sized schools—student spends some time in special class and also in regular class; suggest one day a week in special class and the other days in regular class.

(c) Smaller schools—both handicapped and nonhandi-

Physical Inspection

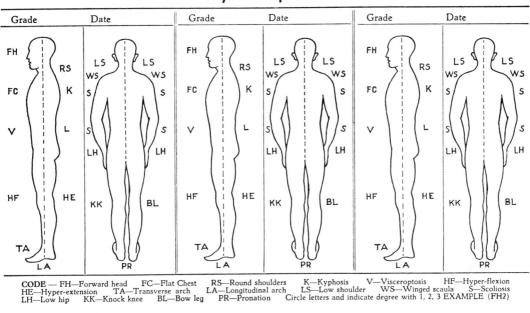

CODE — FH—Forward head   FC—Flat Chest   RS—Round shoulders   K—Kyphosis   V—Visceroptosis   HF—Hyper-flexion
HE—Hyper-extension   TA—Transverse arch   LA—Longitudinal arch   LS—Low shoulder   WS—Winged scaula   S—Scoliosis
LH—Low hip   KK—Knock knee   BL—Bow leg   PR—Pronation   Circle letters and indicate degree with 1, 2, 3 EXAMPLE (FH2)

Physical inspection. (Long Beach, Calif., Public Schools.)

PE 27 3M 7-56 9912

LONG BEACH UNIFIED SCHOOL DISTRICT
PERMANENT INDIVIDUAL EXERCISE CARD — DEPARTMENT OF PHYSICAL EDUCATION

Name_____Grade_____Semester_____Year_____Period_____

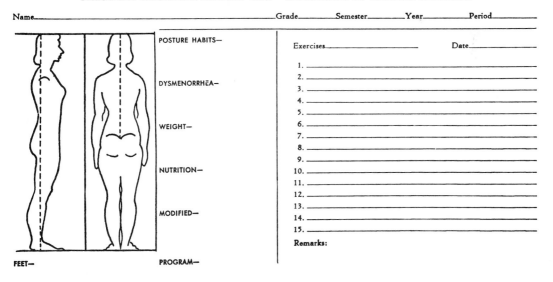

POSTURE HABITS—

DYSMENORRHEA—

WEIGHT—

NUTRITION—

MODIFIED—

FEET—

PROGRAM—

BODY ALIGNMENT—

Exercises_____   Date_____

1. _____
2. _____
3. _____
4. _____
5. _____
6. _____
7. _____
8. _____
9. _____
10. _____
11. _____
12. _____
13. _____
14. _____
15. _____

Remarks:

Permanent individual exercise card. (Long Beach, Calif., Public Schools.)

capped in same class but program is modified and adapted to meet the needs of the handicapped within the regular group of normal students.

5. *Phases of the adapted program.* The program may involve three areas:

(a) Special conditioning—includes developmental exercises to meet student needs such as to increase muscle power, help postural deviations, or improve range of motion.

(b) Aquatics—aquatic activities to meet student needs, such as those concerned with remedial, recreational, and adjustment factors.

(c) Recreational sports—sports are considered the best type of physical activity. Students should be transferred from exercise therapy to active sports therapy or placed directly in adapted sports program in preference to exercises. Recreational sports may contribute in such areas of development as adjustment and socialization.

6. *Evaluation of progress.* Evaluation can be accomplished through the utilization of such techniques as tests, conferences, standards of behavior, etc. Objective measures, if available, should receive first consideration.

7. *Records.* A record that contains data on the handicapped condition, physician's recommendations, program objectives for the student, recommended activities, record of special treatments, consultations, progress rating, and other pertinent information should be kept.

8. *Relationships.* An effective adapted program recognizes the importance of harmonious working relationships between medical and nursing personnel, the home, the school administrators, and other teachers.

ADMINISTRATIVE PRINCIPLES

The following statement was prepared for general use in schools and colleges rather than for special schools for handicapped children. It was approved by the Board of Directors, American Alliance for Health, Physical Education, and Recreation, and endorsed in principle by the Joint Committee on Health Problems in Education, American Medical Association, and National Education Association:

It is the responsibility of the school to contribute to the fullest possible development of the potentialities of each individual entrusted to its care. This is a basic tenet of our democratic faith.

1. *There is a need for common understanding regarding the nature of "adapted physical education."*

Adapted physical education is a diversified program of developmental activities, games, and sports suited to the interests, capacities, and limitations of students with disabilities who may not safely or successfully engage in unrestricted participation in the vigorous activities of the general program.

2. *There is a need for "adapted physical education" in schools and colleges.*

The number of children of school age in the United States with physical handicaps is alarmingly high. Of the 33,500,000 in the age groups five to nineteen, approximately 4,000,000 children have physical handicaps which need some kind of special educational consideration. (Of these, 65,000 are blind or partially seeing; 335,000, orthopedic disabilities; and 500,000 each, deaf or hard of hearing, organic heart disease, and delicate or undeveloped.) The major disabling conditions each affecting thousands of children are cerebral palsy, poliomyelitis, tuberculosis, traumatic injuries, and heart disease. Further evidence indicates that, on the college level, there is a significant percentage of students who require special consideration for either temporary or permanent disabilities.

3. *"Adapted physical education" has much to offer the individual who faces the combined problem of seeking an education and overcoming a handicap.*

"Adapted physical education" should serve the individual by:

(a) Aiding in discovering deviations from the normal and making appropriate referrals where such conditions are noted.

(b) Guiding students in the avoidance of situations which would aggravate their conditions or subject them to undue risks of injury.

(c) Improving general strength and endurance of individuals who are poorly developed and of those returning to school following illness or injury.

(d) Providing opportunities for needed social and psychological adjustment.

4. *The direct and related services essential for the proper conduct of adapted physical education should be available in our schools.*

These services should include:

(a) Adequate and periodic health examinations.

(b) Classification for physical education based on the health examination and other pertinent tests and observations.

(c) Guidance of individuals needing special consideration with respect to physical activity, general health practices, recreational pursuits, and vocational planning.

(d) Arrangement of appropriate physical education programs.

(e) Evaluation of progress through observations, appropriate measurements, and consultations.

(f) Integrated relationships with other school personnel, medical and its auxiliary services, and the family to assure continuous guidance and supervisory services.

(g) A cumulative record for each individual, which should be transferred from school to school.

5. *It is essential that adequate medical guidance be available for teachers of adapted physical education.*

Programs of adapted physical education should not be attempted without the diagnosis, written recommendation, and supervision of a physician. Problems of correction may be very profound. Where corrective measures are deemed necessary, they must be predicated upon medical findings and accomplished by competent teachers working with medical supervision and guidance. There should be an effective referral service between physicians, physical education, and parents, aimed at proper safeguards and maximum student benefits.

6. *Teachers of adapted physical education have a great responsibility as well as unusual opportunity.*

Physical educators engaged in teaching adapted physical education should have adequate professional education fitting them for this work. They must be motivated by the highest ideals with respect to the importance of total student development and satisfactory human relationships. They must have the ability to establish rapport with students who may exhibit social maladjustment as a disability. It is essential that they be professionally prepared to implement the recommendations provided by medical personnel for the adapted physical education program.

7. *Adapted physical education is necessary at all school levels.*

The student with a disability faces the dual problem of overcoming a handicap and acquiring an education which will enable him to take his place in society as a respected citizen. Failure to assist a student with his problems may sharply curtail the growth and development process. Offering adapted physical education in the elementary grades, and continuing through the secondary school and college, will assist the individual to improve function and make adequate psychological and social adjustments. It will prevent attitudes of defeat and fears of insecurity. It will be a factor in his attaining maximum growth and development within the limits of the disability. It will help him face the future with confidence. *

ADAPTED PHYSICAL EDUCATION—AN ESSENTIAL

Physical education programs should give increasing attention to the educational needs of individual children and youth, including those who are physically handicapped or who otherwise deviate from the normal. Physical education programs can offer remedial work as well as modify the program so that each boy and girl receives maximum benefit from participation. Furthermore, by providing an adapted program, students can be expected to be present for each class period and not excused or allowed to observe from the sidelines because of some atypical condition.

In order to have an effective adapted program, the physical education administrator and his or her staff must work harmoniously with the school and college medical staff, parents, and community agencies. Through cooperative effort each student can learn to live at his or her highest level of health.

---

*Committee on Adapted Physical Education, American Association for Health, Physical Education, and Recreation.

Questions and exercises

1. What is meant by the term *adapted physical education?*
2. What are the objectives of the adapted physical education program?
3. What is the relationship between the principle of individual differences and the adapted physical education program?
4. How should students be classified for the adapted program?
5. What are the various methods of scheduling students for the adapted program? List the advantages and disadvantages of each.
6. What qualifications does the teacher of physical education need to work in the adapted program?
7. Outline an adapted physical education program for a high school or college.
8. Read three references on adapted physical education and give a report to the class on these readings.
9. How can the physical educator best adapt his program to the needs of the mentally retarded student?
10. What special physical education needs does the creative student have?
11. To what other resources can the physical educator turn when he or she needs assistance in understanding and working with the atypical student?

Reading assignment in *Administrative Dimensions of Health and Physical Education Programs, Including Athletics:* Chapter 6, Selections 28 to 33.

Selected references

A clarification of terms, Journal of Health, Physical Education, and Recreation **42**:63, 1971.

Activity programs for the mentally retarded, Journal of Health, Physical Education, and Recreation **37**:24, 1966.

Adapted physical education, Journal of Health, Physical Education, and Recreation **40**:45, 1969.

American Association for Health, Physical Education, and Recreation: Project on recreation and fitness for the mentally retarded, Challenge, 1968.

Arnheim, D. D., and others: Principles and methods of adapted physical education, ed. 2, St. Louis, 1973, The C. V. Mosby Co.

Auxter, D.: Integration of the mentally retarded with normals in physical and motor fitness training programs, Journal of Health, Physical Education, and Recreation **41**:61, September, 1970.

Blatt, B.: Public policy with the education of children with special needs, Exceptional Children **38**:537, 1972.

Carlson, R. E.: A diagnosis and remediation plan for physical education for the handicapped, Journal of Health, Physical Education, and Recreation **43**:73, 1972.

Conant, J. B.: Slums and suburbs, New York, 1964, The New American Library, Inc.

Cratty, B. J.: Social dimensions of physical activity, Englewood Cliffs, N. J., 1967, Prentice-Hall, Inc.

Daniels, A. S., and Davies, E. A.: Adapted physical education, ed. 2, New York, 1965, Harper & Row, Publishers.

Drowntzky, John N.: Physical education for the mentally retarded, Philadelphia, 1971, Lea and Febiger.

Duggar, M. P.: Dance for the blind, Journal of Health, Physical Education, and Recreation **39:**28, 1968.

Ersing, W. F.: Current direction of professional preparation in adapted physical education, Journal of Health, Physical Education, and Recreation **43:**78, 1972.

Fait, H. F.: Special physical education: adaptive, corrective, developmental, Philadelphia, 1972, W. B. Saunders Co.

Fantani, M. D., and Weinstein, G.: The disadvantaged: challenge to education, New York, 1968, Harper & Row, Publishers.

Frankel, E. C.: Toward a rebirth of creativity, Journal of Health, Physical Education, and Recreation **38:**65, 1967.

Harvat, R. W.: Physical education for children with perceptual-motor learning disabilities, Columbus, Ohio, 1971, Charles E. Merrill Publishing Co.

Kalakian, L. H., and Motan, J. M.: Physical education and recreation for the mentally retarded and emotionally disturbed, Minneapolis, 1973, Burgess Publishing Co.

Logan, G. A.: Adapted physical education, Dubuque, Iowa, 1972, William C. Brown Co.

Riessman, F.: The culturally deprived child, New York, 1962, Harper & Row, Publishers.

Soane, M.: Handbook of adapted physical education equipment and its use, Springfield, Ill., 1973, Charles C Thomas, Publisher.

Stein, J. U.: A practical guide to adapted physical education for the educable mentally handicapped, Journal of Health, Physical Education, and Recreation **33:**30, 1962.

Tillman, K.: Recreational activities reinforce learning experiences for the disadvantaged student, Journal of Health, Physical Education, and Recreation **43:**32, 1972.

Vedola, T.: Individualized physical education program for the handicapped child, Englewood Cliffs, N. J., 1972, Prentice-Hall, Inc.

Wienke, P.: Blind children in an integrated physical education program, The New Outlook for the Blind **60:**73, 1966.

Winnick, J.: Issues and trends in training adapted physical education personnel, Journal of Health, Physical Education, and Recreation **43:**75, 1972.

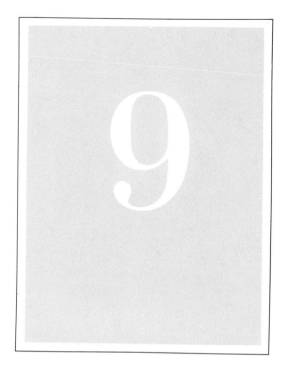

The intramural and extramural programs

In some schools and colleges, intramurals and extramurals in the past have received little emphasis in a school or college physical education program. However, this concept has undergone rapid changes in recent years. Some of the reasons for the increased interest in intramurals are as follows:

1. Many institutions have had to reduce their varsity team play because of increased financial pressures and reduced student interest.
2. Innovative programs for intramurals have been introduced, including emphasis on corecreational activities.
3. Girls and women have become increasingly involved in intramural activities.
4. Community and students are involved in the planning, participation, and teaching of intramural and extramural play.
5. As a result of the energy crisis many schools and colleges have had to curtail intercollegiate and interscholastic sports events.

Before discussing these programs further, a definition of intramurals and extramurals should be established. In this text they refer to that phase of the school or college physical educa-

tion program that is geared to the abilities and skills of the entire student body, and consists of voluntary participation in games, sports, and other activities. They offer intramural activities within a single school or college and such extramural activities as "play" and "sports" days that bring together participants from several institutions.

OBJECTIVES

The objectives of intramural and extramural activities are compatible with the overall objectives of physical education and also with those of education in general. The objectives as listed by the University of Connecticut men's *Intramural Sports Handbook* are presented here in adapted form:

1. To provide the students at the institution with opportunities for fun, enjoyment, and fellowship through participation in sports.
2. To provide the students at the institution with opportunities that will be conducive to their health and physical fitness.
3. To provide the students at the institution with opportunities for release from tensions and aggressions and to provide for a feeling of achievement through sports participation, all of which are conducive to mental and emotional health.

The objectives of the intramural and extramural programs may be classified under four headings: (1) health, (2) skill, (3) social development, and (4) recreation. Each objective will be discussed briefly.

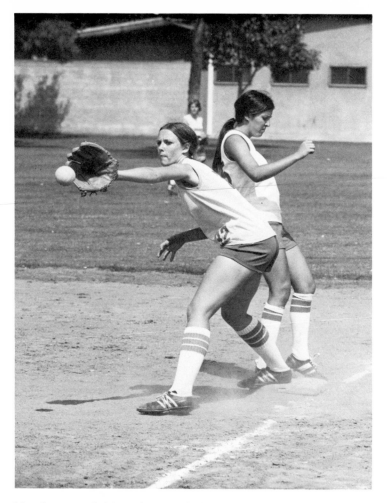

There is increased involvement of girls and women in intramural activities. These girls are participating in intramurals as part of the Youth Services Section of the Physical Education Program in the Los Angeles City Schools.

Health

Intramural and extramural activities contribute to the physical, cognitive, social, and emotional health of the individual. They contribute to physical health through participation in activity that affords healthful exercise. Such characteristics as strength, agility, speed, body control, and other factors that prove their worth in day-to-day living are developed. They contribute to cognitive health by providing opportunities for interpretive thinking, making decisions under highly charged emotional situations, and keeping one's mind occupied in worthwhile pursuits. They contribute to social health through group participation and working toward the achievement of group goals. They contribute to emotional health by helping one to achieve self-confidence and in improving one's self-concept.

Skill

Intramural and extramural activities offer the opportunity for every individual to display and develop his or her skill in various physical education activities. Through specialization and voluntary participation they offer an opportunity to excel and to experience the thrill of competition. It is generally agreed that an individual enjoys those activities in which he or she has developed skill. Participation in athletics offers the opportunity to develop proficiency in various activities in group situations where individuals are equated according to their skill, thus providing for equality of competition. This helps to guarantee greater success and more enjoyment of participation. In turn there will be a carryover into adult living of skills that will enable many to spend leisure moments in a profitable and enjoyable manner.

Social development

Opportunities for social development are numerous in intramural and extramural activities. Through many social contacts, coeducational experiences, playing on teams, and other situations desirable qualities are developed. Individuals learn to subordinate their desires to the will of the group, develop sportsmanship, fair play, courage, group loyalty, social poise, and other desirable traits. Voluntary participation exists in such a program, and students who desire to play under such conditions will live by group codes of conduct. These experiences offer good training for citizenship, adult living, and human relations that are so essential in present-day living.

Recreation

Intramural and extramural programs help to establish a permanent interest in many sports and physical education activities. This interest and enthusiasm will carry over into adult living and provide the basis for many happy leisure hours. These programs also provide the basis for recreation during school days, when idle moments have potentialities for fostering antisocial as well as constructive social behavior.

RELATION TO INTERSCHOLASTIC AND INTERCOLLEGIATE VARSITY ACTIVITIES

Both intramural and extramural activities and interscholastic and intercollegiate varsity athletics are integral phases of the total physical education program. As has been pointed out, the total physical education program is made up of the basic instructional class program, the adapted program, the intramural and extramural program, and the interscholastic and intercollegiate varsity athletic programs. Each has an important contribution to make to the achievement of physical education objectives. The important thing is to maintain a proper balance so that each phase enhances and does not restrict the other phases of the total program.

Whereas intramurals and extramurals are for the entire student body, interscholastic and intercollegiate varsity athletics are for those individuals who are skilled in various physical activities. Intramurals and extramurals are conducted primarily on a school and college basis, while interscholastic and intercollegiate varsity athletics are conducted, as the name implies, on an interschool or intercollege basis.

There is no conflict between these two phases of the program if the facilities, time, personnel, money, and other factors are apportioned according to the degree to which each phase achieves the educational outcomes desired, rather than the degree of public appeal and interest stimulated. One should not be designed as a training ground or farm system for the other. It should be possible for a student to move from one to the other, but this should be incidental in nature, rather than planned.

If conducted properly, each phase of the program can contribute to the other, and through an overall, well-balanced program the entire student body will come to respect sports and the great potentials they have for improving physical, mental, social, and emotional growth. When a physical education program is initially developed, it would seem logical to first provide an intramural program for the majority of the students, with the interscholastic or intercollegiate varsity athletic program coming as an outgrowth of the former. The first concern should be for the many or majority, and the second for the few or minority. This is characteristic of the democratic way of life. Although the intramural and extramural athletic programs are designed for every student, in practice they generally attract the poor and moderately skilled individuals. The skilled person finds a niche in the program for those of exceptional skill. This has its benefits in that it is an equalizer for competition.

A PHILOSOPHICAL MODEL FOR INTRAMURALS*

In the past, and to some degree in the present, the philosophical model depicted below *(A)* formed the basis for the placement of intramurals in physical education programs. This triangular model asserts an interdependency and a building of skills from the instructional level to the intramural level and finally to the "top" or athletic level of attainment. This model serves to convey the philosophy that instruction is basic to the other programs and that intramural skills are essential to producing the athletic skills found in varsity play. This model also represents the relative importance of the three phases of the physical education program. This of course is a mistake, because all phases of the program should serve all students and each phase is equally important in the total program.

The model *(B)* depicted below is suggested because of its practical implications for viewing the phases of the physical education program as both interdependent and equal. It also establishes each phase as independent of the others. Intramural and athletics are placed in their

---

*Adapted from Jones, T. R.: Needed: a new philosophical model for intramurals, The Journal of Health, Physical Education, and Recreation **42:**34, 1971.

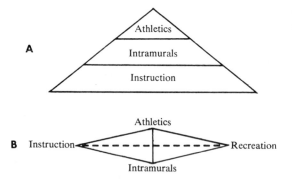

A, The traditional triangular conception of physical education and intramurals. *B*, A modern conceptualization of physical education and intramurals. (From Jones, T. R.: Needed: a new philosophical model for intramurals, Journal of Health, Physical Education, and Recreation **42:**34, 1971.)

model position because each is related to each other more closely than recreation and instruction are related to each other. Recreation has been added to the model because of its contribution to intramural activities and because both have as a primary objective the satisfaction derived from participation.

GENERAL ADMINISTRATIVE POLICIES FOR ORGANIZATION AND ADMINISTRATION OF INTRAMURAL AND EXTRAMURAL PROGRAMS

Some general administrative policies for the organization and administration of the intramural and extramural programs follow.

General administration

Intramural and extramural activities should be centered in the physical education program. However, they should be separate divisions of the overall program, receiving equal consideration with the instructional and interscholastic or intercollegiate athletics divisions in respect to staff, finances, facilities, equipment, supplies, and other essentials. There should be one staff member who has direct responsibility for this program. Such an individual should be one who is well trained in physical education and whose chief interest is intramural and extramural activities. This may not be possible in some smaller schools or colleges. However, it is necessary that the person in charge have adequate time and a sincere interest to do a commendable job in this area. Along with the director there should be assistant directors, supervisors, student managers, and other staff members as needed, depending upon the size of the school or college. There should also be adequate provision for officials. These should be selected and trained with care because of their importance to the program. Varsity players when carefully selected make good officials. Also, varsity coaches, staff members, and student managers should be considered for this work. A list of policies governing the various features of the program should be prepared in written form and well publicized. Sometimes these are effectively publicized through a handbook.

An important feature of the overall administration of an intramural or extramural program is the establishment of a council. This is usually an elected council with representatives from the students, central administration, intramural staff, health department, and faculty. This body could be most influential in the establishment of policy and practices for a broad program of athletics for all students.

A significant development on the national scene was the establishment of the National Intramural Sports Council as a joint project of the Division of Men's Athletics and the Division of Girls' and Women's Sports of the American Association for Health, Physical Education, and Recreation. The purpose of creating the organization was to provide national leadership for intramural programs across the country.

Matthews has developed a set of intramural administration principles that will be helpful to schools and colleges alike in establishing and administering sound intramural and extramural programs. These principles in adapted form are as follows:

1. Policies relative to intramurals should have rapport with the total welfare of the educational institution. Example: they should complement and supplement the academic program. Units of competition should not reflect racial or religious groupings.

2. Good human relationships and attitudes should be stressed. Example: rating plans, supervision, officiating, meetings, rules, etc. should stress sportsmanship.

3. Student planning and management should be encouraged. Example: the administrative council represents an opportunity for student involvement. Team manager, captains, scorers, etc. offer such opportunities as well.

4. The health and welfare of all participants should be protected. Example: periodic physical examinations are mandatory, and constant and close inspection of facilities and equipment is a must.

5. Competition should be equalized so that all participants experience success. Example: a constant loser will soon drop from intramurals and for this as well as other reasons competition should enable all participants to be successful in this phase of the educational program.

6. A variety of activities should be offered. Example: students should be consulted and activities should reflect strenuous and nonstrenuous, team and individual, and also corecreational activities. At least five different sports should be offered.

7. The officiating should be carefully selected and supervised. Example: a program that involves training and orientation for the officials as well as testing and observation is important.

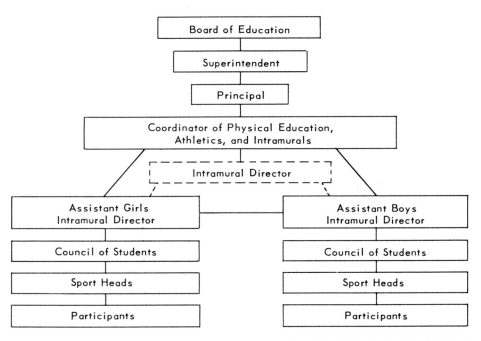

Suggested organization chart for intramurals. (From Intramurals for senior high schools, The Athletic Institute, Chicago.)

8. Grievances and protests should receive fair and equal treatment. Example: channels for grievances should be established, thus helping to assure some degree of satisfaction and success for all concerned.

9. Rules of eligibility and procedures should be established and publicized. Example: committees or the council should carefully establish the rules and see that all concerned are provided with copies of the same.

10. The program should be financed in a manner consistent with school policy. Example: the intramural program is an important part of total educational program and therefore should be subsidized financially through monies allocated by the board of education or central administration. *

Coordinator of intramurals

Many universities and colleges have coordinators of intramurals in departments of recreation that are independent of departments of physical education. Since intramural activities are more closely allied to recreational activities, they are placed under the supervision of the recreation department. This placement allows for increased student participation and greater funding than if the program were in competition

---

*Matthews, D. O.: Intramural administration principles, The Athletic Journal **46**:82, 1966.

with physical education and varsity programs.

Many public and private schools have also established an intramural director or coordinator for many of the same reasons. An intramural director can devote all of his or her time to establishing programs, getting adequate funding, involving the community, and developing innovative methods.

Student involvement in administration of intramurals and extramurals

Student involvement in all phases of education has been steadily increasing. Involvement in the administrative aspects of intramurals and extramurals is happening in high schools and on college campuses. For example, many colleges have "drop-in" centers where student supervisors are on hand to establish programs, reserve equipment, and arrange for the gym or swimming pool to be open for additional hours. Some colleges have student managers who supervise intramural activity.

Another phase of active student involvement is the *sports club* that is managed by the students and may or may not have a nonstudent

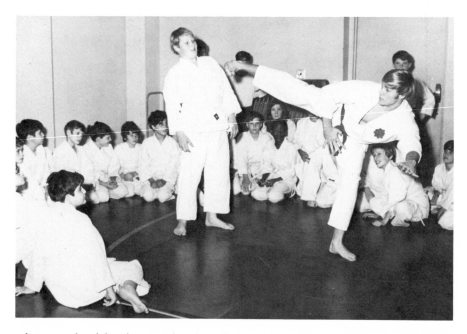

Jiu jitsu makes a popular club or intramural or recreational activity. (Courtesy Department of Parks and Recreation, Hempstead, N. Y.)

AN INTRAMURAL PROGRAM EVALUATION CHECKLIST*

A program can be evaluated in terms of the stated principles and objectives or according to prevalent acceptable standards.

How does the intramural program measure up to the acceptable minimum standards? By taking a few minutes to check off the items listed below, a quick evaluation can be made of the present status of the excellence of the program.

	Yes	No
Philosophy and objectives		
1. Is a written philosophy or a set of objectives available to the participants?		
Organization and administration		
1. Is the director professionally qualified to administer the program?		
2. Does the director devote at least 7.5 hours per week to administering his program?		
3. Are students included in the management of the program?		
4. Is there an advisory committee composed of students and faculty?		
Units of competition		
1. Are students classified according to ability, age, height, or weight within the competitive unit?		
2. Within the basic unit, are students permitted to choose the members of their teams?		
Program of activities		
1. Does the director consult with the students to make sure that their interests are of prime consideration in the choice of activities in the program?		
2. Are there both strenuous and nonstrenuous sports in the program?		
3. Are there both team and individual sports in the program?		
4. Are there at least five different sports making up the program?		
5. Does at least one corecreation activity make up part of the program?		
Time periods		
1. Does the hour immediately after school receive top priority for scheduling?		
2. Is the noon hour utilized as a time period for intramurals?		
Methods of organizing competition		
1. Is the round robin tournament used whenever possible in preference to others?		
Point system of awards		
1. Is recognition of any kind given to the participants for their achievements?		
2. Is the award primarily for achievement instead of incentive for participants?		
Rules and regulations		
1. Are the rules defining such things as eligibility, health, safety, forfeits, postponements, and team membership distributed to all participants?		
2. Is the lack of good sportsmanship regarded as a rule violated?		
3. Is equipment provided for all the activities offered?		
Publicity		
1. Is there a special bulletin board for intramural information?		
Finances		
1. Does the board of education through the school budget provide funds for the operation of the program?		

Rating scale

A "yes" answer must be given in each category if a program is to be considered *good* or *excellent*.

Excellent	15 to 22
Good	13 to 14
Fair	10 to 12
Poor	9 or below

*From Matthews, D. O.: Intramural administration principles, The Athletic Journal **46**:82, 1966. Reproduced courtesy The Athletic Journal.

advisor. These clubs are usually devoted to one activity such as tennis, skiing, or mountain climbing, and they encourage students at all levels of skill to participate. Instruction is provided by skilled members, advisors, or community members. These clubs are popular in schools and colleges, and in some colleges they provide the major thrust of intramural activity.

Evaluation of intramurals

One of the most important functions of the administrator in reference to intramurals is the evaluation of the program. The program must be continually evaluated to see if its goals are being met. It must also be evaluated in terms of budget and numbers of students participating in programs. If a program has few participants and a relatively high cost of operation, it may have to be phased out.

Evaluation techniques will differ, but it can be generally stated that the process should include: (1) definition of program objectives; (2) data collection and evaluation including participation count, team numbers, and games played and forfeited; (3) appraisal forms, including player ratings, scores, and team surveys; (4) study groups and consultant advice; and (5) student opinion about specific activites.

Recent forms of evaluation have utilized consultants on a voluntary, advisory basis. Consultants are usually objective and can provide information without prejudice. Evaluation score cards, such as Ridgeway's Scorecard for Evaluation of Mens' Intramural Sports Programs in Colleges and Universities, have also been found to be functional. In addition, many schools have used computers in evaluating intramural programs. In some cases the cost of computers for evaluations is not practical.

Health examinations

Health examinations should be required of all participants as a safeguard to their health. Sometimes this is taken care of through the annual health examination and at other times through special examinations given before a seasonal activity starts.

Finances

The finances involved in intramural and extramural programs are raised in various ways. Since these programs have as many contributions to make to educational objectives as other parts of the educational program, or more, they should be financed out of board of education and central administration funds, just as other phases of the program are financed. They should be included in the regular physical education budget and supported through regularly budgeted school or college income.

There is another method of financing the programs that has proved quite satisfactory in some high schools and colleges. This plan incorporates the cost of running the programs in the regular activity fee that includes such student activities as dramatics, the interscholastic athletic program, musicals, and band concerts. This allows for stable funds that are in proportion to the student enrollment and can be anticipated in advance. Also, this method eliminates any additional charges to the student.

Other methods of financing that are utilized but that are questioned in some quarters are using money taken from athletic gate receipts, charging spectators to see the games, requiring an entry fee, and special fund-raising projects like athletic nights, carnivals, and presentation of talented athletic and other groups. Some of the arguments against such practices are that they create an overemphasis on gate receipts and result in many problems, that they discourage spectators from attending and students from participating, and that they require special projects to raise money, which should not be necessary for such a valuable phase of the educational program.

Publicity and promotion

It is essential that the student body, faculty, and public in general understand the intramural and extramural programs, the individuals they service, the activities offered, and the objectives they attempt to attain. Such information can be disseminated to the right individuals only through a well-planned and organized publicity and promotion program.

The newspapers should be encouraged to give appropriate space to these activities. Brochures, bulletin boards, and the school newspaper can help to focus attention on the program. Notices can be prepared and sent home to parents in the elementary and secondary schools. A handbook can be prepared that explains all the various aspects of the total program and given to all students and others who are interested. Record boards can be constructed and placed in conspicuous settings. Clinics can be held in the various sports. Orientation talks and discussions can be held in school and college assemblies and at other gatherings. Special days can be held with considerable publicity and such catch slogans as "It Pays to Play" can be adopted. Through utilizing several devices and techniques, a good job of publicity and promotion can be done, with consequent greater participation among the student body and better understanding among the public.*

Scheduling

The time when intramural and extramural activities are scheduled will depend upon the school or college level, facilities, season of year, community, faculty availability, student needs, budget requirements, and other factors.

One of the most popular and convenient times in many schools is late afternoon. This has proved best for elementary and junior and senior high schools. For some seasons of the year—namely, spring and fall—it has also been popular in college. It is a time that is economical, does not require lights, and has the outdoors available. It also ensures faculty supervision to a greater degree.

Evenings have been used quite extensively at the college level during the winter. This is not recommended at the elementary or junior and senior high school levels.

Some schools utilize hours within the school day. However, it should be remembered that the physical education class is primarily an instructional period, and to use this period for such a program does not seem to be in conformance with the standards set by the profession. However, some schools have satisfactorily utilized free, activity, and club periods for the program where facilities would allow.

Noon hour has been popular in some schools, especially at the elementary and secondary levels, and particularly in rural schools where

students do not go home for lunch. Since students will be active anyway, such a period offers possibilities in selected situations, if strenuous activities are not offered.

Recess periods in the elementary school have proved to be a good time for many communities to conduct some of their intramural activities.

Saturdays have also been utilized in some situations. Although the weekend has proved to be a problem in some localities because many individuals have to work or have planned this time to be with their families, it has worked successfully in many communities.

The time before school in the morning has also proved satisfactory in a few schools. Getting up early in the morning does not seem to be a handicap to some individuals.

Special days are set aside in some schools for "field days" when classes are abandoned by administrative decree and all the students participate in a day or a half-day devoted entirely to activities that comprise the program.

In recent years, the computer has been used with greater frequency in the scheduling of intramural events. Most schools, especially colleges, have a computer for use in registration or financial procedures, and this computer may also be used for scheduling purposes. Some schools have made use of the computer in assigning officials to intramural games. This is another aspect of scheduling that can become very complex when there are a large number of intramural events. The use of the computer has greatly simplified this very tedious task.

ACTIVITIES

The activities that comprise the intramural and extramural programs represent the substance that will either attract or divert attention. Therefore, it is important that the right activities be selected. Some administrative guides that may be listed to help in the selection of these activities are as follows:

1. Activities should be selected in accordance with the season of the year and the conditions and influences that prevail locally.
2. Activities should be presented in a progressive manner from the elementary through the college level.
3. Activities should be selected in accordance with the needs and interests of the students.

---

*See also Chapter 20 on public relations for more information on publicity and promotion.

4. Activities that have implications for adult living should be given a prominent place in the program.
5. Corecreational activities should be provided.
6. The activities that are included in the physical education class program should have a bearing on the activities that are included in the intramural and extramural programs. The latter should act as a laboratory for the former.
7. Many desirable activities require little special equipment and do not require long periods of training in order to get the participant in physical condition.
8. Consideration should be given to such activities as field trips, story-telling, dramatics, hiking, handicraft, and others of a more recreational nature.
9. Activities in the elementary school should be selected with special attention to the ability of the child.

The following lists of activities are identified in a publication of The Athletic Institute:*

Individual and dual sports

Achievement tests	Physical fitness
Archery	Rope climbing
Badminton	Scuba diving
Basketball goal	Shooting
and foul	Shuffleborad
Billiards	Skiing
Bowling	Swimming
Deck tennis	Table tennis
Golf	Tennis
Gymnastics	Track and field
Handball	Tumbling
Horseshoes	Weight raining
Paddle tennis	Wrestling

NOTE: Boxing is not approved as an activity.

Club or group activities

Camping and cookouts	Hosteling
Canoeing	Ice skating
Cycling	Marching tactics
Dance—social, folk,	Outdoor skills
square, and modern	Rifle
Figure skating	Roller skating
Fishing	Rowing
Fly or bait casting	Sailing
Hiking	Tumbling
Horseback riding	

Team sports

Baseball	Speed-a-way
Basektball	Speedball
Blooper ball	Swimming
Field hockey	Touch (or flag)
Gymnastics	football
Ice hockey	Track and field
Kick ball	Volleyball
Lacrosse	Water games (water
Soccer	polo, water basket-
Softball	ball)

*Matthews, D. O.: Intramurals for the senior high school, Chicago, 1964, The Athletic Institute.

NOTE: Tackle football for boys may be included in team sports only if the proper conditioning and training, instruction, coaching, officiating, and supervision are provided and the recommended protective equipment is used.

Corecreational activities

Badminton	Ice skating
Bowling	Picnics and outings
Canoeing	Roller skating
Curling	Shuffleboard
Cycling	Skiing
Dance—social, folk,	Softball
square, and modern	Swimming
Deck tennis	Table tennis
Golf	Tennis
Horseback riding	Volleyball

UNITS AND TYPES OF COMPETITION FOR INTRAMURAL AND EXTRAMURAL ACTIVITIES

The careful selection of appropriate units and types of competition will help to enhance the values that accrue from intramural and extramural activities.

Units of competition

There are many ways of organizing competition for the intramural and extramural programs. The units of competition should be such as to lend interest, create enthusiasm, and allow for identity with some group where an esprit de corps can be developed and where a healthy flavor is added to the competition.

At the elementary level, the classroom provides a basis for such activity. It may be desirable in some cases to organize on some other basis, but the basic structure of the homeroom lends itself readily to this purpose.

At the junior and senior high school levels, several units of organization are possible. Organization may be by grades or classes, homerooms, age, height, weight, clubs, societies, residential districts, physical education classes, study groups, or the arbitrary establishment of groups by staff members. The type of unit organization will vary from school to school and from community to community. The staff member in charge of the program should try to determine the method of organization best suited to the local situation.

At the college or university level there are also several possible units for organization. It can be on the basis of fraternities or sororities, classes, colleges within a university, departments, clubs, societies, physical education classes, boarding clubs, churches, residential districts, geographic units or zones of the campus, dormitories, marital status, social organizations, assignment by lot, honorary societies, or groups set up in an arbitrary manner. Again, the best type of organization will vary from situation to situation.

Types of competition

There are several different ways of organizing competition. Three of the most common are on the bases of leagues, tournaments, and meets. These methods of organization take many forms, with league play popular in the major sports, elimination tournaments utilized to great extent after league play has terminated, and meets held to culminate a season or year of sports activity.

Individual and group competition may be provided. Individual competition is adaptable to such activities as tennis, wrestling, and skiing, whereas group competition is adaptable to such team activities as basketball, softball, and field hockey.

Various types of tournament competition have been widely written up in books specializing in intramurals and other aspects of sports. For this reason only a brief discussion of these items will be included here.

The round robin tournament is probably one of the most widely used and one of the best types of competition, since it allows for maximum play. It is frequently utilized in leagues, where it works best when there are not more than eight teams. Each team plays every other team at least once during the tournament. Each team continues to play to the completion of the tournament and the winner is the one who has the highest percentage, based on wins and losses, at the end of scheduled play.

The elimination type of tournament does not allow for maximum play; the winners continue to play, while the losers drop out. A team or individual is automatically out when it or he or she loses. However, this does represent the most economical form of organization from the standpoint of time in determining the winning player or team.

The single or straight elimination type of tournament is set up so that one defeat eliminates a player or team. Usually there is a drawing for positions, with provisions for the seeding of the better players or teams on the basis of past experience. Such seeding provides for more intense competition as the tournament moves toward the finals. Under such an organization, byes are awarded in the first round of play whenever the number of entrants does not equal a multiple of two. Although such a tournament is a timesaver and is quick, it is

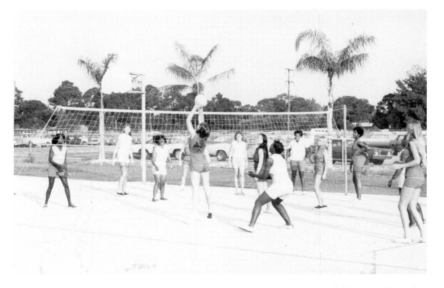

Intramural competition for girls at Central High School, Fort Pierce, Fla.

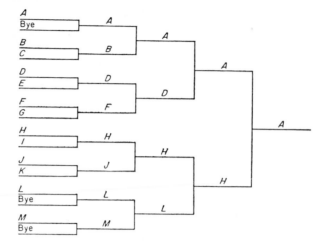

Single-elimination tournament.

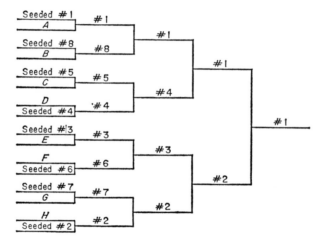

Single-elimination tournament with seedings.

weak in the respect that it does not adequately select the second- and third-place winners. The actual winner may achieve the champhionship because another player who is better has a bad day. Another weakness is that the majority of participants play only once or twice in the tournament.

The double elimination tournament does not have some of the weaknesses of the single elimination because it is necessary for a team or individual to have two defeats before being eliminated. This principle is also characteristic of various types of consolation elimination tournaments that permit the player or team to play more than once.

In some consolation tournaments all the players who lose in the first round and those who, because they received a bye, did not lose until the second round get to play again to determine a consolation winner. In other similar tournaments they permit any player or team who loses once, irrespective of the round in which the loss occurs, to play again. There are also other tournaments such as the Bagnall-Wild Elimination Tournament that places emphasis on second and third places.

I. 1 vs. 5
   2 vs. 6
   3 vs. 7
   4 vs. 8

II. 1 vs. 2
   3 vs. 5
   4 vs. 6
   8 vs. 7

III. 1 vs. 3
   4 vs. 2
   8 vs. 5
   7 vs. 6

IV. 1 vs. 4
   8 vs. 3
   7 vs. 2
   6 vs. 5

V. 1 vs. 8
   7 vs. 4
   6 vs. 3
   5 vs. 2

VI. 1 vs. 7
   6 vs. 8
   5 vs. 4
   2 vs. 3

VII. 1 vs. 6 Round-robin rotation for an eight-team league.
    5 vs. 7
    2 vs. 8
    3 vs. 4

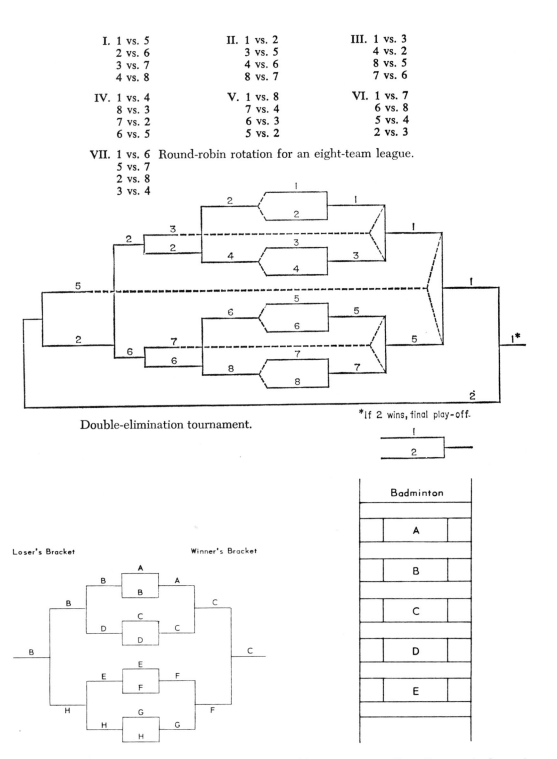

Double-elimination tournament.

*If 2 wins, final play-off.

Consolation tournament—8 teams. (From Intramurals for senior high schools, The Athletic Institute, Chicago.)

Ladder tournament. (From Intramurals for senior high schools, The Athletic Institute, Chicago.)

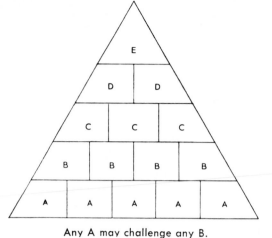

Any A may challenge any B.
Any B may challenge any C.
Any C may challenge any D.
Either D may challenge E.

Pyramid tournament. (From Intramurals for senior high schools, The Athletic Institute, Chicago.)

The ladder type of tournament adapts well to individual competition. Here the contestants are arranged in ladder or vertical formation with rankings established arbitrarily or on the basis of previous performance. Each contestant may challenge the one directly above or in some cases two above, and if he or she wins the names change places on the ladder. This is a continuous type of tournament that does not eliminate any participants. However, it is weak from the standpoint that it may drag and interest may wane.

The pyramid type of tournament is similar to the ladder variety. Here, instead of having one name on a rung or step, there are several names on the lower steps, gradually pyramiding to the top-ranking individual. A player may

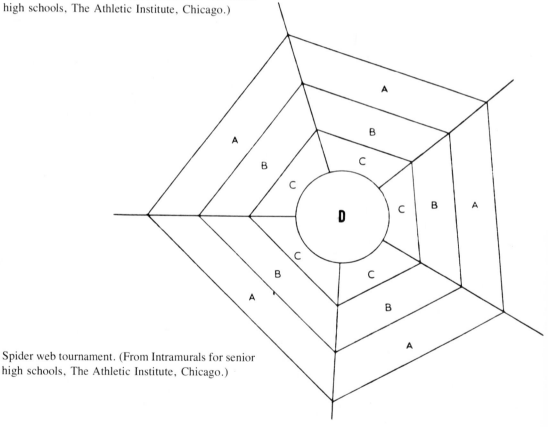

Spider web tournament. (From Intramurals for senior high schools, The Athletic Institute, Chicago.)

Note: Any A may challenge any B.
Any B may challenge any C.
Any C may challenge D.

challenge anyone in the same horizontal row and then the winner may challenge anyone in the row above him or her.

The spider web tournament takes its name from the bracket design, which is the shape of a spider's web. The championship position is at the center of the web. The bracket consists of five (or any other selected number) lines drawn radially from the center and the participant's names are placed on concentric lines crossing these radial lines. Challenges may be made by persons on any concentric line to any person on the next line closer to the center. This type of tournament provides more opportunity for activity.

The type of tournament organization adopted should be the one that is best for the group, activity, and local interests. The goal should be to have as much participation as possible for the facilities and time available. Tournaments make for more student interest and enthusiasm and are an important part of intramural and extramural athletic programs.

INTRAMURAL AND EXTRAMURAL PROGRAMS IN THE ELEMENTARY SCHOOL

The intramural and extramural programs in the elementary school should be outgrowths of the instructional program. They should consist of a broad variety of activities including stunts, rhythmic activities, relays, and tumbling. They should be suited to the age and interests of children at this level. They should be carefully supervised. The younger children in the primary grades probably will benefit most from free play. In the upper elementary grades, recess periods and afterschool activity can take place on both intragrade and intergrade bases. The programs should be broad, varied, and progressive in nature, with participants similar in maturity and ability.

Guidelines for intramural and extramural programs at the elementary school level are as follows:

A basic instructional offering that is geared to the needs, interests, and growth and development levels of

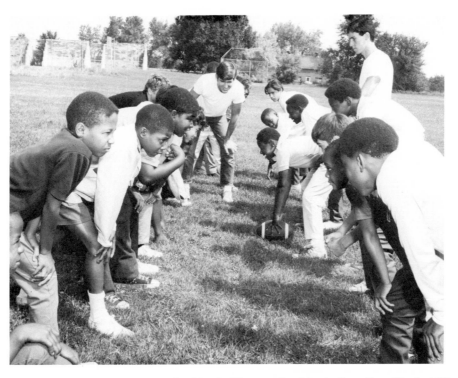

Intramural competition at the elementary school level. (Courtesy President's Council on Physical Fitness and Sports.)

elementary school children should be prerequisite to and foundational for intramural and extramural programs.

Qualified leadership should be provided, which includes competencies involving understanding of the physical, mental, emotional, and social needs of elementary school children.

Competition should only involve children where there is comparability of maturity, size, and ability.

Intramurals and extramurals should be limited to grades four through six in the elementary school. In grades kindergarten through three the regular basic instructional physical education program provides sufficient competition.

Desirable social, emotional, physical, and health outcomes for students should be the aim of intramural and extramural programs.

Activities such as tackle football and boxing should not be permitted.

The planning of the program should involve the students, parents, and community.

INTRAMURAL AND EXTRAMURAL PROGRAMS IN THE JUNIOR HIGH SCHOOL

In the junior high school the main concentration in athletics should be on intramurals and extramurals. It is at this particular level that students are taking a special interest in sports, but at the same time their immaturity makes it unwise to allow them to engage in a highly organized interscholastic program. The program at this level should provide for both boys and girls, appeal to the entire student body, have good supervision by a trained physical educa-

tion person, and be adapted to the needs and interests of the pupils.

Many authoritative and professional groups have gone on record in favor of broad intramural and extramural programs and against a varsity interscholastic, competitive program. They feel this is in the best interests of youth at this age level.

The junior high school provides a setting for giving students fundamental skills in many sports and activities. It is a time of limitless energy when physiologic changes and rapid growth are taking place. Youth in junior high schools should have proper outlets to develop themselves in a healthful manner.

INTRAMURAL AND EXTRAMURAL PROGRAMS IN THE SENIOR HIGH SCHOOL, COLLEGE, AND UNIVERSITY

At both the high school and college levels the intramural and extramural programs should receive a major emphasis. At this time the interests and needs of boys and girls require such a program. These students want and need to experience the joy and satisfaction that are a part of playing on a team, excelling in an activity with one's own peers, and developing skill. Every high school, college, and university should see to it that a broad and varied program is part of the total physical education plan.

The intramural and extramural programs

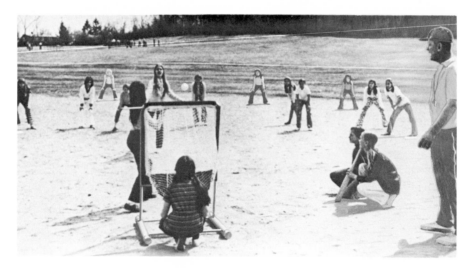

Intramural competition at the junior high school level. (Courtesy Jafro Corporation, Waterford, Conn.)

should receive more emphasis than they are now getting at the senior high school and college levels. They are basic to sound education. They are settings where the skills learned and developed in the instructional program can be put to use in a practical situation, with all the fun that comes from such competition. They should form a basis for the utilization of skills that will be used during leisure time, both in the present and in the future.

There should be adequate personnel for such programs. Good leadership is needed if the programs are to prosper. Each school should be concerned with developing a plan where proper supervision and leadership are available for afterschool hours. Qualified officials are also a necessity in order to ensure equal and sound competition. Facilities, equipment, and supplies should be apportioned on an equitable basis for the entire physical education program. There should be no monopoly on the part of any group or any program.

The college and university level offers an ideal setting for play and sports days for both men and women.

Sports clubs should be encouraged in those activities having special appeal to groups of students. Through such clubs greater skill is developed in the activity and the social experiences are well worthwhile. Sports clubs are discussed in greater detail in the section on Ideas for Intramural and Extramural Programs.

Corecreational activities should play a prominent part in the programs. Girls and boys need to participate more together. Many of the activities in the high school and college programs adapt themselves well to both sexes. Such activities include volleyball, softball, tennis, badminton, table tennis, folk and square dancing, bowling, swimming, and skating. In some cases the rules of the games will need to be modified. The play and sports days that are conducted also offer a setting where both sexes can participate and enjoy worthwhile competition together. Corecreational programs are also

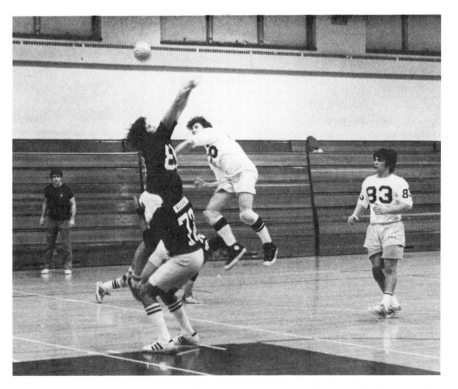

High school boys engaging in intramural team handball competition. (Courtesy North Castle Department of Parks and Recreation, Wilmington, Del.)

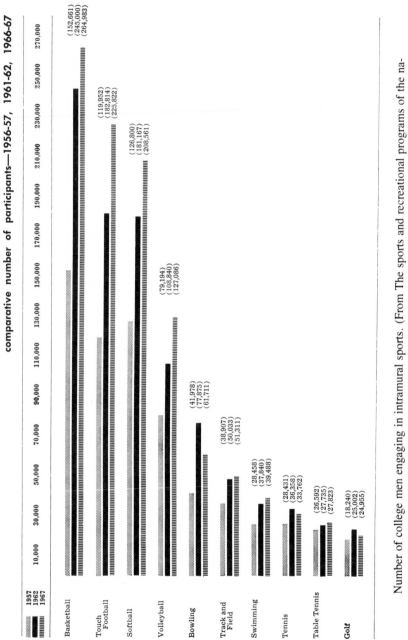

comparative number of participants—1956-57, 1961-62, 1966-67

Number of college men engaging in intramural sports. (From The sports and recreational programs of the nation's universities and colleges, National Collegiate Athletic Association.)

discussed in greater detail in the section on Innovations in Intramural and Extramural Programs.

INTRAMURAL AND EXTRAMURAL PROGRAMS FOR GIRLS AND WOMEN

Most of what has been discussed thus far is applicable to girls and women as well as to boys and men. The objectives, activities, units of competition, and programs at the various institutional levels have been discussed with both sexes in mind. However, in some schools and colleges women's intramurals and extramurals are not given equal representation, facilities, and equipment. Women's activities may be more limited than the men's programs, and play is frequently scheduled at odd hours and with inadequate facilities. A strained budget puts added pressure is women's intramural and extramural programs.

Physical educators and administrators must make a deliberate effort to stop any inequalities concerning women's representation in intramural and extramural activities. Women should be encouraged to participate in women's teams and in corecreational activities. In addition, women should officiate at their own games and be active in the administrative leadership of intramural and extramural programs.

PLAY, SPORTS, AND INVITATION DAYS

Play, sports, and invitation days are rapidly growing in popularity and deserve a prominent place in the extramural athletic program of any school or college. Although they have been utilized mainly by girls' and women's physical education programs, they are equally important for boys and men at the elementary, junior high school, senior high school, and college levels. They have received the endorsement of AAHPER, the National Association for Girls and Women in Sport, and many other prominent associations concerned with physical ed-

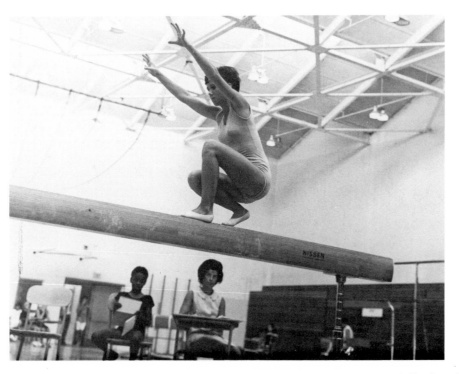

Girl gymnastic champion on the balance beam. Championships conducted by the Youth Services Section, Los Angeles City Schools.

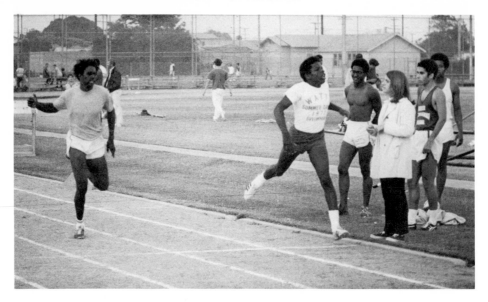

Sports day conducted by the Youth Services Section, Los Angeles City Schools.

ucation. They are an innovation that should receive more and more stress in those places where overemphasis on athletics, highly competitive sports for children of elementary and junior high school ages, and the desire to win at any cost are threatening the accomplishment of the goals of physical education programs.

Sports days refer to that phase of the program where one or several schools or colleges participate in physical education activities. Schools or colleges may enter several teams in various sports. When organized in this manner, each team is identified with the institution it represents. Sports days may also be used to culminate a season of activity for participants within the same school or college. When several schools or colleges participate in a sports day, the number of activities may range anywhere from one to eight, although it is generally agreed that having too many activities sometimes works to a disadvantage rather than an advantage. There are no significant awards for the various events and the publicity is not of a nature that builds up the desire to win.

Play days usually refer to a day or part of a day that is set aside for participation in physical education activities. It may be for students from the same school or college, from several institutions in the same community, or from many schools and colleges in various communities. In the play day each team is composed of individuals from different educational organizations. Here the organization loses its identity, whereas it is maintained in the sports day. The teams are usually labeled by distinctive colored uniforms, arm bands, numbers, or some other device. The activities can be individual as well as team in nature and competitive or noncompetitive. It would be noncompetitive, for example, if several students desired to engage in an activity like horseback riding, not for the purpose of competing against one another but simply for the sociability of the occasion.

An *invitation day* is informal in nature, as are the sports and play days. In this event two schools or colleges usually meet for competition in an activity. This practice has worked out successfully at the end of a seasonal activity, when the winning intramural team or representatives from several teams compete against a similar group from another school or college. The emphasis, however, is not on placing selected, highly skilled players on one team in order to enhance the chances of winning but on the social benefits and fun that can be gained from the occasion.

The advantages of play, sports, and invitation days are very much in evidence. They offer

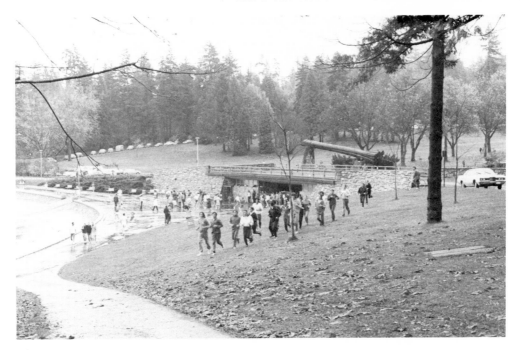

Community involvement in a cross-country run in Vancouver, B. C. (Courtesy Board of Parks and Public Recreation.)

opportunities for the entire student body to participate in wholesome competition, regardless of skill. They offer the student an opportunity to participate in many and varied activities in a spirit of friendly rivalry. They stress both social and physical values. They eliminate the pressures and undesirable practices associated with highly competitive athletics. They are available to the entire student body. They are especially adaptable for immature youngsters who should not be exposed to the practices and pressures of high-level competition. They add interest to student participation and offer innumerable opportunities for leadership.

IDEAS FOR INTRAMURAL AND EXTRAMURAL PROGRAMS

Intramural and extramural programs are expanding with the aid of program innovations. Students today expect and deserve greater involvement in program planning and administration. Many of the programs discussed in this section are "involved" programs where students, faculty, parents, and community come together in the healthy environment of play.

"Lighted school" concept

This concept identifies the school as an activity center that welcomes involvement by the families of the students and the community in general. In turn, the school hopes to use community members and resources as an adjunct to its activity programs. Increased demands on intramural programs encourage innovative concepts such as the "lighted school" (open day and night). Additional new concepts that are compatible with the "lighted school" are discussed in the paragraphs that follow.

Community involvement. The members of the community are a valuable resource for intramural and extramural programs. Volunteers, especially those proficient in a particular activity, can aid in lecturing, teaching, coaching, and officiating. In addition, community recreation areas may be utilized for intramural activities. The school should also be available to the community for supervised recreational activities. By the school and community working together in this manner, the school is able to elicit much needed community support.

Student-parent involvement. Students and

parents should be encouraged to participate together in intramural programs at the school. Father-son or mother-daughter leagues and activity events are very popular especially on the upper elementary and junior high school levels.

Faculty-student involvement. A good way to encourage communication between teachers and students is through participation in intramurals. Such play should be scheduled during the school day and occur every month or twice a month. This is an excellent method of establishing rapport between students and teachers.

Providing for all students. All students should be equally provided for in intramural and extramural programs. This means that the student who is an excellent athlete should be as involved as the student who shows little athletic ability. All too often, programs are devised that prohibit the varsity athlete or outstanding athlete from involvement in intramural events in a particular area. The excellent athlete can advise and instruct other students in such areas as skills, strategy, and rules.

To provide equally for all students, women's intramural programs must be recognized, adequately funded, and given appropriate schedules and use of facilities. Frequently women's intramurals run second place to the men's programs. Intramurals and extramurals for women should be encouraged and publicized.

Sports clubs

Sports clubs provide interested participants an opportunity for social group experiences and the enjoyment of a particular sports activity. Clubs have many different interests including water ballet, table tennis, boating, and ice skating. Most sports clubs provide for student administration and financing. Financing may be derived from the student body through student fees, dances, exhibition games, and the like. The club should provide for some relationship to the athletic administration of the institution. Procedures and policies clarifying this relationship should be a part of the club's by-laws. Such a relationship is necessary in matters of equipment and facility use, eligibility insurance, travel, injuries, and program assistance.

Corecreational programs

Corecreational intramurals have increased greatly in recent years. This type of activity has added new interest to many faltering intramural programs. The potential for coeducational intramural play is tremendous and includes such activities as softball, volleyball, badminton, flag football, and bowling.

Recently, the University of Iowa, Iowa City introduced a "guys and gals" program that has met with great success. During the first year, competition was held in eight sports with more than 600 students participating in a flag football league. Other interesting statistics include a 15-team softball league with 225 participants, and a 27-team volleyball league with 405 student participants.* Competition also took place in basketball, tennis, and paddleball.

Using volunteers in intramurals

In many schools intramural programs have problems in finding persons to supervise activities. Physical educators are often involved with coaching and departmental matters and do not have sufficient time to give to the intramural program. This problem can be solved by enlisting the services of other faculty members. By using a questionnaire, faculty members may be asked to state their interests and experience in sports or related activities. Many faculty members show great enthusiasm at being asked to sponsor a program in which they have a particular interest.

Intromurals

Yes, the spelling is *intro* not *intra* and refers to a new program introduced at the University of San Francisco. Intromurals differ from intramurals in that while intramurals usually emulate athletic competition of a varsity nature, intromurals are devoted to a play ethic and include sports, recreation, and games for all students. The students have complete responsibility for their own activities, eliminating the need for authoritarian figures such as officials or coaches.

The program has been very successful, re-

*Gehrke, Delbert: Guys and gals intramurals, Journal of Health, Physical Education, and Recreation **43**:73, 1972.

sulting in a 70% participation of the 7,000 members of the university community. The programs are both traditional and innovative. The traditional programs provide for coeducational activities including touch football, volleyball, and tennis, and all male-all female team activities. The innovative activities include off-campus trips to observatories, amusement parks, and camping areas. Sports clubs are active in card games, cycling, and jogging. In addition, there are clinic periods where one can receive instruction in yoga, dance, archery, sailing, and diet. This type of program is particularly effective for schools with limited budgets and apathetic student involvement in recreational activities.

AWARDS, POINT SYSTEMS, RECORDS, AND ELIGIBILITY

Awards, point systems, records, and eligibility requirements may present problems in the organization and administration of intramural and extramural competition.

Awards

There are arguments pro and con in respect to awards for intramural and extramural competition. Some of the arguments for awards are that they stimulate interest, serve as an incentive for participation, and recognize achievement. Some of the arguments against awards are that they make for a more expensive program, a few individuals win most of the awards, and they are unnecessary, since individuals would participate even if no awards were given. Leaders who oppose awards also stress the ideas that there should be no expectation of awards for voluntary, leisure-time participation; it is difficult to make awards on the basis of all factors that should be considered; the incentive is artificial; and the joy and satisfaction received are reward enough in themselves.

One study indicates that approximately four out of five intramural directors give awards. Letters, numerals, and similar awards are used most frequently in the junior high schools.

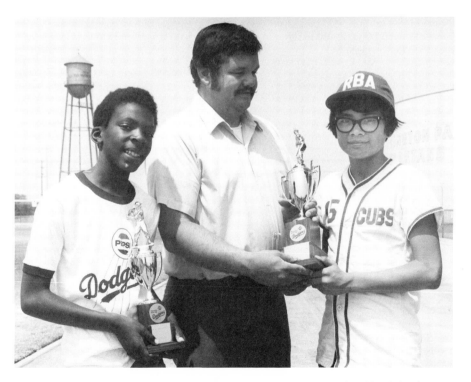

Trophies being awarded by Youth Services Section, Los Angeles City Schools.

Medals and trophies are given more extensively on the junior college and college levels.

When awards are given, they should be inexpensive. They can take the form of medals, ribbons, certificates, plaques, cups, or letters.

Point systems

Most intramural programs have some type of point system that is cumulative in nature and many times figured on an all-year basis. The keeping of such points makes for continued interest and enthusiasm over the course of the school year. It also encourages greater participation.

A system of keeping points should be developed that takes into consideration those factors that stimulate wholesome competition over a period of time, maintain continued interest, and are in conformance with the objectives sought in the total program. The system should be readily understood by all and easy to administer. Under such conditions points should be awarded on the basis of such considerations as contests won, championships gained, standing in a league or order of finish, participation, sportsmanship, and contribution to the objectives of the program.

A point system used by one school system is based on the following items:

Each entry: 10 points
Each win: 2 points
Each loss: 1 point
Forfeits: 0 points
Each team championship: 10 points
Second-place team championship: 6 points
Third-place team championship: 3 points
Each individual championship: 6 points
Second-place individual championship: 4 points
Third-place individual championship: 3 points
Each game an official works: 3 points
Being homeroom representative: 10 points
Each meeting attended by homeroom representative: 2 points

Records

Efficient administration of the program will necessitate the keeping of records. These should not be extensive but should contain the information needed to determine the worth of the program and the progress being made.

Such records allow for comparison with other schools of a similar nature. They show the degree to which the program is providing for the needs of the entire student body and the extent to which students are participating. They show the activities that are popular and the ones that are not as popular. They focus attention on the best units of competition, needs of the program, administrative procedures that are effective, and leadership strengths and weaknesses. Record keeping is an important phase of the program that should not be overlooked.

Eligibility

There is a need for a few simple eligibility rules. These should be kept to a minimum, since the intramural and extramural programs should render a contribution to the vast majority of the student body.

It is generally agreed that there should be no scholarship rules. There should be rules that forbid players from participating in activities when they are on the varsity team or squad. Professionals should be barred from those activities in which they are professional. A student should be allowed to participate on only one team in a given activity during the season. Students, of course, should be regularly enrolled in the school and carrying what the institution rules is a normal load. Unsportsmanlike conduct should be dealt with in a manner that is in the best interests of the individual concerned, the program, and the established goals. Certain activities by their very nature should not be engaged in by individuals with certain health problems. Therefore, such individuals should be cleared by the health department of the school before participation is allowed in such activities.

The eligibility rules established by one college that have implications for high schools as well as colleges are as follows:

1. All students of the college (school) in good standing shall be eligible to compete in any activity promoted by the Intramural Department, except as provided later in these articles.
2. A varsity team member is one who is retained by the coach after the final cut has been made.
3. The varsity and freshman coaches are requested to pass on the list of their respective squads. Participation on these squads will automatically make an individual ineligible for intramural athletics in that particular sport.

4. An individual may represent one team in a given sport in a given season.

5. A team shall forfeit any contest in which an ineligible player was used. The director shall eliminate any points made by an ineligible person in meets. These infractions of the rules must be discovered within 48 hours after the contest.

6. Members of the freshman or varsity squads who become scholastically ineligible in any particular sport shall be ineligible to participate in any allied intramural activity.

7. The director may declare an individual ineligible to participate in intramural athletics for unsportsmanlike conduct toward officials or opponents.

8. An individual receiving a varsity award is ineligible to participate in that particular intramural sport until one complete season has passed since earning his or her letter. *

Questions and exercises

1. What is the place of intramural and extramural programs in the total physical education plan of a school or college? How do they complement and supplement the other phases of the total program?

2. To what extent are the objectives of intramurals and extramurals compatible with those of general education? Give specific evidence to support your answer.

3. Survey at least three schools on either the high school or the college level to determine if there is proper balance between the intramural and extramural and the interschool programs. Prepare a statement of findings.

4. Discuss the importance of evaluation techniques for intramural programs. What general process of evaluation should be followed?

5. Why have sports, play, and invitation days increased so much in popularity during the last few years?

6. Develop a set of principles that could be used as guides for the selection of activities in intramural and extramural programs.

7. Do some research into the women's intramural program at your school or one with which you are familiar. Discuss the activity program, facilities, equipment, and funding.

8. Identify the following: round robin tournament, unit of competition, straight elimination tournament, and ladder tournament.

9. Briefly discuss some of the innovations in intramural and extramural programs. Do you have any to add to this discussion?

10. Develop what you consider to be ideal intramural and extramural programs at the elementary, junior high school, senior high school, or college level.

11. What are some important considerations in administering athletic programs for girls and women? Discuss in detail.

Reading assignment in *Administrative Dimensions of Health and Physical Education Programs, Including Athletics:* Chapter 7, Selections 34 to 38.

Selected references

The Athletic Institute: Intramurals for the senior high school, Chicago, 1964, The Athletic Institute, Inc.

Bucher, C. A.: Field days, The Journal of Health and Physical Education **19:**22, 1948.

Bucher, C. A.: Foundations of physical education, ed. 7, St. Louis, 1975, The C. V. Mosby Co.

Bucher, C. A., and Cohane T.: Little league baseball can hurt your boy, Look, August 11, 1963, p. 74.

Bucher, C. A., and Dupee, R. K., Jr.: Athletics in schools and colleges, New York, 1965, The Center for Applied Research in Education, Inc. (The Library of Education).

Educational Policies Commission: School athletics—problems and policies, Washington, D. C., 1954, National Education Association.

Gehrke, D.: Guys and gals intramurals, Journal of Health, Physical Education, and Recreation **43:**75, 1972.

Gerou, N.: Intramurals and recreation belong together, Journal of Health, Physical Education, and Recreation, **44:**28, 1973.

Jones, T. R.: Needed: a new philosophical model for intramurals, Journal of Health, Physical Education, and Recreation **42:**34, 1971.

Leider, F.: Intramural in the junior high school, Journal of Health, Physical Education, and Recreation **44:**71, 1973.

Matthews, D. O.: Intramural administration principles, The Athletic Journal **46:**82, 1966.

Mueller, P.: Intramurals, programming and administration, New York, 1971, The Ronald Press Co.

National Council of Secondary School Athletic Directors, Division of Men's Athletics, American Association for Health, Physical Education, and Recreation: Evaluating the high school athletic program, Washington, D. C., 1973, American Association for Health, Physical Education, and Recreation.

Rule books for all boys' sports. Available from the National Federation of State High School Athletic Associations, 7 South Dearborn Street, Chicago, Ill.

Rule books for all girls' sports. Available from the Division for Girls' and Women's Sports, American Association for Health, Physical Education, and Recreation, 1201 16th Street, N. W., Washington, D. C.

Stumph, P.: The expanded intramural concept, Journal of Health, Physical Education, and Recreation **44:**55, 1973.

Taylor, J. L.: Intromurals: a program for everyone, Journal of Health, Physical Education, and Recreation **44:**44, 1973.

The Division of Girls and Women's Sports, American Association for Health, Physical Education, and Recreation: 1973 Guidelines for interscholastic athletic programs for high school girls, 1973 Guidelines for interscholastic athletic programs for junior high school girls, 1973 Guidelines for intercollegiate athletic programs for women, Washington, D. C., 1973, American Association for Health, Physical Education, and Recreation.

---

*Adapted from the Handbook of intramural athletics, Michigan State College.

The interscholastic and intercollegiate varsity athletic programs

Interscholastic and intercollegiate athletic programs have always been an integral part of the physical education learning process. However, in recent years certain problems regarding these programs have been brought to the attention of directors of athletic programs, physical education administrators, as well as the general public. Problems requiring immediate solutions include: austerity budgets, unfair treatment of women in athletic programs, alcohol and drug abuse among athletes, certification of coaches, and crowd control. These and other problems will be discussed in this chapter with the hope that interscholastic and intercollegiate athletics can make their essential contribution to a well-rounded physical education program.

The executive secretary of the Missouri State High School Activities Association* indicates that school athletic programs should include the development of the following goals for its youth. They are presented here in adapted form:

1. An appreciation of why the school provides an athletic program
2. A knowledge of the values of athletics to the individual and society
3. An understanding of the rules essential to playing the game
4. The ability to think as an individual and as a team member
5. Faith in and respect for the democratic processes
6. An appreciation of the values of group ideals
7. The development of motor skills
8. Health and physical fitness
9. An understanding and appreciation of what constitutes wholesome recreation and entertainment
10. The desire to be successful and excel
11. Moral and ethical standards
12. Self-discipline, emotional maturity, and self-control
13. Social competence
14. Recognition of the importance of conforming to the rules
15. Respect for the rights of others and those in authority
16. Good human relationships

An era of great expansion in athletics started in the post-World War II period. The physical defects revealed by the draft, the value of sports in building morale, and the emphasis on physical fitness during the war and during periods of national emergency have combined to en-

*Keller, I. A.: School athletics—its philosophy and objective, American School Board Journal 153:22-23, 1966. Reprinted, with permission, from the American School Board Journal, August, 1966. Copyright assigned 1967 to The National School Boards Association. All rights reserved.

courage athletics to a degree that has never been equaled in the history of this country.

The emphasis on athletics has been the focus of much attention and controversy, and consequently the program should be considered carefully by all interested in administration. Interscholastic and intercollegiate athletics have a definite place in high school and college programs of physical education. Such competition can help players achieve a higher standard of mental, moral, social, and physical fitness, provided the overall objectives of physical education are kept in mind.

RELATIONSHIP TO TOTAL PHYSICAL EDUCATION PROGRAM

Varsity interscholastic and intercollegiate athletics represent an integral part of the total physical education program. They should develop out of the intramural and extramural athletic programs.

Athletics, with the appeal they have to youth, should be the heart of physical education and should aid in achieving goals that will help to enrich living for all who participate.

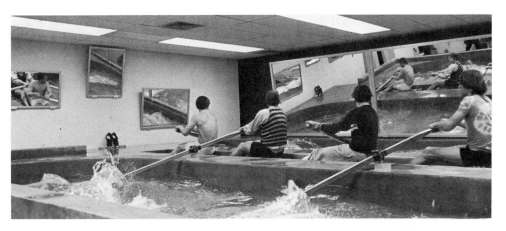

Varsity crew in rowing tank with mirrors. (Trinity College, Hartford, Conn.)

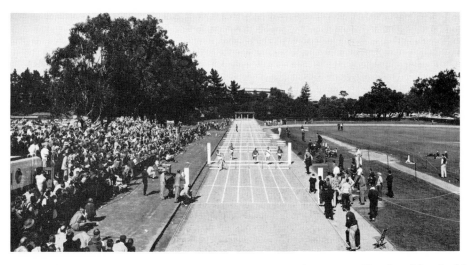

Angell Field, Stanford University, with an intercollegiate dual meet in progress. The rim of Stanford Stadium is visible in the center background.

The challenge of providing sound educational programs in varsity interscholastic and intercollegiate athletics is one that all physical education personnel should recognize. The challenge can be met and resolved if physical educators aggressively bring to the attention of administrators, school and college faculties, and the public in general the true purposes of athletics in a physical education program. It is important to stress that there is a need for having an athletic program that meets the needs of all; that such a program is organized and administered with the welfare of the individual in mind; that it is conducted in the light of educational objectives that are not compromised when exposed to pressures from sports writers, alumni, and community members; and that it provides leadership trained in physical education.

In actual practice the organization of athletics takes two forms. At times they are organized as an integral part of the physical education structure and at other times as a separate unit apart from physical education. Some departments of athletics that operate as separate units evolved from the nineteenth century, when they were not considered an integral part of education. If athletics are looked upon as intrinsically related to education, they should be a part of the physical education program.

THE ATHLETIC COUNCIL

Most colleges and many schools have some type of athletic council, board, or committee that establishes athletic policies for the institution. It may involve only faculty members or it may also involve students. Such councils, boards, or committees are responsible for giving the athletic program proper direction in the educational program.

The composition of such committees or councils varies widely from school to school and college to college. In a school, the principal may serve as chairman, or this position may be held by the director of physical education or other faculty member. The committee may include coaches, members of the board of education, faculty members, students, or members of the community at large. In a college or uni-

versity, the composition of the committee may consist of administrators, faculty members, students, athletic director, coaches, and others.

THE ATHLETIC DIRECTOR

The athletic director implements the athletic policies as established by the council, board, or committee. Responsibilities of the athletic director include preparing the budget for the sports program, purchasing equipment and supplies, scheduling athletic contests, arranging for officials, supervising eligibility requirements, making arrangements for transportation, seeing that medical examinations of athletes and proper insurance coverage are adequate, and supervising the program in general.

A question that is continually asked concerns whether athletic directors should also act as coaches. Very often athletic directors at small community or junior colleges are asked to coach along with their other responsibilities. In an attempt to answer this question, David Poorman, athletic director of Lakeland Community College, Mentor, Ohio, surveyed 206 athletic directors and coaches in junior and community colleges with enrollments ranging from 3,000 to 5,000 students. *

The coaches and athletic directors were asked to respond to the following question: ''Should athletic directors at 2-year junior or community colleges be involved in coaching an intercollegiate sport?'' Responses were obtained from 30 athletic directors, 22 persons who did not specify their athletic position, and 91 coaches. A summary of the responses indicated that 50% of the athletic directors indicated that they should not coach, whereas 27% felt they should coach, and 23% were undecided. Of the coaches responding, 53% indicated that athletic directors should coach, 41% felt they they should not coach, and 6% were undecided. Of the persons responding with unspecified athletic positions, 41% felt that athletic directors should coach, 36% felt that they should not coach, and 23% were undecided.

In general, most athletic directors felt that they should not coach but because of budgetary

---

*Poorman, A. W.: Should A. D.'s Coach? Juco Review **25:**10, 1973.

RATING CARD FOR ATHLETIC DIRECTORS FOR EVALUATING THE ADMINISTRATION OF AN ATHLETIC PROGRAM

A high school rating card has been adapted from Kelliher's college criteria.* These evaluation items assist the athletic director in checking the effectiveness of his program.

The actual rating card includes a column for evaluating each of these thirty-six items. The column is headed "Performance in this Area Is Given: Great Attention; Moderate Attention; Little Attention."

A. Financial soundness
   1. He operates on a sound financial basis.
   2. There is equitable balance in the budget for all sports.
B. Organization of the department
   3. He handles the business of the department efficiently and promptly.
   4. All members of the department handle their work assignments efficiently.
   5. He operates effectively without waste of time or materials.
   6. He develops close cooperation between all members of his staff.
   7. Policies and procedures are written out and are made clear to both players and staff members.
   8. He cooperates with other departments of the school and maintains good relations with the administration.
   9. He is fair and firmly in control of his staff and never fails to recognize organizational channels.
   10. He is easily available to anyone with an interest in the athletic program.
C. Professional status of the staff
   11. His operations are in harmony with the philosophy and objectives of the school and of the physical education department.
   12. His operations are in harmony with the spirit and rules and regulations of interscholastic athletics as established by the state high school athletic association.
   13. He is able to justify the athletic program as an important phase of education.
   14. The director is an educator. His status in the school is comparable to other department heads and is considered high.
   15. He cooperates with the administration; he works with the faculty and keeps them well informed.
D. Well-being of the staff
   16. He has developed a high degree of espirit de corps among all members of his department.
   17. He cooperates with the administration in the selection of staff members who believe in high standards of competitive athletics.
   18. He develops a staff of men with high professional standards and education.
   19. He is loyal to the administration and to his staff and gets facts before making a move.
E. Well-being of the students
   20. The health protection of athletes is rated high.
   21. He insists that athletes strive to keep up with their class.
   22. The best possible education for the boy is the most important criterion.
   23. He produces a program that appeals to a large number of participants.
   24. He considers the after-graduation success of former athletes a measure of success of the athletic department.
   25. He prefers that athletes carry on a career program.
   26. He has understanding of and cooperates with general student body interests.
   27. Students assigned to work in the department give reasonable service for experience and credit earned.
F. Public relations
   28. There is an efficient program of public relations.
   29. He maintains friendly relations with press and radio.
   30. He conducts athletics in an efficient, crowd-pleasing manner.
   31. He insists that squad members are school representatives at all times and that they conduct themselves accordingly.
   32. The activities of the department are well received by the administration, faculty, and community.
   33. The record of sportsmanship of all competitive teams under his administration is high.
G. Care of property and equipment
   34. Teams are well equipped, neat, and clean.
   35. The equipment of the department is cared for in an excellent manner and according to sound procedures.
   36. The buildings and grounds under the supervision of the director are kept in excellent condition.

*Kelliher, M. S.: Successful athletic administration, Journal of Health, Physical Education, and Recreation **30**:31, 1959.

problems, coaching became necessary. The coaches, many of whom expected to eventually enter administration, felt they would like to continue coaching after becoming administrators and thought athletic directors should coach. The unspecified athletic administrators indicated that if athletic directors coached, they would not have adequate time to complete administrative functions.

A rating card was developed by Kelliher for the evaluation of the effectiveness of the athletic director. It is reproduced here for the benefit of the reader.

THE COACH

One of the most popular phases of physical education professional work is that of coaching. Many students who show exceptional skill in some interscholastic sport such as basketball, baseball, or football feel that they would like to become members of the profession so that they may coach. They feel that since they have proved themselves outstanding athletes in high school, they will be successful in coaching. This, however, is not necessarily true. It may seem paradoxic to the layman, but there is insufficient evidence to show that exceptional skill in any activity necessarily guarantees success in teaching that activity. Many other factors such as personality, interest in youth, knowledge of human growth and development, psychology, intelligence, integrity, leadership, character, and a sympathetic attitude carry great weight in coaching success.

Coaching should be recognized as teaching. Because of the nature of the position, a coach may be in a more favorable position to teach concepts that make for effective daily living than any other member of a school faculty. Youth, with their inherent drive for activity and action and their quest for the excitement and competition found in sports, look up to the coach and in many cases feel that he or she is the type of individual to be emulated. Therefore, the coach should recognize his or her influence and see the value of such attributes as character, personality, and integrity. Although a coach must know thoroughly the game he or she is coaching, these other characteristics are of equal importance.

The coach of an athletic team has within himself or herself the power to build future citizens who possess traits that are desirable and acceptable to society, or citizens who have a false conception as to what is considered acceptable behavior. The coach is sometimes tempted to seek outcomes not educational in nature by the insecurity of his or her position, the emphasis on winning teams, student and alumni pressure, the desire for lucrative gate receipts, and the publicity that goes with winning teams. Unless the coach is an individual of strong character and is willing to follow an unswerving course in the direction of what he or she knows to be right, many problems arise.

Coaching is characterized in some schools and colleges by insecurity of position. Whether a coach feels secure depends to a great extent upon the school, college, community, and the administration. Coaching offers an interesting and profitable career to many individuals. However, one should recognize the possibility of finding himself or herself in a situation where the pressure to produce winning teams may be so great as to cause unhappiness, insecurity, and even the loss of a job.

Coaching is only one phase of the physical education profession, and coaching is teaching. Because of this close relationship with physical education and the education field in general, a coach should be thoroughly qualified as a physical educator. The coach needs a background in physical and biologic science, skills, behavioral sciences, education, and the humanities. Only in this way can he or she best serve youth who are interested in athletics.

There are four qualifications that are found in the outstanding coach. First, this person has an ability to teach the fundamentals and strategies of the sport; he or she *must* be a good teacher. Second, there is a need to understand the boy or girl who is a player. The coach needs to understand how a youth functions at a particular level of development—with full appreciation of skeletal growth, muscular development, and physical and emotional limitations. Third, he or she understands the game coached. Thorough knowledge of techniques, rules, and similar information is basic. Fourth, the coach has a desirable personality and character. Patience, understanding, kindness, honesty, sportsman-ship, sense of right and wrong, courage, cheer-fulness, affection, humor, energy, and enthusi-asm are imperative, since the youngsters will be idolizing and emulating his or her every move.

Too often coaches are chosen because of one qualification—they have played the game. Most principals, superintendents of schools, and college presidents would be flattered to have an All-American coaching their football teams. In terms of the welfare of youth, however, the other qualifications are even more important, and the administration will be most likely to find a coach with these qualifications in a per-son who has been trained in physical education.

Professional preparation of the coach

About one-fourth of all coaches in the junior and senior high schools in this country have no professional preparation, and the percentage is much higher among college coaches. The only qualification many coaches have is the fact that they have played the game or sport in high school, college, or the professional ranks. It is generally recognized that the best preparation that a coach can have is training in the field

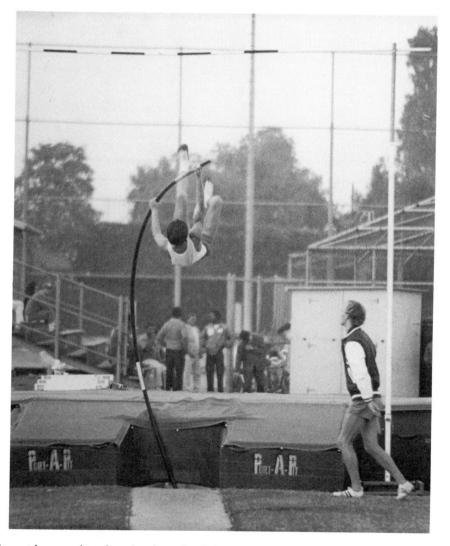

The coach must be a good teacher. A pole vaulter being coached in track in the Youth Services Section, Los Angeles City Schools.

of physical education. In light of this fact, several states are attempting to see that coaches, particularly at the precollege level, have at least some training in the field of physical education.

The single most important factor influencing the participant in a sport's activity is the coach. His or her influence affects the participant in all aspects of life, including personality development, philosophy, and character traits. For these reasons and others many persons feel that the coach should be certified so that his or her course work and training will suit the leadership role entrusted to a coach.

Standards for coaching certification were identified by the American Alliance of Health, Physical Education, and Recreation (AAHPER) through their Task Force on Certification of High School Coaches. The essential areas identified by the Task Force were: (1) medical aspects of athletic coaching, (2) sociologic and psychologic aspects of coaching, (3) theory and techniques of coaching, (4) kinesiologic foundations of coaching, (5) physiologic foundations of coaching.

The Division of Men's Athletics (DMA) Planning Committee further developed these areas in their 1973 Professional Preparation Conference. They strongly feel that all coaches should possess concepts and competencies in these areas in order to fulfill their coaching responsibilities.

The present practice of secondary school administrators hiring coaches who may teach other subject areas is a strong recommendation for training in coaching in undergraduate work. The University of Illinois at Urbana-Champaign has already implemented a minor in physical education for those are are not physical education majors. Other Illinois universities are also studying the inclusion of such a minor area of study.

The Illinois Association for Professional Preparation in Health, Physical Education, and Recreation believes that the state should establish certification standards for teachers in other areas who desire to coach. These standards would also be intended to apply to future coaches. The proposed certification standards are as follows:

1. Coaches should have a major or minor in physical education or a major or minor in coaching.
2. Fifteen semester hours should be taken in each of the following areas:
   a. Medical aspects of athletic coaching
   b. Principles and problems of coaching
   c. Theory and techniques of coaching
   d. Kinesiologic foundations of coaching
   e. Physiologic foundations of coaching

Coaches presently working in school and college positions should be encouraged to seek training even if certification standards have not yet been required by their particular state. The trend toward certification is growing, but more importantly the thorough training of all coaches is essential to the health and performance of school and college athletes.

SOME ADMINISTRATIVE CONSIDERATIONS IN VARSITY ATHLETIC PROGRAMS

There are many administrative considerations pertinent to the conduct of an interscholastic

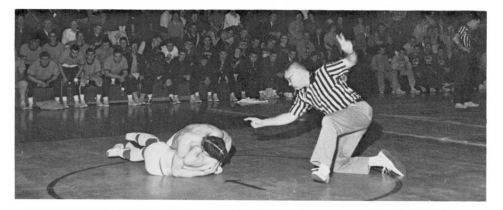

Interscholastic wrestling. (Richwoods Community High School, Peoria Heights, Ill.)

APPROACHES TO CROWD CONTROL*
Summary of reports: small group discussions

The nature and seriousness of the problems in crowd control have recently become more drastic and bizarre as they have occurred in increasing frequency. They take on the collective character of a deliberate attempt either to ignore or confront the system. This social problem may be impossible to eliminate completely, but an attempt must be made to cope with the immediate symptoms. Our only hope is for imaginative and coordinated efforts by the school administration, the majority of students, and community authorities to promote standards of conduct conducive to continuing spectator sports in comparative tranquility. The alternatives are to allow a disruptive element to completely negate the nature of school athletics, to play with no spectators, or to abandon the activity.

The following will present some causes of crowd control problems and some approaches to solutions.

Some causes of problems
Lack of anticipation of, and preventive planning for, possible trouble
Lack of proper facilities
Poor communication resulting in lack of information
Lack of involvement of one or more of the following: school administration, faculty, student body, parents, community, press, and law enforcement agencies
Lack of respect for authority and property
Attendance at games of youth under the influence of narcotics
Increased attitude of permissiveness
School dropouts, recent graduates, and outsiders

Some approaches to solutions
Develop written policy statements, guidelines, and regulations for crowd control.
1. Consult the following before writing policy statements or promulgating regulations: school administration, athletic director, coaches, faculty members involved in the school sports program, school youth organizations, local police departments.
2. Properly and efficiently administer regulations and provide for good communications.
3. Constantly evaluate regulations and guidelines for their relevance and effectiveness.
4. Make guidelines and regulations so effective that the director of athletics who follows them is secure in knowing he has planned with his staff for any eventuality and has sufficient help, appropriately brief, for any situation that may arise.

Provide adequate facilities.
1. Plan and design stadiums, fieldhouses and gymnasiums for effective crowd control.
2. Provide for adequate rest room facilities.
3. Establish a smoking area when indoor contests are held.
4. Complete preparation of facilities before game time.

Teach good sportsmanship throughout the school and the community.
1. Begin education in good sportsmanship in the earliest grades and continue it throughout the school life.
2. Make frequent approving references to constructive and commendable behavior.
3. Arrange for program appearances by faculty members and students jointly to discuss the true values of athletic competition including good sportsmanship.
4. Make use of all news media through frequent and effective television, radio, and press presentations and interviews, commentaries, and frequent announcement of good sportsmanship slogans.
5. Distribute a printed Code of Ethics for Good Sportsmanship.
6. Include the good sportsmanship slogan in all printed programs at sports events.
7. Urge the use of athletic events as an example in elementary school citizenship classes, stressing positive values of good conduct at games, during the raising of the flag and singing of the national anthem; courtesy toward visitors.
8. Involve teachers in school athletic associations, provide them with passes to all sports events, and stress the positive values of their setting an example of good sportsmanship.

Intensify communications prior to scheduled games.
1. Arrange for an exchange of speakers at school assembly programs; the principals, coaches, or team captains could visit the opposing school.
2. Discuss with appropriate personnel of the competing school the procedures for the game, including method and location of team entry and departure.

*From Sixth National Conference of City and County Directors, American Association for Health, Physical Education, and Recreation: Crowd control, Washington, D. C., 1968, The Association, pp. 17-22.

Continued.

APPROACHES TO CROWD CONTROL—cont'd

Intensify communications prior to scheduled games—cont'd

3. Provide superintendent or principal, athletic director, and coach with a copy of written policy statement, guidelines and regulations.
4. Meet all game officials and request them to stress good sportsmanship on the field.
5. Meet with coaches and instruct them not to question officials during a contest; stress the importance of good sportsmanship and the fact that their conduct sets the tone for spectator reaction to game incidents.
6. Instruct students what to expect and what is expected of them.
7. Schedule preventive planning conferences with local police to be assured of their full cooperation and effectiveness in spectator control.

Inform the community.

1. Request coaches and athletic directors to talk to service groups and other community groups.
2. Stress the need for exemplary conduct of coaches at all times.
3. Invite community leaders (non-school people) to attend athletic events.
4. Post on all available notice boards around town, in factories and other public places, posters showing the Sportsmanship Code of Ethics and Guidelines in brief.
5. Release constructive information and positive statements to news media and request publication of brief guidelines on sports pages.
6. Provide news media with pertinent information as to ways in which the community may directly and indirectly render assistance in the crowd control problem.

Involve law enforcement personnel.

1. Police and other security personnel should be strategically located so as to afford the best possible control.
2. Law enforcement professionals should handle *all* enforcement and disciplining of spectators.
3. Strength in force may be shown by appearance of several policemen, motorcycles, police cruise cars, et cetera, at and near the site of the game.
4. Women police may be stationed in women's rest rooms.
5. Civil Defense organizations could patrol parking areas.
6. A faculty member from the visiting school may be used as a liaison with police and local faculty in identifying visiting students.
7. Attendants, police, county sheriffs, deputies should be in uniform. Uniformed authority figures command greater respect.

Use supervisory personnel other than police.

1. Select carefully teacher supervisors who are attentive and alert to signs of possible trouble.
2. Identify faculty members by arm bands or other means.
3. Provide for communication by means of walkie-talkie systems.
4. Assign some faculty members to sit behind the visiting fans; this reduces verbal harassment of visitors.
5. Employ paid ticket takers and paid chaperones to mingle strategically among the crowd and to remain on duty throughout the game, including half-time.
6. Issue passes to junior high physical education teachers to provide more adult supervision.

Plan for ticket sales and concession stands.

1. Arrange for advance sale of student tickets to avoid congestion at the gate.
2. Sell tickets in advance only to students in their own schools, and avoid sale of tickets to outsiders and non-students.
3. Provide for a close check at the gate or entrance.
4. Arrange for concession stands to be open before the game, during half-time, and after the game, but closed during actual play.
5. Channel the flow of traffic to and from concession stands by means of ropes, or other means; keep traffic moving.

Prepare spectators and contestants.

1. Encourage as many students as possible to be in the uniforms of the athletic club, pep club, booster clubs, band, majorettes, cheer leaders.
2. Bus participants to and from the site of the game.
3. Have participants dressed to play before leaving for a game or contest.
4. Adhere to established seating capacity of stadiums and gymnasiums.
5. Request home team fans to remain in their own stands until visiting team fans have left.
6. Try to arrange for a statewide athletic association regulation prohibiting all noise makers including musical instruments except for the school band or orchestra under professional supervision.
7. Request the assistance of visiting clubs.
8. Educate cheerleaders, student leaders, band captains, pep squads, and faculty supervisors by means of a one day conference program.

APPROACHES TO CROWD CONTROL—cont'd

9. Keep spectators buffered from the playing area as much as practical.
10. Request that elementary school children be accompanied by an adult.

Miscellaneous.

1. Inform and involve school superintendents fully when problems arise in connection with sports events.
2. Impose severe penalties on faculty and student leaders guilty of poor conduct.
3. Publish the identity of offenders at games and notify parents, if possible; any penalties inflicted should also be noted. (Note: If the offense leads to Juvenile Court action, care should be taken not to contravene laws about publishing names of juvenile offenders.)
4. Consistently enforce rules and regulations; this is a necessity.
5. Work toward the assumption of responsibility for strong regulation and enforcement of team behavior on the part of the state athletic associations.
6. Attempt to work with the courts toward greater cooperation.
7. Avoid overstressing the winning of games.
8. Discontinue double headers and triple headers.
9. After-game incidents away from the proximity of the stadium or gymnasium are out of the control of school officials, but cause bad public reaction.

Summary

Sound safety controls and crowd controls at school athletic functions are a must! Greater concentration on treating the causes of the problem is essential. Preliminary groundwork is the key to good crowd control. Coordination and cooperation of school and law enforcement agencies is the key to success.

Youth should be taught to know what to expect and what is expected of them. Consistent enforcement of rules and regulations is a necessity if youth is to respect authority. Adult behavior should be such that it may be advantageously and admirably emulated by youth whose actions hopefully may result in deserving praise instead of negative criticism and disapproval.

The athletic program is a constructive and valuable school activity. It should be permitted to function in a favorable, healthful, and friendly environment.

---

or intercollegiate varsity athletic program. Some of the more important of these are: (1) crowd control, (2) health of the players, (3) contracts, (4) officials, (5) protests and forfeitures, (6) game management, (7) schedules and practice periods, (8) awards, (9) records, and (10) transportation. Each will be discussed in the following paragraphs.

Crowd control

Crowd control at athletic contests is becoming of increasing importance in light of recent dissent, riots, and disturbances on both high school and college campuses and in public gathering places. The elimination of night athletic activities has been on the increase, particularly in large cities. School districts and college authorities are taking increased precautions to avoid any disturbances. More police are being brought in to help supervise the crowds at athletic contests, sportsmanship assemblies are being held, townspeople are being informed, administrators are discussing

the matter, and careful plans are being developed.

The Sixth National Conference of City and County Directors of the AAHPER, which was held in Washington, D. C., in December, 1968, spent considerable time on the subject of crowd control at athletic contests. A summary of their discussions as reported in their proceedings is reproduced here.

In 1971, the California Interscholastic Federation—Southern Section published crowd management guidelines after several years of research into crowd control problems in southern California. The suggested guidelines were general in nature and were not strictly applicable to all communities. Civic leaders were urged to meet first with local school administrators to precisely determine in what activities during athletic events civic group assistance would be most helpful. The guidelines would then be expanded or revised to suit the situation. The entire California Interscholastic Federation report on crowd management may be obtained by sending 25 cents (to cover postage) to: Crowd Management Handbook, California Interscholastic Federation, Southern Section, P. O. Box 488, Artesia, California 90701.

Health of the players

Interscholastic and intercollegiate athletics should contribute to the health of the players. Through wholesome physical activity the participant should become more physically, mentally, emotionally, and socially fit.

Medical examination.* One of the first requirements for every participant in an athletic program should be a medical examination to determine physical fitness and capacity to engage in such a program. The strenuous nature of athletics and the demands placed upon the participant make it imperative that a thorough medical examination be required. This should be a practice in all schools and colleges and for all individuals.

The medical examination may be conducted by the family, school, or college physician. The trend appears to be to have the examination given by the family physician. However, the best method of administering the examination should be determined in light of local conditions. The school or college physician should review the examination results and health histories or otherwise determine if there are any defects or other conditions that would be aggravated by participation. No student should be permitted to participate unless a physician can state that he or she is fit for such competition.

Safety. Everything possible should be done to ensure that the safety of the participant is provided for. Only well-trained and qualified coaches should be permitted to be on the staff. Such a coach will always conduct the program with the health of the players in mind. He or she will have a knowledge of first aid and will be continually alert to stop players from further participation if they are unduly fatigued; have received head, spine, or neck injuries; or are dazed. He or she will not allow a player who has been unconscious as a result of injury to resume play until a thorough check and

approval have been given by a qualified physician. The coach will also work closely with the team or school physician, trying to make every effort possible to guard the health of the players.*

Proper conditioning and training should take place before any player is subjected to competition. Such conditioning and training should be progressive in nature and allow for gradual achievement of a state of acceptable physical fitness. There should always be enough players on the squad to allow for substitutions in the event a person is not physically or otherwise fit for play.

Proper facilities and equipment should be available to guard the safety and health of the players. This means that facilities are constructed according to recommended standards in respect to size, surfacing, and various safety features. Protective equipment should be provided as needed in the various sports. If desirable facilities and equipment are not available, such competition should not be provided.

Games should be scheduled that result in equal and safe competition. The desire of small schools to defeat larger schools, where the competition is not equal, often brings disastrous results to the health and welfare of the players. Under such circumstances, one often hears the remark, ''They really took a beating.'' Competition should be as equitable as possible.

Prompt attention should be given to all injuries. Injured players should be examined by a physician and given proper treatment. There should be complete medical supervision of the athletic program. The trainer is not a substitute. A medical doctor should be present at all games and practices, if at all possible. The doctor should be the one to determine the extent of injury. A player after being ill or hurt should not be permitted to participate again until the coach receives an approved statement from the family, school, or college physician.

Proper sanitary measures should be taken. Individual towels and drinking cups should be provided. The day of the ''team'' towel and the ''team'' drinking cup has passed. Equipment and uniforms should be cleaned as often as

---

*See also Chapter 13.

*See Chapter 13 concerning health services.

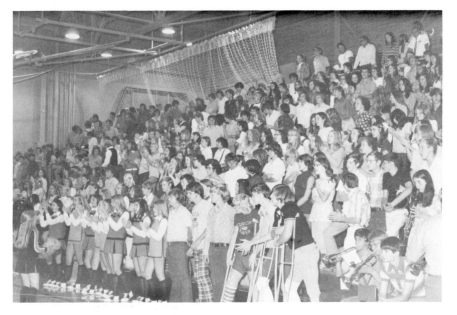

Guidelines exist to help in controlling crowds at sporting events. Students at a pep assembly at Prairie Senior High School, Cedar Rapids, Iowa.

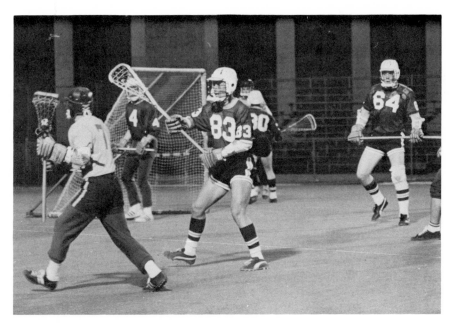

Everything possible should be done to guard the safety of players. NCAA championship competition in lacrosse on the Astro Turf of Hofstra Stadium, New York. (Courtesy NCAA.)

necessary. Locker, dressing, shower, toilet, and other rooms that are used by players should be kept clean and in a sanitary condition. Playing areas should be kept clean and safe. Gymnasiums should be properly heated, and every measure taken to ensure as nearly ideal conditions as possible for students engaging in the athletics program.

Injuries and insurance. * The state athletic association in many states sponsors an athletic insurance plan. Such plans pay various medical, x-ray, dental, hospitalization, and other expenses according to the terms of the plan. There are also some private insurance companies that have such plans. The Wisconsin Interscholastic Athletic Association with its Athletic Accident Plan, recognized as one of the better types of athletic insurance, was a pioneer in the field. This plan covers injuries incurred during practice for or participation in interscholastic athletics. It has a premium rate for "all sports" coverage and also one for all sports except football. As pointed out by this association, the purpose of the plan is to provide enrolled athletes with benefits that will help to meet the cost of medical, dental, and hospital care in the event of accidental injury resulting from participation in physical education or athletics sponsored by a participating school. The amount of any payment for an injury shall be only in the amount of the actual expenses incurred but not in excess of the amounts listed in the schedule of allowance for such injury. In order to collect benefits, plan requirements must be met.

The insurance covered by various state and independent plans usually includes benefits for accidental death or dismemberment, hospital expenses, x-ray fees, physicians' fees, and surgical and dental expenses. Dental benefits may or may not be included in the schedule of surgical benefits. In some plans, catastrophe benefits are also available for injuries requiring extensive medical care and long-term hospitalization. Coverage is normally provided on a deductible basis, with the insurance company paying 75% to 80% of the total cost over the deductible amount up to a maximum of $2,500 to $5,000.

*See also Chapter 18.

After the Wisconsin High School Athletic Association inaugurated its school athletic insurance in 1930, several other state high school athletic associations followed suit. The number of such athletic insurance plans reached twenty-five in the 1940's. However, the commercial insurance industry, seeing the promise and need for athletic insurance, gradually came into the market, some of them providing many attractive policies. Many school administrators were sympathetic to this type of coverage. Increasingly, the commercial insurance people have gained a strong foothold in the school athletic insurance program and today many schools and colleges utilize their policies.

State high school athletic associations in a few states still operate successful benefit plans, primarily by adopting many of the benefits utilized by the insurance industry, namely, nonallocated benefits, catastrophic coverage, and nonduplication of benefits.

California is the only state in this country that by law requires schools to furnish accident insurance for pupils. However, most school districts voluntarily purchase athletic insurance or make it available to parents.

Every school and college should have a written policy in regard to financial and other responsibilities associated with injuries. The administrator, parents, and players should be thoroughly familiar with the responsibilities of each in regard to injuries.

Drug abuse. Drug abuse among high school and college students is a reality—one that must be recognized and treated. The athlete is no exception to the growing use of drugs among students. Many coaches and physical educators labor under the assumption that the rigid training and health requirements of athletes somehow protect them from drug abuse. However, it must be recognized that athletes are a part of the whole school social environment and intense peer group pressures are exerted on them just as they are on other students.

It is important that programs be developed to come face-to-face with the drug problem. Some suggestions in formulating an antidrug abuse program include:

1. A major effort for the coordination and exchange of information concerning drug

abuse by universities and professional organizations is vitally important.

2. Teacher training programs should provide physical educators and coaches with knowledge of adolescent psychology and human development.

3. Athletic administrators should demonstrate to their respective communities the fact that athletic activities contribute to an effective anti–drug abuse program.

4. Support must be elicited from community members and public service groups in the fight against drug abuse.

5. It is important to involve a student's family in activities to aid in cementing family relationships. Athletic activities may be enjoyed by all family members and help to bridge the communication gaps that may exist.

In addition to drug abuse, alcohol abuse has once again appeared as a threat to our young people. Many students who have lost interest in drugs or have become fearful of the effects of drugs have started drinking alcohol in large quantities. Athletic administrators should be aware of alcohol abuse and conduct staff information programs to acquaint physical and health educators and coaches with the aspects of the problem. An antialcohol campaign should be introduced in all physical education and health education classes and should be fully discussed with all athletes.

Contracts

Written contracts are usually essential in the administration of interscholastic and intercollegiate athletics. On the college level, in particular, games are scheduled many months or years in advance. Memories and facts tend to fade and become obscure with time. In order to avoid misunderstanding and confusion, it is best to have in writing a contract between the schools or colleges concerned.

Contracts should be properly executed and signed by official representatives of both schools and colleges. Many athletic associations provide specially prepared forms for use of member schools or colleges. Such forms usually contain the names of the schools, dates, and circumstances and conditions under which the contest will be held. Furthermore, they usually provide for penalties if the contract is not fulfilled by either party.

Officials

The officials will greatly influence the interscholastic or intercollegiate athletic program and determine whether it is conducted in a manner that will be of most benefit to the players and the schools or colleges concerned. Officials should be well qualified. They should know the rules and be able to interpret them accurately; recognize their responsibility to the players; be good sportsmen; and be courteous, honest, friendly, cooperative, impartial, and able to control the game at all times.

In order to ensure that only the best officials are utilized, machinery should be established to register and determine those who are qualified. Officials should be required to pass examinations on rules and to demonstrate their competency. Rating scales have been developed that aid in making such estimates. Most athletic associations have some method of registering and certifying those acceptable officials whom they wish to use. The National Association for Girls and Women in Sport of AAHPER has a rating committee that certifies officials. In some states the officials who are used, in turn, rate the schools or colleges as to facilities, environment, and circumstances surrounding the game.

Subject to contract differences, officials usually are chosen by the home team with approval of opponents. The practice of the home team selecting officials without any consideration of the wishes of other schools or colleges or regard for impartial officiating has resulted in relations that have not been in the best interests of players or of athletics in general. A growing practice of having the conference or association select officials to be used has many points in its favor.

Officials should be duly notified of such details as the date and time of the contests to which they have been assigned. Officials' fees usually vary from school to school and from college to college, although some associations have set up standard rates. It is usually considered best to pay a flat fee that includes

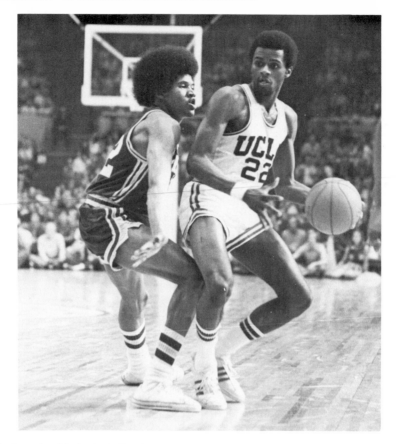

NCAA championship basketball. (Courtesy NCAA.) (Photograph by Malcolm W. Emmons.)

salary and expenses, rather than to list both separately.

Protests and forfeitures

There should be a set procedure for handling protests and forfeitures in connection with athletic contests. Of course, there should be careful preventive action beforehand in order to avoid a situation where such protests and forfeitures will occur. Proper interpretation of the rules, good officiating, elimination of undue pressures, and proper education of schools, colleges, and coaches on the objectives of interscholastic and intercollegiate athletics will act as preventive measures against such action.

However, the essential procedure for filing protests and forfeitures of contests should be established. This procedure should be clearly stated in writing and contain all the details, such as the person to whom the protest should

be sent, time limits involved, person or group responsible for action, and any other information that is necessary. A frequent reason for a protest is the utilization of ineligible players. Most associations require the forfeiture of any game in which ineligible players participate.

Game management

Since there are so many details in connection with game management it is possible to include only a brief statement of the more important items. In order to have an efficiently conducted contest, it is important to have good organization. There must be someone responsible. Attention must be given to details. There must be planning. Many details must be attended to before the game, during the game, and after the game. Some of these details include: (1) before-game preparation, (2) game responsibilities, (3) after-game responsibilities, and

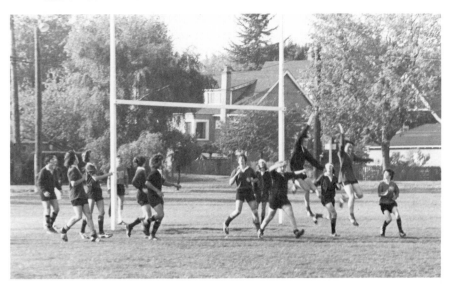

Practice periods are important but should not intrude on students' time excessively. High school rugby at Balaclava Park in Vancouver. (Courtesy Board of Parks and Public Recreation, Vancouver, B. C.)

(4) preparation for out-of-town games. Before a home game, such details as contracts, eligibility records, equipment, facilities, tickets, public relations, medical supervision, officials, and physical examinations must be thoroughly checked. Game responsibilities at home games include such items as supplies and equipment, entertainment, tickets and ushers, scoreboards, public-address system, presence of physician, and quarters for visiting teams. The responsibilities after a home game consist of such items as payments to officials and visiting school, records of receipts, record of officials, and participation records. When preparing for an out-of-town game, such important details as parents' permissions, transportation, funding, contracts, personnel, and records must be attended to.

Schedules and practice periods

The trend in athletics is to limit the length of seasons for various sports. If this is not done, overemphasis often results with a particular sport monopolizing the time of students and allowing only little time for other activities. Football has often been accused of this with its fall practice before school or college starts, postseason games that run into the new year, spring practice, and summer work in

preparation for the fall season. Such a schedule is not in the interests of the students' general welfare.

There should be defined limits in respect to the length of seasons. These should have the approval of school and college authorities. The length of seasons should be so arranged that they interfere as little as possible with other school and college work. They should provide for adequate practice before the first game so that the players are in good physical condition. There should be limits on the total number of games, depending upon the sport, and also on the number of games played in any one week. Postseason games are not considered advisable by many educators. Teams that are as nearly as possible of equal ability and equal skill should be scheduled.

Awards

The basis for awards in interscholastic and intercollegiate athletics is the same as that for intramural and extramural athletics. As pointed out, there are arguments for and against giving awards. Some individuals feel that the values derived from playing a sport—joy and satisfaction, physical, social, and other values—are sufficient in themselves and that no awards should be given. Others point to the fact that awards are symbolic of achievement and are traditional in this culture and should be given.

The policy that will be adopted in respect to awards should be determined locally. A definite policy should be established that cuts across all the affairs of the school or college. At the present time the practice of giving awards in the form of letters, insignia, or some other symbol is almost universal. It is recommended that when awards are given they should be very simple and of very little monetary value. Some state athletic associations, for example, have stated that the award should not cost more than $1.00. Furthermore, it seems wise not to distinguish between so-called major and minor sports when giving awards. They should be treated on an equal basis.

Below is the statement of the philosophy and principles for administering athletic awards used in one school system.

Records

The good administrator and coach will keep accurate records of all the details concerned

---

STATEMENT OF PHILOSOPHY REGARDING AWARDS

There are arguments pro and con in respect to awards for athletic participation. Some of the arguments for awards are: they stimulate interest, they serve as an incentive for participation, and they recognize achievement. Some of the arguments against awards are: they make for a more expensive program, a few individuals win most of them, they are unnecessary since students would participate even if no awards were given, it is difficult to make awards on the basis of all factors that should be considered, and the incentive is artificial since the joy and satisfaction received are enough reward in themselves.

Although the conferring of awards is overdone in many cases, the practice of giving out valuable awards indiscriminately cannot be justified educationally or financially. The responsibility of the physical education department is to teach boys and girls to play for the "love of playing" without any thought of an award. It is the feeling of this committee that the human desire for recognition is most natural. The receiving of an award for achievement in athletics in the form of a ribbon, emblem, certificate, or simple medal fosters personal pride in accomplishment. Academically, we recognize students with high grades. We select valedictorians and members of local and national honor societies.

Awards are symbols of achievement and should not be recognized as a prize. In Greek times the olive wreath given to a victor was the most coveted award that could be obtained by a Greek athlete. The importance of such an award was not its material value, but what it symbolized. The custom of awarding insignia or letters by school and college authorities to athletic teams in order to foster school spirit and personal pride in accomplishment and set up high ideals of sportsmanship is almost universal. Because of the long tradition of granting awards and because of the fact that this is a common practice in other activities of life, simple awards—mere symbols of achievement with little or no monetary value—seem to be justifiable.

The school should consider such factors as attitude, dependability, school citizenship, scholarship, participation, and improvement, as well as athletic prowess, in establishing a policy for the conferring of awards. Such a practice would make it advisable for many school officials to be involved in the determination of who receives awards. Furthermore, the basis for students receiving awards should be broadened to include as many levels and kinds of achievement as possible while still keeping the award meaningful as a form of recognition.

Principles for administering athletic awards

1. Awards should have little or no monetary value and should serve as a symbol of achievement.
2. Awards should not detract from the primary goal, namely, the enjoyment of the activity for the activity itself.
3. Opportunities should be provided for all students to obtain awards.
4. Good sportsmanship, scholarship, character, attitude, and citizenship should be considered along with participation and achievement in the conferring of awards.
5. Awards should be presented as a culminating activity of the physical education program.
6. Money for awards should come from the budgeted school funds and not be secured through clubs, alumni, and civic organizations.
7. Awards and dinners or other events given in honor of athletes, should be sponsored *only* by school authorities and not by clubs, alumni, or civic organizations.
8. There should be no major and minor distinction in presenting awards.

with the administration of interscholastic or intercollegiate athletics. There should be records of students' participation, for eligibility purposes and to show the extent of the program; records of the conduct of various sports from year to year so that they can be compared over a period of time and also compared with other schools and colleges; statistical summaries of player and game performance that will help the coach to determine weaknesses in game strategy or identify players' performances and other items essential to well-organized play; records of equipment and supplies; officials' records; financial records, and other items in connection with the conduct of the total program. Good business and good administration demand good record keeping.

Transportation

Transporting athletes to games and contests presents many administrative problems. Such questions arise as; Who should be transported? In what kind of vehicles should athletes be transported? Is athletics part of a regular school or college program? Should private vehicles or school- and college-owned vehicles be used? What are the legal implications involved in transporting athletes in school- and college-sponsored events?

It appears that the present trend is to view athletics as an integral part of the educational program so that public funds may be used for transportation purposes. At the same time, however, statutes vary from state to state, and persons administering athletic programs should examine carefully the statutes in their own state.

The energy crisis has presented a problem in the area of transportation. Because of the shortage and increased expense of fuel many interscholastic and intercollegiate programs are being curtailed or dropped from the calendar. It is recommended that schools try to conduct athletic activities on school days, use public transportation, and utilize carpools wherever possible.

The feeling among many administrators in regard to transportation is that athletes and representatives of the school or college concerned, such as band and cheerleaders, should travel only in transportation provided by the educational institution. Where private cars belonging to coaches, students, or other persons are used, the administrator should be sure to determine whether the procedures are in conformity with the state statutes regarding liability. Under no circumstances should students or other representatives be permitted to drive unless they are authorized drivers and recognized as such by the state statutes. Under most circumstances it is recommended that students not be used as drivers.

SOME ADMINISTRATIVE PROBLEMS

There are many problems with which the administration of any interscholastic or intercollegiate athletic program has to contend. Some that are particularly prominent at the present time are those concerned with (1) gate receipts, (2) tournaments and championships, (3) eligibility, (4) scholarships, (5) recruitment, (6) proselyting, (7) scouting, and (8) austerity budgets.

Gate receipts

Gate receipts are the source of many unfortunate practices in athletics. Too often they become the point of emphasis rather than the valuable educational outcomes that can accrue to the participant. When this occurs, athletics cannot justify existence in the educational program. Furthermore, the emphasis on gate receipts results in a vicious cycle—the money increases the desire for winning teams so that there will be greater financial return, which in turn results in greater financial outlays to secure and develop even better teams. This goes on and on, resulting in a false set of standards forming the basis for the program.

Throughout the country interscholastic and intercollegiate athletics are financed through many different sources. These include gate receipts, board of education and central university funds, donations, special projects, students' fees, physical education department funds, magazine subscriptions, and concessions. In high schools a "general organization" quite frequently handles the funds for athletics.

Some colleges finance part of the program through endowment funds.

It has long been argued by leaders in the physical education profession that athletics have great educational potentials. They are curricular in nature rather than extracurricular. This means they contribute to the welfare of students like any other subject in the curriculum. Upon this basis, therefore, the finances necessary to support such a program should come from board of education or central university funds. Athletics should not be self-supporting or used as a means to support part or all of the other so-called extracurricular activities of a school or college. They represent an integral part of the educational program and as such deserve to be treated in the same manner as other aspects of the program. This procedure is followed in some schools and colleges with benefits to all concerned and should be an ideal toward which all should strive.

Tournaments and championships

The question frequently arises as to whether postseason tournaments and championship playoffs should be conducted as part of an athletic program. It is generally agreed by physical education leaders that all the educational values that can be derived from athletics can be gained without ever playing a tournament or championship game. The main purposes of such ventures are usually to make money, to entertain the public, and to crown a winner. Furthermore, many problems enter the picture when tournaments and championships are conducted. As a result of such contests the emphasis on winning becomes more pronounced, participation often results in physical and emotional strain on players, spectator pressure increases, gambling often enters the picture, and the emphasis is on a few individuals.

Eligibility

Standards in regard to the eligibility of contestants are essential. These should be in writing, disseminated widely, and clearly understood by all concerned. They should be established well ahead of a season's or year's play so that the student, coaches, and others will not become emotional when they suddenly realize

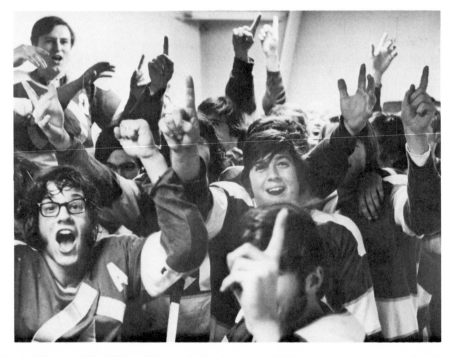

The College of Dupage, Glen Ellyn, Ill., varsity hockey team celebrates winning the state championship and receiving a bid to the National Tournament.

they will lose their chance to win a championship because they cannot use a star player who is ineligible.

Standards of eligibility in interscholastic circles usually include an age limit of not more than 19 or 20 years; a requirement that an athlete be a bona fide student; rules on transfer students that frequently require their being bona fide residents in the community served by the school; satisfactory grades; a limit of three or four on number of seasons of competition allowed (playing in one game usually constitutes a season); regular attendance at school; permission to play on only one team during a season; and a requirement that the participant have a medical examination, amateur status, and parent's consent. These regulations vary from school to school and from state to state.

The National Federation of State High School Athletic Associations considers a student ineligible for amateur standing if (1) he or she has accepted money or compensation for playing in an athletic contest, (2) he or she has played under an assumed name, (3) he or she has competed with a team whose players received pay for their playing, and (4) he or she has signed a contract to play with a professional team.

Eligibility requirements at the college and university level include rules in respect to such items as residence, undergraduate status, academic average, amateur status, limits of participation, and transfer. In some cases players must have been in residence for at least 1 year, whereas in others they can play as freshmen. Furthermore, they must be bona fide, fully matriculated students carrying on a full program of studies; have a satisfactory grade-point average; and have had only so many years of competition. Also, a student cannot participate after the expiration of four consecutive 12-month periods following the date of initial enrollment in an institution of higher learning. Amateur status is also a requirement.

Scholarships

Should athletes receive scholarships or special financial assistance in schools and colleges? This subject is argued pro and con and is mainly a problem at the college level. Those in favor

of scholarships and financial assistance claim that a student who excels in sports should receive aid just as much as one who excels in music or any other subject area. They claim that such inducements are justified in the educational picture. Those opposed point to the fact that scholarships should be awarded on the basis of the need and general academic qualifications of a student, rather than skill in some sport. Another controversy concerns the right of women to also receive athletic scholarships.

One solution is to have a list of criteria drawn up for the purpose of making such grants and have them handled by an all-school or all-college committee. This plan is based on the premise that scholarships and student aid should not be granted to the athletic or to any other department. Instead, they should be handled on an all-school or all-college basis and given to students who need them most and are best qualified. In this way, those students who are in need of assistance, regardless of the area in which they specialize, will be the ones who will receive aid.

Recruitment

The recruitment of athletes in order to develop star and winning teams is not condoned for any educational institution. The procedure for admittance should be the same for all students, regardless of whether they are athletes, chemistry students, music students, or others. No special consideration should be shown to any particular group. The same standards, academic and otherwise, should prevail.

Athletic teams should be composed of matriculated students attracted to the school or college because of its educational advantages. Recruitment policies for the primary purpose of developing winning teams should be avoided in all institutions of higher learning. In addition, outside support in the funding and recruitment of athletes indicates a problematic athletic environment.

Proselyting

Proselyting is a term applied to a high school or college that has so strongly overemphasized athletics that it has stooped to unethical behavior to secure outstanding talent for winning teams. High schools are not troubled with this problem as much as colleges, but in some quarters they also have difficulties. There have been incidents where a father was provided employment so that he would move his family to a particular section of a city or a particular community so that his boy would be eligible to play with the local team. However, thanks to vigilant state athletic associations, such incidents have been kept to a minimum. The following represent some of the rules in force in many states to eliminate special inducements to attract athletes. These rules have been established by many state high school athletic associations:

1. Only acceptable forms of recognition should be presented to athletes. These usually include letters, monograms, or school insignias.
2. The educational institution or athletic association should be the only source of awards to athletes.
3. No student should be the recipient of special treatment from any outside organization.
4. Complimentary dinners (from local organizations) may be accepted by athletic teams if approved by the superintendent of schools.

Scouting

Scouting has become an accepted practice at high school and college levels. By watching another team perform, the formations and plays used will be known and certain weaknesses will be discovered. One coach said that his scouting consisted of watching players to determine little mannerisms they had that would give away the play that was going to be used.

Many schools and colleges are spending considerable money in this manner. Some schools and colleges scout a rival team every game during the season. Some use three or four persons on the same scouting assignment, and such schools and colleges take moving pictures at length so that the opponent's play can be studied in great detail. Such money, it is felt by some physical educators, could be spent more wisely if used to enhance the value of the game for the participants, rather than to further any all-important effort to win.

Many unethical practices have entered into scouting. Coaches have been known to have scouts observe secret practice sessions and utilize other unethical methods. Scouting is considered unethical under any circumstances except by means of observing regularly scheduled games. If scouting does occur, the head coach at the institution has direct responsibility for the action.

Many coaches feel that the only reason they want to scout is that they themselves are being scouted. Therefore, they feel it will work to their disadvantage unless they follow the same procedure. If something could be done to eliminate or restrict scouting, considerable time and money could be put to much more advantageous use.

Austerity budgets

A recent survey indicates that one out of every five U. S. primary and secondary schools has cut back athletic programs or may soon do so, as a result of budgetary difficulties. Declining athletic support has also resulted in lessened support for other nonacademic activities. This survey, conducted by Compass-Competitive Athletics in Service to Society, polled 1,543 athletic directors in all 50 states in order to determine the current status of school athletic programs.* Some of the results indicated by the survey are:

1. Bond issue and tax levy referendums had a success rate of only 54.4%, as compared to 74.7% in 1964 to 1965.
2. Twenty-six percent of the directors polled indicated they had no local support for rebuilding community interest in sports programs.
3. One of every seven athletic directors was not aware of any method to aid in boosting public support for athletic programs.
4. Of athletic directors with jeopardized programs, 27% reported cutbacks in their schools' coaching staff, sometimes along with salary reductions among employed coaches.

It is interesting to note that this survey indicated a notable increase in organized athletic activity for girls, even in schools facing financial cutbacks. Almost 90% of all athletic directors responded that organized girls' athletics had increased. In schools not suffering financial problems, more than 98% reported an increase in girls' sports.

---

*School athletes face austerity budgets, Sportscope, September-October, 1973.

Financial problems in school districts are apparent throughout the country in large and small communities alike. Some examples of austerity budgets and their implications for school athletic programs are discussed here.

Philadelphia, Pennsylvania. Because of a $30 million deficit, the Philadelphia School Board cut all athletic programs in Philadelphia schools in the school year 1971 to 1972. Only after a public outcry did a deficit program go into effect to restore most of the cut programs.

San Francisco, California. Budget cuts in the 1971 to 1972 school year deprived San Francisco public school students of interscholastic athletics at the junior high school level and intramural activities at the high school level.

Waldwick, New Jersey. In order to keep this community within an austerity budget, the school board proposed the elimination of all interscholastic sports, saving $70,000 in expenses.

These are only a few of the countless communities that are suffering under austerity programs. It is unfortunate that athletic programs are often the first to be cut. Athletic administrators have an urgent responsibility to make their programs known to the public and to generate community and school administrative support for the continuance of athletic programs.

INTERSCHOLASTIC ATHLETICS AT THE ELEMENTARY AND JUNIOR HIGH SCHOOL LEVELS

Since athletics were first introduced into the educational picture, there has been a continual pushing downward of these competitive experiences into the lower education levels. Educational athletics started at the college level with a crew race between Harvard and Yale in 1852. Then other sports were introduced to the campuses throughout the United States. As higher education athletic programs expanded and gained recognition and popularity, the high schools felt that sports should also be a part of their educational offerings. As a result, most high schools in America today have some form of interscholastic athletics. In recent years, junior high schools have also felt the impact of

interscholastic athletic programs. A survey made by the National Association of Secondary-School Principals, and including 2,296 junior high schools, showed that 85.2% had some program of interscholastic athletics while 14.8% did not.

There should not be any interscholastic athletics at the elementary school level. In kindergarten to grade six physical activities should be geared to the developmental level of the child. Starting with grade four it may be possible to initiate an intramural program on an informal basis. However, there should not be undue emphasis on developing skill in a few sports or requiring children to conform to adult standards of competition.

The special nature of grades seven through nine, representing a transition period between the elementary school and the senior high school and between childhood and adolescence, has raised a question in the minds of many educators as to whether an interscholastic athletic program is in the best interests of the students concerned.

Many of the guidelines of the American Academy of Pediatrics listed below apply to the junior high school level, as well as to the elementary school level, and to the type of athletic competition that should be offered:

1. All children should have opportunities to develop skill in a variety of activities.
2. All such activities should take into account the age and developmental level of child.
3. a. Athletic activities of elementary school children should be part of an over-all school program. Competent medical supervision of each child should be ensured.
   b. Health observation by teachers and others should be encouraged and help given by the physician.
4. Athletic activities outside of the school program should be on an entirely voluntary basis without undue emphasis on any special program or sport, and without undue emphasis upon winning. These programs should also include competent medical supervision.
5. Competitive programs organized on school, neighborhood and community levels will meet the needs of children twelve years of age and under. State, regional and national tournaments; bowl, charity and exhibition games are not recommended for this age group. Commercial exploitation in any form is unequivocally condemned.
6. Body-contact sports, particularly tackle football and

boxing, are considered to have no place in programs for children of this age.

7. Competition is an inherent characteristic of growing developing children. Properly guided it is beneficial and not harmful to their development.

8. Schools and communities as a whole must be made aware of the needs for personnel, facilities, equipment and supplies which will assure an adequate program for children in this age group.

9. All competitive athletic programs should be organized with the cooperation of interested medical groups who will ensure adequate medical care before and during such programs. This should include thorough physical examinations at specified intervals, teaching of health observation to teachers and coaches, as well as attention to factors such as: (a) injury; (b) response to fatigue; (c) individual emotional needs; and (d) the risks of undue emotional strains.

10. Muscle testing is not, per se, a valid estimate of physical fitness, or of good health.

11. Participation in group activities is expected of every child. When there is a failure to do so, or lack of interest, underlying physical or emotional causes should be sought.

12. Leadership for young children, should be such that highly organized, highly competitive programs would be avoided. The primary consideration should be a diversity of wholesome childhood experiences which will aid in the proper physical and emotional development of the child into a secure and well-integrated adult.

The research in regard to a highly organized athletics at the junior high school level indicates points of substantial agreement, as listed in the following section:*

1. The junior high school educational program should be adapted to the needs of boys and girls in grades seven, eight, and nine. This is a period of transition from elementary school to senior high school and from childhood to adolescence. It is a time when students are trying to understand their bodies, gain independence, achieve adult social status, acquire self-confidence, and establish a system of values. It is a time when a program of education unique to this age group is needed to meet the abilities and broadening interests of the student.

2. The best educational program at the junior high school level is one that provides for pro-

gram enrichment to meet the needs of students in grades seven through nine, rather than using the senior high school or other educational level as a blueprint to follow.

3. There is need for a distinct and separate educational climate for these grades in order to ensure that the program will not be influenced unduly by either the elementary or the senior high school.

4. There is a need for teachers (including coaches) whose full responsibilities involve working with grades seven, eight, and nine and whose training has included an understanding of the needs of these students and of the educational program required to meet those needs.

5. The junior high school should provide for exploratory experiences with specialization delayed until senior high school and college.

6. The junior high school should provide for the mental, physical, social, and emotional development of students.

7. Out-of-class as well as in-class experiences should be provided.

8. There should be concern for the development of a sound standard of values in each student.

9. The principal and other members of the administration have the responsibility for providing sound educational leadership in all school matters. The type of physical education and athletic programs offered will reflect the type of leadership provided.

10. The physical education program at the junior high school level should consist of a class program, an adapted program, and intramural and extramural programs (the interscholastic athletic program is controversial).

11. The interscholastic athletics program, if offered, should be provided only after the prerequisites of excellent physical education class, adapted, and intramural and extramural programs have been developed, and only as special controls in regard to such items as health, facilities, game adaptations, classification of players, leadership, and officials have been provided.

12. The physical education program should be adapted to the needs of the junior high school student. There is a need for a wide variety of activities, based on physical and neuromuscular

---

*New York State Education Department: Interscholastic athletics at the junior high school level, Albany, 1965, The Department. (Charles Bucher, consultant, New York State Department of Education.)

maturation, that will contribute to the development of body control, enable each student to experience success, provide for recognition of energy output and fatigue, and take into consideration the "growth spurt" of early adolescence.

13. The physical education program should represent a favorable social and emotional climate for the student. There should be freedom from anxiety and fear, absence of tensions and strains, a feeling of belonging for each student, a social awareness that contributes to the development of such important traits as respect for the rights of others, and an atmosphere that is conducive to growing into social and emotional maturity.

14. Personal health instruction should be closely integrated into the physical education program.

15. Coeducational activities should be provided.

16. All physical activities should be carefully supervised medically and conducted under optimal health and safety conditions.

17. Students who are not physiologically mature should not engage in activities where there is danger of body contact, a high degree of skill is required, great amounts of endurance are necessary, and highly competitive conditions are present.

18. Physiologic maturity is the best criterion for determining whether a student is physiologically ready for participation in most interscholastic athletic activities.

19. Competition itself is not the factor that makes athletics dangerous to the physiologically mature student. Instead, such items as the manner in which the program is conducted, type of activity, facilities, leadership, and physical condition of the student are the determining factors.

20. Physiologic fitness can be developed

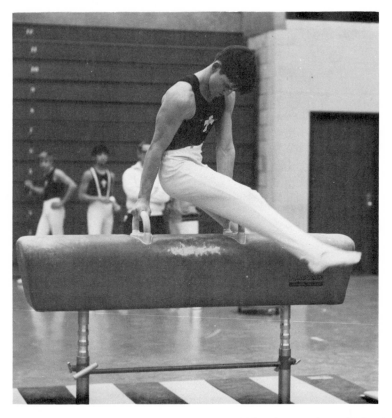

Interscholastic athletics in gymnastics at Thornwood High School, South Holland, Ill.

without exposure to an interscholastic athletic program.

21. Competitive athletics, if properly conducted, have the potential for satisfying such basic psychologic needs as recognition, belonging, self-respect, and feeling of achievement, as well as providing a wholesome outlet for the physical activity drive. However, if conducted in the light of adult interests, community pressures, and other questionable influences, they can prove psychologically harmful.

22. Interscholastic athletics, when conducted in accordance with desirable standards of leadership, educational philosophy, activities, and other pertinent factors, have the potential for realizing beneficial social effects for the student, but when not conducted in accordance with desirable standards they can be socially detrimental to the student.

23. Of all competitive activities, tackle football, ice hockey, and boxing are subject to most criticism as being of questionable value for junior high school students.

INTERSCHOLASTIC ATHLETICS AT THE HIGH SCHOOL LEVEL

The responsibility of the school for the interscholastic athletic program is one that cannot be avoided. Therefore, it is essential that all administrators be aware of the best practices recommended for the various phases of the total program. These are listed in the checklist of recommended standards on p. 245.

ATHLETICS IN TWO-YEAR COLLEGES

In order to determine the status of athletics at 2-year colleges, a survey was recently conducted among 448 junior colleges. * The survey was concerned about physical education, intramurals, athletics, and administration. An analysis of the survey results indicates that 2-year colleges utilize facilities, staff, and funds to their finest potential in all programs.

---

*Yarnell, D.: Implications of a recent survey of physical education and athletics in two-year colleges, JUCO Review **23:**20, 1971.

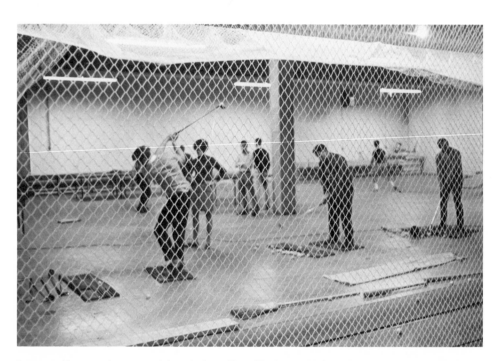

Second year college students practicing their golf at Florissant Valley Community College in St. Louis. (Photograph by LeMoyne Coates.)

The following checklist provides an evaluation aid in determining the relationship of the high school athletic program to the total educational program.

	Yes	No
1. Athletic program an integral part of total curriculum		
a. The sports are an outgrowth of the physical education program.		
b. A variety of sports is available for all students.		
c. The educational values of sport are foremost in the philosophy.		
d. All students have an opportunity to participate in a sport.		
e. Athletics are used appropriately as a school's unifying force.		
f. Athletes are not excused from courses, including physical education, because of athletic participation.		
2. Coaches as faculty members		
a. Coaches have an adequate opportunity to exercise the rights and privileges of other faculty members in determining school and curricular matters.		
b. Coaches attend, and they are scheduled so they may attend, faculty meetings.		
c. Coaches are not expected to assume more duties of a general nature than are other faculty members.		
d. Teaching tenure and other faculty privileges are available to athletic personnel.		
e. Assignments for extra duties are made for coaches on the same basis as for other teachers.		
3. Participants encouraged by activities to perform adequately in academic areas		
a. Athletes are held accountable scholastically at the same level as other students.		
b. Practices are of such length and intensity that they do not deter students' academic pursuits.		
c. Game trips do not cause the students to miss an excessive number of classes.		
d. Counseling services emphasize the importance of academic records in regard to career education.		
e. Athletes are required to attend classes on days of contests.		
4. Meeting philosophy of school board		
a. New coaches are made aware of the board policies, and informed that they will be expected to follow them in spirit as well as letter.		
b. All coaches are regularly informed by the principal and athletic director that they must practice within the framework of board policy.		
c. A procedure is available for the athletic director and coaches to make recommendations regarding policy change.		
d. Noncoaching faculty members are made aware of board policy regarding athletics so they may discuss it from a base of fact.		
e. The philosophy of the board is written and made available to all personnel.		
5. Awards		
a. Only those intrinsic awards authorized by local conferences and state athletic associations are given.		
b. Diligence is exercised to insure that outside groups do not cause violations of the award regulations.		
c. Care is taken to assure that athletes are not granted privileges not available to the general student body.		
6. Projected program outcomes		
a. It is emphasized that participation in athletics is a privilege.		
b. Development of critical thinking as well as athletic performance is planned into the program.		
c. Development of self-direction and individual motivation is a real part of the athletic experience.		
d. The athletes are allowed to develop at their own cognitive, psychomotor and effective readiness level.		
e. The accepted social values are used as standards of behavior both on and off the playing area.		
7. Guarding against student exploitation		
a. The student is not used in athletic performance to provide an activity that has as its main purpose entertainment of the community.		

Continued.

	Yes	No
b. The student's academic program is in no way altered to allow him to maintain eligibility with less than normal effort on his part.	_____	_____
c. The student is not given a false impression of his athletic ability through the device of suggesting the possibility of a college scholarship.	_____	_____
d. The athletes are not given a false image of the value of their athletic prowess to the material and cultural success within the school and community.*	_____	_____

*National Council of Secondary School Athletic Directors: Evaluating the high school athletic program, Washington, D. C., 1973, American Association for Health, Physical Education, and Recreation.

The extent of the athletic program appears to be directly related to the size of the school and the method of financing. Community colleges and branches of state universities exhibited the most athletic teams and had the largest student bodies. Private junior colleges had smaller enrollments and fewer athletic teams. Eligibility requirements were usually based on certain academic standards, class attendance, amateur status, and health status. The majority of junior colleges belong to the National Junior College Athletic Association (NJCAA) and accept their rules of eligibility.

This survey indicated that most 2-year colleges prefer professionally trained coaches with the exception of technical schools. Coaches are usually drawn from the physical education staff and other faculty members. Compensation is given for coaching in the form of extra pay, including coaching in the base salary, and by reduced teaching loads.

The survey also indicated that physical education is an integral part of the 2-year college curriculum, with more than 80% of the schools polled requiring physical education. In addition, most colleges had intramural programs, usually financed by student activity fees. It is interesting to note here that women were not found to be as involved in athletics as often as men. Approximately one-fourth of the reporting schools indicated varsity teams for women, whereas approximately 50% indicated that extramurals were provided for women.

This report on women leads us to a more recent survey* concerned with women's intercollegiate athletic programs at junior colleges in the United States. This survey polled 355

*Boojarma, L. M., and Messing, A.: A survey of women's intercollegiate athletic programs at junior colleges in the United States, JUCO Review 25:37, 1973.

junior colleges and received a 57% return of its questionnaires. The objectives of the survey were to ascertain the status of intercollegiate athletic programs in 2-year colleges and to also determine the need for national intercollegiate athletic competition among 2-year colleges in the United States.

Some of the results of the survey are given here:

In 87% of the schools, men and women worked under the same department chairman, and in 81% of the schools this person was a man.

In 67% of the responding schools, a women's intercollegiate athletic program is maintained, and 74% of the programs are under the direction of women.

The mean allocation of funds for women's intercollegiate athletic programs was $4,000, as opposed to the men's allocations of $25,000.

In some schools where the enrollment is 50% female, male physical educators outnumber women by a ratio of 2:1.

This survey suggests that women's intercollegiate athletic programs are expanding, but their continued success is dependent on (1) hiring more qualified women, (2) providing adequate facilities, and (3) giving women the opportunity for self-rule and direction.

ATHLETICS IN 4-YEAR COLLEGES AND UNIVERSITIES

It is at the college and university level that overemphasis has taken place to the largest extent in the field of varsity athletics. Commercialization flourishes when 60,000 people gather for a sports spectacle, the cost of tickets ranges from $2.00 to $8.00, and large stadiums, long trips, and many scholarships predominate. A few colleges have established "easy courses" in the curriculum so that athletes will not have to meet the usual academic standards. Records have been falsified to enable some to meet entrance requirements. Others have been given tuition, board, spending money, and sometimes even cars to attract them. Players have been recruited from various sections of the country through unethical means. Alumni pressure for winning teams, the firing of coaches, and other undesirable practices have been in evidence in some quarters.

Some of the responsibility for athletic abuses lies in the academic areas where student athletes are often encouraged to take so-called ''snap'' courses and generally perform according to subcollege standards. In addition, abuses occur when athletic events are turned into spectacles that are alien to university functions. Athletics should not be a major source of revenue or means of securing public support. Too great an emphasis on athletics can detract from the academic superiority of an institution and encourage many types of athletic abuses.

Bucher and Dupee have surveyed the standards for high school and collegiate athletics and summarized the selected recommended standards for these educational levels. They are presented here for the information and reference of the reader.

Summary of selected recommended standards for varsity interscholastic and intercollegiate athletics*

1. Organization
   a. The wholesome conduct of the athletic programs should be the ultimate responsibility of the school administration.
   b. Athletic policy should be adopted, evaluated, and supervised by a faculty committee.
   c. Athletic policy should be implemented by the director of physical education and the director of athletics.
   d. Athletics should be organized as an integral part of the department of physical education.
2. Staff
   a. All members of the coaching staff should be members of the faculty.
   b. All coaches should be hired on their qualifications to assume educational responsibilities, and not on their ability to produce winning teams.
   c. All coaches should enjoy the same privileges of tenure, rank, and salary which are accorded other similarly qualified faculty members.

*Bucher, C. A., and Dupee, R. K., Jr.: Athletics in schools and colleges, New York, 1965, The Center for Applied Research in Education, Inc. (The Library of Education), pp. 99-101.

   d. All public school coaches should be certified in physical education.
3. Finances
   a. The financing of interscholastic and intercollegiate athletics should be governed by the same policies that control the financing of all other educational activities within an institution.
   b. Gate receipts should be considered an incidental source of revenue.
4. Health and safety
   a. An annual physical examination should be required of all participants; a physical examination on a seasonal basis would be preferable.
   b. Each school should have a written policy for the implementation of an injury-care program.
   c. Each school should have a written policy concerning the responsibility for athletic injuries and should provide or make available athletic accident insurance.
   d. All coaches should be well qualified in the care and prevention of athletic injuries.
   e. A doctor should be present at all contests at which injury is possible.
   f. Only that equipment offering the best protection should be purchased.
   g. Proper fitting of all protective equipment should be insured.
   h. Competition should be scheduled only between teams of comparable ability.
   i. Games should not be played until players have had a minimum of three weeks of physical conditioning and drill.
   j. Playing fields should meet standards for size and safety.
5. Eligibility
   a. All schools should honor and respect the eligibility rules and regulations of respective local, state, and national athletic associations.
   b. A student who is not making normal progress toward a degree or diploma should not be allowed to participate.
6. Recruiting
   a. The athletic teams of each school should be composed of bona fide students who live in the school district or who were attracted to the institution by its educational program.
   b. All candidates for admission to a school should be evaluated according to the same high standards.
   c. All financial aid should be administered with regard to need and according to the same standards for all students. The recipient of financial aid should be given a statement of the amount, duration, and conditions of the award.
7. Awards
   a. The value of athletic awards should be limited.
   b. There should be no discrimination between awards for different varsity sports.
   c. The presentation of all-star, most valuable player, and most improved player awards should be discouraged.

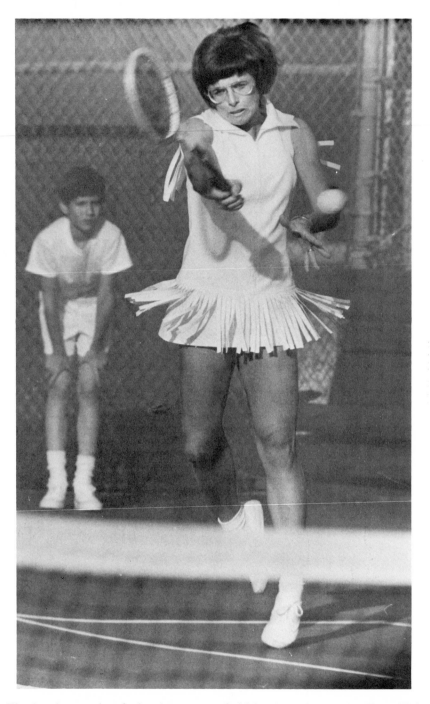

Billie Jean King has done much to further the progress of girls' and women's sports. (From Klafs, C. E., and Lyon, M. J.: The female athlete: conditioning, competition, and culture, St. Louis, 1973, The C. V. Mosby Co.)

GIRLS' AND WOMEN'S ATHLETICS

Girls and women have suffered in some school and college athletic programs. They have had limited access to many athletic activities and have often been subjected to poor equipment and dilapidated facilities. The arguments used by physical educators and administrators to justify discrimination against women in sports often centered around their supposed delicacy, health, and femininity. Recent studies indicate that women can participate in active sports, just as their male counterparts.

The women's movement and other proponents of equality in women's athletics have

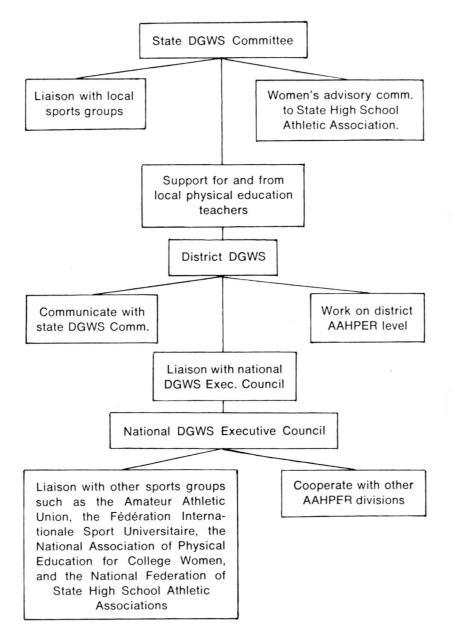

Relations of DGWS to other sports and policy-making groups. Note that DGWS in 1974 became the National Association for Girls and Women in Sport (NAGWS). (From Philosophy and standards for girls' and women's sports, American Association for Health, Physical Education, and Recreation, 1969, p. 51.)

altered the concept of women's sports in recent years. Women are becoming more and more accepted as athletes, with a full right to experience all types of sports activities. Many persons wrongly interpret this kind of statement to mean that women want to compete with men in all sports activities. This is certainly not the case. While women may compete with men in certain coeducational activities (bowling, tennis, volleyball), they generally want separate but equal athletic programs, including equal funding, equipment, and facility use.

The National Association for Girls and Women in Sport (NAGWS) of AAHPER subscribes to the belief that teams should be provided for all girls desiring competitive athletic participation. Adequate funds, facilities, and staff should be provided for these programs. This organization considers that while the exceptional woman athlete may derive a positive experience from competing with males, this does not generally hold true. The reason for this NAGWS position is that women do differ from men in physical strength and power. Women who are well trained athletes will still achieve less muscular strength that their trained male counterparts. For these reasons, it is important that women participate on *separate but equal teams*.

Procedures and practices in respect to interscholastic and intercollegiate athletic competition for girls vary from state to state. Some schools and colleges have broad programs of interscholastic athletics, others do not have any, and some have modified programs. In those having modified programs, play days, sports days, invitation games, and telegraphic meets are increasingly playing a more prominent part. Most states do not set up specific requirements for girls' athletics but feel that their established regulations apply to both girls and boys. A few states have athletic associations for girls that are similar to those for boys.

The National Association for Girls and Women in Sport (NAGWS) of AAHPER is the most influential organization affecting athletics for girls and women. This organization is comprised of leaders in the field of physical education and recreation. The purpose of the organization is to develop, promote, and super-

vise desirable sports programs for girls and women. In order to accomplish this purpose, guiding principles and standards have been developed and publicized. The NAGWS also publishes many official guides in various sports, scorebooks, pamphlets on desirable practices, and special publications concerned with such matters as menstruation, teaching materials, audiovisual resource list, and special events for girls' and women's programs.

Guiding principles and standards established by the NAGWS are concerned with the sports program, leader, and participant. The organization feels that the program should be developed on the basis of such factors as individual differences among girls and women and the environment in which the activity is conducted. The leaders of these programs should have a full understanding of the needs and interests of girls and women and be exemplary in their conduct. The participant should develop skill and other characteristics in accordance with her potential, and the activities in which she engages should contribute to her health and welfare. Competition should be so designed to enable each player to participate at the level of her ability. Officials should understand the role of girls and women in sports, and the rules of the NAGWS should be the official rules of all contests.

Recommendations of the National Association for Girls and Women in Sport

The recommendations of the National Association for Girls and Women in Sport with regard to competitive sports for various age level groupings represent a definitive statement of standards for girls' and women's athletics.

During the junior high school years, girls should have the time and opportunity to explore a great variety of sports. Because of growth and development patterns, this is an age when many goals can be accomplished through team sports and a time when skills of individual sports should also be sampled and developed. Therefore, the junior high school sports program for girls should involve opportunities to participate in many kinds of sports and in a variety of sports situations.

It is also recognized that some girls with high skill potential will wish to extend their training and competitive experiences under competent leaders outside the jurisdiction of the school.

A wide variety of activities should be offered and made available to all students in the school instructional and intramural programs. Opportunities for interschool competition may be provided in the form of a limited number of sport days at the end of the intramural season. The following guidelines are recommended:

1. Competitive sports opportunities for junior high school girls should be planned as a program separate and different from the program of competitive athletics for senior high school girls, whether or not the state high school athletic organization includes the junior high school level.

2. Sports competition should be planned for the values offered to the participant rather than as a spectator sport or as a training program for senior high school teams.

3. Extramural programs may be a valuable supplement to broad instructional and intramural programs, provided sufficient time, facilities, and personnel are available for these programs.

4. The responsibility for leadership of the local girls' interscholastic program should be delegated to the women physical education teachers. The school administration should delegate to them the major responsibility for planning, organizing, coaching, and supervising the program with the understanding that the ultimate authority remains in the hands of the administration.

5. The program, based on the needs and interests of the girls, should include those individual and team activities for which qualified leadership, financial support, and adequate facilities are available.

6. The entire financing of the girls' sports program should be included in the total school budget. Any monies collected should go into the general fund.

7. DGWS-recommended guidelines should be used in all sports. It is strongly recommended that DGWS rules be used in those sports in which DGWS publishes rules.

8. The administration should provide a healthful, safe, and sanitary environment for all participants. *

Competitive sports are an important part of the total physical education program for high school girls. A program of intramural and extramural participation should be arranged to augment a sound and inclusive instructional program in physical education. The interscholastic program should not be promoted at the expense of the instructional or the intramural programs.

As the interscholastic program is expanded, the State High School Activities Association will be the regulatory body for its member schools. For schools that are not members, a regulatory body may need to be formed. The state Department of Education should be involved.

1. Existing legislative administrative bodies for interscholastic athletic programs will retain ultimate control of the total program for girls within the state. However, a women's advisory board composed mainly of women high school physical educators should be formed to propose policies to these administrative and legislative groups and to review policies approved by them.

2. Total responsibility for the administration and supervision of the local interscholastic athletic program is vested in the local school administration and the appropriate persons designated by the administration.

3. The responsibility for leadership of the local girls interscholastic program should be delegated to the women physical education teachers. The school administration should delegate to them the major responsibility for planning, organizing, coaching, and supervising the program with the understanding that the ultimate authority remains in the hands of the administration.

4. The program, based on the needs and interests of the girls, should include those individual and team activities for which qualified leadership, financial support, and adequate facilities are available.

5. All-star teams are not appropriate for girls' sports programs.

6. The entire financing of the girls' sports program should be included in the total school budget. Any monies collected should go into the general fund.

7. DGWS-recommended guidelines should be used in all sports. It is strongly recommended that DGWS rules be used in those sports in which DGWS publishes rules.

8. The administration should provide a healthful, safe, and sanitary environment for all participants. *

The intercollegiate athletic programs should be specifically designed for women, and administration and organization should be the responsibility of the women in physical education. It is also the responsibility of the physical education faculty women to recommend and formulate policy for the expanded program to be submitted to the appropriate policy-approving authority of the institution.

1. Intercollegiate participation should not interfere with primary educational objectives.

   (a) A girl should participate on only one competitive team during a season.

   (b) Participation on more than one team includes participation on an additional team outside an institution. In unusual circumstances such participation may be permitted provided it contributes to the welfare of the participant and does not place excessive demands and pressures upon her.

2. The athletic schedule should not jeopardize the student's class and study time.

   (a) The length of the season and the number of games should be established and agreed upon by the participating schools.

---

*The Division for Girls' and Women's Sports: 1973 Guidelines for interscholastic athletic programs for junior high school girls, Washington, D. C., 1973, AAHPER.

*The Division for Girls' and Women's Sports: 1973 Guidelines for interscholastic programs for high school girls, Washington, D. C., 1973, AAHPER.

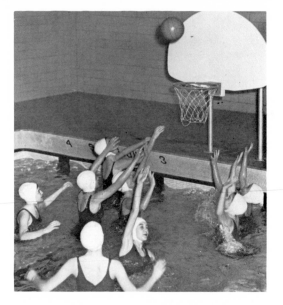

Junior high school. (Waterloo, Iowa.)

(b) The length of the season will vary according to the locale and sport and should not be so long that the educational values for the student in terms of the total program are jeopardized (approximately 12-14 weeks). This season should include conditioning and instruction.

(c) The season may be lengthened to include opportunities for participation in state, regional or national tournaments or meets for which individuals or teams qualify.

3. Teams for girls and women should be provided for all who desire competitive athletic experiences. While positive experiences for the exceptional girl or woman competitor may occur through participation in boys or men's competitive groups, these instances are rare and should be judged acceptable only as an interim procedure for use until women's programs can be initiated.

4. Any woman who is presently enrolled as a full-time undergraduate student in a college, junior college, or university, and who maintains the academic average required for participation in all other major campus activities at her institution shall be eligible to participate.

5. Transfer students are immediately eligible for participation following enrollment in the institution.

6. Students may not participate in the same annual event for more than four years.

7. All participants must have amateur status. Amateur status is maintained in a sport if a player has not received and does not receive money, other than expenses, as a participant in that sport. A participant may receive money from her own school to pay for housing, meals, and transportation providing such funds do not exceed actual costs. For open or inter-national competition governed by the respective sports governing body, a student may lose amateur status if she receives remuneration in excess of her expenses for playing, coaching, or officiating. Scholarships allowed by AIAW will not jeopardize a student's amateur status for DGWS-AIAW competition.

8. A medical examination is a prerequisite to participation in intercollegiate athletics. This examination should be given within the school year prior to the start of the sport season. Where health examinations are done by the family physician, a covering letter explaining the program of activities and an examination which would include the information needed are suggested. Written permission by the physician should be required for participation after serious illness, injury, or surgery. *

Recently the Association for Intercollegiate Athlethics for Women (AIAW) Executive Board and member schools along with the DGWS Executive Council changed their policy on athletic scholarships. Both of these associations revised their policies to allow women athletes to receive financial aid as long as abuses are avoided and certain guidelines are followed. The DGWS guidelines are as follows:†

1. The enrichment of life should be the main objective of athletic programs.

2. Adequate funding for athletic programs should receive priority over money assigned for financial aid.

3. Staff time and budget should be devoted to programs not recruitment.

4. Students should be free to choose a college on the basis of programs offered rather than the scholarship offered.

5. Financial aid should not show favoritism to participants in certain sports.

6. Students should be encouraged to participate in athletic programs for reason other than financial aid.

The NAGWS cooperates with many national sports organizations. This is becoming increasingly common as the desire for more desirable competitive sports experiences for girls and women becomes a part of our culture. A few of the cooperative relationships are Council for National Cooperation in Aquatics, Women's National Aquatics Forum, United States Field Hockey Association, United States Women's Lacrosse Association, United States Volleyball Association, International Joint Softball Rules Committee, National Federation of State High

*The Division for Girls' and Women's Sports: 1973 Guidelines for Intercollegiate Athletic Programs for Women, Washington, D. C., 1973, AAHPER.

† Adopted from: Policies on women athletes change, Journal of Health, Physical Education, and Recreation **44**:51, September, 1973.

School Athletic Associations, Amateur Athletic Union, United States Track and Field Federation, United States Gymnastics Federation, United States Olympic Development Committee, College Women in Sports, and the National Association for Physical Education of College Women.*

Criteria for the evaluation of programs in girls' and women's sports

The accompanying criteria have been established by the Division for Girls' and Women's Sports to assist administrators and others in determining if their program meets acceptable standards.

*Crawford, E.: DGWS cooperates with national sports organizations, Journal of Health, Physical Education, and Recreation **36:**25, 1965.

ATHLETIC ASSOCIATIONS

An individual school or college, by itself, finds it difficult to develop standards and control athletics in a sound educational manner. However, by uniting with other schools and colleges such a project is possible. This has been done on local, state, and national levels in the interest of better athletics for high schools and colleges. By establishing rules and procedures well in advance of playing seasons, the necessary control for conducting a sound athletic program is provided educators, coaches, and others. It aids them in resisting pressures of alumni, students, spectators, townspeople, and others who do not always have the best interests of the program in mind.

There are various types of athletic associations. The ones that are most prevalent in high

---

CRITERIA FOR EVALUATION *

Standards and guidelines established by the Division for Girls' and Women's Sports should be used to evaluate program on local, regional, and national levels.

The sports program should be evaluated frequently according to criteria based on sound educational philosophy and scientific research.

Frequent evaluation of the program is necessary to ascertain if the objectives are being realized. The following list of criteria may be of help in this evaluation:

1. The administrator assumes responsibility for the realization of the values and objectives of the sports program.
2. Professionally qualified teachers and leaders are selected and delegated appropriate responsibility and authority to administer the program.
3. The objectives and policies which govern the sports program are determined by competent professional leaders.
4. The objectives of the program are concerned with the total growth and development of the individual.
5. Educational objectives take precedence over matters of expediency.
6. The educational and recreational aims of the school or sponsoring agency are realized through the sports program.
7. In all situations the spirit of fair play predominates.
8. The program is planned using knowledge based on current research.
9. The program is planned and conducted with primary concern for the welfare of the individual player.
10. The program is considered to be both worthwhile and enjoyable by the players and the leaders alike.
11. Sports experiences are so conducted that maximum values are realized by the participant.
12. Participants in sports activities have a voice in the planning and execution of the program.
13. The diversity within the program meets the needs of all age and skill levels.
14. Qualified women direct, coach, and officiate the program.
15. Trained officials are used in the program.
16. The most recent DGWS rules, standards, skills, and tactics of specific sports are used; where these are not specified, the leader employs professional judgment.
17. The participant meets her responsibility in perpetuating the spirit of good sportsmanship.
18. The total sports program includes instruction, intramurals, and extramurals.
19. Established DGWS standards and guidelines are used in frequent evaluations of the program.
20. Financing of the total sports program is included in the school recreational budget.

*From Division for Girls' and Women's Sports: Philosophy and standards of girls' and women's sports, Washington, D. C., 1969, American Association of Health, Physical Education, and Recreation, pp. 26-27.

schools and colleges are student athletic associations, local conferences or leagues, state high school athletic associations, National Federation of State High School Athletic Associations, National Collegiate Athletic Association, Association for Intercollegiate Athletics for Women (AIAW), and various college conferences.

The student athletic association is an organization within a school that is designed to promote and participate in the conduct of the athletic program of that school. It is usually open to all students in attendance. Through the payment of fees it often helps to support the athletics program. Such associations are found in many of the high schools throughout the country. They can be very helpful in the development of a sound athletic program.

There are various associations, conferences, or leagues that bind together athletically several high schools within a particular geographic area. These are designed in the main to regulate and promote wholesome competition among the member schools. They usually draw up schedules, approve officials, handle disputes, and have general supervision over the athletic programs of the member schools.

The state high school athletic association that now exists in almost every state is a major influence in high school athletics. It is open to all professionally accredited high schools within the state. It has a constitution, administrative officers to conduct the business, and a board of control. The number of members on the board of control varies usually from six to nine. Fees are usually paid to the association on a flat basis or according to the size of the school. In some states there are no fees, since the necessary revenue is derived from the gate receipts of tournament competition. State associations are interested in a sound program of athletic competition within the confines of the state. They concern themselves with the usual problems that have to do with athletics, such as rules of eligibility, officials, disputes, and similar items. They are interested in promoting good high school athletics, equalizing athletic competition, protecting participants, and guarding the health of players. They are an influence

for good and have won the respect of educators in the various states.

The National Council of Secondary School Athletic Directors

The American Alliance for Health, Physical Education, and Recreation recently established the National Council of Secondary School Athletic Directors. The increased emphasis in sports and the important position of athletic directors in the nation's secondary schools seemed to warrant an association where increased services could be rendered to enhance the services given to the nation's youth. The membership in the National Council is open to members of the AAHPER who have primary responsibility in directing, administering, or coordinating interscholastic athletic programs. The purposes of the Council are as follows:

> To improve the educational aspects of interscholastic athletics and their articulation in the total educational program
> To foster high standards of professional proficiency and ethics
> To improve understanding of athletics throughout the nation
> To establish closer working relationships with related professional groups
> To promote greater unity, good will, and fellowship among all members.
> To provide for an exchange of ideas
> To assist and cooperate with existing state athletic directors' organizations
> To make available to members special resource materials through publications, conferences, and consultant services

The National Federation of State High School Athletic Associations

The National Federation of State High School Athletic Associations was established in 1920 with five states participating. At the present time nearly all the states are members. The National Federation is particularly concerned with the control of interstate athletics. Its constitution states this purpose:

> The object of this Federation shall be to protect and supervise the interstate athletic interests of the high schools belonging to the state associations, to assist in those activities of state associations which can best be operated on a nationwide scale, to sponsor meetings, publications and activities which will permit each state association to profit by the experience of all other member associations,

and to coordinate the work so that waste effort and unnecessary duplication will be avoided.

The National Federation has been responsible for many improvements in athletics on a national basis, such as doing away with national tournaments and working toward a uniformity of standards.

The National Collegiate Athletic Association

The National Collegiate Athletic Association was formed in the early 1900's. The alarming number of football injuries and the fact that there was no national control of the game of football led to a conference of representatives of universities and colleges, primarily from the eastern section of the United States, on December 12, 1905. Preliminary plans were made for a national body to assist in the formulation of sound requirements for intercollegiate athletics, particularly football, and the name Intercollegiate Athletic Association was suggested. At a meeting March 31, 1906, a constitution and by-laws were adopted and issued. On December 29, 1910, the name of the association was changed to National Collegiate Athletic Association. The purposes of the NCAA are to uphold the principle of institutional control of all collegiate sports; to maintain a uniform code of amateurism in conjunction with sound eligibility rules, scholarship requirements, and good sportsmanship; to promote and assist in the expansion of intercollegiate and intramural sports; to formulate, copyright, and publish the official rules of play (in eleven sports); to sponsor and supervise regional and national meets and tournaments for member institutions; to preserve athletic records; and to serve as headquarters for collegiate athletic matters of national import.

National Association of Intercollegiate Athletics

Also on the college and university levels is the National Association of Intercollegiate Athletics, which has a large membership, especially among the smaller schools. This organization has recently become affiliated with the American Alliance for Health, Physical Education, and Recreation.

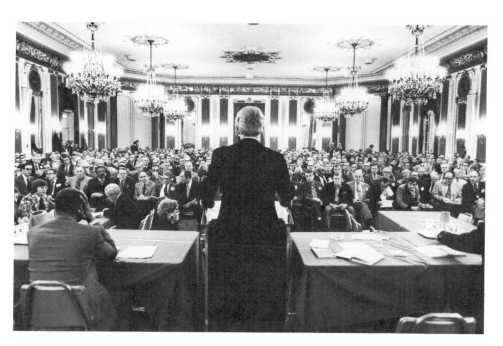

NCAA's Sixty-Eighth Annual Convention in Chicago.

The National Junior College Athletic Association

The National Junior College Athletic Association is an organization of junior colleges who sponsor athletic programs. It has nineteen regional offices with an elected regional director for each. Regional business matters are carried on within the framework of the constitution and bylaws of the parent organization. The regional directors hold an annual legislative assembly in Hutchinson, Kansas, are run by an executive committee, and determine the policies, program, and procedures for the organization. The *Juco Review* is the official publication of the organization. Standing and special committees are appointed each year to cover special items and problems that develop. Membership, which costs $75.00 annually, entitles each member to the services provided by the NJCAA.

National championships are conducted in such sports as basketball, cross country, football, wrestling, baseball, track and field, golf, and tennis. National invitation events are also conducted in such activities as soccer, swimming, and gymnastics.

The NJCAA is affiliated with the National Federation of State High School Athletic Associations and the National Association of Intercollegiate Athletics. It is also a member of the United States Track and Field Federation, Basketball Federation, the United States Collegiate Sports Council, United States Olympic Committee, United States Gymnastics Federation, National Basketball Committee, and American Alliance for Health, Physical Education, and Recreation.

Some of the services offered by the NJCAA to its members include an insurance plan for athletics, recognition in official records, publications, film library, and participation in events sponsored by the association.

Other organizations

In higher education, there are in addition many leagues, conferences, and associations formed by a limited number of schools for athletic competition. Examples are the Ivy League and the Big Ten Conference. These associations regulate athletic competition among their members and settle problems that may arise in connection with such competition.

EXTRA PAY FOR EXTRA SERVICES *

A frequent topic of discussion at school meetings is: Should teachers receive extra pay for extra services? Parents, taxpayers, and school boards have been trying to decide whether or not athletics, coaches, band leaders, dramatics supervisors, publication consultants, and others who do work in addition to their teaching load should receive additional compensation for such services.

A sensible solution to this problem is essential to the good morale of a school staff. Besides, since school systems are demanding more and more services, some policy must be formulated to cover the extra duties that are being heaped on the shoulders of teachers.

To help solve the extra-pay delimma, many surveys, studies, and conferences have been conducted during recent years. The National Education Association, the American Alliance for Health, Physical Education, and Recreation, several state organizations, local boards of education, and other groups have been busy gathering data on the problem. They have found that many communities give extra pay for extra services. However, this is by no means standard procedure.

My own study has indicated that practices in selected school systems across the country generally fall into five groups:

Extra pay is provided for all school activities that require work beyond the normal school day.

Extra pay is given only in the area of athletics.

Released time is provided for extra work.

Supplemental teachers are hired.

All school activities are considered part of the normal teaching load, and no additional pay is given.

Practices across the country

The public schools in one school system in South Dakota pay for all extra activities. The

---

*National Congress of Parents and Teachers: PTA guide to what's happening in education, New York, 1965, Scholastic Book Services, pp. 203-210.

EXTRA PAY FOR EXTRA SERVICES*

$$\frac{\text{Number of hours spent in activity per day}}{\text{Number of hours in school day}} \times \frac{\text{Length of activity per school years (days, weeks, months)}}{\text{Length of normal school year}} = \frac{\text{Basic time index}}{}$$

Example 1. High school basketball coach who spends 2 hours per day with his squad. Season lasts 5 months in 10-month year with an 8-hour day.

$2/8 \times 5/10 = $ basic index $ = .125$

Example 2. High school chemistry teacher spends 1 hour, twice a month with science club. School operates on 8-hour day and 200-day year.

$1/8 \times 20/200 = $ basic index $ = .0125$

These time indices may be applied on a B.A. base, base of degree held, step on B.A. scale, or step on teacher's basic salary scale.

*From Thurston, J. P.: Secondary school athletic administration: a new look, Report of the Second National Conference on Secondary School Athletic Administration, Washington, D. C., January 12-15, 1969, pp. 82-83.

---

assistant football coach receives $350 a year and the ticket manager, $150. Intramural activities pay $75 per sport. The band director gets $600; the supervisor of school publications, $300; the staff member in charge of the school radio program, $200; and the printing instructor, $300. In a school system in Tennessee extra pay is given at varied rates, ranging all the way from $25 a month for a special teacher of handicapped children to $150 a month for a senior high school coach.

In a community on Long Island, New York, extra pay for extra work is based on five criteria: the time required for the activity, the number of students involved, the pressure to which a teacher may be subjected by public performances, the closeness with which the activity is related to the curriculum, and the extent to which the activity is a teaching rather than a supervisory or an advisory function. On the basis of these criteria, each extracurricular activity is placed in one of five categories, each carrying its own rate of pay. The pay ranges from $360 to $880 a year for the various kinds of activity.

The State College Area School District in Pennsylvania established a rating method for extra pay for extra duty that involved nine criteria. An illustrated version of this rating method is seen in Table 10-1.

Many schools faced with the extra-pay problem pay for coaching duties only. A city in Utah follows this practice. There the annual pay for senior high school athletic coaches is $500 more than that of other teachers with similar training and experience, except for teachers of special education, who receive the same rate as coaches. In a Kentucky city some athletic coaches receive as much as $1,000 in extra compensation, but the board of education has not supplemented the salaries of teachers in charge of band, dramatics, and other activities. A few individual schools give some of these teachers part of the proceeds from plays and other activities that they supervise. A city in New York pays its athletic instructors supplementary salaries ranging from $600 for the football coach to $3.00 an hour for athletic league coaches in grade schools.

Some schools throughout the country do not give extra pay. Instead, released time is provided. As a former superintendent of schools in Chicago, pointed out: "In our salary schedule we do not provide extra pay for extra services. We make an exception for teachers who work beyond the normal school day—that

Table 10-1. Rating method—extra pay for extra duty*†

I. All athletics and nonclass-related activities

Criteria	A	B	C	D	E	F	G	H	I		
Possible rating scores	1-10	1-10	1-5	1-5	1-5	1-20	1-20	1-5	1-5		
Weighted value	4	4	3	2	2	3	2	1	2		
Example	5	3	2	2	0	0	2	0	0	Raw rating	
Activity xx (rating X value)	20	12	6	4	0	0	4	0	0	Weighted rating 46	Final rounded 45

CRITERIA	A&B: Hours–550-600	rating 10	C: Students	
	500-549	9	150 pupils or more	5
A *Hours*—total out of school	450-499	8	100-149	4
B *Weekend*—vacation hours—Friday 3—Sunday	400-449	7	50- 99	3
C *Students*—directly involved	350-399	6	25- 49	2
D *Experience*—training necessary	300-349	5	under 25	1
E *Injury risk*—to pupil (other than normal classroom risk)	250-299	4		
F *Pressures*—crowd, spectator, community, faculty, administration	200-249	3		
G *Responsibility*—equipment, facilities, funds	150-199	2		
H *Environmental influence*—outdoor, indoor weather conditions	100-149	1		
I *Travel supervision*—bus trips, etc.	under 100	5		

II. Rating method—class-related activities

Criteria	A	B	C	D	E	F	G	H	I
Possible ratings	1-10	1-10	1-5	1-5	1-5	1-20	1-20	1-5	1-5
Weighted value	4	4	1	1	2	1	1	1	2

*From Solley, P. M.: Extra pay for extra duty, Today's Education, **58**:54, 1969.
†State College Area School District Guide, "Extra Pay for Extra Duty."

is, those who have additional classes because of the shortage of space. We pay extra compensation for this extra time. In regard to the coaching of athletics, we adjust the teaching schedule to compensate for this work."

In one city in California, junior college supplemental teachers are hired to take on certain activities. The supervisor of personnel research reports that the supplemental teachers are assigned to an afterschool activity that is not part of the full day's program and that requires up to 40 hours a month. The activity may be in drama, music, stagecraft, journalism, yearbook, speech, or other areas. Such teachers receive $6.16 an hour.

Finally, there is the great mass of schools where coaching, band, orchestra, and similar activities are considered part of the normal

teaching load and no additional pay is provided. The school system of a community in Missouri is typical of this group. These schools "believe in paying all teachers well," writes a member of the school administration. "In turn, they expect teachers to do the work for which they are hired. No . . . teacher has been paid above schedule. . . . A full explanation of the situation is given at the time of employment." In a town in Connecticut, pressure for extra pay has been exerted by coaches and other groups. The board of education has held, however, that their duties are part of their regular job.

Roundup of suggestions

The many-faceted problem of extra pay and extra services concerns a large number of educators, administrators, and laymen. Various

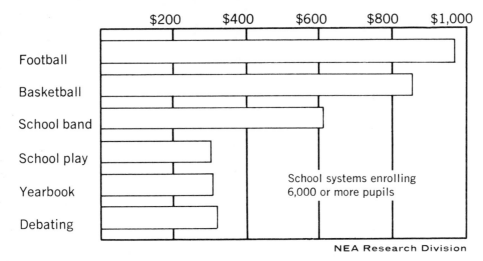

Average maximum annual supplements 1967-1968 for selected pupil-participating activities. (From NEA Research Bulletin **46**:79, 1968.)

ideas of solving it have been advanced, of which the following are perhaps the most pertinent.

The educational program in all school systems should rest on a sound financial base. Teachers' salaries should be sufficient to provide a comfortable living. Faculty members should not have to seek extra work in school or elsewhere to make ends meet.

If possible, there should be enough staff members in every school to make it unnecessary for anyone to take on an extra load.

Extra work means loss of efficiency. A teacher can perform at his or her best for only a certain number of hours a day, then the law of diminishing returns sets in.

All teachers work beyond the school day. They prepare teaching assignments, grade papers, keep records, and take on other professional responsibilities. It is difficult, therefore, to determine what is "extra work."

Extra work in education is not comparable to extra work in business or industry. Professional ethics dictate that positions in public service cannot be categorized in the same way as can those involving only personal gain.

Teaching loads should be equalized as far as possible. If inequalities exist that cannot be corrected through extra staff, extra pay is justified.

Where extra pay is provided, it should be distributed equitably for all who work beyond a normal school day. Teachers should perform extra work only in areas where they are qualified.

The most acceptable form of compensation for additional duties appears to be extra salary. The practice of released time does not seem to meet the wishes of most teachers.

The problem of extra pay for extra service is not an easy one to resolve. Convincing arguments can be given for or against the views that have been presented. Since local needs differ, a nationwide solution cannot be prescribed. However, any community that is wrestling with this problem may well be guided by the foregoing points. They represent the thinking of many teachers and administrators throughout the country.

CONCLUDING STATEMENT ON ATHLETICS

The standards for athletics at school and college levels have been clearly stated. There should be no doubt in any individual's mind as to the types of interscholastic and intercollegiate programs that are sound educationally and in the best interests of students who will participate in them. It is the responsibility of administrators and others concerned with such programs to implement the various standards that have been established. *In every case, it is not a question of deemphasis but a question of reemphasis along educational lines. Good leadership will make the interscholastic program a force for good in education that has no equal.*

Athletics are a part of the total physical education program. The objectives that have been stated earlier in this book for physical education also apply to interschool and intercollegiate athletics. The administrator can evaluate his or her program in terms of the extent to which the listed objectives are being achieved. There should be no question as to where a school stands.

Questions and exercises

1. Develop a set of standards that could be used to appraise an athletic program at the high school or college level.
2. Have a debate on the question: Resolved: that all gate receipts for interscholastic athletic contests should be abolished.
3. Write a profile of what you consider to be the ideal coach.
4. Write a brief essay concerning the question of whether athletic directors should coach.
5. What are some essential points to keep in mind in respect to each of the following: (a) contracts, (b) officials, (c) protests and forfeitures, (d) game management, (e) schedules, (f) awards, (g) records, and (h) medical examinations?
6. Describe in detail how athletic insurance works.
7. As a Director of Athletics, what administrative policy would you recommend in respect to each of the following: (a) gate receipts, (b) tournaments and championships, (c) eligibility, (d) scholarships, (e) recruiting, (f) proselyting, and (g) scouting?
8. What is the role of the Athletic Association in the conduct of athletics?
9. Develop a set of guiding administrative principles for girls' athletics.
10. Discuss standards for coaching certification identified by the American Alliance of Health, Physical Education, and Recreation.
11. Debate the following question: Do national playoffs in sports constitute a desirable activity for children under 12 years of age?
12. What practical suggestions can you make for eliminating the "big business" aspects of intercollegiate athletics?
13. Write a brief essay discussing the effects of austerity budgets on school athletic programs.

Reading assignment in *Administrative Dimensions of Health and Physical Education Programs, Including Athletics:* Chapter 8, Sections 39 to 47.

Selected references

American Association for Health, Physical Education, and Recreation: Approaches to problems of public school administration in health, physical education and recreation, Proceedings of the Sixth National Conference of City and County Directors, Washington, D. C., 1968, The Association.

American Association for Health, Physical Education, and Recreation: Secondary school athletic administration, Washington, D. C., 1969, The Association.

Boojarma, L. M., and Messing, A.: A survey of women's intercollegiate athletic programs at junior colleges in the United States, Juco Review **25:**37, 1973.

Bucher, C. A.: Foundations of physical education, ed. 7, St. Louis, 1975, The C. V. Mosby Co.

Bucher, C. A., and Dupee, R. K., Jr.: Athletics schools and colleges, New York, 1965, The Center for Applied Research in Education, Inc. (The Library of Education).

Bucher, C. A., and Koenig, C.: Methods and materials for secondary school physical education, ed. 4, St. Louis, 1974, The C. V. Mosby Co.

Collison, R.: Master coach certification proposed, the Prep Coach, February, 1972, Publication of Minnesota High School Coaches Association.

Crowd Management Manual: California Interscholastic Federation—Southern Section, Chicago, 1971, Compass.

Division for Girls' and Women's Sports: 1973 guidelines for intercollegiate athletic programs for women, Washington, D. C., 1973, American Association for Health, Physical Education, and Recreation.

Division for Girls' and Women's Sport: 1973 guidelines for interscholastic athletic programs for junior high school and high school girls, Washington, D. C., 1973, American Association for Health, Physical Education, and Recreation.

Educational balance in jeopardy: Sportscope, November-December 1972.

Educational Policies Commission: School athletics—problems and policies, Washington, D. C., 1954, National Education Association.

Fraser, C.: Coaches need a certification program, Texas Coach **25:**26, 1972.

George, J. F., and Lehmann, H. A.: School athletic administration, New York, 1966, Harper & Row, Publishers.

Gilbert, B., and Williamson, N.: Programmed to be losers, Sports Illustrated **38:**60, 1973.

Hixson, C. G.: The administration of interscholastic athletics, New York, 1967, J. Lowell Pratt and Co.

Hult, J.: Separate but equal athletics for women, Journal of Health, Physical Education, and Recreation **44:**57, June, 1973.

Keelor, R. O.: The realities of drug abuse in high school athletics **43:**48, 1972.

Koenig, F.: Did DGWS fail? No—a response from OGWS, Journal of Health, Physical Education, and Recreation **45:**8, 1974.

Maetozo, M., editor: Required specialized preparation for coaching, Journal of Health, Physical Education, and Recreation **42:**12, 1971.

Meinharat, T.: A rationale for certification of high school coaches in Illinois, Journal of Health, Physical Education, and Recreation **42**:48, 1971.

Murphy, E., and Vincent, M.: Status of funding on women's intercollegiate athletics, Journal of Health, Physical Education, and Recreation **44**:11, 1973.

Policies on women athletes change: Journal of Health, Physical Education, and Recreation **44**:51, 1973.

Poorman, D.: Should A. D.'s coach? Juco Review **25**:10, 1973.

Razor, J. E.: Variables in crowd control, The Athletic Journal **52**:30, 1971.

Rule books for all boys' sports. Available from the National Federation of State High School Athletic Associations, 7 South Dearborn St., Chicago, Ill.

Rule books for all girls' sports. Available from the Division for Girls' and Women's Sports, American Association for Health, Physical Education, and Recreation, 1201 16th St. N. W., Washington, D. C., 10036.

Rushall, B. S., and Siedentop, D.: The development and control of behavior in sports and physical education, Philadelphia, 1972, Lea & Febiger.

School athletics face austerity budgets, Sportscope, September-October, 1973.

Stutzman, S. J., and McCullough, C.: Did DGWS fail? Yes—a steady refusal to change, Journal of Health, Physical Education, and Recreation **45**:6, 1974.

Talamini, John T., and Page, C. H.: Sport and society—an anthology, Boston, 1973, Little, Brown and Co.

Yanall, D.: Implications of a recent survey of physical education and athletics in two-year colleges, Juco Review **11**:20, 1971.

Administering physical fitness programs

The desire to be physically fit doesn't just happen. It must be stressed during a student's school and college years in order for a person to maintain fitness as an adult. A recent survey concerning adult fitness revealed that millions of adult Americans do not engage in physical activity in order to stay physically fit. This study will be discussed in detail later in this chapter.

The administration of physical fitness programs must be concerned with the community as well as with the students. Community and family fitness are essential factors in the administration of any school or college fitness program. A person who is physically fit tends to derive greater enjoyment and fulfillment from his or her life and tends to share these feelings with friends and family. Fitness should be a primary objective of physical education programs.

A fit person is one who (1) *physically* has a strong organic base, exhibits vigor, is active, is skilled in some physical activities, and enjoys a sense of well-being; (2) *socially* recognizes the principle once stated by Justice Stone that "no man can live unto himself alone" and, therefore, understands and respects the rights of others, likes people, practices service above self, and makes satisfactory group adjustments; (3) *mentally* has a healthy outlook on life, thinks independently and constructively, has good judgment, is resourceful, and wants to be fit; and (4) *emotionally* has stability and self-control, faces reality in an honest manner, and has high ethical standards.

PHYSICAL FITNESS

Physical fitness, as one aspect of total fitness, involves three important concepts. It is related to the tasks the person must perform, his or her potential for physical effort, and the relationship of physical fitness to the total self. The same degree of physical fitness is not necessary for everyone. It should be sufficient to meet the requirements of the job, plus a little extra as a reserve for emergencies. A football player or a foot soldier in the Army needs a different type of physical fitness from that required by a train conductor or a stenographer. The question of "fitness for what" must always be asked. Furthermore, discussion of the physical fitness of a person must be within the context of his or her own human resources and not to those of others. It depends on one's potentialities in the light of one's own physical makeup. Finally, physical fitness cannot be considered by itself but, instead, as it is affected by mental, emotional, and spiritual factors as well. Human beings function as a whole and not in segmented parts.

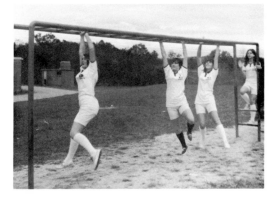

Henderson County Schools, Hendersonville, N. C.

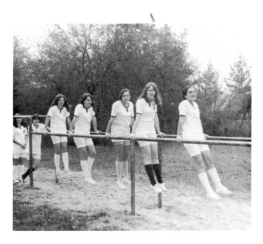

Henderson County Schools, Hendersonville, N. C.

Components of physical fitness

The attempt to define and break down the term *physical fitness* has led to the identification of certain specific components that collectively make up physical fitness. Such factors as resistance to disease, or the ability of the body to keep its disease-fighting equipment in good shape; muscular strength, or the ability to exert force against a resistance; muscular endurance, or the ability to repeat activities involving resistance; and cardiorespiratory endurance, or the ability of the circulatory and respiratory systems to support activities requiring sustained effort, such as distance running or swimming— these make up the components of physical fitness set forth by most authorities.

Larson and Yocom* list ten components of physical fitness—namely, resistance to disease, muscular strength and endurance, cardiovascular-respiratory endurance, muscular power, flexibility, speed, agility, coordination, balance, and accuracy. McCloy and Young† list components such as the speed of muscular contraction, dynamic energy, ability to change direction, agility, dead weight, and flexibility. Cureton‡ appraises physical fitness in terms of physique and organic efficiency, which he says implies anatomic and physiologic soundness, and adds a component that he calls "motor fitness." This motor fitness, according to Cureton, includes endurance, power, strength, agility, flexibility, and balance.

Morehouse and Miller§ include a psychologic component that to them implies possession of necessary emotional stability, drive or motivation, intelligence, and educability.

As can be seen from these statements of leaders in the field of physical education, there is not complete agreement on what physical fitness is and what its components are. Research is needed to obtain more valid evidence about this important aspect of health and physical education work.

Developing physical fitness

The question of how to obtain physical fitness is controversial. Since we do not know exactly what it is and what its components may be, the answer as to how one obtains it is also somewhat nebulous. We do know, however, that heredity plays an important role. The form and structure of the body are determined largely by genetic factors. Heredity sets certain direction and limitations to development. Good nutrition is essential. Good health habits—such as having proper rest, relaxation, and sleep and otherwise

*Larson, L. A., and Yocom, R.: Measurement and evaluation in physical, health, and recreation education, St. Louis, 1951, The C. V. Mosby Co., p. 162.

†McCloy, C. H., and Young, N. D.: Tests and measurements in health and physical education, ed. 3, New York, 1954, Appleton-Century-Crofts, pp. 4-5.

‡Cureton, T. K.: Physical fitness appraisal and guidance, St. Louis, 1947, The C. V. Mosby Co., p. 21.

§Morehouse, L. E., and Miller, A. T., Jr.: Physiology of exercise, ed. 5, St. Louis, 1967, The C. V. Mosby Co., p. 268.

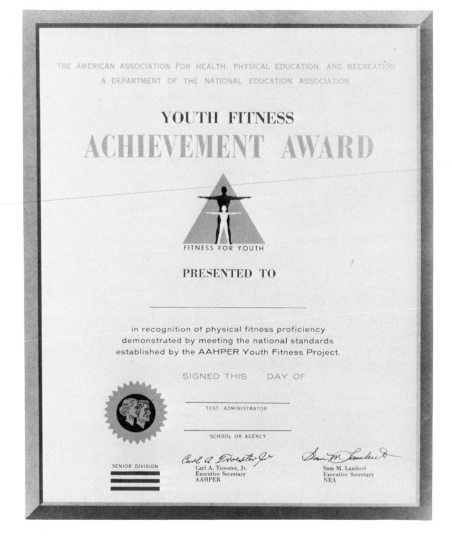

Youth Fitness Achievement Award. (Courtesy American Alliance for Health, Physical Education, and Recreation.)

providing good care for the body—are necessary. The important contributions of mental, emotional, spiritual, and social health must be considered. In addition, there is increasing recognition of the importance of physical activity. The value of exercise in developing many of the components of physical fitness and, in addition, in contributing to mental, social, and emotional well-being is an important factor.

Methods of developing physical fitness. Some of the methods of utilizing physical activity in the development of physical fitness

include circuit training, interval training, weight training, weight lifting, isometric exercises, and the Exer-Genie.

Circuit training involves a series of exercises, usually around ten, that are performed in a progressive manner. Physical activity is performed at each of the ten stations. The training is done on a time basis and progress is checked against the clock. The length and nature of activities performed can be changed as the performer becomes stronger.

Interval training requires physical activity involving distance to build endurance, an increase of speed, an increase in the number of repetitions, and the rest or recovery period. As the performer becomes stronger the recovery interval is reduced. Its main contribution is in the area of cardiovascular endurance development.

Weight training utilizes resistance exercises, taking into consideration the number of repetitions of resistance exercises and also the duration and intensity of the exercises being performed.

Weight lifting involves the lifting of weights and usually involves only a few repetitions.

Isometric exercises are exercises whereby muscles contract and build up tension and hold without any shortening or lengthening. (*Isometric* is derived from the words *iso,* meaning same, and *metric,* meaning length.) They are valuable in developing strength.

In *calisthenic exercises* the muscles contract so that they shorten and the ends are brought together (concentric), or the muscles lengthen and the ends go away from the center, as in the beginning of a pull-up when one lowers himself into a hanging position (eccentric) (isotonic).

The *Exer-Genie* can utilize either isometric or isotonic exercises. It is an instrument sold commerically that involves rope and handles. The amount of strength required to pull the ropes in various positions can be adjusted, thus enabling a progressive development of strength and endurance.

HISTORICAL BACKGROUND OF CURRENT PHYSICAL FITNESS EMPHASIS

The subject of fitness is not new to the American educational system. There have been numerous times during the educational history of this country when educators have been called upon to upgrade the fitness of American youth. World Wars I and II both caused the pendulum to swing toward more emphasis in this direction.

During recent years there has been a renewed stress on the subject of fitness. Results of some physical fitness tests have revealed the poorer physical condition of American children and youth as compared to children and youth in other countries. Although some of these tests have been criticized by many physical education leaders as not possessing validity, they have stirred up considerable interest in the area of physical fitness. The information forthcoming from these tests was noted by the President of the United States, with the result that a program of action was established in high government circles.

A President's Conference on Fitness of American Youth, held at the United States Naval Academy, Annapolis, Maryland, June 18-19, 1956, initiated a government-sponsored program in fitness that was destined to influence considerably the fields of health education and physical education. It was attended by 150 leaders in sports, education, medicine, public relations, government, and other areas. Most of the conferees were presidents, directors, or other top officials of organizations interested in the fitness of American youth. At the closing session of the conference the Vice-President announced that a President's Council on Physical Fitness, composed of members of the Cabinet, would be established to help improve the mental and physical health of the nation's young people. The President also announced that a President's Citizens' Advisory Committee on the Fitness of American Youth would be established. These committees have been functioning since their formation. The Advisory Committee, according to the President, ''is to examine and explore the facts and, thereafter, to alert America on what can and should be done to reach the much-desired goal of a happier, healthier, and more totally fit youth in America.''

A summary of some of the recommendations resulting from group discussions at this conference shows the challenge that fitness had at that time and still has for the schools:

1. There is a need for more research.
2. An agency or commission on fitness for American youth should be created.
3. Much is being done at the present time for the fitness of American youth. However, it is not enough and what is being done is very poorly coordinated.
4. Youth must be involved in much of the planning.
5. Programs must be fitted to the needs of the individual child and they must reach *all* the children.

6. Better school health examinations are needed.

7. The fitness of this nation is based on the fitness of its people. If there is something we need and know we need—this nation should have it!

8. There should be more and better leadership.

9. Leaders should themselves believe in fitness and provide a fitting example for the youth of this country.

10. Community leadership should be drawn from schools, recreation agencies, parents, law enforcement agencies, labor, management, youth groups, and the whole gamut of community life.

11. Higher salaries and other inducements for attracting qualified leadership into this work should be provided.

12. Families should make the best possible use of their own resources. Home space should be provided for children's play.

13. School facilities should receive maximum use. Other facilities, such as camps, fairgrounds, parks, etc., should also be used.

14. Foundations should be urged to contribute to the support of fitness endeavors.

15. Colleges and universities and mass communication media can help gain public support.

16. Parents must be impressed with the importance

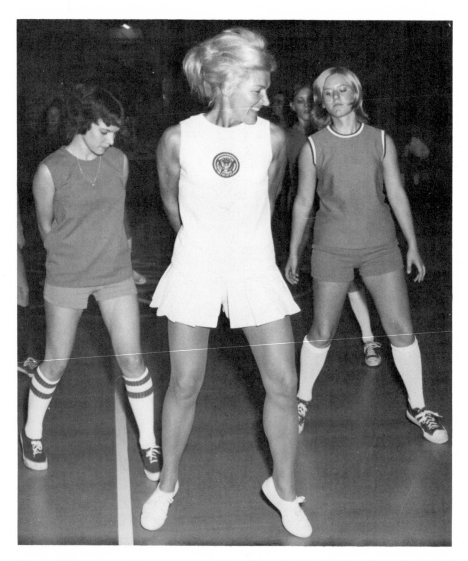

Physical Fitness Clinic conducted by a representative of the President's Council on Physical Fitness and Sports.

of taking an active interest in fitness of children—spending time with them, teaching sportsmanship, loyalty, spirit, etc.

17. Youth must be sold on the importance of being physically fit.
18. Fitness programs should begin in the home, and all members of the family should engage in these activities.
19. The schools do not represent the only facet of community life that should have a role in building fitness—churches, social agencies, veterans groups, government agencies, sports groups, and others can play an important part.
20. Girls should receive as much attention as boys.
21. Greater financial support is needed for better and larger programs.

The present administration has emphasized the role of the schools and colleges in physical fitness. The recommendations of the President's Council on Physical Fitness and Sports are discussed later in this chapter.

PHYSICAL ACHIEVEMENT AND THE SCHOOLS

In the last decade the President's Council on Physical Fitness and Sports indicates there was much progress in improving the physical achievement standards of American youth—for example: 9.2 million children are participating in school physical activity programs; four out of every five pupils now successfully pass standardized physical fitness tests (only two out of three passed in 1961); 68% of all schools have strengthened their physical activity programs; the number of parochial schools providing physical education instruction has doubled; seventeen states have raised their school physical education requirements; and teaching positions for health and physical education have increased by 27%—school enrollments have increased 11%.

Although much progress has been made in recent years, there is much left to be done—for example: 14% of children in school today do not participate in any physical activity program, and an additional 27% participate only 1 or 2 days per week; only four schools in ten provide physical education programs 5 days per week; and 23% of the schools have administered the American Alliance of Health, Physical Education, and Recreation seven-item physical achievement test, but on this test only 57% of

the boys and 51% of the girls were reported to have scored "satisfactory" on all items.

WHAT SCHOOLS AND COLLEGES CAN DO

Education in its broadest sense means preparation for life. It should help each individual to become all he or she is capable of being. Therefore, it is inexorably tied in with fitness. Education must be concerned with developing in each individual optimal health, vitality, emotional stability, social consciousness, knowledge, wholesome attitudes, and spiritual and moral qualities. Only as it accomplishes this task will it achieve its destiny in the American way of life.

Schools and colleges have the responsibility for providing many opportunities for understanding and developing fitness. Of all the agencies involved in carrying out the President's fitness program, the schools and colleges are the focal point. The fact that some 60

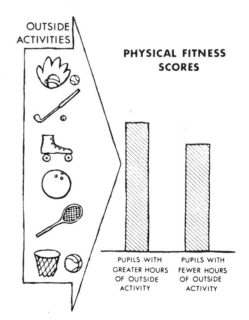

Those students who participated more in activities outside the school had higher fitness scores than those pupils with fewer hours of physical activity outside the school. (Physical fitness achievement in selected physical education programs, Albany, 1965, The University of the State of New York.)

million children and youth can be reached through them is an important reason for recognizing their worth. The schools and colleges also have the needed facilities and their teachers are trained for carrying out such a program. The school and college can instill children and youth with a desire for fitness. Education can likewise equip youngsters with the necessary tools to attain and maintain fitness throughout life. Their qualified teachers can also provide leadership in community programs that have valuable contributions to make.

The schools and colleges should be fitness conscious. Programs must be so constituted that experiences and services contribute to fitness. This means that health knowledge, attitudes, and practices are stressed; that protective health services are provided; that physical activities are available to and engaged in by *all*—not just the few who are skilled; that necessary facilities are provided; that the environment is conducive to proper growth and development; that experiences in every area stress proper social and ethical behavior.

Leadership in the schools and colleges should exemplify fitness—fitness is the responsibility of all disciplines and all teachers and staff. It should permeate the entire program and all persons connected with it. It is not the responsibility of only one area and just a few people.

The schools and colleges represent only one force for developing a fit populace. The home, church, recreational agency, volunteer groups, and other persons and organizations also have major contributions to make. Schools and colleges should work closely with and play a leading role in mobilizing the entire resources of each community to do the job.

Children and youth must want to be fit. Unless the desire to be fit is instilled in each child, the way of life that results in fitness will not be achieved. By the time students leave school and college to enter into adult life, the importance of fitness in achieving personal ambitions and desires, in feeling well and happy, in living most and serving best, and in contributing to a strong nation must be inculcated in every boy and girl who attends our schools and colleges.

This is a responsible role for the schools and colleges to pursue but a very necessary one.

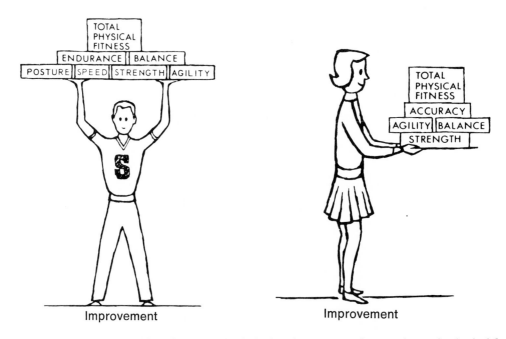

Boys and girls who participated in high quality physical education programs improved more in physical fitness than did those pupils participating in minimum programs. (Physical fitness achievement in selected physical education programs, Albany, 1965, The University of the State of New York.)

It is a challenge we must take up if we are not to become a nation of "softies" and unfit individuals.

Health education and physical education can contribute much to the development of total fitness. Many benefits accrue to those persons who have experiences in these specialized fields. They possess an understanding of the human body—its needs and its limitations—the ability to discriminate fad from scientific fact, the interest and desire to be physically fit, the resources to spend leisure hours in a manner that contributes to fitness, and the skill in activities that provide release from strains and tension associated with modern living. They are also provided with experiences that contribute to wholesome personal and group adjustments and opportunities for creative expression. These are only a few of the many benefits that can be listed. These values, however, do not automatically accrue. Leadership is the key to their fulfillment.

Leaders in health, physical education, and recreation must never lose sight of the fact they are working with the "whole" individual. Programs should make provision for the selected activities that best develop all aspects of self. They should also be concerned with the contributions their respective fields can make, individually and collectively, to this "whole" development.

More specifically, some essential points that school and college health and physical education and recreation programs must consider if they are to adequately promote the health and well-being of boys and girls who attend our schools are listed here:

1. School and college health and physical education programs must be available to *all* children and youth and based on their individual differences.

2. Every student should have one period of each school day devoted to the physical education program. College youth should have a required and a voluntary program to meet their needs. Anything less is inadequate.

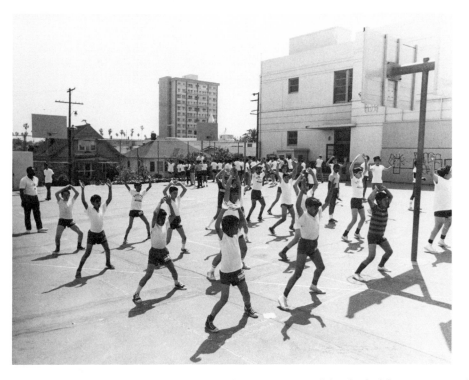

An elementary school physical education class doing calisthenics as part of the physical fitness program. (Courtesy President's Council on Physical Fitness and Sports.)

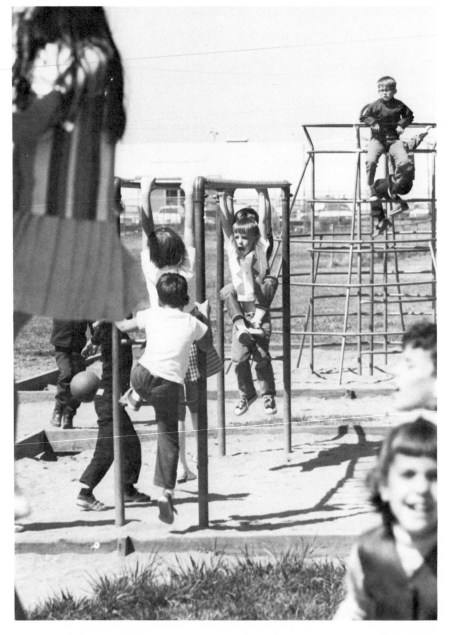

As shown here, elementary school youngsters enjoy utilizing apparatus as a means of developing physical fitness.

3. Sports and games should not be limited to only the varsity squads in football, basketball, or baseball. Every student should participate, whether skilled or not, weak or strong, boy or girl.

4. Boys and girls need professionally trained teachers in the fields of health and physical education. Furthermore, the ratio of teachers to students in such classes should be the same as for academic subject areas.

5. Children and youth should participate in physical education programs that include class periods, intramurals, play, sports, and field days, adapted activities, and scholastic and collegiate sports.

6. Physical activities contribute to physical fitness as they are planned around the following three essentials: *Frequency*—regular daily workouts are needed to develop and maintain a state of optimal health. *Intensity*—big muscles must be vigorously used, with resulting stimulation of the heart and breathing rates. As many muscles should be put into action as possible. *Duration*—1 hour a day, with frequent rest periods, should be devoted to physical activity.

7. In addition to the benefits received from the physical activity program, young people should also understand the importance of being in good health and the factors that build fitness. There should be a comprehensive program of health instruction for all pupils based on their interests and needs.

8. Many health services are essential to promoting physical fitness in the schools and colleges. Most important is a good medical examination in which health defects can be uncovered and steps taken to ensure their correction.

9. There should be coordination between school, college, and community programs to ensure the conduct of sound out-of-school and college programs of recreation, sports, and athletics. Efforts to expand public and private facilities such as YMCA's, Boys' Clubs, and playgrounds must be continued. Present facilities meet only about 15% of public needs.

10. A healthful environment is essential to fitness. Safe, sanitary, and attractive facilities and equipment, plus an atmosphere that is conducive to optimal mental and emotional health, are necessary.

11. Motivation for fitness must be developed. Students and the public must be oriented as to the importance of fitness for living. People will change only if sufficiently motivated.

12. There should be homework in physical activities. It cannot all be done in the gymnasium, swimming pool, or playground. Activities must be taught that may be enjoyed away from the conventional gymnasium and athletic fields. The program should include many kinds of home activities that can be conducted in backyards or basements.

13. If the schools and colleges are going to build strong bodies, they need the necessary equipment and facilities. Taxpayers and administrators must recognize the importance of this work and supply the necessary funds.

14. Health and physical education should receive equal recognition with other subjects in the curriculum. This means credit and other considerations should be given. Participation in musical organizations, military training, driver education, or other activities should not be permitted to serve as a substitute for physical education.

15. Health and physical education classes should be scheduled early in the program if the needs of students are to be met. In many cases this means they will be scheduled before other subjects. Other things being equal, the school subjects that have the greatest number of pupils enrolled should receive first consideration. The number of staff members and teaching stations are also considerations.

16. Utilization of valid techniques to determine which students are below par in physical fitness is needed, so that special programs may be provided.

17. A progressive program should be provided in health and physical education from kindergarten through college.

ADULT FITNESS

The importance of adult physical fitness cannot be overlooked. Tomorrow's adults are today's students, and their concepts of physical

---

A PHYSICAL FITNESS CHECKLIST*

Medical aspects   Yes   No

1. Thorough dental and health examination each year   _____ _____
    (a) Fit heart and circulatory system, digestive system, nervous system, etc.   _____ _____
    (b) Proper body development, according to age and sex (height and weight, etc.)   _____ _____
2. Correction of remedial health defects, i.e., vision, hearing, overweight etc.   _____ _____

Physical activity

1. At least 1½ to 2 hours a day spent in vigorous physical activity, preferably outdoors _____ _____
2. Adequate muscular strength and endurance   _____ _____
3. After running 50 yards, heart and breathing return to normal rates within 10 minutes _____ _____
4. Average skill in running, jumping, climbing, and throwing   _____ _____
5. Control of body in activities involving balance, agility, speed, rhythm, accuracy   _____ _____

Posture

1. When standing upright, string dropped from tip of ear passes through shoulder and   _____ _____
    hip joints and middle of ankle
2. When sitting in a chair, trunk and head are erect, weight balanced over pelvis, or   _____ _____
    trunk slightly bent forward
3. When walking, slumping is avoided, body is in proper balance, and excessively   _____ _____
    wasteful motions of arms and legs are eliminated

Health habits

1. Rest: at least 8 hours of sleep each night   _____ _____
2. Diet: consists of four servings daily from each of the four basic food groups   _____ _____
    (a) Meat, poultry, fish, and eggs
    (b) Dairy products
    (c) Vegetables and fruits
    (d) Bread and cereals
3. Cleanliness:
    (a) Daily bath   _____ _____
    (b) Teeth brushed after every meal   _____ _____
    (c) Clean hair, nails, and clothing   _____ _____
4. Abstain from use of tobacco and alcohol   _____ _____

*From Bucher, C. A., and Koenig, C., Methods and materials for secondary school education, ed. 4, St. Louis, 1974, The C. V. Mosby Co.

---

fitness should be inculcated while in school and college. In addition, the physical educator and administrator should be involved in the community and be aware of the fitness needs of that community.

The National Adult Physical Fitness Survey was recently conducted for the President's Council on Physical Fitness and Sports by the Opinion Research Corporation of Princeton, New Jersey. The study was national in scope, utilizing a representative sampling of personal interviews with 3,875 men and women, aged 22 years and over, in 360 communities throughout the United States.

The survey indicated that 45% of all adult Americans (approximately 49 million of the 109 million adult men and women) do not engage in physical activity for the purpose of exercise. These Americans tend to be older, less well educated, and less affluent than those who do exercise. The survey also cited that walking was the most popular form of exercise, followed by bicycle riding and swimming. Adults who were school or college athletes tend to be more active than those adults who did not participate in sports during their school years. Of those who do exercise regularly, nearly one-half do so for health reasons. It is interesting to note that most adults reported that the federal government has been the major source of their awareness of physical fitness. Other sources indicated included: insurance companies, "Y's," and the American Medical Association. Television was cited as the major method of communication concerning fitness. Schools and colleges were not frequently mentioned in this regard.

A major question raised by this survey is what are educational institutions doing to impart fitness information to their students, adults, and the public in general? Educators are involved today in communicating information about such topics as drugs, mental health, nutrition, and sex to the community. Isn't it also important to communicate relevant facts about how a person can develop and maintain physical fitness throughout his or her lifetime and the role physical activity plays in achieving this goal? Why have physical educators shirked this responsibility? They do a great job communicating with each other through professional literature and at conventions and conferences, but physical educators have been remiss in reaching students and the public in general. Is this because they are so occupied with game and sports programs that they have forgotten about communicating the foundations for and

importance of exercise and physical fitness? Is it because they are so concerned with the present fitness level of our students that the important role of securing future fitness is overlooked? Physical educators must recognize that what happens to their students after they graduate from school and college will determine the real worth of the physical education program to which they were exposed.

Physical educators in schools and colleges should be concerned with much more than getting their boys and girls involved in physical exercise while they are students. Equally or more important is having them understand and appreciate why they should be physically active all of their lives and the impact this activity will have upon their biologic, psychologic, and sociologic welfare. To accomplish this goal, physical education should meet in the classroom as well as the gymnasium, have physical education textbooks for students as well as bats and balls, and graduate physically educated rather than merely physically trained individuals. In addition, the profession must extend its efforts and influence into the larger community of which schools and colleges are a part.

Only a little over half of the general public feel they get enough exercise

The data show that while many people feel they do not get enough exercise (40%), more say they do get enough (57%). The percentage of people saying they do not get enough exercise translates to about 44 million people.

In particular, the older respondents are more inclined to say they get enough exercise than are the younger respondents.

Amount of exercise

"Do you feel that you get enough exercise or not?"

	Get enough (%)	Do not (%)	No opinion (%)
Total public	57	40	3
Men	61	37	2
Women	54	43	3
22 to 29 years old	46	52	2
30 to 39	49	49	2
40 to 49	53	45	2
50 to 59	62	36	2
60 or older	71	25	4
Exercise now	53	46	1
Do not exercise now	63	33	4

Most people who exercise do so for reasons related to health

Among those people who exercise, a number say they exercise for good health, to lose weight (primarily among women), and because they feel exercise is generally a good thing. Some respondents also find exercise enjoyable.

Those people who do not exercise (45%) were asked why. Their reasons include: not enough time (13%); they feel they get enough exercise by working (11%); there are medical reasons (8%); and age (5%).

Reasons for exercising

"What are some of the reasons why you exercise?"
(Asked only of those who exercise)

Asked (%)	Total public 55%	Men 56%	Women 55%
For good health:			
Good for my heart; to keep in shape; to stay in good physical condition; I can breathe better	23	26	20
Good for you in general:			
Makes me feel better; good for me; I feel like it's good for me	18	8	12
To lose weight:			
To keep slim; I like to keep my shape; I'm a little on the heavy side; to flatten my stomach	13	9	17
Enjoyment:			
I like doing it; for pleasure and relaxation; for recreation	12	13	11
Doctor told me to	3	4	3

PHYSICAL EDUCATION
Most people have taken physical education at some time while they were in school

About three-fourths of the general public report having taken physical education and there is little, if any, difference between men and women. Note, however, that age is a factor, probably reflecting the increasing incidence of physical education programs in our school systems. Nearly everyone under 40 has had physical education classes. This proportion drops to under half among those 60 years old or over.

As might be expected, participation in physical education depends somewhat on the amount of time spent in the educational system. Those who did not finish high school are less likely to have taken physical education classes than are those who have attended college.

Physical education

"Did you ever take physical education or gym class while you were in school?"

	Yes (%)	No (%)	Not reported (%)
Total public	71	28	1
Men	70	29	1
Women	71	28	1
22 to 29 years old	93	7	*
30 to 39	89	10	1
40 to 49	74	25	1
50 to 59	67	32	1
60 or older	39	58	3
High school incomplete	45	53	2
High school complete	87	12	1
Some college	93	7	*

*Less than 0.5%.

Most people who have taken gym classes feel that physical education is beneficial

Among the 70% of the general public who have taken physical education, a strong majority say it was good for them. Only a few say it made no difference and almost no one believes gym classes were detrimental.

Effects of physical education

"Do you feel that gym classes were good for you, bad for you, or didn't they make any difference?" (Asked only of those who had physical education or gym class in school)

	Asked (%)	Good (%)	Bad (%)	No difference (%)	Don't know (%)
Total public	70	60	1	8	1
Men	70	62	1	7	1
Women	71	59	1	10	1

There is strong support for physical education at all grade levels

Majorities of both men and women feel that people should have physical education in school. This support is across the board and comes from all subgroups. Only a few people in any age, economic, or social class say people should not have physical education.

Should people have physical education?

"Do you feel that most people should have physical education in elementary school *or shouldn't they?"*

"Do you feel that most people should have physical education in junior high, senior high, *or* college *or shouldn't they?"*

	Total public (%)	Men (%)	Women (%)
Elementary school			
Yes	90	89	90
No	4	5	3
Makes no difference	4	4	4
Other/no opinion	2	2	3
Junior high, senior high, or college			
Yes	91	91	90
No	2	2	2
Makes no difference	4	4	4
Other/no opinion	3	3	4

People who took physical education are more likely to participate in noncompetitive sports now than are those who did not take physical education

"Looking at this card, please tell me which of these sports (other than the ones you already mentioned) you now participate in or *participated in during the last season on a* noncompetitive *basis–that is, either by yourself, or with friends?"*

	Participation in physical education	
	Yes (%)	No (%)
Swimming	22	4
Bowling	15	4
Golf	8	2
Tennis	7	1
Volleyball	6	1
Baseball	5	2
Softball	5	1
Basketball	5	*
Football	4	1
Water skiing	4	*
Snow skiing	3	*
Gymnastics	2	1
Handball	2	*
Track and field	1	*
Wrestling	1	*
Soccer	1	0
Other	4	1

*Less than 0.5%.

As mentioned earlier, people who participated in school sports are more likely to be participating in noncompetitive sports now than are people who did not participate in school sports

"Looking at this card, please tell me which of these sports (other than the ones you already mentioned) you now participate in or participated in during the last season on a noncompetitive basis—that is, either by yourself, or with friends?"

	Participation in school sports		
	More than one (%)	One (%)	None (%)
Swimming	26	14	11
Bowling	17	7	9
Golf	11	5	4
Tennis	8	5	3
Basketball	8	3	2
Baseball	7	3	3
Softball	7	3	3
Volleyball	7	3	3
Water skiing	7	2	1
Football	6	2	1
Snow skiing	5	2	1
Handball	3	1	1
Gymnastics	2	*	1
Wrestling	2	*	*
Track and field	1	*	*
Soccer	1	0	*
Other	5	3	3

*Less than 0.5%.

Community physical fitness

Many schools and colleges are beginning to become involved with community needs for fitness. One such college is Brookdale Community College in Monmouth County, New Jersey. Brookdale provides opportunities for community participation in many athletic interests. Wrestling was one program recently offered to community residents. Participants in programs are not excluded by age, sex, or skill level. Brookdale also has a walk-in recreation program where community members can participate in fitness activities under the supervision or instruction of the physical education department. This program is scheduled during lunch hours, early afternoons, evenings, weekends, and summer. The fitness learning laboratory, providing a fitness profile and other resources, is open to the community on a drop-in basis, 60 hours a week.

Family fitness

A nationwide campaign to promote family fitness was recently launched by the President's Council on Physical Fitness and Sports and the Travelers Insurance Companies. This company declared a commitment to furthering the goals of the Physical Exercise Pays (PEP) program that embraces a wide range of activities involving fun, family, and physical fitness. Some of the activities in the PEP program include badminton, swimming, bicycling, skating, cross-country skiing, and jogging. Family fitness provides an opportunity for the family to do something enjoyable together while building physical fitness. It is important for a family to allow a certain amount of time each week to participate in some physical activity together. It can be time for communication, fitness, and fun.

Industrial fitness

The Adult Physical Fitness survey cited earlier in this chapter is a definite indictment of the exercise habits of adults. One of the chief areas of industrial incentive *could* be and *should* be American industry. If industrial employees could be motivated toward physical activity on a regular basis, adult exercise patterns would definitely improve. In order to achieve this goal, industrial officers must make a commitment to employees and their health and fitness. Such a commitment will represent a sound investment in the organization.

The hidden costs to American industry of the physical degeneration of its employees are staggering. For example, loss of production in the United States as a result of premature death caused by chronic cardiovascular disease alone, according to Dr. Roy J. Shephard of the University of Toronto's Department of Physiological Hygiene, is $19.4 billion per year. In addition, there are other losses: in terms of illness—$5 billion; disruption of homelife—$5 billion; hospital and other services—$3 billion. Heart attacks alone cost industry about

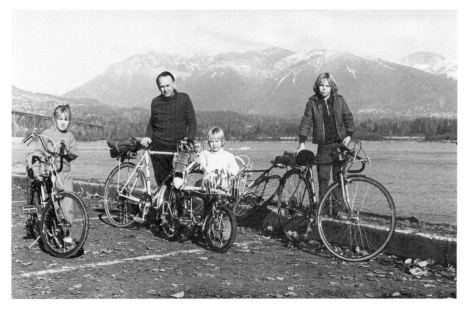

Bicycling is an excellent way to encourage family fitness. A family on a bicycle trip in Vancouver. (Courtesy Board of Parks and Public Recreation, Vancouver, B. C.)

132,000,000 workdays yearly or approximately 4% of the gross national product. Backaches, which many doctors feel are caused by physical degeneration, cost American industry $1 billion each year in lost goods and services and another $225 million in workmen's compensation, according to the National Safety Council. Such statistics do not take into consideration other important factors such as shortened work days caused by workers' fatigue and minor aches and pains, or absenteeism for several days from illness caused by lowered physical resistance to disease.

The values, on the other hand, that would accrue to American industry by instituting fitness programs in their establishments will pay hugh dividends, not only for the nation but also for industry itself. Research studies have shown that companies with fit employees have higher performance, greater production, improved morale among their workers, reduced absenteeism, more creative ideas, and better cooperation between labor and management.

W. W. Keeler, Chairman of the Board of Phillips Petroleum Company, who recently was presented with a certificate recognizing that he had jogged 400 miles in one year, was thinking of many psychologic as well as physical bene-

fits of fitness programs when he pointed out, "For most of us, the benefits of a physical conditioning program go beyond our personal well-being. They accrue to the businesses with which we are associated. When our employees are gaining physical fitness through regular exercise they become more productive and happier individuals. . . ."

Executives, in particular, should recognize the value of being physically fit, since it may provide them with a larger salary check. A survey conducted among 50,000 executives by the Robert Half Personnel Agencies and reported in *The Wall Street Journal* found that fitness and company position were related. About one out of three of those persons in the $10,000 to $20,000 salary bracket was overweight by more than 10 pounds, whereas in the $25,000 to $50,000 bracket only one out of ten was overweight by the same amount.

The fact that fitness is good business and pays dividends was shown in a study conducted by the National Aeronautics and Space Administration in cooperation with the U. S. Public Health Service. The study included 259 executives, ranging in age from 35 to 55 years, who volunteered to exercise regularly as part of their daily routine. After 1 year, the results showed that: 93% of the persons who participated in the study reported feeling better, more than 60% lost weight, 89% had greater stamina, 15% of those who smoked cut down, one out of two became more diet conscious and involved in more physical activity beyond the required program. In addition, among the subjects in the study, there were improved work performance, a more positive attitude toward the job, and their enthusiasm caused other persons outside the study with whom they associated to become interested and involved in fitness activities.

Many leading American corporations, recognizing the importance of fitness, have developed programs and provided facilities and other incentives for their employees.

North American Rockwell Corporation has one of the best industrial fitness programs in the

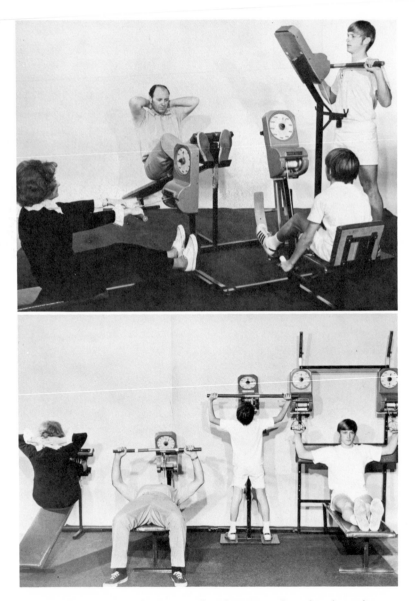

Some industrial fitness programs use various types of equipment, such as that shown here, to encourage employees to exercise. (Courtesy Mini-Gym, Independence, Mo.)

country at El Segundo, California. Begun in 1960, it has as its goal to have each employee and family member participate daily in the many physical activities that are provided. E. A. Emmick, manager of Employee Services, and Ken White, personnel representative, spent 7 years selling the values of the program within the company and the community.

The American Rockwell program requires each participant to first have a medical examination and then be tested for such components of fitness as cardiovascular efficiency and lung capacity. The test results determine the person's level of fitness and accordingly he is placed in one of five color squads: *green* (novice), *red* (average), *blue* (better), *gold* (good), and *purple* (outstanding). Employees are encouraged to try and progress from one squad to a higher level of fitness. A typical session, of which there are three to five per week for each squad, includes warmup exercises for 10 to 20 minutes, then very vigorous exercising for 5 to 30 minutes, and finally tapering off exercises for 5 to 15 minutes. Charts are posted on the walls where the performance of each participant is recorded for all to see. The activities are tailored to the needs of each individual, and competition is avoided because of the danger that some persons may overextend themselves and harm themselves physically.

Special awards may be earned in several activities by persons who reach the blue or higher division: *Running*—by jogging 1,200 miles in one year or 75 miles in 1 week; *swimming*—by swimming 500 miles in one year or 26 miles in two weeks; *bicycling*—by pedaling 5,000 miles in one year or 200 miles in 2 days, and *hiking*—by covering 50 miles in 2 days.

Executives as well as workers participate at El Segundo. As North American Rockwell's Vice President for Marketing Services, Jim Daniell, says, "When the workers see their bosses out there huffing and puffing, and sweat streaming down their faces, they say to themselves, 'There's got to be something to this physical fitness, or these fellows wouldn't be working so hard at it.'"

The Metropolitan Life Insurance Company has developed an effective physical fitness program in their home office in New York City for men aged 20 to 40. Dr. William Cunnick, Medical Director, who believes he is working with people in a vulnerable age, since it is a time when men increase their caloric input and cut down on their physical activity, developed a program that includes a physical fitness test involving jogging, rowing, bicycling, and sit-ups. The test determines how the subject's pulse rate responds to exercise. The yardstick is the length of time it takes the pulse to return to normal after exercise—the longer it takes, the poorer physical condition the person is in. After the testing is over, subjects are informed of their physical status, provided with literature on the importance of keeping fit, and encouraged to exercise regularly. A special motivating device is that each participant is given a leaflet entitled, *Measure Up To Par,* which gives the distance from various locations throughout New York City to the Metropolitan office and provides a scoring system for covering distances in a certain amount of time.

The Xerox Corporation has invested large sums of money in its fitness program at Webster, New York, where its superb facilities include an executive fitness laboratory, putting green, skating rink, and jogging paths. The company also has an executive fitness program in downtown Rochester. Clubs are organized for the employees in such sports as sailing, skiing, scuba diving, horseback riding, judo, and square dancing. Men's and women's physical fitness classes are also offered at various times of the day throughout the year. Part of the program's success is the result of the fact that it has become a prestige factor to participate—there is always a waiting list and only as participants drop out can new persons be added. To remain on the list an employee must participate at least five times every 2 weeks and no less than two times in any one week. This regulation reaffirms a basic belief that fitness level begins to deteriorate in a short period of time if training is interrupted.

Although any company desiring to develop a physical fitness program for its employees doesn't necessarily have to spend large amounts of money on facilities, it should strive to meet six other criteria developed by Glenn Swengros,

Director of Program Development for the President's Council on Physical Fitness and Sports:

> The program should be an adjunct of the company's health program.
>
> It should include a medically oriented screening test as a criterion for participation.
>
> A person skilled in prescribing exercise should direct it.
>
> Exercise should be tailored to the individual participant, and should be progressively more strenuous, in order for him to benefit from it.
>
> Activities should be noncompetitive; that is, individuals should compete only against other participants in the program.
>
> A system of periodic evaluation should be included to measure progress and to aid in program design.

THE PRESIDENT'S COUNCIL AND PHYSICAL FITNESS*

The President's Council on Physical Fitness and Sports continues to be active in promoting the cause of physical fitness throughout the United States. For example, in one year it attracted more than 10,000 persons to physical fitness clinics that were conducted by Council staff members and outstanding sports and physical education experts. It continues to award the Presidential Physical Fitness Awards to boys and girls who qualify. The number of young people receiving the award exceeds 100,000 in a year. It has established over 130 schools throughout the nation as physical fitness demonstration centers. It has been active in poverty areas in organizing programs of swimming, basketball, and other sports. These are only a few of the projects the Council is undertaking.

The President's Council on Physical Fitness and Sports, an extension of the President's Council on Youth Fitness established in 1956, came into being by Executive Order on March 4, 1968. Its purpose is to "expand opportunities to engage in exercise, active recreation and sports."

The President of the United States has urged the adoption of the recommendations of his Council by the schools in order to ensure a basic program of physical developmental ac-

tivity. A summary of these recommendations and the suggestions for implementing them follow.

Health appraisals

It is suggested that every child have continuing medical supervision from his or her family physician and dentist. This should also include periodic examinations of any disabilities. These health resources should be supplemented by school and community services. Health appraisal procedures should include:

1. Identification of students with corrective orthopedic and other health problems and subsequent referral to medical services.
2. Students' posture should be checked, including foot examination. Problems of an acute nature should be referred to medical services.
3. Height and weight measurements should be individually interpreted, and problem areas should be referred to medical supervision.
4. Other means of health appraisal and follow-through should be included as necessary.

Identification of the physically underdeveloped child

Physical performance tests are needed to identify the physically underdeveloped student. The screening tests suggested below will assist in identifying low levels of fitness. Once problems are identified, a program of developmental activities should be implemented.

Students should be screened at the beginning of the school year and retested every 6 weeks on test items failed until they pass. The recommended screening tests measure levels of cardiovascular endurance, muscular strength, and agility. The tests are:

1. Recovery index test (cardiovascular endurance)
2. Pull-ups and flexed arm hang (arm and shoulder strength)
3. Sit-ups (abdominal strength)
4. Squat thrust (agility)

Skillful observation

It is important that the physical educator is alert to all unusual signs and symptoms in order for effective screening to take place. The following signs demand medical supervision:

1. *Excessive breathlessness.* This indicates breathlessness that persists long after exercise has been completed.

---

*President's Council on Physical Fitness and Sports: Youth physical fitness—suggestions for school programs, Washington, D. C., June, 1973, The Council.

2. *Bluing of the lips*. Except in a cold, damp environment, bluing of the lips and nail beds is an unusual reaction to exercise.
3. *Pale or clammy skin*. If normal temperatures prevail, cold sweating is unusual following exercise.
4. *Unusual fatigue*. Lack of endurance or failure to maintain moderate activity suggests medical referral.
5. *Persistent shakiness*. Shaking that continues for more than 2 minutes after exercise is reason for medical attention.
6. *Muscle twitching or tetany*. Muscular contractions, localized or generalized, may occur as an unusual reaction to exercise. These should be medically checked.

Other symptoms related to exercise may also call for medical referral. These symptoms may not be a cause for alarm but should be checked:

1. Headache
2. Dizziness
3. Fainting
4. Interrupted night's sleep
5. Digestive problems
6. Pain not associated with injury
7. Undue pounding or uneven heartbeat
8. Disorientation or personality changes

FURTHER RECOMMENDATIONS OF PRESIDENT'S COUNCIL FOR EMPHASIZING PHYSICAL FITNESS IN HEALTH AND PHYSICAL EDUCATION PROGRAMS

Programs of health education and physical education recommended by the President's Council should include the following items.

Health and safety education

Direct instruction relating to specific health concepts and problems should be provided at every grade level. The topics treated should be in keeping with the interests, needs, and maturational level of the children as they progress grade by grade. Such direct instruction would be augmented by the teaching of healthful and safe behavior through the health appraisal procedures, by capitalizing on interest-arousing events, by correlating health and safety with other subjects, and by other means.

Grades 1 to 3; ages 6 to 8. At this level, much of the child's health learning relates to developing good practices in daily living at home, in the school, and in the community. Health needs include attention to cleanliness; nutrition; sleep, rest, and relaxation; heathful physical activities; acquaintance with the dentist, nurse, and physician; learning about community health agencies; care of the eyes, ears, and teeth; and elementary concepts of prevention and control of disease.

Grades 4 to 6; ages 9 to 11. Increasing attention is

given to the understanding of *why* health practices should be followed. Elementary treatment of the scientific bases of healthful and safety behavior is carried forward. New units are introduced on the body structure and function, simple first-aid procedures, elementary principles of mental and emotional health, and other topics.

Grades 7 to 9; ages 12 to 14. Direct instruction in health and safety should amount to at least one semester of five regular periods per week during the 3 years. At this level, heavier emphasis should be given to the physiological and other scientific bases and to the use of scientific methods in solving health and safety problems. The focus should be on problems of adolescence and should include units on: growth and development; differences in rate of growth; physical maturation; acne and skin disorders; effects of maintaining an adequate diet; use of tobacco, alcohol, and other drugs; getting along with parents; establishing friendships; desirable relationships with the opposite sex; introduction to vocations, including health careers; importance of exercise and physical forms of recreation; and other related topics.

Grades 10 to 12; ages 15 to 18. Instruction centers around problems of adult living and of family and community health. Important topics include: emotional health; chronic disease, such as heart disease, cancer, diabetes, and mental illness; instruction concerning consumer health (intelligent utilization of health services and products); national and international health organizations; health careers; health and safety aspects of civil defense; safety in the home, in transportation, recreation; more advanced first aid; the role of exercise in developing and maintaining health and fitness; exercise and weight control; health problems relating to alcohol, tobacco, and narcotics.

Adequate coverage of these topics requires, at a minimum, the equivalent of a full semester of daily periods of regular length. Two full semesters are recommended.

Physical education

The physical education curriculum should include a core of physical fitness activities designed to develop strength, speed, agility, balance, coordination, flexibility, muscular endurance, good posture and body mechanics, and organic efficiency. Activities and exercises should affect all parts and systems. The curriculum should also include a broad scope and balance of physical activities that promote well-rounded physical, social, and intellectual development. Activities should become progressively more complex in organization and skills, and more demanding of physical development and control grade by grade.

The programs should be adapted to the needs, interests, and capacities of each child and youth, including those pupils who, for physical and other reasons, are unable to participate safely and successfully in the general program. All pupils should be motivated to achieve high levels of physical fitness, compatible with their capabilities.

Grades 1 to 3; ages 6 to 8. Emphasis should be placed upon learning the fundamentals of movement and building a foundation of physical fitness.

Walking, running, hopping, skipping, balancing,

jumping, sliding, catching, climbing, hanging, throwing; elementary rhythmical activities, creative movement experience, and simple games which set the stage for later, more complicated activity skills; activities on the jungle gym and other types of playground equipment; simple stunts and tumbling; elementary swimming wherever possible—all of these activities and more should be included. Active participation and vigorous movement should be highlighted.

Grades 4 to 6; ages 9 to 11. The "fitness core" should have continued emphasis, giving particular attention to development of the back, chest, shoulders, and arms. This age group is ready for elementary calisthenics. Class instruction should include fundamentals of sports skills in several team sports, track and field, and simple forms of individual and dual sports. Opportunity to practice the skills and to gain knowledge in organized games should be provided.

Folk dances and other rhythmical activities are important as are relays, simple games involving running, tumbling, and simple gymnastics. Vigorous outdoor activities such as skating and cycling should be encouraged.

Screening for physical capacity as well as physical achievement testing should begin at this level and continue periodically thereafter. Simple tests of skills and knowledge should also be used.

Grades 7 to 9; ages 12 to 14. The physical fitness core should include advanced conditioning and developmental activities, e.g., weight-resistance exercises, and the activities should increase in intensity, frequency, and distance. The wide range of individual differences among these youngsters in prepubertal and pubertal stages of development should be noted and programs adjusted accordingly.

The curriculum should include a broad range of offerings in sports and other activities. Emphasis should be given to skillful participation in team sports and increasing attention to individual and dual sports that carry over to recreation hours. Intramural and extramural sports programs should be conducted.

Folk, square, and social dancing are important activities for this age group. Also to be highlighted are stunts, tumbling, gymnastics, and trampolining; aquatics (whenever feasible), with emphasis on survival tactics; combative activities, e.g., wrestling (for boys); and outing activities, e.g., hiking, camping, and hunting.

Grades 10 to 12; ages 15 to 18. The fitness core continues to be stressed with more opportunities for individual leadership provided.

The broad program is carried forward with particular emphasis on sports, rhythmics, and other activities that carry over into recreation hours throughout life. Specialization in such activities should be encouraged. Ways of maintaining physical fitness at various age levels under

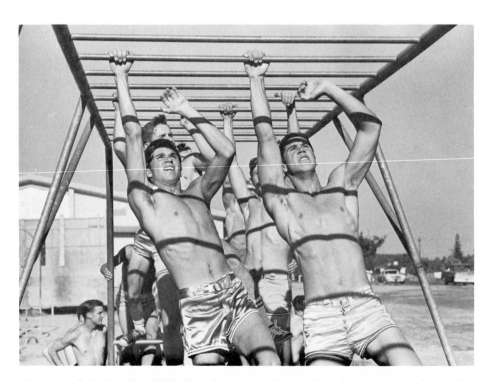

The development of the shoulder girdle through such exercises as these is important to the development of muscular strength. (Courtesy President's Council on Physical Fitness and Sports.)

varying circumstances should be taught. Additional attention should also be given to outing activities and recreational activities for the family unit, particularly those that promote physical aspects of fitness. *

PHYSICAL FITNESS TESTING

The history of physical fitness testing goes back many years. It probably started as part of the physical education profession at the time when anthropometry was utilized. Anthropometry involved the measuring of the body and its parts, since size seemed to be related to strength. Then there was the emphasis on strength testing, often through use of dynamometers. The work of Dudley A. Sargent and his development of the Intercollegiate Strength Test are characteristic of this early era. It was soon realized, however, that strength testing alone could not measure the functional capacity of individuals. This realization led to cardiorespiratory testing. Schneider expressed this concept when he said:

Physical exertion overtaxes the circulatory mechanism long before it exhausts skeletal musculature; and while it is not easy to overwork the muscles, the heart can quite

readily be overworked. The convalescent from infectious disease is limited in his exercise not by what his muscles can do but by the strength of his heart. Hence today the general opinion is that strength tests do not permit us to draw satisfactory conclusions regarding the efficiency of the entire body. *

As a result of this emphasis on functional capacity, many tests were developed, most of which involved changes in frequency of heart rate and blood pressure as a result of exercise. Examples of these are Tuttle's Pulse Ratio Test, McCurdy-Larson's Organic Efficiency Test, Carlson's Fatigue Test Curve, and Brouha's Step Test.

In 1925 strength testing was revived by Frederick Rand Rogers with his emphasis on physical capacity tests in the administration of physical education. More recent developments in strength testing have been accomplished by Harrison Clarke, who developed the tensiometer for use with orthopedic disabilities and by Hans Kraus and Ruth P. Hirschland, who devised a six-item test of "minimum muscular fitness" that appraises flexibility as well as strength.

---

*President's Council on Physical Fitness and Sports: Youth physical fitness—suggestions for school programs, Washington, D. C., June, 1973, The Council.

*Schneider, E. C.: Physical efficiency and the limitations of efficiency tests, American Physical Education Review **28:**405, 1923.

GIRLS' PHYSICAL FITNESS TEST RECORD

Name _____ Grade _____ Period _____

School _____ Age ____ Ht. ____ Wt. ____ Test 1 Classification _____

Age ____ Ht. ____ Wt. ____ Test 2 Classification _____

Test No.	1		2	
Date				
Event	Score	Percentile	Score	Percentile
Modified Pull-Ups				
Sit-Ups (Max 50)				
Broad Jump				
50-yd. Dash				
Shuttle Run				
Modified Push-Ups				
600-yd. Run-Walk				
Softball Throw				
P.F.I.—Average percentile of 5 events				

During World War II, when physical fitness was a major objective, several performance type tests were developed. Some of these were the Army Air Force Test, the Army Physical Efficiency Test, the Navy Standard Physical Fitness Test, and the Victory Corps Test.

Several tests with which to measure physical fitness are available today. Some of these have been scientifically validated, whereas others have been presented without objective evidence of validity. Validity and reliability are important criteria of a test, but administrative efficiency may place one test ahead of another. Validity, however, is the weak point in most physical fitness tests today.

Not all physical fitness tests measure the same kind of physical fitness. The evidence is that tests of physical fitness do not correlate very highly. Therefore, when selecting a fitness test, it is necessary to select one that measures the kind of fitness the program is aiming to achieve.

It is difficult to identify the items we want to measure in physical fitness. Many experts feel we are a long way from having an all-purpose test and that it would be better to test component parts of physical fitness (posture, strength, balance, endurance), by means of several tests of each component. Then, through a partial correlation process it would be possible to determine the most valid test of each component. In turn, these most valid tests could be combined into a battery. Most physical fitness tests measure component factors that are not truly comprehensive. They stress primarily arm strength, leg strength, and endurance. However, there are other considerations. For example, a husky body requires more strength for one pull-up than does a slight one. In addition to body build, physiologic age (when dealing with children) should also be considered. These and similar factors may account for the difficulty in validating tests.

The possibility of a universal battery of tests is remote because of disagreement among experts as to the nature of physical fitness. How much of it is esthetic and how much is a matter of health or expediency? Many physical education leaders feel it is important that the profession consider the adoption of a single tool of measurement. They feel this is of utmost importance if we are to propose a program that will become widely adopted and provide an answer to the present demand for an emphasis on physical fitness.

Tables 11-1 and 11-2 list the physical fitness components and tests that measure these components, as well as the selected tests of physical fitness.

The American Alliance for Health, Physical Education, and Recreation* has developed its own physical fitness test for national use.

---

*AAHPER youth fitness test manual, American Association for Health, Physical Education, and Recreation, 1201 16th St. N.W., Washington, D. C. 20036.

Table 11-1. Physical fitness components and tests*

Component	Selected tests
Arm and shoulder strength	Pull-ups, push-ups, parallel bar, dips, rope climb
Speed	50-yard dash, 100-yard dash
Agility	Shuttle run, agility run
Abdominal and hip strength	Sit-ups, sit-ups with knees flexed, 2-minute sit-ups
Flexibility	Trunk flexion standing, trunk flexion sitting, trunk extension (prone position)
Cardiorespiratory endurance	600-yard run, half-mile run, mile run, 5-minute step test
Explosive power	Standing broad jump, vertical jump
Static strength	Grip strength, back lift, leg lift
Balance	Bass test, Brace test, tests on balance beam
Muscular endurance	Push-ups, chest raisings (prone position, hands behind neck, legs held down), V-sit (against time)

*From Hunsicker, P.: Physical fitness—what research says to the teacher, Washington, D. C., 1963, National Education Association, p. 17.

It consists of seven basic items plus a swimming test:

1. Pull-ups (modified for girls to flexed arm hang); to test arm and shoulder girdle strength
2. Sit-ups; to test strength of abdominal muscles and hip flexors
3. Shuttle run: to test speed and change of direction
4. Standing broad jump: to test explosive power of leg extensors
5. 50-yard dash: to test speed
6. Softball throw for distance: to test skill and coordination
7. 600-yard walk or run: to test cardiovascular system
8. Swimming test (jump into water, rest, and swim 15 yards): to test protective powers in the water

Norms have been established for girls and boys in grades five through twelve and for college students and may be obtained from the Alliance. A manual gives, in addition, complete directions for testing each item.

The State Department of Education of New York State* is an example of many state groups that have developed their own physical fitness tests for local use. The New York test consists of seven components that are measured to obtain a total physical fitness score:

1. Posture—evaluated by means of a posture rating chart
2. Accuracy—measured by means of a target throw, utilizing a softball and a circular target
3. Strength—evaluated by pull-ups for boys and modified pull-ups for girls
4. Agility—evaluated by means of the side-step
5. Speed—evaluated by means of the 50-yard dash

*New York State physical fitness test, The University of the State of New York, The State Education Department, Albany, New York.

Table 11-2. Selected tests of physical fitness*

Test	Source
AAHPER Youth Fitness Test	American Association for Health, Physical Education, and Recreation, 1201 16th St. N.W. Washington, D. C. 20036.
AAHPER-U. S. Office of Education Committee on Physical Fitness for Girls	Journal of HPER, pp. 308-311, 354-355, June, 1945.
All-around Muscular Endurance	Anderson, John E.: Endurance of young men, Society for Research in Child Development, vol. X, serial No. 40, No. 1, Washington, D. C., 1958, American Association for Health, Physical Education, and Recreation.
Army/Air Forces Physical Fitness Test	AAHPER Research Quarterly **15:**12-15, March, 1944.
Army Physical Fitness Test	War Department, FM 21-20, 1945.
California Physical Fitness Test	California State Department of Education, Feb., 1948.
Harvard Step Test	AAHPER Research Quarterly **14:**31-36, March, 1943.
Illinois Physical Fitness Test for High School Boys	Illinois State Department of Public Instruction, Bulletin No. 6, 1944.
Indiana High School Physical Condition Test	Indiana State Office of Public Instruction, Bulletin No. 136, Sept., 1944.
The JCR Test	AAHPER Research Quarterly **18:**12-29, March, 1947.
Kraus-Weber Test of Minimum Muscular Fitness	AAHPER Research Quarterly **25:**178-188, May, 1954.
Larson Muscular Strength Test	AAHPER Research Quarterly **11:**82-96, Dec., 1940.
McCloy Strength Test	McCloy, H. C., and Young, N. E.: Tests and measurements in health and physical education, ed. 3, New York, 1954, Appleton-Century-Crofts, pp. 128-152.
Navy Standard Physical Fitness	Bureau of Naval Personnel, Training Division, Physical Fitness Section, 1943.
New York State Physical Fitness Test	New York State Education Department, 1948.
Youth Physical Fitness	President's Council on Youth Fitness: Youth physical fitness, Washington, D. C., 1961, United States Government Printing Office.
Rogers Strength Test	Clarke, H. Harrison: Application of measurement to health and physical education, ed. 3, New York, 1959, Prentice-Hall, Inc. pp. 182-213.

*From Hunsicker, P.: Physical fitness—what research says to the teacher, Washington, D. C., 1963, National Education Association, p. 17.

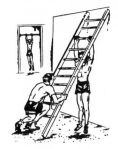

Improvised equipment for pull-up.

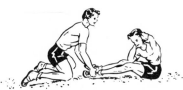

Final position for sit-up.

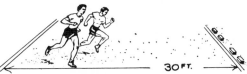

Starting the shuttle run.

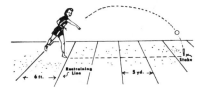

Measuring the softball throw for distance.

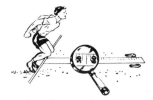

Measuring the standing broad jump.

Test items from AAHPER Youth Fitness Test Manual. (From NEA Journal **51**:33, 1962.)

6. Balance—evaluated by means of the squat-stand
7. Endurance—evaluated by means of the treadmill

Norms have been established and are listed in a manual, together with a description of the test.

In recent years studies have been written that question the validity of fitness testing. One of the tests questioned is the AAHPER Youth Fitness Test.* One may ask the question of the test, "Is it really a fitness test or a test of fitness-motor capability?" If students possess little skill in ball throwing, then of what value is measuring arm and shoulder strength through the use of the softball throw? Should the 50-yard dash be used as a measure of fitness? The ability to run fast is not really a fitness component. Some very "unfit" persons may run very fast, whereas "fit" people may do poorly on such a test. In addition, the standing broad jump requires a high degree of body coordination but does not necessarily indicate fitness. The validity of most currently used physical fitness tests should be carefully researched and tested by experts in this field. All such tests need frequent updating in the light of current scientific information.

Questions and exercises

1. Outline what you consider to be an effective physical fitness program for a high school.

---

*Smith, C. O.: Fitness testing: questions about how, what, and with what, Journal of Health, Physical Education, and Recreation **43**:37, 1972.

2. Discuss the health appraisal and identification of the physically underdeveloped child policies of the President's Council on Physical Fitness and Sports.
3. What are some of the recommendations of the President's Council regarding physical education programs?
4. Develop your own definitions of fitness and physical fitness.
5. Discuss industrial fitness in detail, outlining its objectives, advantages, and disadvantages. Interview an officer of a local corporation in order to determine the extent of industrial fitness programs at this corporation.
6. Evaluate the statement of fitness made by the American Association for Health, Physical Education, and Recreation.
7. What are some of the tests for physical fitness? Evaluate each in the light of criteria in the chapter on Measurement and Evaluation.

Reading assignment in *Administrative Dimensions of Health and Physical Education Programs, Including Athletics:* Chapter 5, Selection 27.

Selected references

AMA and AAHPER Joint Committee: Exercise and fitness, Journal of Health, Physical Education, and Recreation **35:**5, 1964.

American Association for Health, Physical Education, and Recreation: Youth fitness test manual, Washington, D. C., 1961, The Association.

Annarino, A. A.: Developmental conditioning for physical education and athletics, St. Louis, 1972, The C. V. Mosby Co.

Barney, V. S.: Conditioning exercises, St. Louis, 1973, The C. V. Mosby Co.

Bucher, C. A.: Highlights of President's Conference on Fitness of American Youth, unpublished paper, 1956.

Bucher, C. A.: Foundations of physical education, ed. 7, St. Louis, 1975, The C. V. Mosby Co.

Collins, G. J., and Hunter, J. S.: Physical achievement and the schools, Bureau of Educational Research and Development, Office of Education Bulletin, 1965, No. 13.

Cureton, T. K.: Physical fitness and dynamic health, New York, 1973, Dial Press.

Espenschade, A.: Restudy of relationships between physical performances of school children and age, height, and weight, Research Quarterly **34:**144, 1963.

Gallagher, J. R., and Brouha, L.: Physical fitness, Journal of the American Medical Association **125:**834, 1944.

Hatch, C.: Physical fitness: a practical program, Rutland, Vermont, 1970, C. E. Tuttle.

Hunsicker, P.: Physical fitness—what research tells the teacher, Washington, D. C., 1963, National Education Association.

Johnson, W. P., and Kleva, R.: The community dimension of college physical education, Journal of Health, Physical Education, and Recreation **44:**40, April, 1973.

Johnson, W. R., editor: Science and medicine of exercise and sports, New York, 1960, Harper & Row, Publishers.

Journal of the American Association for Health, Physical Education, and Recreation, Sept., 1957, entire issue.

Kraus, H., and Hirschland, R. P.: Minimum muscular fitness tests in school children, Research Quarterly **25:**178, 1954.

Newsletter: National adult physical fitness survey, President's Council on Physical Fitness and Sports, May, 1973.

Newsletter: The Travelers, President's Council joins forces to promote family fitness, President's Council on Physical Fitness and Sports, April-May, 1973.

President's Council on Youth Fitness: Suggestions for school programs, Washington, D. C., September, 1973, The Council.

Report of the National Conference on Fitness of Secondary School Youth: Youth and fitness: a program for secondary schools, Washington, D. C., 1958, American Association for Health, Physical Education, and Recreation.

Ricci, B.: Physical and physiological conditioning for Journal of Health, Physical Education, and Recreation **41:**28, March, 1970.

Ricci, B.: Physical and Physiological conditioning for men, Dubuque, Iowa, 1972, William C. Brown Co.

Roy, H.: Physical fitness for schools, New York, 1971, International Publications Service.

Smith, C. D.: Fitness testing: questions about how, why, and with what, Journal of Health, Physical Education, and Recreation **43:**37, February, 1972.

Vitale, F.: Fitness in a changing world, Englewood Cliffs, N. J., 1972, Prentice-Hall, Inc.

Vitale, F.: Individualized fitness programs, Englewood Cliffs, N. J., 1973, Prentice-Hall, Inc.

PART THREE

Health programs
for students

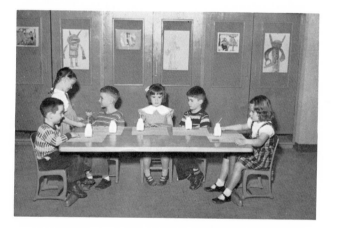

The health science instruction program–with implications for physical education*

Some persons may question the need for health instruction in the 1970's. These people often feel that health materials are widely disseminated through the media, and certain controversial health topics are best left alone. However, there are many sound reasons that health instruction should be offered to school and college students. Some of these reasons are as follows:

1. Healthful living should be inculcated at an early age so persons may live their lives in the best possible manner.
2. Health should be a primary objective of education, and health-directed behavior should be established early in life.
3. In our ever-shrinking world, the possibility of contracting disease increases, and health education can aid in anticipating and solving this problem.
4. Health problems encompass our daily lives, and we should be educated in such areas as drug, alcohol, and tobacco abuse; obesity; heart disease; nutrition; environmental problems, and accidents. These are ony a few of the situations with which we must learn to deal adequately.
5. Numbers of mental health problems reach new high figures each year. An important

aspect of health instruction includes mental and emotional well-being.
6. The need to understand human sexuality, marriage, problems of divorce and children of divorced parents, and family-life education are essential to the well-being of a person growing up in today's society.

Our communities, schools, and individual families have a responsibility to educate young people in health-related matters. The school provides only one facet of health instruction, and health education should not be limited to young people. Society in general needs to be made aware of new health developments and how they affect us as individuals. Health education is for all people of all ages.

Throughout the history of education the schools and colleges have indicated an interest in health. In 1918 the report of a commission on education of the National Education Association listed health as its first objective. The Educational Policies Commission, an important policy-making group in education, pointed out that an educated person understands basic facts concerning health and disease, protects his or her own health and that of his or her dependents, and strives to improve the health of the community. The American Council on Education, an-

---

*The school and college attempt to promote health in children and youth through a specialized program that contributes to the understanding, maintenance, and improvement of the health of students and school personnel, including health services, health science instruction, and healthful school living. The healthful school and college living phase of the health program will be considered in Chapters 14 and 15. The health services phase of the total health program will be considered in Chapter 13.

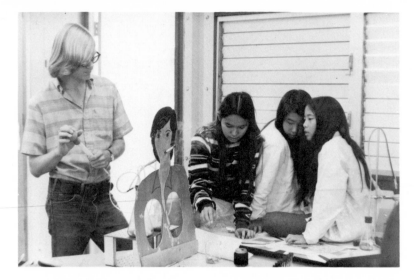

In health studies class at Kaiser High School in Honolulu, Hawaii, students of Japanese, Hawaiian, and American backgrounds analyze the effects of smoking. (Courtesy Ed Arrigoni.)

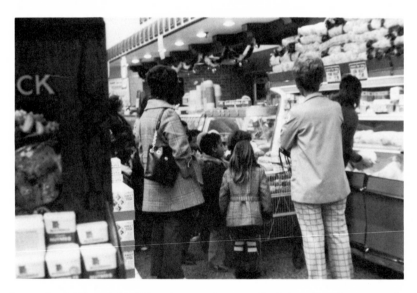

Health education teacher in Greenbelt, Md., takes her class on a food shopping trip as part of a nutrition unit. (Courtesy Eileen Cleinman Forman.)

other policy-making group, has encouraged schools and colleges to help pupils improve and maintain their health. White House Conferences on Education have stressed physical and mental health as important educational objectives.

There are well-supported reasons for these statements emphasizing the importance of health in education. Research has shown that the healthy person has a better chance to be a suc-

cess in school and college, to be more effective scholastically and academically, and to be more productive. In addition to these factors, it should be noted that the school acts in loco parentis and, as such, has a legal as well as a moral responsibility to concern itself with the health of the student.

If schools and colleges accept their responsibility for, and do an effective job in, health

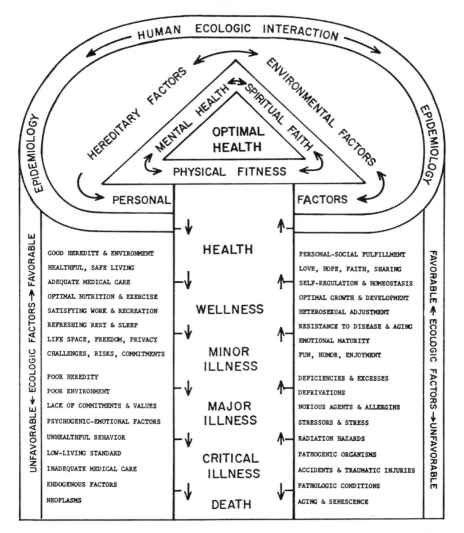

An ecologic model of health and disease. Examples of favorable and unfavorable dynamic, interacting, hereditary, environmental, and personal ecologic factors and conditions that are determinants of the levels of health and disease on a continuum extending from zero health (death) to optimal health. (From Hoyman, H. S.: Journal of School Health **35**:113, 1965.)

science instruction, the program should result in the following:

1. Students will become concerned about health matters and relate their knowledge to themselves, their families, and their communities.

2. Students will have a better understanding of the values of health, the necessity of maintaining good health, and the contributions that good health makes to human effectiveness and happiness.

3. Students will be aware of available health services and effective health consumption.

They will not be taken advantage of by quick-cure claims and other fraudulent health schemes.

Many children and youth with different kinds of health problems and disabilities are attending schools and colleges, and few live at their optimal level of physical and emotional efficiency. Students are involved in accidents caused by carelessness. They suffer from remediable physical defects. They find it difficult to be realistic in respect to the demands of their environment. They contract needless diseases and infections.

A recognition of the need for health science

instruction in the schools and colleges has developed through the years, as educators and the lay public have come to realize the importance of providing learning experiences that will result in healthful living for more people. Furthermore, they have come to see more clearly the relationship of knowledge, attitudes, and practices in respect to health.

The importance of health has been taught by educators since early times. Older generations tell about how they received instruction in physiology, learned how to trace the flow of blood through the body, and memorized long definitions of various anatomic and physiologic aspects of the human body. This approach to health education has changed over the years. Toward the end of the nineteenth century some new ideas were introduced into school and college curricula. This resulted from a feeling on the part of certain individuals that students should be taught about the evil effects of alcoholic beverages. They also felt there should be a greater emphasis on the hygienic aspects of living. As a result, these concepts became an important part of health teaching, especially in colleges.

This emphasis continued until the early twentieth century. Then, the impact of World Wars I and II gave health education the impetus it needed to become firmly embedded as an important part of school and college programs. The public became aroused, for example, by the number of health defects discovered in young men through Selective Service examinations. The results of such a disclosure included passing state laws, developing courses of study, publishing textbooks concerned with health education, and providing for the training of special teachers in this area. Today, there is increased recognition that health education can play a very important role in helping to make individuals aware of their responsibility for their own health and also that of others. Health is regarded as "everybody's business."

There is increased emphasis upon health teaching in schools and colleges today and upon such topics as drugs, ecology, sex and family life education, alcohol, tobacco, personality development, and accident prevention. Professional preparation institutions are placing greater emphasis on instructing teachers about their responsibilities in this area. There is closer cooperation between the school or college and community health officers. Medical doctors, dentists, and other representatives of professional services are taking more interest in health. School and college administrators and their teaching and professional staffs are voicing concern about students and their health. More research is providing new and better directions to help the schools and colleges in changing the health behavior of many boys and girls.

THE NATURE AND SCOPE OF HEALTH SCIENCE INSTRUCTION

One of the revealing studies in the area of health education and the schools was the School Health Education Study. This study determined the nature and scope of health education in the public schools of the United States, the kind of instruction students receive, how much boys and girls know about health matters, who teaches these pupils, how the subject is organized and scheduled in the school program, the health content areas that need to be emphasized, and many other factors of importance to all educators and persons interested in health. As a result of this study and professional efforts in the field, great improvements have been made in health science instruction. The project involved such procedures as a survey of 135 public school systems regarding the health practices of approximately 16 million students in more than 1,000 elementary schools and 359 secondary schools. The following represents a sampling of some of the findings in this study:

Most health instruction in the elementary schools is taught by the classroom teacher, without supervisory assistance, and is included in the curriculum in combination with other subjects.

On the average, in those districts with secondary grades, a separate class in health education is offered in grades 7 and 8 by 61.2 percent of the large, 69.1 percent of the medium, and 48.0 percent of the small school districts. The average percentage of districts scheduling a separate class of health education in grades 9 through 12 is 52.2 percent of the large, 43.1 percent of the medium, and 31.8 percent of the small school districts.

On the average, health education is a required subject for all students in grades 7 and 8 in 55.6 percent of the large, 62.2 percent of the medium, and 48.0 percent of the small school districts of the sample group of districts that included secondary grades; in grades 8 through 12, 25.0 percent of the large, 37.5 percent of the medium, and 24.9 percent of the small districts require health education of all students.

In all districts, two-thirds or more of the health classes in grades 7, 8, and 9 and 90 percent or more in grades 10, 11, and 12 in all districts are taught by the teacher with a combined major in health and physical education, or with specialization in physical education only. The percentage reported varied by grades and within districts.

In the majority of secondary schools, boys and girls are separated for health instruction. In those instances where combined classes are scheduled, these tended to be the pattern more frequently in grades 7 and 8 than in the upper grades. Percentages of responses vary throughout the grades and among the districts. The majority of responses indicate that separate classes in health education for boys and girls are held because of staff, space, and scheduling problems. The nature of the subject matter as a reason for a separation was mentioned to a far lesser extent and then mainly by the medium and small districts only.

At the secondary level the large districts rely to a far greater extent than do the medium or small districts on local curriculum guides and local community influence in determining course content. The small districts depend heavily on the state course of study as a resource for deciding what to teach in health education. *

Some instructional problems involved with health science instruction, as cited by school administrators in the School Health Education Study, are ineffectiveness of instructional methods, parental and community resistance to certain health topics, insufficient time allocated for health instruction, lack of coordination, inadequate professional staff, lack of interest among teachers, and neglect of the health education course when combined with the physical education experience.

The School Health Education Study revealed that many health misconceptions exist among students. A brief sampling of these misconceptions includes the following:

1. Commercial medicines are safe to purchase if the label clearly indicates the dose and contents, or if recommended by a pharmacist.
2. The use of "pep" pills and sleeping pills does not require medical supervision.
3. The purpose of fluoridating water supplies is to purify water and make it safe to drink.

4. Unrefrigerated chicken salad is not a potential source of food poisoning.
5. Chronic diseases can be transmitted from person to person.
6. Venereal disease can be inherited.

In respect to the basic health science course in colleges and universities, a survey conducted a few years ago showed that better than 80% of the institutions included in the survey offered a personal health course for their students. In some cases the course was offered on an elective basis, in other cases it was required. Teacher preparatory programs, in particular, provided the setting for most of the required courses.

The college survey also showed that in most cases the basic health science course was offered by the Health and Physical Education Department. However, in other cases it was offered by Departments of Biology or Zoology, Science Department, Department of General Education, Home Economics Department, College Health Service, College of Medicine, and College of Nursing.

The college survey further showed that the basic health science course was offered on the average for two or three semester or quarter hour credits and was taught by a variety of persons including health educators, physical educators, biologists, and physicians. Some of the topics covered in the courses included mental health, family health, nutrition, reproduction, tobacco, alcohol, narcotics, preparation for marriage, personal appearance, disease control, health appraisal, and care of the body.

The School Health Education Study and other more recent research findings indicate more and more the need for health science instruction in schools and colleges. The growth and development characteristics of students, the social demands of dating, the preparation for marriage, and the pressures of the peer group are important considerations. Youth must be helped to make informed choices in meeting the pressing problems they face each day of their lives. These studies have shown that students are weak in health content concerning fatigue, sleep and rest, mental health, and habit-forming substances; that exposure to alcohol tends to occur first at 13 to 14 years of age; that dietary practices become increasingly worse throughout the

*School Health Education Study: A summary report, Washington, D. C., 1964, National Education Association.

teen-age years; that the greatest number of smokers begin smoking between 10 and 15 years of age; and that annually venereal diseases infect one out of every 250 young persons 15 to 19 years of age.

Tables 12-1 and 12-2 indicate the training that teachers of health in one state have had. As the tables show, physical educators play a major role in teaching health in today's schools.

TEACHER CERTIFICATION IN HEALTH EDUCATION

In recent years there has been a trend among school systems to employ full-time health in-

Table 12-1. Undergraduate majors of teachers of health *

Major	Teachers	Major	Teachers
Physical education	775	Psychology	4
Health education and	289	Business	4
physical education		Nursing	4
Science	173	Education	3
Biology	100	Special education	3
Home economics	99	Recreation	3
Social studies	32	Physiology	2
English	24	Physics	2
History	18	Guidance	2
Social science	16	Music	2
Health education	15	Industrial arts	1
Elementary education	13	French	1
Chemistry	8	Theology	1
Mathematics	6	Speech	1
Art	5	Political science	1
Physical science	4		

*From Michigan Department of Education: Patterns and features of school health education in Michigan public schools, East Lansing, 1969, Michigan State Department of Education, p. 7.

Table 12-2. Undergraduate minors of teachers of health *

Minor	Teachers	Minor	Teachers
Health education	258	Driver education	4
Physical education	128	Art	3
Science	68	Natural science	2
Biology	58	Spanish	2
Social studies	39	Physiology	2
English	34	Psychology	2
History	32	German	1
Social science	32	French	1
Mathematics	16	Journalism	1
Home economics	15	Conservation	1
Physical science	8	Economics	1
Elementary education	7	Political science	1
Business	7	Dance	1
Education	6	Language	1
Speech	6	Guidance	1
Geography	5	Commercial	1
Chemistry	5	Literature	1
Recreation	5	Nursing	1
Industrial arts	5	Zoology	1

*From Michigan Department of Education: Patterns and features of school health education in Michigan public schools, East Lansing, 1969, Michigan State Department of Education, p. 7.

structors. Schools have come to recognize the specialized nature of health instruction and are seeking teachers who have special college preparation in health education.

This trend is reflected in the growth of professional preparation programs for school health educators in the colleges and universities of the United States. In the years from March, 1961, to January, 1970, the number of schools offering majors in health education doubled from 43 to 87. As of January, 1970, 104 institutions offered degree programs in school health education.* In 1974 there were 165 institutions.

There are no national standards for health certification requirements. Many health teachers are not adequately prepared to teach health. Certification for specific requirements in order to teach health education should be the prerequisite for being employed as a health teacher. The scope of health education continues to expand, and the most qualified persons are needed to teach in this area.

What can be done to improve the current situation regarding health certification? Some suggestions follow:

1. Standards of health education certification should be set according to competence and performance levels.
2. Guidelines leading to reciprocity in certification should be established.
3. Efforts to establish certification requirements should be coordinated with appropriate health-oriented organizations and agencies.

COMPETENCY BASED PROFESSIONAL PREPARATION IN HEALTH EDUCATION

Temple University's new competency based program is "primarily designed to prepare school health educators whose basic role is to conduct programs of classroom instruction of various developmental and learning levels. In addition, it serves to enable the individual to become involved in some phase of program leadership by developing competencies in curriculum design, administration, evaluation, and human relationships."*

The program at Temple University takes into consideration that health education majors must also have appropriate preparation in general studies. The four general education areas include: humanities, social sciences, natural sciences and mathematics, and human performance. The general competencies stressed include:

1. Personal qualities of self-direction, self-actualization, communication, and decision-making
2. Understanding humans as thinking, creative organisms
3. Understanding humans in a social context
4. Understanding humans as functioning organisms

The professional education component of the health major program at Temple University includes 80 semester hours, or approximately 60% of the 4-year program. The areas studied include: health sciences, theoretical practice, learning theory and teaching, and research, evaluation, and measurement. Additional alternative methods of achieving competencies in the health program include an independent guided study program and a field work experience. The guided study program enables the student, working with the major field advisor, to select specific readings, research activities, and independent projects (related to health science) and carry them through to fruition. Field work provides for laboratory, clinical, or actual work experiences as a method of developing professional competencies.

In order to evaluate professional competencies for graduation and certification, four examinations are conducted to assess competencies in the professional education program. These examinations are given in health science, theoretical practice, learning theory and teaching, and research, evaluation, and measurement. The competency examinations may be taken at any time during the student's program in the health education curriculum.

---

*Statistics adapted from report: Institutions offering programs of specialization in health education, School Health Education Study, Washington, D. C., 1970.

*Levy, M., Greene, W., and Jenne, F.: Competency based professional preparation: School Health Review **3:**26, 1972.

ADMINISTRATION OF THE HEALTH SCIENCE INSTRUCTION PROGRAM

The manner in which health science instruction is administered will vary with the local situation. At the outset, however, it should be recognized that health education should be taught by individuals who are trained in the methodology of teaching. An individual who has studied educational psychology and other subjects that yield knowledges and techniques important to effective teaching is better prepared to do a good job of instruction in health than is the individual who does not have such training. This does not exclude using representatives of the health department and voluntary health agencies as consultants and resource persons. They can be invaluable in drawing up courses of study and in the presentation of various phases of the health education program.

Local administration will again determine where health science instruction should be located within the school or college structure. In some schools and colleges it is placed in such areas as physical education, science, and home economics. In other schools and colleges it is a separate area by itself. In most schools and colleges health is administratively located in the health and physical education department. In the larger schools especially, and in colleges and universities, there may be a separate health education department with full-time personnel who have been trained in the area of health education. Such an administrative arrangement is conducive to good interrelationships between the school and college and public health agencies, to the development of a health council, and to a well-coordinated and well-integrated health program. In smaller and medium-sized schools and colleges, there should also be full-time health educators charged with this important responsibility.

The physical education person many times is assigned such responsibilities as coaching, intramurals, and special events in addition to physical education classes. If the responsibility for health education is given to a teacher of physical education, in addition to these numerous other duties, some responsibility is going to suffer. In many cases, with pressure for winning teams, the class instruction program is neglected. School and college administrators should recognize that health education is a very important part of the school or college offering. It should be assigned only to qualified persons and should receive ample time and facilities to make it effective.

Every school and college, regardless of size, should have someone on its staff assigned to coordinate the various aspects of the health program. In larger schools and colleges this might be a full-time position. In smaller schools and colleges it could be the principal, chairman of the health department, or some qualified staff member who has interest and responsibility in this area.

The administration of the health education program should also include a health council or committee. The *health council* would be composed of representatives from the central administration, subject matter areas, students, parents, professional groups, community members, custodial staff, and others whose duties have particular bearing on the health of the student. Such a group of individuals, regardless of type or size of school, can play an important part in planning and carrying out the health education program. They can be instrumental in providing the necessary funds, materials, staff, and experiences that make for an outstanding program. They would have as a major responsibility the identification and solution of health problems.

ADMINISTRATIVE PROBLEMS ENCOUNTERED IN SCHOOL HEALTH PROGRAMS

The area of health education involves problems of integrating departments to achieve the best possible health continuum in dealing with students and parents concerning sensitive health issues. These and other problems are mentioned here for consideration:

1. How should the health education curriculum be decided upon? Who should be involved in this decision?
2. Who should teach health education courses and should health certification be mandatory?
3. What materials should be utilized in teaching health courses? Who should decide upon the use of these materials?
4. How should community resources be utilized, and which ones should be used?

Statistical
Bulletin
January
1974

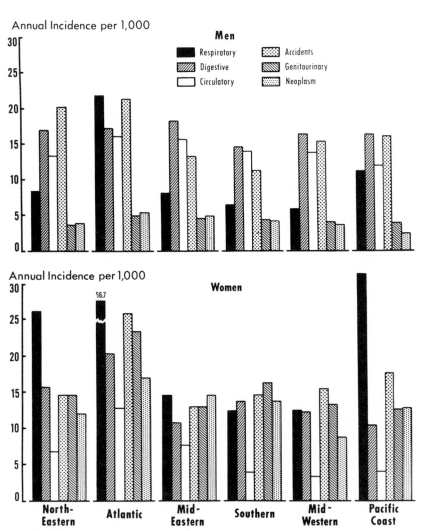

The incidence of health disabilities, many of which can be prevented, is one indication of the need for health science instruction. (Courtesy Metropolitan Life Insurance Company. From Metropolitan Life Insurance Company Statistical Bulletin, January, 1974, New York.)

5. How can health educators and physical educators work together cooperatively?
6. How should such topics as human sexuality and drug abuse be dealt with?
7. How should the administration handle pregnancy among its students?
8. What is the best method of working with physicians, dentists, nurses, and other community health personnel?
9. How can students become more involved in planning for health education programs?
10. How can the effectiveness of health education programs be evaluated?

THE SCHOOL HEALTH TEAM

The following paragraphs discuss those persons who are participants in the school health team.

Teacher of health. The teacher of health is a key person if the health science program is to be effective. This person should possess an understanding of what constitutes a well-rounded health program and the teacher's part in it. Preparation should include a basic understanding of the various physical, biologic, and behavioral sciences that help to explain the importance of health to the optimal functioning of the individual, including understanding of such areas as structure and growth of the human body, nutrition, and mental health. The teacher should be interested in the health needs and interests of pupils, possess personal characteristics that exemplify good health, and acquire knowledge and skill for presenting health knowledge in a meaningful and interesting manner to all students. The teacher should be competent to organize health teaching units in terms of the health needs and interests of students, motivate the child to be well and happy, and be aware of the individual differences of the pupils. The teacher should also be able and willing to interpret the school health program to the community and enlist its support in solving health problems.

Health coordinator. The health coordinator is a person on the staff who has special qualifications that enable him or her to serve as a coordinator, supervisor, teacher, or consultant for health education. He or she is concerned with developing effective working relationships with school, college, and community health programs and coordinating the total school or college health program with the general educational program. A health coordinator can render valuable service in seeing that a well-rounded health program exists. Health instruction can be more carefully planned. In addition to the direct health teaching, there can also be provision for the correlation and integration of health instruction with many subject matter areas. Resource materials can be provided for the classroom and other teachers involved in health teaching. School, college, and community relationships can be developed. The total health program can be guided to function as an integrated whole. Each administrator should recognize the importance of the position of health coordinator and designate a person qualified for such a responsibility. The Nebraska State Departments of Health and Education outline the responsibilities for the health coordinator in the panel below.

School or college administrator. The school or college administrator is a key figure in making important decisions in regard to health programs, such as the personnel appointed to teach health courses, the methods of instruction, the topics to be covered, and the budget essential to having the necessary equipment and supplies. Therefore, a school or college administrator, to be effective in the health science program, should be sympathetic and interested in meeting the health needs and interests of students, in see-

---

The school health coordinator should:*

Coordinate the health activities of all school personnel.

Provide leadership in the development of a health curriculum based upon the progression of health knowledge, concepts, and activities from kindergarten through high school.

Serve as a liaison person between school, public, and voluntary health agencies to establish desirable working relationships and coordination of school and community health efforts.

Be a resource person for teachers needing help with health education materials, references, teaching aids, and methods.

Establish good relationships with the community's professional medical and dental resources so that the school's program is properly understood.

Promote inservice training for the teaching of health through faculty meetings, small group meetings, workshop shop sessions with nurses and other school health personnel, and individual interviews with teachers.

With the assistance of the school health council, study needs and present activities of the school health program; from the findings make recommendations that will develop an improved program.

*From Health policies and procedures for Nebraska schools, Lincoln, Nebraska Department of Health and the Nebraska Department of Education, p. 8.

ing that the health courses include topics that meet these needs and interests, and in assuring that health is taught by competent faculty members in a way that will motivate behavior.

School or college physician. The school or college physician can be an effective member of the health team by discussing results of medical examinations with teachers, drawing implications from the medical examinations for health science instruction, stressing to administrators and the community in general the need for instruction in health, visiting classes, and periodically being a visiting lecturer in the health classes.

Nurse. The nurse works closely with medical personnel on one hand and with students, teachers, and parents on the other. As the person who engages in such duties as administering health tests, assisting in medical examinations, screening for hearing and vision, holding parent conferences, keeping health records, teaching health classes, helping to control communicable disease, and coordinating school, college, and community health efforts, the nurse can play an effective and important role in giving support and direction to the health instruction program. The school nurse can help in the identification of the topics that need to be covered, emphasizing the health needs of the students, and interpreting to administrators the importance of health in the school or college program.

A recent American Alliance for Health, Physical Education, and Recreation* position statement concerning the school nurse in education recommended that:

1. School nurses should be employed by boards of education implying equal status and benefits with teachers.
2. State licensure as a registered professional nurse and a baccalaureate degree including study in school health should be minimum requirements for employment.
3. School nurse certification should be based on state requirements and recommended standards of professional associations.
4. Guidelines for nurses should be established by local school districts.
5. Nurses should pursue graduate study and be active in professional associations.
6. School nurses should be responsible for supervision

of trained auxiliary personnel in the health services program.

Physical educator. Although the physical educator may not be qualified or interested in teaching health courses, he or she can contribute much to the health program. Training in such areas as first aid and the foundational sciences and direction of the physical education program places the physical educator in a position to impress upon students the importance of gaining desirable health knowledge, developing desirable health attitudes, and forming desirable health practices. Physical education can be a setting for correlated health teaching with the many opportunities that continually arise that are closely related to the health and fitness of students.

Dentist. The dentist employed to work with school children is frequently involved in such duties as conducting dental examinations of pupils, giving or supervising oral prophylaxis, and advising on curriculum material in dental hygiene. The health teacher can be helped by the dentist in the selection of curriculum material for classroom teaching, by discovering dental problems of students, and by participating himself in the classroom experiences of pupils as a resource person.

Dental hygienist. The dental hygienist usually assists the dentist and does oral prophylaxis. The teacher of health can therefore benefit from a close working relationship with this specialist in much the same way as she or he works with the dentist.

Custodian. All aspects of the school or college health program must be carefully coordinated—the health instruction program, health services, and healthful living. Therefore, the cleanliness of the building and a healthful physical environment are contributions to the health program. The custodian can be invited to help plan pertinent aspects of the health curriculum that specifically relate to his area of responsibility, to have the school or college be a model of cleanliness and of good health practices, and to adhere to proper health standards in respect to such items as lighting, ventilation, and heating.

Nutritionist. The nutritionist can contribute to health science instruction by contributing to the subject matter to be covered concerning nu-

---

* AAHPER Position Statement: The school nurse in education, School Health Review **2:**36, 1971.

trition, in speaking about food and nutrition, and in discussing nutritional problems of students.

Guidance counselor. An individual on the school staff that is too frequently overlooked as an effective member of the school health team is the guidance counselor. Since many academic problems are health related and since the guidance counselor is interested in helping each student to have a successful school experience, his or her interest must at times concern itself with areas of health. As such, the guidance counselor can make suggestions for health topics to be discussed in classes and can be an effective guest speaker in health classes to discuss the relationship of health to scholastic and vocational success.

A GUIDE FOR THE DEVELOPMENT OF A HEALTH EDUCATION CURRICULUM

The Curriculum Commission of the School Health Division of AAHPER recently proposed a guide for developing a health curriculum that will meet the needs of individuals associated with schools and school districts. The guide was developed by curriculum directors and others

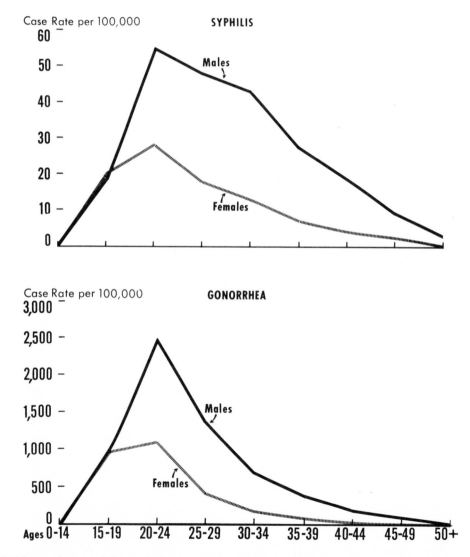

The incidence of venereal disease indicates the need for health education instruction. (Courtesy Metropolitan Life Insurance Company. From Metropolitan Life Insurance Company Statistical Bulletin, November, 1973, New York.)

responsible for health curriculum development.

The guide proposed certain steps to be taken in developing a local curriculum. These steps are summarized in the following paragraphs.

Preplanning. In order for a program to succeed, it must have community support as well as support from the administration and staff. A written policy should include funds, time allocations, class space, class day, and material.

Two committees should be formed. The first would be an in-school steering committee consisting of representation from the students, teachers, administrators, parents, school nurses, and special interest or ethnic groups. A second or advisory committee would be out-of-school and consist of community personnel (counselor, lawyers, doctors, health specialist, and others) and representatives from the PTA and other organizations.

The basic considerations necessary in the development of any curriculum include: (1) meeting all state and local requirements; (2) identification of behavioral objectives; (3) meeting the needs of community members, students, and specific community requirements; (4) developing a health education philosophy; (5) considering controversial areas; (6) developing a work schedule; and (7) exploring fully all sources of funding.

Review of existing school health education program. The status of the present health education program should be evaluated in terms of pupil knowledge and behavioral objective standards as well as staff, policies, budget, and facilities. The conclusions and recommendations should be thoroughly discussed and evaluated.

Broad content areas. Content areas should be based on student needs and opinions of the steering and advisory committees. In addition, student health records and absences might also be evaluated.

Format. The format of the curriculum guide should include the specific content area, behavioral or instructional objectives, concept, student learning experiences, student and teacher resources, and evaluation techniques for students and teachers.

Field testing. Field testing should be conducted at a variety of levels. Both novice and experienced teachers should be used as well as all types of students: rural, urban, and disadvan-

taged. Changes should be made where indicated.

Implementation. The plan for implementation should be specific in terms of target date and schedule. Administration approval should be included.

Reevaluation. All programs must be reevaluated every 3 to 5 years. Students' needs change over a period of years, and the curriculum must also change to meet these needs.

CONTENT AREAS FOR THE HEALTH SCIENCE INSTRUCTION PROGRAM

There is considerable knowledge and information that may be taught in health education. With all the literature that is available in such forms as textbooks, resource books, pamphlets, and promotional material, it is important that content be selected with care. At present there is little uniformity in the content of health education courses being taught in the schools and colleges throughout the country.

Some basic principles for selecting curriculum experiences in the health science instruction program are as follows:

1. The content of health science instruction should be based on the needs and interests of the students. Such considerations as developmental characteristics of children and youth and psychologic needs of students, such as security, approval, success in athletics, appearance, and peer-group approval, are considerations in relating teaching to the interests of students.

2. The problems and topics covered must be appropriate to the maturity level of the students.

3. The materials used should be current and scientifically accurate. The course should not be a textbook course. Many materials and experiences should be provided.

4. Pupils should be able to identify with the health problems discussed. As such, the problems should be geared to or related to the daily living experiences of the student body.

5. Health should be recognized as a multidisciplinary subject, and, as such, subject matter, projects, and methods of teaching should take cognizance of the new developments in the related sciences.

6. Health science instruction should be taught in light of a rapidly changing society,

new knowledge, and ways of affecting the behavior of human beings.

7. Health teaching should take place in an environment that represents a healthful psychologic and physical environment.

8. The teacher of health science, in order to be most effective in this subject, must exemplify good health, be well informed, and be a happy and successful individual.

9. The basic concepts in health should be identified and taught.

10. The new technologic methods and aids should be utilized in improving visual presentations of health material to students.

11. Considerations should be given to students' previous health experiences.

12. Planning for health science instruction should be a total school or college endeavor with students, teachers, specialists, and consultants participating. Furthermore, health instruction should permeate the entire school or college curriculum.

13. Objectives of the school or college health program, including knowledge, attitudes, practices, and skills, need to be reviewed and the program planned intelligently and meaningfully in light of these goals.

14. The community should be involved in health science instruction, including personnel from the health department, voluntary health associations, medical and dental professions, and other health associations and agencies.

15. School health science instruction should be closely integrated with home conditions.

16. New methods of organizing for teaching, including the nongraded school, team teaching, individualized instruction, and programmed instruction, should be considered.

17. Constant research and evaluation of the program should take place to provide the best instructional program for the students concerned.

18. Health instruction in general should share the same prestige and respect in the eyes of school or college administrators, teachers, and students as other respected school or college offerings, with time allotments and other considerations receiving equal attention.

Student health needs and interests

It has been pointed out that content areas in health education should be selected on the basis of the needs and interests of the students being served. Therefore, the question arises as to how such interests and needs can be determined. Some ways in which this vital information may be obtained include an analysis of the health records that every school and college should keep in a cumulative manner and that contain such valuable information as the results of health appraisal and health counseling. Teacher observations offer some indication of student interests, desires, and health problems. Tests of knowledge, attitudes, and habits uncover superstitions and other health problems, together with the accuracy of the health knowledge possessed by the student. Conferences with parents, teachers, and students reveal many health interests and needs. A student interest survey will offer valuable information. A study of current literature concerned with scientific information in the field of health is essential. New knowledge and new health problems are revealed each day through experimentation and research on the part of the medical and other professions. Finally, a study of the community will show the health problems that are peculiar to the local setting.

The Joint Committee on Health Problems of the National Education Association and the American Medical Association suggested several years ago, and this still holds true today, the following bases for determining needs and problems of students:

An analysis of biological needs of human beings.
An analysis of the characteristics of children of different age levels: their growth and developmental needs.
Health problems are revealed through a study of mortality records by age groups.
Health status by age groups as revealed on health records, accident and illness records, special studies, and surveys.
Analysis by age groups of activities related to health in which the majority of boys and girls engage.
Analysis of environmental health hazards at school and in the home and community.
Analysis of citizenship responsibilities relating to health.
Analysis of major social trends relating to health.
Analysis of vocational opportunities in health education.*

Although the specific health course of study will vary from community to community, it is

---

*Joint Committee on Health Problems in Education of National Education Association and American Medical Association: Health education, Washington, D. C., 1961, National Education Association, pp. 127-129.

still necessary to recognize that the basic health needs of students and the general content areas of health education are similar. To a great degree, what takes place is the specific adaptation of these general areas to local situations.

It seems important for the general information of the reader to point out some of the basic health needs of students and also the general health content areas, as listed by leaders in the field. Finally, it seems essential to discuss briefly some of the controversial content areas.

A Denver, Colorado, research project, concerned with a study of health needs, examined textbooks and programs of health in use throughout the United States and discussed health needs of students with teachers and physicians. The study resulted in the following list of eighteen broad areas that represented health needs of students:*

1. Keeping physically fit
2. Group health
3. Cause of disease
4. Protection from disease
5. Structure and function of the body
6. Dental health
7. Good eating habits
8. Selection and composition of food
9. Stimulants and narcotics
10. Rest and relaxation
11. Personal appearance
12. Personality development

*Corliss, L. M.: A report of the Denver research project on health interests of children, The Journal of School Health **32:**355, 1962.

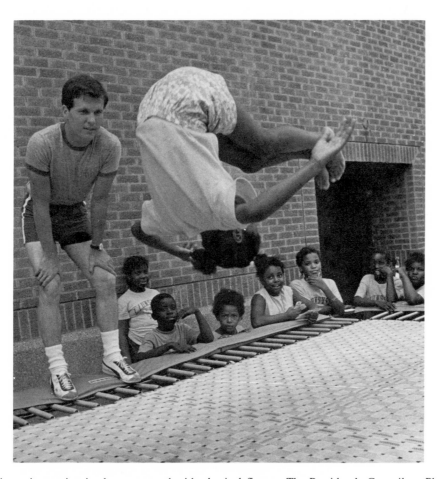

Health science instruction is also concerned with physical fitness. The President's Council on Physical Fitness and Sports promotes healthful living through its National Summer Youth Sports Program. (Courtesy President's Council on Physical Fitness and Sports.)

13. Social health
14. Heredity and eugenics
15. First aid
16. Home nursing
17. Safety
18. Vocations in health

Health content areas based on needs and interests of students

The Joint Committee on Health Problems in Education of the National Education Association and the American Medical Association* suggested the following areas of health content at the junior high school educational level:

Physical growth and development
Living practices
Health maintenance and improvement
Food and nutrition
Mental health
Personality development
Family life
Sex adjustment
Safety and first aid
Community health

For the senior high school educational level the Joint Committee on Health Problems in Education of the National Education Association and the American Medical Association suggested the following areas of health content:

1. Structure and function of the human body; scientific concepts relative to normal and abnormal function; contributions of scientific research and medical practice to information relative to maintenance of normal function.

2. The balanced regimen of food, exercise, rest, sleep, relaxation, work, and study; evaluation of individual health needs.

3. Mental health, personal adjustment, development of emotional maturity, establishment of maturing sex roles, boy-girl relations.

4. Preparation for marriage, family life, child care; health implications of heredity and eugenics; good budgeting; health aspects of housing; budgeting for health insurance, medical and dental services; spending the health dollar wisely.

5. Communicable and noncommunicable diseases with emphasis on adolescent and adult disease problems; prevention and control of disease and illness including heart disease, cancer, diabetes, mental illness, alcoholism.

6. Consumer health education: choosing health products and services; scientific health care as contrasted with fads,

quackery, and charlatanism; evaluating sources of information; awareness of nature of advertising appeals and "gimmicks" used to sell products.

7. Personal and community programs and practices in accident prevention and emergency care; driver education; recreational and occupational safety; fire prevention; civil defense and disasters.

8. Protection from hazards of poisons, drugs, narcotics; environmental hazards of radiation, air pollution, water contamination; chemical hazards in food production, processing, and distribution.

9. Community health: local, state, national, and international; tax-supported and voluntary health agency programs; contributions of individual citizens to community health.

10. Health careers in medicine, dentistry, nursing, public health, teaching, hospital administration, laboratory services, dietetics, physical therapy, occupational therapy, and allied professions.*

In Table 12-4 Hoyman presents a schematic health science spiral curriculum for kindergarten to grade twelve.

The health education content areas and the number of schools that include this area in their health science course, as reflected in a survey in which 810 schools returned the questionnaire, are shown in Table 12-3.

The content and basic aims of the New York State Health Education Programs include five strands to be covered in grades kindergarten through twelve: Physical Health, Sociological Health Problems, Mental Health, Environmental and Community Health, and Education for Survival (see diagram on p. 308 for more details).†

The health education program in Los Angeles includes the following topics and units in their junior high and senior high school programs.‡

Junior high school
    Unit 1—Introduction to health science
    Unit 2—Growing and maturing
    Unit 3—Achieving personal health
    Unit 4—Food for growth and health
    Unit 5—Addicting, habit-forming, and other dangerous substances
    Unit 6—Progress in community health
    Unit 7—First aid and safety

---

*Joint Committee on Health Problems in Education of National Education Association and American Medical Association, op. cit., pp. 204-205.

*Joint Committee on Health Problems in Education of National Education Association and American Medical Association, op. cit., pp. 234-235.
†New York State Department of Education, New York State Program in the Health Sciences, Albany.
‡Langan, J. J.: Health education in Los Angeles schools, National Association of Secondary Schools Bulletin, March, 1968.

Table 12-3. Health education content areas *

Subject area	Schools	Subject area	Schools
Personal health	263	Hit and miss	5
Smoking, tobacco	155	Child care	4
Drugs	150	Menstruation	4
Sex education	150	Civil defense	3
Alcohol	148	Heart	3
Anatomy and physiology	113	Sanitation	3
First aid	112	Self-help	3
Communicable disease	109	Those required by	3
Nutrition	81	state law	
Mental health	52	Sight and hearing	3
Safety	41	Genetics	2
Growth and development	37	Major health problems	2
Physical fitness	30	School health	2
Marriage and family living	20	Immunization	1
Public and community health	19	Psychology	1
All areas	10	Recreation	1
Dental health	9	Young adult problems	1
Cancer	6	Regular physical examination	1
Personality	6	Daily shower in physical	1
Personal relations	5	education	

*The Department of Education: Patterns and features of school health education in Michigan public schools, East Lansing, 1969, Michigan State Department of Education, p. 9.

Senior high school
   Unit 1—Orientation to health needs
   Unit 2—Guidelines for improved nutrition
   Unit 3—Transitions to maturity
   Unit 4—Narcotics, alcohol, tobacco, and other harmful
     substances
   Unit 5—Progress in public health
   Unit 6—Consumer health protection
   Unit 7—Essentials of first aid

The Pennsylvania Department of Education lists such topics as the following for junior and senior high school health content areas: alcohol, anatomy, consumer health, dental health, disease control, drugs and narcotics, family relationships, health careers, heredity and environment, human sexuality, mental health, nutrition, physical fitness, physiology, safety, and smoking.*

A UNIFIED APPROACH TO HEALTH TEACHING

The American Alliance for Health, Physical Education, and Recreation (AAHPER) prepared a position statement concerning a unified

*Pennsylvania State Department of Education: Conceptual Guidelines for School Health Programs in Pennsylvania, Harrisburg, 1970, Pennsylvania State Department of Education.

approach to health teaching.* They found, in many cases, that current health topics (drugs, venereal disease, sexuality) were hastily treated to "solve" a specific problem, and frequently these topics would be forgotten the following year.

The recommendations of the AAHPER Position Statement included the following points:

1. There should be scope and sequence from kindergarten through grade twelve in a unified approach to health instruction.
2. Curriculum development should include the identification of specific courses including conduct, learning activities, and evaluation techniques.
3. Curriculum content in health courses should be correlated and integrated with other subject areas.
4. The health curriculum should represent the thinking of school personnel, curriculum directors, state and federal consultants, and voluntary and official health agencies.
5. Teachers of health should be specifically prepared and have a genuine interest in health education.

HEALTH CONCEPTS

The concept approach to teaching various subject matter fields of specialization has won much acclaim in educational circles in recent

* AAHPER Position Statement: A unified approach to health teaching, The Journal of School Health **41:**171, 1971.

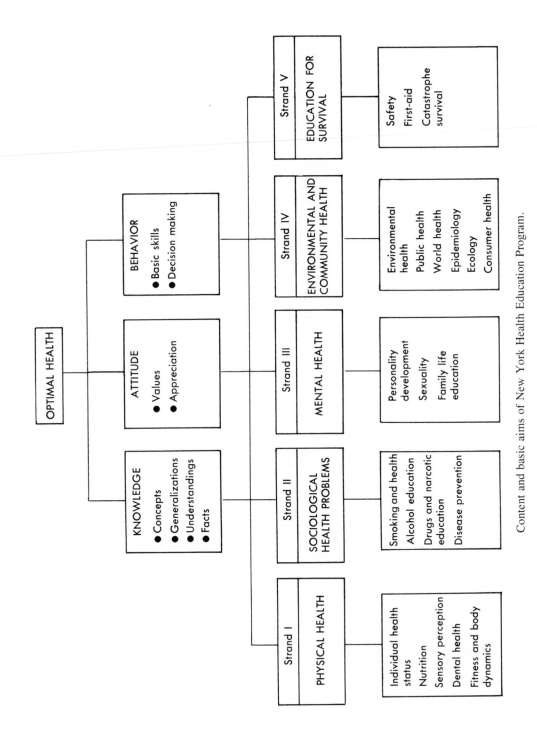

Content and basic aims of New York Health Education Program.

Table 12-4. A schematic health science spiral curriculum for kindergarten to grade twelve*†

Major health instruction areas	Primary grades				Intermediate grades			Junior high grades			Senior high grades		
	K	1	2	3	4	5	6	7	8	9	10	11	12
1. Human ecology and health, disease, longevity	X	X	X	X	X		X		X				X
2. Human growth, development, maturation, aging	X	X	X	X	X		X		X				X
3. Healthful living and physical fitness	X	X	X	X	X		X		X				X
4. Nutrition and personal fitness	X	X	X	X	X		X		X				X
5. Alcohol, tobacco, and narcotics	X	X	X	X	X		X		X				X
6. Prevention and control of disease	X	X	X	X		X			X			X	
7. Community and environmental health	X	X	X	X		X			X			X	
8. Consumer health education	X	X	X	X		X			X			X	
9. Rise of modern scientific medicine	X	X	X	X		X			X			X	
10. Safety education	X	X	X	X	X		X	X		X			X
11. First aid and home nursing	X	X	X	X		X			X		X		X
12. Personality development and mental health	X	X	X	X		X		X			X		X
13. Family-life and sex education	X	X	X	X		X		X				X	X
14. Current health events and problems	X	X	X	X	X	X	X	X	X	X	X	X	X

*From Hoyman, H. S.: An ecologic view of health and health education, The Journal of School Health **25:**118, 1965.
†In kindergarten to grade three the X's denote topics, in grades four to twelve, units, or major parts of combined units.

Note: Separate health courses may be scheduled at the junior and senior high school levels as a part of the health science spiral curriculum where this method of scheduling is preferred.

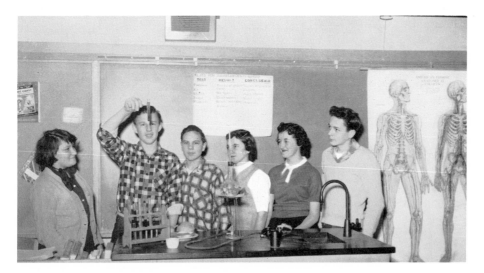

Nutrition instruction as part of the health education program.

years. It is felt that the decisions that people make and their behavior patterns are determined largely by their concepts. Concepts that evolve can have an impact on cognition (knowledge, intellectual abilities, and skills) and values, attitudes, and appreciations.

Recognizing the value of the concept approach, the School Health Education Study developed an outline entitled *A Conceptual Approach to Health Education.*

The concept approach outlined by the School Health Education Study recognizes the three dimensions of health—mental, physical, and social. These are closely interwoven. Furthermore, it stresses the triad of health education—the unity of human beings in respect to their physical, mental, and social aspects; the knowledges, attitudes, and practices as factors important to influencing health behavior; and the focus of health education upon the individual, family, and community. All these components of the triad are interdependent and constantly interacting.

The study identified three key concepts, ten conceptual statements, and thirty-one substantive elements that represent the conceptual framework for health. The ten concepts into which the key concepts are delineated are:

> Growth and development influences and is influenced by the structure and functioning of the individual.
> Growth and development follows a predictable sequence, yet is unique for each individual.
> Protection and promotion of health is an individual, community, and international responsibility.
> The potential for hazards and accidents exists, whatever the environment.
> There are reciprocal relationships involving man, disease, and environment.
> The family serves to perpetuate man and to fulfill certain health needs.
> Personal health practices are affected by a complexity of forces, often conflicting.
> Utilization of health information, products, and services is guided by values and perceptions.
> Use of substances that modify mood and behavior arises from a variety of motivations.
> Food selection and eating patterns are determined by physical, social, mental, economic, and cultural factors.*

*From Sliepcevich, E. M., and Nolte, A. E.: The school health education study, The National Elementary Principal **47**:43, 1968.

SEX EDUCATION, DRUGS, AND OTHER CRITICAL CONTENT AREAS IN HEALTH SCIENCE INSTRUCTION

The question often arises as to whether such critical subjects as sex, narcotics, or alcohol education should be provided for in the health science instruction program. The fact that some of these problems are more pronounced in certain communities, and possibly restricted to some population groups, together with the fact that such education might tend to stimulate curiosity, are reasons put forth for not including them in courses of study.

On the other hand, instruction in regard to the ill effects of narcotics and alcohol is required by law in many states. Furthermore, it is felt that if children and youth are provided with the facts, intelligent instruction in these subjects will act as a preventive measure. In the area of sex education, it is believed that the term *sex education* creates opposition among many parents and church groups and consequently should not be used. If it is introduced in the natural process of instruction without undue emphasis, much good can be done.

Some of the best thinking in the field emphasizes the fact that the nature of the instruction will depend upon the local situation. Where a narcotics or alcohol problem exists, there should be provision in the school curriculum for the presentation of sociologic, physiologic, and psychologic facts, as well as the legal aspects of such a problem. Students should understand these facts and be guided intelligently in making the right decisions and establishing a sound standard of values.

Health education is not the only area in which discussions of sex, narcotics, and alcohol should take place. Social studies, biology, general science, physical education, and other classes also have a responsibility. Many phases of these subjects logically fit into certain aspects of these courses. Teachers must appreciate the importance of such instruction and the need for treating these subjects objectively on the basis of the facts. It is not necessary for the teacher to take a definite stand on the subject. Instead, if students obtain the necessary facts through re-

Table 12-5. Suggested treatment of drugs in state health education curriculum guides (eleven states included)*

State	Grade level	Outline of content
A	7-12	Suggests collecting popular magazine articles on drugs and discussing reasons for A.M.A. acceptance or rejection (sic). Suggests pointing out the dangers to consumer health of over-gullibility to patent medicine advertising, and that the danger of patent medicines is delay in proper diagnosis and treatment. One of twelve content areas deals with stimulants and depressants.
B	1-12	Primary level—dangers in the incorrect use of medicines Junior high level—effects of alcohol, drugs, and tobacco on body and social functions Senior high level—analyzing effects of narcotics, drugs, tobacco and alcohol, and the use of patent medicines
C, D, E	7-12	Grades 7-9—suggests discussion of hazards of self-diagnosis and self-medication, review of medicine chest contents, evaluation of drug advertising Grades 10-12—suggests more comprehensive practice of the above and guest lectures on drugs by physicians and pharmacists
F	7-12	Discusses the importance of following prescription directions under the topic "Home Nursing." Mentions narcotics and stimulants with alcohol.
G	K-12	Defines the responsibility of informing students of dangers of drug abuse
H	K-12	Mentions narcotic drugs only in conjunction with alcohol and tobacco
I, J, K	1-12	Nothing on drugs

*From Smith, M. C., Mikeal, R. L., and Taylor, J. M.: Drugs in the health curriculum: a needed area, The Journal of School Health **39:**334, 1969.

search or some other method and then interpret them intelligently, the right answers will be clear. The students make their own decisions, not on the basis of the teacher's position but on the basis of the facts they have collected.

In regard to sex education, the emphasis should be on the psychologic and sociologic aspects rather than only on the biologic aspects. The end result should be to have students recognize what is desirable behavior and what constitutes a healthy sexuality rather than only to become acquainted with a body of factual knowledge such as that concerned with the reproductive organs. Sex education should not be a separate course but should be included and discussed in every course where its various aspects arise during regular discussions. Parents and representative community groups should be consulted and asked to participate in any discussions relative to the planning for instruction in this area. It is very important to have well-trained and qualified teachers handling such instruction. If the right type of leadership is provided, the result can be very beneficial to all concerned, but if poor leadership exists, many harmful results can come from such discussion.

A resource unit in family life and sex education has been developed by the Committee on Health Guidance in Sex Education of the American School Health Association. The subunit

RESOLUTIONS

Drug abuse education

Whereas, Drugs and medicines make a positive contribution to personal and community health, and

Whereas, A large segment of our population looks to drugs to alleviate a host of physiological, psychological and social discomforts, and

Whereas, The best deterrent to drug abuse is the individual's value system and his assessment of the consequences associated with drug involvement, and

Whereas, Those who develop school policies must be fully informed regarding the nature of drugs, psychosocial motivations, legal considerations, and the content and process of their communities' teacher inservice training and student instructional programs, and

Whereas, The nature of the problem is such that the school program must draw together the students, the total staff, and the community.

Be it Resolved:

1. That schools develop intensive inservice programs with assistance from specialists with experience and background in developing educational programs, including specialists in group process training and communications,
2. That planned programs be developed to involve and inform parents and community leaders regarding their roles in preparing young people to mature successfully in our culture,
3. That school programs for students be developed having these elements:
    a. a sequential plan beginning in the elementary years,
    b. emphasis on the decision-making process and why people use drugs,
    c. increasing understanding of the social conditions that promote drug use and abuse,
    d. a total institutional attitude which encourages acceptance of all children and an understanding that their individual needs, when frustrated, may lead to drug abuse,
4. That drug misuse education should be an important part of the total health education curriculum.

Sex education

Whereas, Problems related to family life, sex education, and related interpersonal relationships are of concern to children and youth and have a bearing on their present and future welfare, and

Whereas, Children and youth need reliable information and interpretation from competent adults on issues bearing on their emotional and social well-being, and

Whereas, They learn best when there are cooperative relationships among families, schools, and communities, and

Whereas, There is concern that both critics and proponents have presented sex education issues in a sensational manner which inhibits the further development of a sound program,

Be it Resolved:

1. That a total institutional approach to human sexuality be initiated in the schools,
2. That schools develop sequential K-12 health education programs which encompass family life and sex education,
3. That schools assume leadership in involving parents and other responsible community leaders in the development and interpretation of school programs in family life and sex education,
4. That schools employ competent staff professionally prepared to assume leadership in the development and direction of comprehensive health education programs,
5. That inservice programs for better understanding of the schools responsibility be developed.

Adopted by the Representative Assembly of the American Association for Health, Physical Education, and Recreation, meeting at the 84th Anniversary Convention, Boston, Massachusetts, April 15, 1969.

titles for grades seven to twelve are listed here:

Grade 7
    Unit 1. Understanding ourselves
    Unit 2. The family
    Unit 3. Review of male and female reproductive process
Grade 8
    Unit 1. Emotions and behavior
    Unit 2. Dating
    Unit 3. The family
    Unit 4. Review of the female reproductive process
    Unit 5. Review of the male reproductive process
Grade 9
    Unit 1. Mental and emotional health
    Unit 2. Family relationships
    Unit 3. Boy-girl relationships
Grades 10 and 11
    Unit 1. Psycho-social development
    Unit 2. Boy-girl relationships in light of both immediate and long-range goals
    Unit 3. Family planning
    Unit 4. Growth and reproduction
Grade 12
    Unit 1. Preparation for marriage
    Unit 2. Adjustments in marriage
    Unit 3. Planning for parenthood
    Unit 4. Family living
    Unit 5. Attitudes toward sex and sexual behavior*

HEALTH SCIENCE INSTRUCTION AT THE PRESCHOOL AND ELEMENTARY SCHOOL LEVELS

The committee on Health Education for Pre-School Children of the American School Health Association lists the following as a topical outline of content for preschool children:

Cleanliness and grooming
Dental health
Eyes, ears, nose
Rest and sleep
Nutrition
Growth and development
Family living
Understanding ourselves and getting along
Prevention and control of disease safety†

For each of these topics the committee has identified key concepts, suggested learning experiences, and means of evaluation.

Health education at the elementary level is aimed primarily at having the child develop good health habits and health attitudes, and at helping him or her live happily, healthfully, and safely. This is achieved in great measure by adapting good health practices to the regular routine of school and home living, rather than by dispensing technical, factual knowledge concerning health. The responsibility for the guidance, planning, and stimulation of good health practices and attitudes falls upon the classroom teacher. He or she is the guiding influence and his or her understanding of good health will determine to a great degree the effectiveness of such a program.

The type of health program offered should be adapted to the child's level and planned in accordance with his or her interests and needs. It should also be remembered that health education is a continuous process and cannot be compartmentalized within a definite subject area or within a class period. It embraces all activities and subjects that are part of the child's life.

It is difficult to prescribe the amount of time that should be devoted to the teaching of health on the elementary level because the needs and interests of pupils vary. However, the amount of time devoted to health education should be equal to the other major areas of the curriculum.

At the primary grade level the emphasis should be more on the child and his or her daily routine as it is affected by certain health practices and attitudes. The child's various routines and associations at school and at home form the basis for the health emphasis. The importance of a healthful classroom environment is stressed. Such items as cleanliness, eating, use of lavatories, safety, and good mental hygiene are brought out as the child plays, eats, and performs those many experiences that are common to all youngsters of his age.

The committee on Health Education for Elementary School Children of the American School Health Associations lists the following as a topical outline of content for this age group:

Grades 1, 2, and 3
    Cleanliness and grooming
    Rest and exercise
    Sleep and rest
    Growth
    Posture
    Role of physician and dentist
    Individual responsibility for one's health

---

*As quoted from Mayshark, C., and Irwin, L. W.: Health education in secondary schools, ed. 2, St. Louis, 1968, The C. V. Mosby Co., pp. 136-137.

†Health instruction: suggestions for teachers, The Journal of School Health **39:**11, 1969.

Responsibility for the health of others
Dental health
Vision and hearing
Babies
Nutrition
Making new friends
Being alone sometimes
Family time
Protection from infection
Food protection
Safety
Grades 4, 5, and 6
Health care
Cleanliness and grooming
Vision and care of eyes
Hearing and care of ears
Heart
Teeth
Exercise, rest, and sleep
Nutrition
Growth and development
Family living
Understanding ourselves
Getting along with others
Making decisions
Environmental health
Prevention and control of diseases
Safety and first aid*

For each of these topics the committee has identified key concepts, suggested learning experiences, and means of evaluation.

The Joint Committee on Health Problems in Education of the National Education Association and the American Medical Association† has suggested areas for health teaching in the kindergarten and primary grades. These areas pertain to school and home experiences relating to: food and nutrition; exercise, rest, and sleep; eyes, ears, and teeth; clothing; cleanliness and grooming; mental and emotional health; communicable disease control; safety; home, schools, and neighborhoods.

In the upper elementary years the values of certain health practices are brought out. A planned progression in instruction is developed. Although there is still stress on the actual practices and attitudes concerned with the daily routines and associations, more factual information is incorporated to form the basis for such habits. Furthermore, more and more responsibility is

---

*Health instruction: suggestions for teachers, The Journal of School Health **39:**22, 34, 1969.

†Joint Committee on Health Problems in Education of National Education Association and American Medical Association, op. cit., p. 149.

placed on the child for his or her own self-destruction and self-control.

The utilization of trips and textbooks that point up the value of healthful living, interesting and inspiring stories, visual aids, class discussions, and projects can become a part of the experiences of each child so that the need for certain behavior is dramatically and effectively stamped upon his or her mind and total being.

Since health experiences should be based on the needs and interests of the child, the wise teacher will utilize various means of obtaining accurate information about these needs and interests. Such techniques as talks with parents and pupils, observations of children under various situations, a perusal of health records, a study of the home environment and community together with scientific measuring devices that have been developed to determine health knowledge and attitudes will be utilized. A health education program that is not based on accurate knowledge of needs and interests will fail to accomplish its objective of helping individuals to live a happier and healthier life.

HEALTH INSTRUCTION ACTIVITIES FOR THE ELEMENTARY SCHOOL

The Joint Committee on Health Problems in Education of the National Education Association and the American Medical Association has listed some of the health instruction activities in which pupils in intermediate and elementary grades can engage:

1. Conducting animal feeding experiments and experiments to test for food nutrients
2. Taking field trips to local dairies, markets, restaurants, bakeries, water supply and sewage treatment plants, and housing projects
3. Visiting museums
4. Preparing charts and graphs for visualizing class statistics, such as absence due to colds or school accidents
5. Making pin maps of sources of mosquitoes, rubbish depositories, and slum areas
6. Making health posters
7. Setting up room and corridor health exhibits
8. Preparing health bulletin boards and displays
9. Making murals and dioramas
10. Maintaining class temperature charts
11. Arranging a library corner of health materials on the subject being studied
12. Using sources of printed material—reference books, texts, bulletins, newspapers, and magazines—for the study of a particular topic

13. Giving reports in various ways—chalkboard talks, dramatizations, role-playing, panels
14. Serving on the safety patrol
15. Joining the bicycle safety club
16. Participating in a home or school cleanup campaign
17. Planning menus
18. Preparing meals for class mothers or other guests
19. Sharing health programs with primary grades
20. Securing a health examination
21. Having all dental corrections made
22. Taking inoculations
23. Keeping records of growth through charts or graphs
24. Keeping diaries of health practices
25. Studying text or references to find answers to problems
26. Thinking through solutions to problems
27. Applying in daily practices health principles learned*

Health suggestions for the classroom teacher

The classroom teacher is the key school person involved in the health of the elementary school child. The organization of the school with the self-contained classroom enables him or her to continually observe the pupils and to note deviations from normal. Continuous contact with the same children over a long period of time also makes it possible to know a great deal about their physical, social, emotional, and mental health. The teacher can help them develop the right knowledge, attitudes, and practices. Some of the responsibilities of the classroom teacher in regard to the health of the pupils are:

1. Possess an understanding of what constitutes a well-rounded school health program and the teacher's part in it.
2. Meet with the school physician, nurse, and others in order to determine how he or she can best contribute to the total health program.
3. Become acquainted with parents and homes of students and establish parent-school cooperation.
4. Discover the health needs and interests of his or her pupils.
5. Organize health teaching units that are meaningful and in terms of the health needs and interests of his or her students.
6. See that children needing special care are referred to proper places for help.

7. Be knowledgeable in first-aid procedures.
8. Participate in the work of the school health council. If none exists, interpret the need for one.
9. Provide an environment for children while at school that is conducive to healthful living.
10. Continually be on the alert for children with deviations from normal behavior and signs of communicable diseases.
11. Provide experiences for living healthfully at school.
12. Help pupils assume an increasing responsibility for their own health as well as for the health of others.
13. Set an example for the child of what constitutes healthful living.
14. Motivate the child to be well and happy.
15. Be present at health examinations of pupils and contribute in any way helpful to the physician in charge.
16. Follow through in cooperation with the nurse to see that remediable health defects are corrected.
17. Interpret the school health program to the community and enlist its support in solving health problems.
18. Provide a well-rounded class physical education program.
19. Help supervise various activities that directly affect health—school lunch, rest periods.
20. Become familiar with teaching aids and school and community resources for enhancing the health program.
21. Be aware of the individual differences of pupils.

HEALTH SCIENCE INSTRUCTION AT THE SECONDARY LEVEL

Since many aspects of health education at the secondary level are covered in this chapter under the topics of Content Areas for the Health Science Instruction Program, Concentrated, Correlated, Integrated, and Incidental Health Teaching, and Organization of Classes, this discussion will be limited to a brief summary of some of the points of emphasis in health education at the secondary level.

The changes taking place in American society and the research data available emphasize a need to stress certain areas of health instruction.

---

*Joint Committee on Health Problems in Education of National Education Association and American Medical Association, op. cit., pp. 187-188.

These include alcohol education, community health problems, health careers, international health activities, sex education, venereal disease education, tobacco and narcotics, nutrition and weight control, environmental hazards, and consumer health education.

The current status
of health instruction
at the secondary level

A survey* initiated in 1971 had as its primary objective to provide a profile of the current emphasis on health instruction at the secondary level. Letters were written to each state department of education requesting a copy of the state's health education curriculum guidelines and other materials that might affect health instruction in that state. Responses were received from 44 state departments of education, or 88%. From the information received, data was gathered that related to (1) subject matter content, (2) teaching approaches, (3) regulations in regard to instruction. The following paragraphs discuss information derived from this survey.

Curriculum guidelines. Thirty-two of the 44 states responding indicated that they had a curriculum guide to assist teachers with their health instruction programs. Five states indicated that they had no guide at present but guides were in the process of development. States where there were no guidelines indicated that budget cutbacks and other problems had curtailed the development of guidelines although they had a high interest in health instruction.

The health topics most frequently mentioned for instruction at this level were family living (28), nutrition (27), mental-emotional health (26), diseases (25), safety (25), consumer health (24), and drugs and narcotics (22). It is interesting to note that venereal disease and interpersonal relations were only mentioned in three cases and health services in two cases.

Additional materials. Thirty-two of the 44 responding states have materials other than the curriculum guide. These materials usually pertained to such topics as program evaluating

---

*Leigh, T.: Nationwide profile of health instruction, School Health Review **4**:35, 1973.

drugs, family living or sex education, alcohol, venereal disease, and tobacco. Supplementary materials often include position papers and appraisals of state laws governing health instruction.

Teaching strategies. Teaching strategies were a part of many curriculum guidelines or accessory guides. In order of their mention, some of these strategies are: class discussion (24), guest speakers (22), experimentation or demonstration (21), individual reports (21), audiovisual aids (20), role-playing (18), field trips (18), bulletin boards (17), and community or school surveys (17).

Required health instruction. Most states require health education in one form or another. Eleven states indicate that general instruction in health is required some time during the secondary school years. Four states require that only certain topics be taught, and 16 additional states require both specific and general health instruction. Time and grade requirements varied widely from 150 minutes per week each year in grades seven through twelve, and 20 minutes per day in grades nine through twelve, to no requirement at all in reference to time and year level.

Health and the structural organization
of the secondary school

The structural organization of the secondary level differs from the elementary level. At the elementary level, the classroom teacher frequently takes overall charge of a group of children. He or she teaches them in various subjects, stays with them throughout the entire day, and supervises their activities. At the secondary level, the student has many different teachers. These teachers specialize in subject matter to a greater degree than they specialize in pupils. There is departmentalization into such subject matter areas as mathematics, social studies, and English. This structural organization affects health education tremendously.

First, this structural organization points up the need for concentrated courses in health education, such as those found in the other subject matter areas. Health education as a subject should receive equal consideration with the other important subjects in the secondary school offering, in all aspects such as scheduling, facilities, and staff. The minimum time that should be allotted has been stated as a daily period for at least two semesters, at the seventh-, eighth-, or ninth-grade level, and a daily period for two semesters, preferably at the eleventh- or twelfth-grade level.

Second, this structural organization emphasizes the need for a specialist in the teaching of health education. Just as specialists are needed in English and the other subjects offered at the secondary level, so are they needed in the field of health education. The body of scientific knowledge, the training needed, and the importance of the subject make such a specialist a necessity.

Third, this structural organization stresses the need for coordination and cooperation. Health cuts across many subject matter areas, as well as the total school life of the child. In order that it may be properly treated in the various subject matter areas such as science, home economics, and social studies, in order that the physical environment and the emotional environment may be properly provided for, in order that health services may be most effectively administered, and in order that close cooperation and coordination between the school and the rest of the community may be obtained, there is an essential need for some type of coordinating machinery. There is a need for a school health council or committee where individuals representing various interests and groups can pool their thinking and bring about cooperative efforts. There is a need for some individual to act in the capacity of a health coordinator, to spearhead the movement for cooperation and coordination, and to develop good relationships among the various departments and interests represented in the total school situation, as well as with those in the broader community.

In order to have an effective, sound health education program at the secondary level, the central administration must provide the type of leadership that leaves no doubt as to the importance of health in the lives of the many children who attend the schools. Such administrative leadership will reflect itself from the very top to the very bottom of the school structure and be felt at the grass roots of all community enterprises.

The junior high school. The junior high school was created to meet the physical, mental, and socioemotional needs of the preadolescent and early adolescent boys and girls who make up grades seven, eight, and nine. These grades represent a period of transition when the characteristics of growth and development, although varying from individual to individual, form a relatively uniform pattern during the age period of 12 to 14 years.

Junior high school students are in need of knowledge and proper attitudes that will result in desirable health practices. The fact that students may not be interested in such information represents a challenge for the junior high school educational program. The consumption of many sweets as a substitute for essential foods, omission of breakfast, and other undesirable practices, an interest in personal grooming, a need to understand one's bodily makeup, the maturing sexual drive, and other factors make it imperative to get across health information at this time. Health education activities contribute feelings of satisfaction and understanding that may never be possible of accomplishment in the regular academic program.

Health content should be adapted to the needs and interests of the students in this age group. Stress should be on the personal health problems of the students themselves, and how hereditary factors affect their health, how good or poor health is manifested, and how health practices affect the attainment of life ambitions and goals. Such topics as food, rest, exercise, first aid, safety, alcohol and narcotics, mental health, communicable disease, growth and functions of the human body, personality development, family life, and community health would be covered.

The health teaching that takes place in the junior high school should take into consideration the developmental tasks that characterize the early adolescent. These include the desire for independence of adults, self-respect, and peer identification, as well as accepting one's physical makeup, adjusting to the opposite sex, and establishing a standard of values.

The committee on Health Education for Junior High School of the American School Health Association lists the following as a topical outline of content for this age group:

Health status
Cleanliness and grooming
Rest, sleep, and relaxation
Exercise
Posture
Recreation and leisure-time activities
Sensory perception
Nutrition
Growth and development
Understanding ourselves
Personality
Getting along with others
Family living
Alcohol
Drugs
Smoking and tobacco
Environment
Air and water pollutions
Consumer health
Disease*

For each of these topics the committee has identified key concepts, suggested learning experiences, and means of evaluation.

The senior high school. During grades ten, eleven, and twelve, the stress continues to be on many subject-matter areas that were emphasized for the health content in the junior high school years. However, the material and experiences presented would be more advanced and adapted to the age group found in the later high school years. Such topics as the structure and function of the human body could stress more scientific concepts as found through research, evaluation of individual health needs in the light of proper balance in one's daily routine, and the means of attaining proper emotional maturity and mental health.

The committee on Health Education for Senior High School of the American School Health Association lists the following as a topical outline of content for this age group:

Health status
Fatigue and sleep
Exercise
Recreational activities
Sensory perception
Nutrition
Growth and development toward maturity
Family living
Alcohol

Drugs
Smoking and tobacco
Health protection
Noise pollution
Health agencies
Health careers
World health
Safety and accidents*

For each of these topics the committee has listed key concepts, suggested learning experiences, and means of evaluation.

Although personal health receives considerable attention during the high school years, a major part of the teaching is concerned with problems of adult and family living and community health. Such health areas as preparation for marriage and family life, communicable and noncommunicable disease control, evaluation of professional health services, environmental health, industrial health, Civil Defense, consumer health education, accident prevention, emergency care, protection from environmental hazards such as radiation, health agencies at the local, state, national, and international levels, and the various health careers open to high school students receive great stress.

Some students will not be going to college. This means that the senior high school years offer the last opportunity to impress boys and girls with their health responsibilities—to themselves, their loved ones, and the members of their community.

Health education at the secondary level can represent an experience that will have a lasting effect for the betterment of human lives. The leadership provided, the methods used, and the stress placed upon such an important aspect of living will determine in great measure the extent to which each school will fulfill its responsibility.

HEALTH SCIENCE INSTRUCTION AT THE COLLEGE AND UNIVERSITY LEVEL

The college and the university also have responsibilities for health science instruction. Health is important to everyone regardless of the type of work he or she may do.

*Health instruction: suggestions for teachers, The Journal of School Health **39:**48, 1969.

*Health instruction: suggestions for teachers, The Journal of School Health **39:**71, 1969.

Years ago the college and university health education offerings consisted mainly of lectures on various aspects of the anatomy and physiology of the human body. These were usually given by medical personnel and were often a collection of uninteresting facts unrelated to the student's interests and health problems. In more recent years this type of presentation has changed. The emphasis has shifted from the factual medical knowledge to health problems that students themselves encounter in day-to-day living and also to those subjects in which students are especially interested. Consequently, discus-

sions are now held on subjects concerned with family living, personal and community health, mental health, drugs, environmental health, nutrition, the prevention of disease, and related subjects.

The Third National Conference on Health in Colleges recommended major health instruction courses appropriate to special groups of students. It also suggested "a minimum of 45 class hours or three to four semester credits" for a basic or general health course in "personal and community health." Other recommended procedures for college health courses that have been

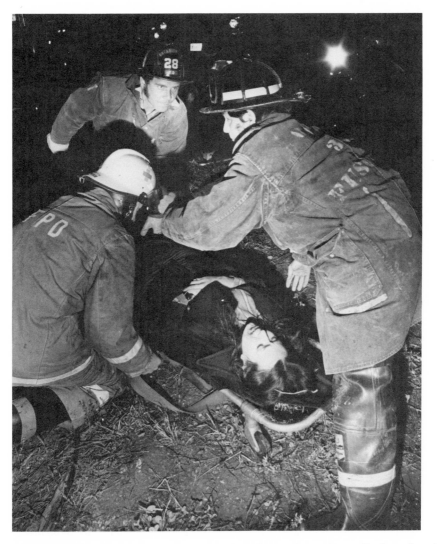

First aid and emergency care are included in the health science instruction program. Students from College of DuPage, Glen Ellyn, Ill., participating in a local emergency rescue unit and hospital emergency procedures.

set forth include (1) the 3- or 5-hour one-semester required or elective course, (2) the 2-hour per week course for two credits, (3) the 2-hour course shared with a physical education requirement, and (4) the 1-hour per week course for one credit. Such a course should meet frequently enough to maintain the student's interest and to cover the subject adequately. Furthermore, the lecture method of presentation should not be the only one used.

The President's Commission on Higher Education stressed the importance of health instruction for college students. It particularly stressed instruction based directly on the practical problems of personal and community health.

The American College Health Association has recommended that every college and university have a requirement in health education for all students who fall below acceptable standards on a college-level health knowledge test.

The junior college is in a particularly strategic position to offer health instruction. The 2-year college reaches a significant segment of the population that does not go on to the 4-year colleges and universities. Furthermore, research has shown that junior college students have demonstrated as much as 25% more interest in health problems than high school students. Junior college students are more mature, and this may be an explanation of their increased interest in health problems. Topics such as sex instruction, marriage, mental health, emotional health, alcohol, tobacco, and narcotics are of particular interest to this segment of the college population.

A recent survey concerning the status of required health education courses in colleges and universities revealed a trend toward eliminating the requirement for health courses in many such institutions.* This survey reviewed 1,200 college and university catalogues (those reviewed closely resembled those 1,200 accredited institutions listed in the ninth edition of *American Universities and Colleges*) and determined that 109 of these schools required health education courses of all students. Of the 109 schools sent survey questionnaires, 81 responded. Three of the responding schools had dropped the require-

ment in the past year and a half. The 78 remaining schools offered the following information about their health requirement:

1. Approximately 15% of schools with this requirement are planning to drop it in the next few years.
2. The number of credit hours required had declined from previous studies.
3. The majority of departments offering the course were not solely responsible for health education.
4. The course content trend seemed to be emphasizing alcohol, drugs, narcotics, mental health, personal adjustment, marriage preparation, and parenthood and child care.

It is generally felt that a health education department should be established to coordinate the instruction in health, that student needs should represent an important consideration for the determination of subject matter content, that only qualified faculty members be permitted to teach health education classes, and that classes be limited to a maximum of thirty-five students. Testing of new students is also recommended, after which those students who fall below desirable standards are required to take the required health education course.

Presently, health education courses offered in colleges and universities are listed in college catalogues under such names as Personal Hygiene, Health Education, Personal and Community Health, Health Science, Hygiene, Healthful Living, Health and Safety, Health Essentials, and Problems of Healthful Living. Courses are taught in such departments as health, physical education, and recreation; health education; biology; education; health and safety; basic studies; psychology; and biologic sciences. Students required to take such courses vary from only those students in schools of education or in departments of health, physical education, and recreation, or elementary education major students, to liberal arts students. In some institutions courses are required for women but not for men.

There is a need for a uniform requirement for all college students to demonstrate that they know basic facts in the field of health. Those students who fail to meet such standards should

*Braza, J. F.: The status and administration of the required health courses, The Journal of School Health **41**:142, 1971.

be required to take a course in this area. Such a requirement is basic to the general education, productivity, and health of each person.

HEALTH EDUCATION FOR ADULTS

Adults are the guiding force in any community. The prestige they have, the positions they occupy, and their interests determine the extent to which any project or enterprise will be a success. Therefore, if the schools are to have an adequate health education program, if the knowledge that is disseminated, attitudes that are developed, and practices that are encouraged are to become a permanent part of the child's being and routine, the adult must be taken into consideration. Unless this is done, the schools' efforts will be of no avail.

There is a great need for parental education and for education in regard to the many health problems that confront any community. Adults are interested not only in children's health problems but also in the causes of sickness and death in the population and ways in which they can live a healthier life. Adult education is increasing in this country. It is important that health education become one of the areas considered in any such program.

Schools and colleges should play a key part in adult education programs through the facilities, staff, and other resources at their disposal. They

---

RESOLUTION NO. 5

adopted by

Joint Committee on Health Problems in Education
National Education Association—American Medical Association

February, 13-16, 1971

Coordination of school-community health programs

Whereas,	The component parts of the health program for schools frequently are fragmented, and
Whereas,	The overall school health program is ineffective if there is no organizational structure to coordinate the component parts of a school health program with all phases of the school system, and
Whereas,	The solution of major child and youth health issues requires the concerted action by the entire community, including schools, therefore be it
Resolved,	That the component parts of a health program in a school system be coordinated by an advisory school health council consisting of representatives of the administration, instructional staff, students, parents, employees, and the health disciplines, and be it further
Resolved,	That local medical and dental societies, advisory school health councils, other educational related organizations, and all health related agencies be encouraged to work together through a Community Health Council or Comprehensive Health Planning Council to coordinate efforts in solving health issues in schools and communities.

(Reprinted with permission of the Joint Committee on Health Problems in Education of the National Education Association and the American Medical Association.)

should cooperate fully with the many official and voluntary health agencies and other interested community groups in the furtherance of health objectives. Adult education programs in the area of health should be designed to discover community health problems, understand the health needs of children, and understand school health programs. Such discovery and understanding should lead to active participation in meeting health needs and in solving health problems. Such a program would also lend itself to growth in respect to health knowledge, attitudes, and practices.

METHODS OF TEACHING HEALTH

Methods of teaching health, such as lecture, recitation, and assignments in the textbook, represent a limited array of approved techniques for the modern health class. Although good textbooks are important and the other methods have value under select conditions, there are many other methods that can motivate students and create interest in health topics.

The methods used should be adapted to the group of students being taught, be in accordance with the objectives sought, be capable of use by the instructor, stimulate interest among the students, and be adaptable to the time, space, and equipment in the school program. Some of the more popular methods for teaching health are discussed in the following paragraphs.

Problem solving is one of the most effective and best methods for teaching health. Health topics can be stated in the form of problems and then a systematic approach can be utilized by the students to obtain an answer. For example, the problem can be stated: ''What are the effects of narcotics on health?'' A systematic approach to this problem might include (1) stating the nature and scope of the problem, (2) defining the various possible solutions to the problem, (3) collecting scientific information to support each of the various aspects of the problem, (4) analyzing the information gathered as to its source, authoritativeness, date of origin, and other pertinent factors, and (5) drawing conclusions for the solution of the problem.

Textbook assignments may be given, followed by class discussions based on the readings.

Field trips can include planned visits to an agency or place where health matters are of importance, such as a hospital, local health department, water purification plant, health clinic, or fire department.

Class discussions on health topics of interest can be encouraged among the members of the class.

Demonstrations are an excellent method to show how something functions or is constructed, such as good and poor forms of posture or first-aid procedures.

Experiments, such as observing the growth of animals when certain types of diet are administered, are informative.

Independent study in which the students are assigned health topics for investigation is helpful.

Resource people, such as doctors, dentists, firemen, or other specialists, can be brought in to speak to health classes.

Audiovisual aids, such as films, network educational television and cable television, filmstrips, slides, radio, and recordings, are helpful in presenting certain types of health material to the students in an interesting and clear manner.

Graphic materials such as posters, graphs, charts, bulletin boards, and exhibits are valuable for motivating students in regard to health matters, arousing interest, attracting attention, and visualizing ideas.

Interviews can be arranged in which students may be assigned to interview such persons as officers of the local health department, representatives of safety councils, members of voluntary health agencies, and heads of medical and dental societies for the purpose of getting the views of specialists and their recommendations on health matters.

Panels can be made up of students for an informal exchange of ideas or points of view regarding pertinent health matters.

Buzz sessions in which a class is organized into small groups of students for the purpose of discussing health topics, permitting each student more opportunity for discussion, is an excellent method.

Class committees can be formed by dividing a class and assigning topics for exploration.

Dramatizations, such as a play or a skit, can

be put on by a class to bring to the pupils' attention a health matter such as the importance of safety on the playground.

Surveys in regard to health problems in the school, college, or community that need investigation and more information as to their solution can be suggested. Survey forms can be constructed by pupils themselves or else standard forms may be available under certain conditions.

Games and quizzes patterned after popular shows on radio or television can provide interesting methods and challenge the thinking of students.

Health aids can be provided in which community health agencies may offer opportunities for students to obtain experience by keeping records or engaging in various types of activities where the jobs do not require experience and special training. Working on a Red Cross blood program is an example.

CONCENTRATED, CORRELATED, INTEGRATED, AND INCIDENTAL HEALTH TEACHING

Four ways of including health education in the school offering are through concentrated, correlated, integrated, and incidental teaching. Each of these will be discussed.

Concentrated health teaching

Concentrated health education refers to the provision in the school offering for regularly scheduled courses that are confined solely to a consideration of health, rather than a combination with some other subject matter area. It implies a scheduled time for class meetings and a planned course of study. It is recommended that such courses be given on the secondary school level. Furthermore, such courses should be held for a daily class period at least one semester during the ninth or tenth grade and also during the eleventh or twelfth grade.

It is the general consensus that concentrated health education is a necessity. If the objectives for which the school health program has been established are to be achieved, time must be made available in the curricular offering of the school. Health has been listed as one of the main objectives in the field of education. Therefore, it would seem logical to assume that in order to achieve such an objective proper provisions must be made.

Concentrated health education courses required of all students result in many educational benefits. There is a specialized body of knowledge to impart that can best be given to students in a concentrated manner, rather than by depending upon some other subject to provide this information. It allows for better planning, teaching progression, and evaluation. It further allows for the giving of credit, such as is given for any other course that is offered separately. It is more likely to result in health instruction by teachers who have specialized in this particular area and who are qualified and interested in participating in such a course. When offered as a separate course it enables boys and girls to be in the same class, as in other subjects. This is not true if it is combined with physical education, where boys and girls are usually in separate groups. It offers greater opportunities for discussion of personal health problems, with guidance and counseling in regard to these problems, and for the utilization of teaching methods appropriate to such a course.

Correlated health teaching

Correlated health education refers to the practice of including health concepts in the various subject matter areas. For example, in the area of history the relationship of the rise and fall of various groups of people could be related to their health and the prevalence of disease, as could the increased speed of transportation and the transfer of disease from one country to the other. In the area of English, a study of the works of literature could be selected with a view to pointing up the health problems of individuals during various periods of history. The relationship of music and of art to mental health could be brought out. Mathematics could be used as a tool to figure the costs of various health projects. Science could bring out the health aspects in relation to the structure and functions of the human body. Home economics provides an excellent setting for teaching such things as nutrition and personal cleanliness. There is hardly a subject matter area that cannot be correlated with health education.

Table 12-6. Health education correlation*

Subject	Schools	Subject	Schools
Science	244	Conservation	1
Physical education	217	Driver education	1
Home economics	183	Educational guidance	1
Biology	165	Elective living	1
General science	34	Home arts	1
Family living	29	Home living	1
Sociology	11	Household mechanics	1
Social studies	10	Life adjustment	1
Psychology	6	Modern problems	1
Orientation	4	Nursing	1
Civic	3	Personal biology	1
Guidance	3	Personal living	1
Reading	3	Physics	1
Art	2	Political science	1
Chemistry	2	Sex education	1
Life science	2	Social living	1
Natural science	2	Teen living	1
Physiology	2		

*From State Department of Education: Patterns and features of school health education in Michigan public schools, East Lansing, 1969, Michigan State Department of Education, p. 4.

Correlated health education should be a part of every school health program. This necessitates definite planning to ensure that such an important subject is emphasized at every opportunity. Schools with health coordinators have found that such a person can perform an outstanding job in this area by meeting with teachers in the various subject matter areas and discussing and planning the contributions they can make to health education. Although correlated health education is very important and should be included in every school, it should not be regarded as a substitute for concentrated health instruction. Even when there is a concentrated health program there should also be a correlated health program that permeates the entire school offering. When both correlated and concentrated health education are provided for, in adequate amounts and in the right manner, the best results are obtained. A survey of Michigan schools shows the various subjects with which health is correlated in that state.

Integrated health teaching

In integrated health teaching, health learnings are integrated into other aspects of the classroom program. Learning experiences are organized around a central objective. Whereas in correlated teaching, health is brought into various subject matter areas, such as physical education and mathematics, in integrated health teaching various parts of a unit of study are related to a central theme. Two such themes might be that of living in a city or planning a visit to a foreign country. Health is one consideration involved in the planning, discussion, and assignments concerning this central theme. Health factors, for example, can be a very important consideration in living in a large metropolitan city or in going to a foreign country. There are problems concerned with water supply, sewage supply, fire prevention, disease control, immunizations, and medical examinations. Integrated health teaching finds its best setting in the elementary school.

Incidental health teaching

Incidental health education refers to that education that takes place during normal teaching situations, other than in regular health classes, where attention is focused on problems concerned with health. Such occasions may arise as the result of a question asked by a student; a problem that is raised in class; a personal problem that confronts a member of the class, a family, or the community; or a sudden illness, accident, or special project. It represents an opportunity for the teacher, physician, dentist, or nurse to provide information that is educational in nature. When a child has his eyes examined or his chest x-rayed, for example, many questions arise and opportunities are afforded to give the child information that will have a lasting and beneficial value. In many cases this will benefit the health of the child more than information given in more formalized, planned class situations. Teachers and others should constantly keep in mind the necessity for continually being alert to these "teachable moments." When a child is curious and wants information, this establishes a time for dynamic health education. Incidental health education can be planned for in advance. Situations and incidents should be anticipated and utilized to their fullest in the interests of good health.

ORGANIZATION OF CLASSES

Many problems arise in connection with the organization of health science classes. Some of the more prevalent of these are concerned with whether boys and girls should meet together or separately, time arrangement, and scheduling.

Class membership

Boys and girls should be scheduled for health classes in a way that is in the best interests of all concerned. This would mean that where health science instruction is a combined program with physical education, and where the boys and girls are in separate classes, it would probably be best to conduct the health classes in a similar manner. On the other hand, if health science and physical education are not combined, it would seem that they should be handled in the same manner as any other subject. This would mean there would be mixed groups. The fact that the subject matter is health science should not mean separation of sexes. It should be pointed out, however, that some leaders in the field maintain this concept is wrong and advocate keeping the sexes separate as a means of getting better organization.

It is generally agreed that if boys and girls meet as a mixed group for health science they should continue as a mixed group throughout the entire course. It does not seem wise to have them meet separately when certain topics are considered. To do so tends to place undue emphasis on certain aspects of health science. It is best to treat all subjects in a natural and educational manner.

Time arrangement

There are many time arrangement patterns being followed in respect to health science. This is true especially on the secondary level.

The *Suggested School Health Policies—A Charter for School Health* recommends that "specific courses in health should be provided for all pupils in both junior and senior high schools. The minimum time allotment for the junior high school health course should be a daily period for at least two semesters, during the seventh, eighth, or ninth grade. The minimum time allotment for the health course in the senior high school should be a daily period for at least two semesters, preferably during the eleventh or twelfth grade. Health courses should receive credit equal to that given for courses in other areas. Health courses should be given in regular classrooms, adequately equipped. The classes should be comparable in size to those in other subject matter areas."*

The Joint Committee on Health Problems in Education of the National Education Association and the American Medical Association reaffirmed this stand when they pointed out that the trend appears to be toward concentrated health courses, one early in the high school, the other late in the senior high school period.

RESOURCES

The teacher or other individuals interested in obtaining help in planning, organizing, and administering a health education program can consult numerous persons and organizations for guidance and help. There are also many materials available for their use. Within the school itself, resource help exists in the form of staff members who possess specialized knowledge, such as the school physician, nurse, and home economics and physical education teachers. The

---

*National Committee on School Health Policies: Suggested school health policies, ed. 3, Chicago, 1962, American Medical Association.

RATING SCALE TO EVALUATE HEALTH EDUCATION MATERIALS *

Suitable material meets all of these criteria	Yes	No
1. Is appropriate to the course of study.		
2. Is a reinforcement of other materials.		
3. Is significantly different.		
4. Is impartial, factual, and accurate.		
5. Is up-to-date.		
6. Is nonsectarian, nonpartisan, and unbiased.		
7. Is free from undesirable propaganda.		
8. Is free from excessive or objectionable advertising.		
9. Is free or inexpensive and readily available.		

Pamphlets

	Excellent	Good	Fair	Poor
1. Readability of type.				
2. Appropriateness of illustrations.				
3. Organization of content.				
4. Logical sequence of concepts.				
5. Important aspects of topic stand out.				
6. Material directed to one specific group such as teachers, pupils, or parents.				
7. Reading level appropriate for intended group.				
8. Based on interest and needs of intended group.				
9. Positively directed in words, description, and actions.				
10. Directed toward desirable health practices.				
11. Minimal resort to fear techniques and morbid concepts.				
12. In good taste; avoids vulgarity, stereotypes, and ridicule.				
Total rating				

Posters

	Excellent	Good	Fair	Poor
1. Realistic and within experience level.				
2. Appeals to interest.				
3. Emphasizes positive behavior and attitudes.				
4. Message clear at a glance.				
5. Little or no conflicting detail.				
6. In good taste.				
7. Attractive and in pleasing colors.				
Total rating				

Recommended for use

1. For use by:

   a. Pupils _____ b. teachers _____ c. parents _____ d. adults _____

2. Appropriate grade level:

   a. primary _____ b. elementary _____ c. junior high school _____ d. secondary _____

   e. college _____ f. adult _____

Not recommended for use and why

Date _____ Evaluated by _____

*From Osborn, B. M., and Sutton, W.: Evaluation of health education materials, The Journal of School Health **34**:72, 1964. (Rating scale prepared by members of the school activities subcommittee.)

community also offers numerous resources that can enrich the health education program immensely. In addition to the school and community, the state and nation also have rich resources that in many cases are available merely for the asking.

The organizations at the local, state, and national levels that offer resources for the field of health education can be listed and discussed under the following headings: (1) professional agencies and associations, (2) official agencies, and (3) commercial organizations.

Professional agencies and associations

Under professional agencies and associations can be listed such organizations as voluntary health agencies, medical, dental, and nursing associations, council of social agencies, and other health education associations. Some of the more prominent are listed here:

Voluntary health organizations

American Cancer Society, 219 E. 42nd St., New York, N. Y. 10017

American Heart Association, 44 E. 23rd St., New York, N. Y. 10010

American National Red Cross, 17th and D Streets, N. W., Washington, D. C. 20006

American Social Health Association, 1740 Broadway, New York, N. Y. 10019

Child Welfare League of America, 67 Irving Place, New York, N. Y. 10003

National Association of Hearing and Speech Agencies, 919 18th Street, N. W., Washington, D. C. 20006

National Association for Mental Health, 1800 N. Kent Street, Rosslyn, Va. 22209

National Foundation–March of Dimes, Box 2000, White Plains, N. Y. 10602

National Safety Council, 425 N. Michigan Ave., Chicago, Ill. 60611

National Society for the Prevention of Blindness, 79 Madison Ave., New York, N. Y. 10016

National Easter Seal Society for Crippled Children and Adults, 2023 West Odgen Ave., Chicago, Ill. 60217

National Tuberculosis and Respiratory Disease Association, 1740 Broadway, New York, N. Y. 10019

Professional associations

American Academy of Pediatrics, 1801 Hinman Ave., P. O. Box 1034, Evanston, Ill. 60204

American Alliance for Health, Physical Education, and Recreation, 1201 16th St. N. W., Washington, D. C. 20036

American Dental Association, 211 E. Chicago Ave., Chicago, Ill. 60611

American Hospital Association, 840 N. Lakeshore Dr., Chicago, Ill. 60610

American Medical Association, 535 N. Dearborn St., Chicago, Ill. 60610

American Nurses Association, 2420 Pershing Rd., Kansas City, Mo. 64108

American Public Health Association, 1015 18th St. N. W., Washington, D. C. 20036

American School Health Association, 515 E. Main St., Kent, Ohio 44240

Child Study Association of America, 9 E. 89th St., New York, N. Y. 10028

National Education Association, 1201 16th St. N. W., Washington, D. C. 20036

National League for Nursing, 10 Columbus Circle, New York, N. Y. 10019

Official agencies

Official agencies, such as state departments of health, state departments of education, and public health departments, offer a rich source of help. They offer guidance and consultant services, disseminate information and materials in various forms for use in health classes, and make available films and other visual aids.

Government agencies on the national level provide resources in various forms, including consultant services, health reports, and grants-in-aid, and publish various materials of interest and use to all those teaching health education.

State colleges and universities, as well as private institutions, should be kept in mind when seeking resources for health. In many such institutions the staffs, with their various specialists, are available for use in the schools. Many times they will conduct workshops and institutes to provide inservice training to local schoolteachers. Many have libraries of films and other materials that may be rented at a nominal fee.

Thought and planning are required in order to use these various resources effectively. The right persons to contact should be known, materials that are borrowed should be returned on time, and consultant services should be handled in a considerate manner.

The names of some official agencies follow:

Atomic Energy Commission, Washington, D. C.

Department of Agriculture, Washington, D. C. (Bureau of Animal Industry and Bureau of Home Economics and Human Nutrition)

Department of Commerce, Bureau of the Census, Washington, D. C.

Department of Health, Education, and Welfare, Washington, D. C. (Office of Education, Office of Special Services, Public Health Service, and Social Security Administration)

Department of the Interior, Bureau of Mines, Washington, D. C.

Department of State, Washington, D. C.

Executive Office of the President, National Security Resources Board, Civilian Defense Office (Federal Civil Defense Administration), Washington, D. C.

Government Printing Office, Superintendent of Documents, Washington, D. C.

State boards of health, located in the state capitals

State departments of education, located in the state capitals

State universities and colleges

Tennessee Valley Authority, Health and Safety Division, Knoxville, Tenn.

World Health Organization, Palais des Nations, Geneva, Switzerland

Commercial organizations

There are many commercial companies that dispense health materials. Although this material should be evaluated with care, much of it will prove helpful in the field of health education. Some of the commercial companies are listed:

The American Institute of Baking, 400 E. Ontario, Chicago, Ill. 60611

The Cereal Institute, 135 S. LaSalle St., Chicago, Ill. 60603

General Mills, Inc., 9200 Wayzata Blvd., Minneapolis, Minn. 55426

The Evaporated Milk Association, 910 17th St. N. W., Washington, D. C. 20006

The Florida Department of Citrus, Lakeland, Fla. 33802

The National Livestock and Meat Board, 36 S. Wabash Ave., Chicago, Ill. 60603

Sunkist Growers, Box 2706, Terminal Annex, Los Angeles, Calif. 90054

The United Fresh Fruit and Vegetable Association, 777 14th St. N. W., Washington, D. C. 20005

The Wheat Flour Institute, 14 E. Jackson Blvd., Chicago, Ill. 60604

EVALUATION

Chapters 17 and 18 discuss in detail the evaluation process concerning school and college health programs. These chapters should be reviewed by the reader for the evaluation of the health science instruction program.

Periodic evaluations of school and college health science instruction programs should provide information on the knowledge achieved by the students, the degree to which student needs are being met, the extent to which objectives are achieved, the value of certain methods of teaching, the effectiveness of the teaching, and the strengths and weaknesses of the program.

Instruments that have been found to be effective in evaluating the health science instruction program include the following:

1. Observation of students in respect to their behavior and skills
2. Checklists
3. Questionnaires
4. Rating scales
5. Interviews with students and parents
6. Tests—standardized and teacher-made
7. Examples of students' work
8. Diaries and other records kept by students
9. Case studies of individual students

CHECKLIST FOR EVALUATING THE HEALTH SCIENCE INSTRUCTION PROGRAM*

General

	Yes	No
1. The school has a clear statement of the philosophy and principles upon which an effective school health instruction program is based.		
2. Teachers on the staff appreciate the importance of health instruction and understand the contributions it makes to the total education program.		
3. The school administration has assigned a qualified person from the staff to coordinate the entire school health program and provides him time to carry out his duties and responsibilities.		

*From State of Ohio Department of Education: a guide for improving school health instruction programs, Columbus, Ohio, 1963, State of Ohio Department of Education, Division of Elementary and Secondary Education.

CHECKLIST FOR EVALUATING THE HEALTH SCIENCE INSTRUCTION PROGRAM—cont'd

	Yes	*No*

4. The school has an active health committee that helps in planning and coordinating the school health program.
5. The school provides a physical environment and an emotional atmosphere that helps to make possible the achievement of the goals of the health instruction program.
6. Teachers and other school staff members set a good example, in terms of good physical and mental health habits and attitudes, as part of the health instruction program.
7. The health instruction program is based upon the health needs, problems, interests, and abilities of the pupils.
8. The school has developed a teaching guide outlining a progressive plan of health instruction from grades 1 through 12.
9. The school has established definite goals of achievement in relation to habits, understanding, attitudes, and skills for each.
10. The school administration promotes the integration of health and safety instruction with all curricular areas and extracurricular activities of the school.
11. The school includes in its in-service education program opportunities for its staff to become better qualified for conducting the health instruction program.
12. The school administration provides adequate materials, such as books, charts, filmstrips, and pamphlets needed for the program.
13. Textbooks used in health classes are authoritative, up-to-date, written in an interesting manner, and suitable for the grade level in which they are used.
14. The school evaluates its health instruction periodically to determine its effectiveness in achieving established goals.

Elementary program

15. In grades 1 to 3 sufficient time is provided during the school day for incidental and integrated teaching of health.
16. In grades 4 to 6 a minimum of three periods a week is allotted for direct health instruction.
17. The planned health instruction is supplemented in the upper grade by incidental teaching, correlation, and integration.
18. Classroom teachers meet the state's minimum standards relative to college preparation in health education.
19. The health instruction program centers around the daily living of the child instead of rote learning of health facts and rules.
20. The program provides many interesting and worthwhile activities that are helpful to the child in solving his health problems related to growth, development, and adjustment.
21. If the school attempts to integrate health instruction with large teaching units, the services of a health educator are utilized in planning those phases of unit dealing with health.
22. The health instruction program includes the major health areas and problems.

Junior and senior high schools

23. The time required for direct health instruction at the junior high school level is equivalent to one full semester of daily classes.
24. The time provided for direct health instruction in the senior high school is equivalent to one full semester of daily classes.
25. In addition to specific health courses, health instruction is correlated with other subject areas and programs.
26. Teachers of health classes in the school have at least a minor in health education or a major in health and physical education.

Continued.

CHECKLIST FOR EVALUATING THE HEALTH SCIENCE INSTRUCTION PROGRAM—cont'd

Junior and senior high schools—cont'd   *Yes*   *No*

27. The health teacher is keenly interested in the health instruction program and atttmpts to achieve the potentialities inherent in the program.
28. The number of pupils assigned to health classes is no greater than those assigned to other classes in the school.
29. The school provides suitable classrooms and adequate facilities for health classes.
30. The teacher utilizes the films, materials, and other resources available to him from local and state health agencies.
31. The content of the program is interesting and meaningful to the pupils and helps them meet their health problems.
32. The school has established definite policies relative to the teaching of controversial areas in health education.
33. The health instruction program in the junior high school includes the health areas recommended by leaders in the field.
34. The health instruction program in the senior high school includes the health areas recommended by leaders in the field.

Questions and exercises

1. What is the relationship of health education to the total school health program?
2. Write an essay of 250 words citing evidence to show the need for health education.
3. What part do the superintendent and principal play in the development of a desirable health education program for the schools?
4. If a physical education person is teaching health education, what should be his or her qualifications in order to do an acceptable job?
5. What is the current status of health education at the secondary level? What is it at the college level?
6. Briefly explain the trend toward certification of health teachers. Write a paragraph or two giving your opinion of this trend.
7. What are eight content areas in health education? Which do you feel are most important in your school? What are the controversial content areas?
8. How does health education vary at the elementary, junior high school, senior high school, and college levels?
9. What are the resources available to individuals in the area of health education?
10. What are some of the administrative problems encountered in school health programs? How can some of these problems be alleviated?

Reading assignment in *Administrative Dimensions of Health and Physical Education Programs, Including Athletics:* Chapter 9, Selections 48 to 54.

Selected references

American Academy of Pediatrics, Committee on School Health: School health policies, Chicago, 1954, The Academy.

AAHPER Position Statement: A unified approach to health teaching, The Journal of School Health **41:**171, 1971.

AAHPER Position Statement: The school nurse in education, School Health Review **2:**36, 1971.

Anderson, C. L.: Health principles and practice, ed. 6, St. Louis, 1970, The C. V. Mosby Co.

Anderson, C. L.: School health practice, ed. 5, St. Louis, 1972, The C. V. Mosby Co.

Braza, J. F.: The status and administration of the required health courses, The Journal of School Health **41:**142, 1971.

Bucher, C. A., Olsen, E., and Willgoose, C.: The foundation of health, New York, 1967, Appleton-Century-Crofts.

Curriculum Commission of the school health division, AAHPER: A guide for development of a health education curriculum, School Health Review **2:**35, 1971.

Fort, J.: Alcohol: our biggest drug problem, New York, 1973, McGraw-Hill Book Co.

Greenberg, J. S.: Emerging educational concepts and health instruction, The Journal of School Health **42:**356, 1972.

Grout, R. E.: Health teaching in schools, ed. 5, Philadelphia, 1968, W. B. Saunders Co.

Hafen, B. Q.: Man, health and environment, 1972, Burgess Publishing Co.

Harris, W. H.: Suggested criteria for evaluating health and safety teaching materials, Journal of Health, Physical Education, and Recreation **35:**26, 1964.

Henkel, B. O., and others: Foundations of health science, Boston, 1971, Allyn & Bacon, Inc.

Hicks, D. A.: Professional preparation of health education in the 70's, The Journal of School Health **42:**243, 1972.

Hoyman, H. S.: An ecologic view of health and health education, The Journal of School Health **35:**110, 1965.

Irwin, L. W., and others: Health for better living, Columbus, Ohio, 1972, Charles E. Merrill Publishing Co.

Johnson, W. R., and Belzer, E. G.: Human sexual behavior and sex education, Philadelphia, 1973, Lea & Febiger.

Joint Committee on Health Problems in Education of National Education Association and American Medical Association: Health education, Washington, D. C., 1961, National Education Association.

Leigh, T.: Nationwide profile of health instruction, School Health Review **4:**35, 1973.

Levy, M., Greene, W., and Jenne, F.: Competence based professional preparation, School Health Review **3:**26, 1972.

Mayshark, C., and Irwin, L.: Health education in secondary schools, ed. 2, St. Louis, 1968, The C. V. Mosby Co.

National Committee on School Health Policies: Suggested school health policies, ed. 2, Washington, D. C., 1966, National Education Association.

Oberteuffer, D., and others: School health education, New York, 1972, Harper & Row, Publishers.

Pollock, M. B.: The significance of health education for junior college students, The Journal of School Health **34:**333, 1964.

Projections of the joint committee on health problems in education of the NEA and AMA: School Health-1985, School Health Review **3:**2, 1972.

Randall, H. B.: School health in the 70's, The Journal of School Health **7:**125, 1971.

Read, D. H., and Greene, W. H.: Health and modern man, New York, 1973, The Macmillan Co.

Report of the Study Committee on Health Education in the Elementary and Secondary School of the American School Health Association: Health instruction—suggestions for teachers, The Journal of School Health **34:** 1964. (Entire issue.)

Schiller, P.: Creative approach to sex education and counseling, New York, 1973, Association Press.

School Health Education Study: A summary report, Washington, D. C., 1964, School Health Education Study, 1201 16th St., N. W.

School Health Education Study: Health education: a conceptual approach, Washington, D. C., 1965, School Health Education Study, 1201 16th St., N. W.

Slocum, H. M.: Teacher preparation in health education, School Health Review **2:**8, 1971.

Smolensky, J., and Bonevchio, L. R.: Principles of school health, Boston, 1966, D. C., Heath & Co.

Sorochan, W. D.: Health instruction—why do we need it in the 70's? The Journal of School Health **41:**209, 1971.

Tuck, M. L., and Grodner, A. B.: Consumer health, 1972, Dubuque, Iowa, William C. Brown Co., Publishers.

Veenket, C. H.: Certification of health educators: a priority for the seventies, School Health Review **2:**3, 1971.

Willgoose, C.: Health education for secondary schools, Philadelphia, 1972, W. B. Saunders Co.

Willgoose, C. E.: Health education in the elementary school, ed. 3, Philadelphia, 1969, W. B. Saunders Co.

Health service programs for students, including athletes

Health services are concerned with the health of all students, including athletes. The health service program is essential to the physical, emotional and social health of all students. The treatment of athletes is an important part of any health service program especially in areas of injury prevention and treatment. If health services are inadequate, the health and safety of students are jeopardized.

Health services cover a broad area. They include the procedures established to:

1. Appraise the health status of students and educational personnel
2. Counsel students, parents, and other persons concerning appraisal findings
3. Encourage the correction of remediable defects
4. Help plan for the health care and education of handicapped (exceptional) children
5. Help prevent and control disease
6. Provide emergency care for the sick and injured
7. Promote environmental sanitation
8. Promote the health of school and college personnel

THE HEALTH OF THE ATHLETE

The health of the athlete is of such importance to the students who read this text that this special section is being included. Although the entire chapter has implications for all who participate in physical education classes, this particular section emphasizes some of the essential health services for athletes. The growth of sports and athletic programs at both school and college education levels supports this emphasis.

Health services for athletes involve continuous medical attention, sound policies and procedures, and the availability of qualified personnel. A close working relationship should exist between coaches, trainers, athletic directors, and school and college administrators and medical society representatives if the athlete is to be adequately protected from injury and harm.

The American Medical Association, through its Committee on the Medical Aspects of Sports, the National Trainers' Association, and such athletic organizations as the National Federation of State High School Athletic Associations, has done an outstanding job in preparing materials, making recommendations to safeguard the health of the athlete, and outlining such procedures as first aid for athletic injuries. A few of the selected materials relating to health services for the athlete are included here. They include a checklist to help evaluate five major factors in the health supervision of athletes, disqualifying conditions for sports participation, and first aid procedures for athletic injuries. Furthermore, a suggested sports candidate's questionnaire, health examination form, and a student partic-

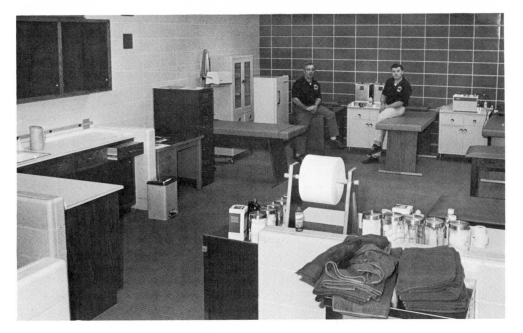

Training room for athletes. (Trinity College, Hartford, Conn.)

ipation and parental approval form are also shown.*

Providing medical services for athletes

Medical supervision is essential for all sports participants. Unfortunately, many athletic contests are not adequately supervised from a medical point of view. Dr. Allan J. Ryan cites his experiences at the University of Wisconsin concerning the lack of medical supervision in high school athletics. In one semester, Dr. Ryan encountered 27 male freshmen enrolled in an adaptive physical education program who were suffering from musculoskeletal system defects. Eighteen of these students incurred the defects as a result of athletic competition in football, basketball, and ice hockey.

---

*A Joint Statement of The Committee on the Medical Aspects of Sports of the American Medical Association and the National Federation of State High School Athletic Associations: Safeguarding the health of the athlete, Chicago, 1965, The American Medical Association.

The Committee on the Medical Aspects of Sports, American Medical Association: A guide for medical evaluation of candidates for school sports, Chicago, 1966, The American Medical Association.

The Committee on the Medical Aspects of Sports, American Medical Association: First aid chart for athletic injuries, Chicago, 1965, The American Medical Association.

There are numerous reports of football fatalities caused by neck and brain injuries and deaths from heat stroke because of inadequate preventative measures. In many cases there is a lack of communication between medical supervisors (physicians) and coaches. Wrestling is another sport where numerous injuries occur. Many reports are cited where boys on wrestling teams endure dramatic weight losses in order to qualify for lower weight class matches.

Medical supervision can be improved in reference to athletes if the administration, physical educators, coaches, and trainers make this a priority commitment. Frequently, coaches are lacking in medical training, and they feel that too much supervision from doctors and nurses will hurt the chances of their team. A philosophy of medical supervision must be adapted that puts the individual athlete first and enables him or her to have the best possible medical attention.

There are other factors inherent in adequate medical supervision. These factors include the following:

1. *Selection of a team physician.* A team physician must be selected with care. He or she must not neglect team responsibilities because of a growing practice or other commitments.

The physician should remain objective and avoid being influenced by students, parents, and coaches. If a physician is needed and there is none available, consult the local medical society for a recommendation of one person or perhaps two doctors who will jointly care for the team.

2. *Maintenance of adequate medical facilities.* Elaborate training rooms and equipment are not essential in high school athletic programs. What is essential is a private examining room with an examining table, a desk, and a few chairs. An injured athlete should not return to play until authorized by the team physician.

Adequate health supervision of sports is essential. Some of the reasons given in support of adequate medical supervision include: (1) the physical, physiologic, and psychologic demands of competition; (2) the problem of treatment and rehabilitation involved in athletic injuries; (3) the increased possibility of infectious diseases caused by lowered resistance; and (4) the close relationship existing between physical activity and disease and injury.

A recent survey* taken to determine the current standards of health supervision and how they were implemented in 2-year college intercollegiate sports concluded that there was much need for improvement in this area. Some of the recommendations of this survey were:

1. There should be centralization of medical control of intercollegiate athletics in the college health service.
2. There should be implementation of nationally and regionally adopted standards governing health aspects of intercollegiate sports. Some of the standards would include: (a) a physical examination and medical history for each athlete, (b) physician coverage at all contact sports, (c) ambulance at all contact sports, (d) availability of communication for emergency purposes, (e) athletic facilities that are safe and meet size

---

*Rolnick, M.: Health supervision of intercollegiate sports in junior and community college, JUCO Review **24:**20, 1972.

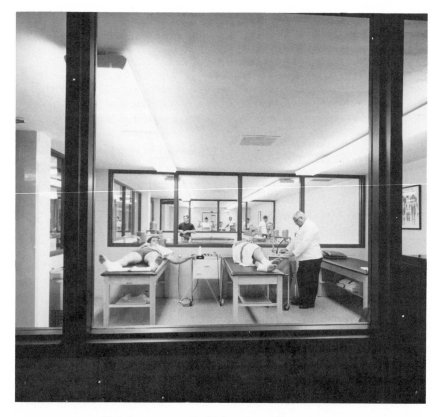

Training room at the University of Notre Dame.

requirements, (f) use of noncaustic materials for marking athletic fields.

3. Certification by National Junior College Athletic Association that health standards have been implemented.
4. Stipulation of medical standards in contracts with competing colleges. Failure to comply would result in forfeiture.

These suggestions for adequate medical supervision are applicable to all schools and colleges with interscholastic and intercollegiate activity programs.

Preventing sports injuries

What is the administrator's responsibility in the prevention of sports injuries? His or her first responsibility is the hiring of physicians, coaches, and trainers who understand the frequency and occurrence of sports injuries and how to treat them. These persons should also be aware of preventative measures necessary for sports safety. This may not be a simple job for the administrator since trained personnel are difficult to find, and the administrator may also run into budget difficulties, proliferation of sports, and established regulations. In addition, schedules may prohibit proper training prior to athletic competition and sports seasons tend to overlap more and more.

In order to prevent injuries, careful medical examinations must be given to each athlete. These examinations should be complete and include blood tests. Athletes who are immature physically, those who have sustained previous athletic injuries, and those who are inadequately conditioned are all prone to sports injuries. Such practices as crash diets and dehydration are very injurious to an athlete's health. Training practices based on sound physiologic principles are the best answer to avoidance of sports injuries. Of course proper protective equipment must be used in appropriate sports.

In general, there must be an intensification of efforts by governmental agencies, nonprofit public service organizations, voluntary associations, and educational institutions toward safety in sports. Facilities and equipment must be developed with safety factors in mind, and sport regulations must be reviewed in reference to safety procedures. In addition, research must be conducted in the area of improving sports safety.

Athletic trainers

The importance of athletic trainers in sports injury prevention and treatment cannot be overlooked. It is unfortunate to note that where athletic trainers are most needed (in the secondary schools), they are poorly represented; only about 100 schools have a full time teacher-athletic trainer. Compounding this situation is the inadequate medical and injury prevention training of most coaches. Even if the coach has been well prepared in these areas, he or she does not have sufficient time to carry out coaching duties as well as the responsibilities of the athletic trainer.

The duties of the athletic trainer include the following:

1. The prevention and care of injuries associated with competitive athletics
2. Preparation and utilization of an athletic conditioning program
3. Administration of first aid as needed
4. Application of devices such as strapping or bandaging to prevent injury
5. Administration of therapeutic techniques under the direction of physician
6. Development and supervision of rehabilitation programs for injured athletes under supervision of team physician
7. Selection, care, and fitting of equipment
8. Supervision of training menus and diets
9. Supervision of safety factors involved in facilities and use of equipment

The professional preparation of athletic trainers consists of course requirements in areas of the sciences, psychology, coaching techniques, first-aid and safety, nutrition, exercise, and other related subjects. The National Association of Athletic Trainers (NATA) has an approved educational program for athletic trainers that stipulates semester hours required in each subject classification. In 1971, there were only six approved undergraduate curricula in athletic training; approximately 30 more were in developmental stages. In addition, a certification examination is also given by the NATA. Information concerning the profession can be obtained through the NATA.

The entry of women into this field is long overdue. Athletic competition among women has greatly increased, and there is a real need for

SAFEGUARDING THE HEALTH OF THE ATHLETE*

A joint statement of the Committee on the Medical Aspects of the American Medical Association and the National Federation of State High School Athletic Associations

A checklist to help you evaluate five major factors in health supervision of athletics.

Participation in athletics is a privilege involving both responsibilities and rights. The athlete's responsibilities are to play fair, to keep in training, and to conduct himself with credit to his sport and his school. In turn he has the right to optimal protection against injury as this may be assured through good conditioning and technical instruction, proper regulations and conditions of play, and adequate health supervision.

Periodic evaluation of each of these factors will help to assure a safe and healthful experience for players. The checklist below contains the kinds of questions to be answered in such an a appraisal.

PROPER CONDITIONING helps to prevent injuries by hardening the body and increasing resistance to fatique.

1. Are prospective players given directions and activities for preseason conditioning?
2. Is there a minimum of three weeks of practice before the first game or contest?
3. Are precautions taken to prevent heat exhaustion and heat stroke?
4. Is each player required to warm up thoroughly prior to participation?
5. Are substitutions made without hesitation when players evidence disability?

CAREFUL COACHING leads to skillful performance, which lowers the incidence of injuries.

1. Is emphasis given to safety in teaching techniques and elements of play?
2. Are injuries analyzed to determine causes and to suggest preventive programs?
3. Are tactics discouraged that may increase the hazards and thus the incidence of injuries?
4. Are practice periods carefully planned and of reasonable duration?

GOOD OFFICIATING promotes enjoyment of the game and the protection of players.

1. Are players as well as coaches thoroughly schooled in the rules of the game?
2. Are rules and regulations strictly enforced in practice periods as well as in games?
3. Are officials qualified both emotionally and technically for their responsibilities?
4. Do players and coaches respect the decisions of officials?

RIGHT EQUIPMENT AND FACILITIES serve a unique purpose in protection of players.

1. Is the best protective equipment provided for contact sports?
2. Is careful attention given to proper fitting and adjustment of equipment?
3. Is equipment properly maintained, and are worn and outmoded items discarded?
4. Are proper areas for play provided and carefully maintained?

ADEQUATE MEDICAL CARE is a necessity in the prevention and control of injuries.

1. Is there a thorough preseason health history and medical examination?
2. Is a physician present at contests and readily available during practice sessions?
3. Does the physician make the decision as to whether an athlete should return to play following injury during games?
4. Is authority from a physician required before an athlete can return to practice after being out of play because of disabling injury?
5. Is the care given athletes by coach or trainer limited to first aid and medically prescribed services?

*From Committee on the Medical Aspects of Sports of the American Medical Association and the National Federation of State High School Athletic Associations: Tips on athletic training. XI. Chicago, Illinois, 1969, The American Medical Association.

female athletic trainers. Administrators and physical educators must be made aware of the need for women trainers, and students interested in physical education should be told about the profession of athletic training.

Sports medicine

A rapidly expanding development relating to health services for athletes is the area of sports medicine. The fact that more than 17 million persons are injured each year in this country in physical activities and sports has accented this new field of endeavor.

Sports medicine is particularly concerned with how these injuries from sports and other physical activities occur, how they can be prevented, and the long range impact they have on a person's performance.

An example of an institute of sports medicine and athletic trauma that has been developed is the one founded by Dr. James Nicholas, orthopedic surgeon at Lenox Hill Hospital in New

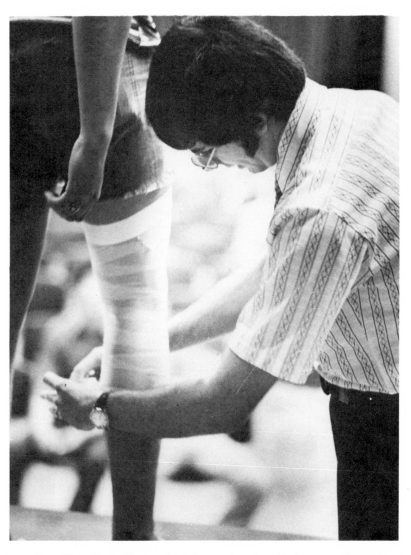

College of DuPage, Glen Ellyn, Ill., held a special 2-day seminar for athletic team trainers, showing techniques and methods to current and prospective team trainers.

York City. The center is concerned with a study of "the mechanics, diagnosis, treatment and rehabilitation of physical injuries sustained in organized and unorganized athletics and recreational activities."

THE PLACE OF HEALTH SERVICES IN SCHOOLS AND COLLEGES

The health services program must be well publicized so that educators, coaches, and the public in general will understand why such services are essential. Only as this need is understood will there be adequate planning and provision for such services.

The Joint Committee of the American Medical Association and the National Education Association* has listed the following as reasons why health services should exist:

1. They contribute to the learning experience and the realization of other educational aims.
2. They facilitate adaptation of school and college programs to individual needs.
3. They help in maintaining a healthful environment.
4. They help children secure the medical or dental care they need.
5. They possess inherent values for increasing students' understanding of health and health problems.

Health services contribute to the realization of educational aims. Educational committees, conferences, and other important groups have continually listed health as one of the objectives of education. Health services are necessary to attain this objective.

Health services minimize the hazards of school and college attendance. They make it possible for the student to attend school and college under safe conditions. Through emergency care, it is possible to greatly reduce the harmful effects of injuries in the event of accidents. Adequate precautions are taken against the spread of communicable disease. Medical examinations identify health defects, making for safer participation in athletics and other school activities. These are only a few of the many hazards that can be removed or minimized through effective health services.

Health services help youth to adapt better to school and college programs. Through careful and regular checking of vision and hearing and general physical condition and correction of defects, students will better assume their responsibilities. Deficiencies, defects, and weaknesses that are prevalent will be noted and provided for.

Health services have potentialities for educating the parents as well as the students. They have potentialities for developing proper attitudes toward health, developing proper habits, and imparting scientific information. Through the medical examination, for example, the teacher, nurse, physician, coach, and others have an opportunity to educate students and parents about various aspects of health.

The forty-seventh annual report of the Health Service Department of the Denver schools* includes a report on the basic functions that this department performs in the education of children and youth in that city. Since this school system has won national recognition for its school health services program, this information is given to provide a better understanding of what all schools should be trying to accomplish in this area:

Health services to assure a safe and wholesome school environment
1. Selection of healthy adult employees
2. Implementation of city health and building regulations
3. Application of control measures to stop the spread of illnesses.
   a. Implementation of official health rules
   b. Prompt attention to ill children and exclusion from school
   c. Immunizations for those who request it
4. Health consultations and periodic evaluations for adult personnel

Health services to detect conditions among pupils that would diminish their most effective participation in educational activities
1. Routine screening tests for vision, hearing, physical growth, and dental health
2. Periodic medical appraisals to evaluate general development and significant physical conditions and defects

---

*Joint Committee of American Medical Association and National Education Association: School health services, ed. 2, Washington, D. C., 1964, National Education Association, pp. 7-8.

*Corliss, L. M.: Forty-seventh annual report, 1971-72. Health Service Department, Denver Public Schools, Denver, Colo.

3. Screening tests on preschool children for hearing and vision

Health services to assist in health instruction for all pupils
1. Cooperative efforts with instruction department on materials and inservice training
2. Educational emphasis on all health procedures
3. Work with faculties for classroom health units
4. Tuberculosis testing

Health services to promote followup care and correction of pupils' health problems and deficiencies
1. Nurse counseling with pupils, parents, teachers, social workers, and other school personnel
2. Intercommunications between school health personnel and private physicians and clinics
3. Cooperation with other community health agencies

Health services to assist with other needs of some pupils
1. Medical appraisal of those with physical, mental, and emotional problems that seem to interfere with learning
2. Placement in special educational classes
3. Contributions of the consultant psychiatrist
4. Help in first-aid care of injuries
5. Medical reports on "battered" children

Additional health service department responsibilities
1. Continual evaluation of department activities
2. Close rapport and administrative planning with medical and dental profession and with official and nonofficial health agencies
3. Continued cooperative programs with other departments within the schools and with community and civic groups
4. Assistance with health, disability, and retirement leaves for adult personnel.

Table 13-1, taken from the Denver Report, indicates the recommended timing and frequency of routine school health services in respect to grades.

THE RESPONSIBILITY FOR SCHOOL HEALTH SERVICES

The question is frequently raised as to whether school health services should fall within the province of school personnel or public health

---

SUGGESTED SPORTS CANDIDATES' QUESTIONNAIRE

(To be completed by parents or family physician)

Name_____Birth date_____

Home address_____

Parents' Name_____Tel. No._____

1. Has had injuries requiring medical attention	Yes	No
2. Has had illness lasting more than a week	Yes	No
3. Is under a physician's care now	Yes	No
4. Takes medication now	Yes	No
5. Wears glasses	Yes	No
contact lenses	Yes	No
6. Has had a surgical operation	Yes	No
7. Has been in hospital (except for tonsillectomy)	Yes	No
8. Do you know of any reason why this individual should not participate in all sports?	Yes	No

Please explain any "Yes" answers to above questions:

_____

_____

9. Has had complete poliomyelitis immunization by inoculations (Salk) or oral vaccine (Sabin)	Yes	No
10. Has had tetanus toxoid and booster inoculation within past 3 years	Yes	No
11. Has seen a dentist within the past 6 months	Yes	No

_____

Parent or Physician

Suggested sports candidates' questionnaire. (From Committee on the Medical Aspects of Sports, American Medical Association: A guide for medical evaluation of candidates for school sports, 1966, The Association, p. 2. Reprinted with permission of the American Medical Association.)

SUGGESTED HEALTH EXAMINATION FORM

(Cooperatively prepared by the National Federation of State High School Athletic Associations and the Committee on Medical Aspects of Sports of the American Medical Association.) Health examination for athletes should be rendered after August 1 preceding school year concerned.

(Please Print) Name of Student _____ City and School _____

Grade_____ Age_____ Height_____ Weight_____ Blood Pressure_____

Significant Past Illness or Injury_____

Eyes_____ R 20/ ; L20 /; Ears_____ Hearing R /15; L /15

Respiratory_____

Cardiovascular_____

Liver_____ Spleen_____ Hernia_____

Musculoskeletal_____ Skin_____

Neurological_____ Genitalia_____

Laboratory: Urinalysis_____ Other:_____

Comments_____

Completed Immunizations: Polio_____ Tetanus_____

                         Date   Date

| Instructions for use of card | Other_____

I certify that I have on this date examined this pupil and find him (her) physically able to compete in supervised activities NOT CROSSED OUT BELOW.

BASEBALL	FOOTBALL	ROWING	SOFTBALL	TRACK
BASKETBALL	HOCKEY	SKATING	SPEEDBALL	VOLLEYBALL
CROSS COUNTRY	GOLF	SKIING	SWIMMING	*WRESTLING
FIELD HOCKEY	GYMNASTICS	SOCCER	TENNIS	OTHERS_____

*Weight loss permitted to make lower weight class: Yes_____ No_____; if "Yes" may lose _____pounds.

Date of Examination: _____ Signed:_____

Physician's Address_____ Examining Physician

                                            Telephone_____

- -

STUDENT PARTICIPATION AND PARENTAL APPROVAL FORM

Name of student:_____ Name of School:_____

               First   Last   Middle Initial

Date:_____ Date of Birth:_____ Place of Birth:_____

This application to compete in interscholastic athletics for the above high school is entirely voluntary on my part and is made with the understanding that I have not violated any of the eligibility rules and regulations of the State Association.

| Instructions for use of card | Signature of Student:_____

PARENT'S OR GUARDIAN'S PERMISSION

I hereby give my consent for the above high school student to engage in State Association approved athletic activities as a representative of his high school, except those crossed out on reverse side of this form by the examining physician, and I also give my consent for the above student to accompany the team as a member on its out-of-town trips.

                         Signature of Parent or Guardian:_____

Date:_____ Address:_____

                                (Street)   (City or Town)

NOTE: This form is to be filled out completely and filed in the office of the high school principal or superintendent of schools before student is allowed to practice and/or compete.

Suggested health examination form. (From Committee on the Medical Aspects of Sports, American Medical Association: A guide for medical evaluation of candidates for school sports, 1966, The Association, p. 3. Reprinted with permission of the American Medical Association.)

department personnel. Both the school and the public health department are vitally interested in seeing that such services are provided. Both have specialized personnel who can render important contributions to the successful administration of health services. The school is especially interested in the educational aspects of such services and the vast potentialities they have for educating the children and the public. It has personnel who are specially trained in educational methods and techniques. In many communities it also has physicians on the staff who perform medical examinations and other health services. On the other hand, the public health department has specialists in sanitation, epidemiology, and other areas pertinent to the health services program.

Since both the school and the public health

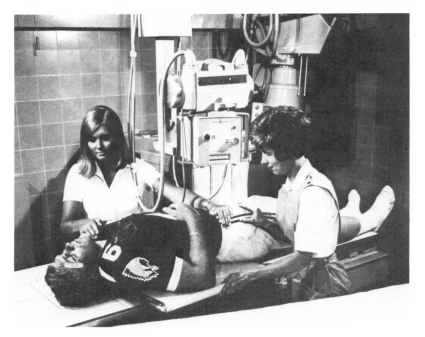

Proper health service techniques provide that athletes are transferred with care. Here is the Spenco Roll-Aid, a lightweight patient transfer device that can easily be manipulated by one person. Length is designed to properly support the shoulders and hips of the patient for easy transfer. (Courtesy Spenco Medical Corporation, Waco, Tex.)

department have interests in health services, each local community should decide how such a program can best be carried out. In some communities the public health department is better staffed and qualified to perform many of the health services. In other communities the school has the better staff and other requisites. In many cases, health services should be a cooperative endeavor, where the health department and the school work together, sharing their resources and cooperatively planning a program.

EDUCATION VERSUS TREATMENT

With the school becoming an increasingly important social organization of the community, the question often arises as to whether it should provide treatment as part of its health services program. The philosophy on which the school program is based establishes it mainly as an agency concerned with education. The educational aspects of the health services program represent the major contribution of the schools. By identifying health defects, making referrals to medical, dental, and other experts, counsel-

ing, providing for emergency care, making special provisions for the handicapped, and establishing and encouraging measures to prevent and control communicable diseases, the school is carrying out its responsibilities in health services. However, in some communities, as a result of agreement and consultation among public health, medical and dental professions, educators, and others, provisions have been made to provide dental treatment, occupational therapy, and other services. Such programs are exceptions to the rule, however, and usually are initiated as a result of a need for expediency and because it is felt that such a practice is the best way to handle certain health problems. Treatment is not usually a part of the school health program.

HEALTH SERVICES

The rest of the chapter will be concerned with a discussion of the various health services: (1) health appraisal, (2) health counseling, (3) correction of remediable defects, (4) care and education of exceptional children, (5) communica-

Table 13-1. Timing and frequency of some routine school health services *

Type of service	Grade												
	K	1	2	3	4	5	6	7	8	9	10	11	12
Vision screening tests													
At certain grades as shown; on all new pupils and referred pupils at other grades	X	X		X		X		X			X		
Hearing screening tests													
At certain grades as shown; on all new pupils, on referred pupils and those with known defects	X	X		X				X					
Dental education and/or inspections													
At grades shown and at about 5-year intervals, high school pupils are inspected and DMF rates ascertained	X	X	X	X	X	X	X	X					
Weight and growth measurements													
On all new and referred pupils (often done cooperatively with P.E. teachers as part of the fitness program)	X	X	X	X	X	X	X						
Medical appraisals													
a. All pupils who participate in varsity sports who do not bring reports from private or clinic physicians											X	X	X
b. Pupils who participate in swimming classes when private or clinic physician reports are not obtained								X	X	X	X	X	X
c. NDCC members if other physician reports are not obtained											X	X	X
Medical and/or nursing appraisals													
a. All pupils with suspected health or learning problems without current reports of family or clinic physicians	X	X	X	X	X	X	X	X	X	X	X	X	X
b. All pupils being considered for placement in special education	X	X	X	X	X	X	X	X	X	X	X	X	X
Special services													
a. Mandatory skin test for those who have not had one within 9 months								X					
b. Scalp ringworm inspection	(as needed)												
c. Other nuisance diseases	(as needed)												
d. Color vision rechecks by the school nurse										X (new pupils here)			

*From Forty-Seventh Annual Report, 1971-1972, Department of Health Services, Denver Public Schools, Denver, Colorado.

DISQUALIFYING CONDITIONS FOR SPORTS PARTICIPATION*

Conditions	Contact†	Noncontact endurance‡	Others§
General			
Acute infections:			
Respiratory, genitourinary, infectious mononucleosis, hepatitis, active rheumatic fever, active tuberculosis, boils, furuncles, impetigo	X	X	X
Obvious physical immaturity in comparison with other competitors	X	X	
Obvious growth retardation	X		
Hemorrhagic disease:			
Hemophilia, purpura, and other bleeding tendencies	X		
Diabetes, inadequately controlled	X	X	X
Jaundice, whatever cause	X	X	X
Eyes			
Absence or loss of function of one eye	X		
Severe myopia, even if correctable	X		
Ears			
Significant impairment	X		
Respiratory			
Tuberculosis (active or under treatment)	X	X	X
Severe pulmonary insufficiency	X	X	X
Cardiovascular			
Mitral stenosis, aortic stenosis, aortic insufficiency, coarctation of aorta, cyanotic heart disease, recent carditis of any etiology	X	X	X
Hypertension on organic basis	X	X	X
Previous heart surgery for congenital or acquired heart disease	X	X	
Liver			
Enlarged liver	X		
Spleen			
Enlarged spleen	X		
Hernia			
Inguinal or femoral hernia	X	X	
Musculoskeletal			
Symptomatic abnormalities or inflammations	X	X	X
Functional inadequacy of the musculoskeletal system, congenital or acquired, incompatible with the contact or skill demands of the sport	X	X	
Neurological			
History or symptoms of previous serious head trauma or repeated concussions	X		
Convulsive disorder not completely controlled by medication	X	X	
Previous surgery on head or spine	X	X	
Renal			
Absence of one kidney	X		
Renal disease	X	X	X
Genitalia			
Absence of one testicle	X		
Undescended testicle	X		

*Committee on the Medical Aspects of Sports, American Medical Association: A guide for medical evaluation of candidates for school sports, Chicago, Illinois, 1966, The Association, pp. 4-5.
†Lacrosse, baseball, soccer, basketball, football, wrestling, hockey, rugby, etc.
‡Cross country, track, tennis, crew, swimming, etc.
§Bowling, golf, archery, field events, etc.

ble disease control, (6) emergency care, (7) environmental sanitation, and (8) health of school and college personnel. Each of these health services will be considered in respect to how it fits into the total health program. Some of the various techniques that are used and administrative problems that arise, together with acceptable procedures to be followed, will be discussed.

Health appraisal

Health appraisal is that phase of health service that is concerned with evaluating the health of the student in as objective a way as possible, through examinations, observations, and records.

The cooperation of many individuals is needed to do an acceptable job in health service. Teachers, administrators, physicians, dentists, psychologists, public health officials, social workers, parents, and lay leaders must all work together. Through the active cooperation of all, the necessary plans will be made for continuous evaluation and appraisal. If a health council exists, this body can play a major role in coordinating the various aspects of the program.

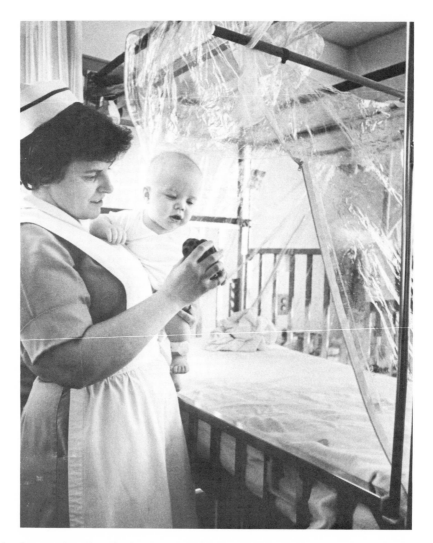

The nurse is a key member of any health services team. The nursing program at College of DuPage, Glen Ellyn, Ill., trains nurses.

Planning should provide for desirable facilities and procedures for health appraisal. There should be provision for privacy and quiet so that the best type of examinations and other techniques can be used in an acceptable manner.

The aims of health appraisal include identifying students in need of medical or dental treatment, those who have problems relating to nutrition, and those who are in need of treatment by a psychiatrist or guidance clinic. In addition, the objectives of health services are to measure the growth of pupils; identify students with nonremediable defects so that modified programs may be provided, such as for crippled or mentally retarded pupils; identify students who need additional examinations, such as x-ray studies; and identify students who need programs apart from the school setting, such as the blind and deaf.

The techniques used in health appraisal that will be discussed here include medical, psychologic, and dental examinations, screening for vision and hearing, teacher observations, and health records.

Examinations. Examinations are effective means of health appraisal.

Medical examinations. There are many important considerations for the administrator to keep in mind if medical examinations are to fulfill their objective. The following are some administrative guides.

TYPES. Both periodic and referral examinations should be given to students. *Periodic* medical examinations are given at stated intervals. *Referral* examinations are those that are given to students who have health problems needing special attention and who have been referred to the proper professional source. Such students may be referred to the physician as a result of teacher's observations, screening examinations, health records, or other indications that special attention is needed. The *examination of athletes* is also a type of medical examination that needs to be considered.

PLANNING. Medical examinations require planning. Young children should be informed of their nature and purposes. The teacher can play an important role in explaining some of these purposes and procedures. Desirable attitudes can be developed so that children and parents look forward to such an event with interest and anticipation. The various instruments that are used, such as the stethoscope, can be shown and discussed. Planning should also take into consideration the provision of adequate facilities, having parents present, and making available the necessary health records.

FREQUENCY. At least four periodic medical examinations should be given during the time a child is in the elementary and secondary schools. There should be a minimum of one examination at the time of entrance to school, one at the intermediate grade level, one at the junior or early high school level when the student is entering the adolescent period, and one toward the termination of the high school period. The desirable procedure, however, would be to have a medical examination each year. Referral examinations should be given at any time that health problems are detected. There is also a need for more medical examinations for students who are engaging in the athletic phase of the physical education program and for those whose health conditions are such that the physician recommends examinations at more frequent intervals.

EXAMINER. It is recommended that the family physician conduct the medical examination. It is felt that through a more complete knowledge of the family history and a closer personal relationship, a better job can be done. However, since some families do not have their own physicians, since it means an additional outlay of funds, and for other reasons, many schools must rely on a school physician to administer the examination. The procedure that is utilized in each community should be a local prerogative and based upon the type of examination that will produce the best results.

PERSONNEL IN ATTENDANCE. The personnel that should be in attendance at the medical examination for young children would include the physician, nurse, child, teacher, and parents. At the secondary school level, the child should have progressed to the point where he or she assumes the responsibility for his own health, and so the need for parents at the examination is not as great. Special attention should be given to sending a written invitation to parents, listing the date and time of the examination. The pres-

HEALTH RECORD

Parents or Guardians—Mr. and Mrs.	
Occupation of Father	Session Teacher
Occupation of Mother Family Doctor	Family Dentist

(Right margin, top to bottom: Last Name · First Name · Address · Telephone)

MEDICAL EXAMINATION		1	2	3	4
1.	Date of Examination				
2.	Age				
3.	Weight				
4.	Height				
5.	Hearing Rt.				
	Lt.				
6.	Eyes Rt.				
	Lt.				
7.	Test with glasses	Yes No	Yes No	Yes No	Yes No
8.	Ring Worm				
9.	Plantar Warts				
10.	Hair				
11.	Personal Hygiene				
12.	Pulse before exercise				
13.	Pulse after exercise				
14.	Heart				
15.	Lungs				
16.	Tremor				
17.	Abdomen				
18.	Hernia				
19.	Ears				
20.	Nose				
21.	Tonsils				
22.	Adenoids				
23.	Teeth				
24.	Thyroid				
25.	Glands				
26.	Nutrition				
27.	Skin				
28.	P. E. Classification				
	Unrestricted (A or B)				
	Partially Restricted (C)				
	Rest Only (D)				
	Permanent Excuse				
	Temporary Excuse				
29.	Swimming				
	Permanent Excuse				
	Temporary Excuse				
Doctor's Initials					

HISTORY OF DISEASE

Chicken Pox	St. Vitus Dance	Diphtheria	Measles	Mumps	Pneumonia	Scarlet Fever	Rheumatic Fever	Whooping Cough	Tonsillitis	Hay Fever	Asthma	Date of Vaccination for Small Pox	T. B. in Family?	Date of Skin Test

Headaches:		Menstruation	
Never		Regular	
Occasionally		Irregular	
Frequently		Dysmenorrhea	

Operations:		Injuries	
Tonsils			
Others:			

Postural Findings	L	R	L	R	L	R	L	R
Scoliosis								
Shoulder High								
Hip High								
Feet: Pronation								
Long. Arch								
Transverse Arch								
Head Forward								
Round Shoulders								
Hollow Back								
Abdomen								
Body Balance								
Posture Grade								
Corrective Gym								

COMMENTS:

Explanation of Terms: "O"—Normal; "X"—Slight Defect; "XX"—Moderate; "XXX"—Marked.

Girl's health record. (Highland Park High School, Highland Park, Ill.)

ence of parents at these medical examinations provides an excellent opportunity for educating them in regard to their child's health, as well as their own.

SETTING. The place where the examination is held should be conducive to good results. The physical and the emotional atmosphere should receive attention. There should be privacy for disrobing, so that interruptions will not occur, and quiet so that distractions will be reduced to a minimum. The examination room should also provide ample space for personnel, equipment, and supplies and should be attractive. Tension, hurry, and excitement should be reduced to a minimum. The entire setting should be friendly and informal.

RECORDS AVAILABLE. Essential health records should be brought up to date and be available at the time of the examination. These would include students' health cards, vision and hearing records, height-weight statistics, accident reports, and any other information that will help the physician to better interpret the results of the examination.

SCOPE. The periodic medical examination will include inspection or examination of such items as the following:

Eyes and lids	Nose
Throat and mouth	Teeth and gums
Heart: before and after exercise	Lymph node and thyroid gland
Nutrition	Lungs
Posture	Scalp and skin
Feet	Bones and joints
Speech	Nervous system
Behavior attitudes	Inguinal and umbilical region for hernia in males
Ears: canal and drums	

TIME. The examination that is administered by the school physician should be of sufficient length to detect any health defects and also make the experience educational in nature. The minimum average time per student should be 15 minutes or four per hour.

Examination of athletes. Administrative guides for athletic examinations are as follows:

1. Medical examinations should be administered to all engaged in athletics previous to actual participation and as they are needed during the time the sport is in progress. This refers to all forms of strenuous athletics, whether inter-

---

H-6 3M 9-36

LONG BEACH CITY SCHOOLS
HEALTH SERVICE DEPARTMENT
ATHLETIC PHYSICAL EXAMINATION REPORT

Name_____ School_____ Class_____

Age_____
Type of Athletic Activity—F. B., Basket Ball, Track, B. B., Class A. B. C.
Height_____Weight_____Standard_____Chest Circum.
In_____ Ex_____

Standing. Posture_____ Musculature_____ Nutrition_____
Skin_____ Superficial Glands_____
Hands_____ Arms_____ Abdomen_____
Hernia_____ Genitalia_____ Leg_____
Feet_____

Sitting: Hair_____Teeth_____Eyes, Reflexes_____
R._____ R._____
Vision— Corrected—
L._____ L._____
R._____
Hearing—_____ Nose_____ Gums_____
L._____
Tongue_____Tonsils_____Pharynx_____
Ears_____Chest_____Heart_____
Pulse, sitting_____ After exercise_____
2 min. later_____ Temp._____ Lungs_____
Blood Pressure Systolic_____ Diastolic_____
Knee Reflexes_____
Urine Analysis: Sp. Grav._____ Alb._____ Sugar_____
Summary
Advice Date_____

Athletic physical examination report. (Long Beach, Calif., Public Schools.)

scholastic, intramural, or part of the class program.

2. There should be adequate provision for medical service at all athletic contests.

3. A physician's recommendation should accompany any athlete returning to competition after a period of illness.

4. Examinations for participation in athletics should preferably be conducted by the family physician. In instances where this is not feasible, the school physician should perform this service.

Psychologic examinations. With the increased emphasis on mental health, various psychologic examinations are being used more extensively. These examinations, however, represent only a very small part of the mental health services that should be available. Mental health programs are concerned with helping students to adjust satisfactorily to the school or college environment, detecting individual behavior problems, aiding the teacher, parent, and others to better understand human behavior, and helping in every way possible to appraise personality and to discover mental handicaps, emotional difficulties, and maladjustments.

Psychologic examinations and tests that appraise such factors as students' abilities, attitudes, personalities, intelligence, and social adjustment offer techniques for obtaining much information. The administration and interpretation of the findings of such techniques should be handled by qualified individuals.

Dental examinations and inspections. Following are administrative guides governing school dental services.

EMPHASIS. The emphasis in school dental services should be on health education. Children and parents should develop proper attitudes toward dental caries and oral hygiene. Periodically, they should consult their family dentist for the necessary examination, care, and advice.

PERSONNEL. The personnel in the school particularly concerned with dental health include the teacher, nurse, physician, and dental hygienist. The staff will depend upon the com-

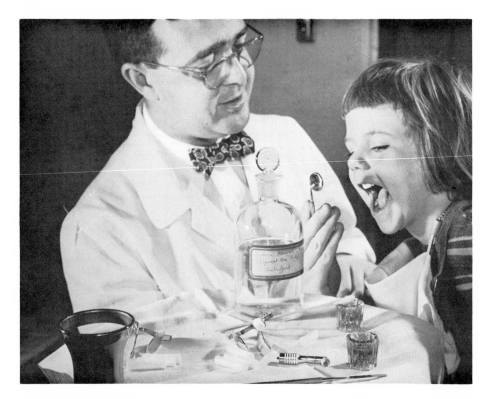

Dental inspection. (Indiana State Department of Health.)

munity philosophy concerning dental care. If the emphasis is upon education, it will be different than if it is on treatment. When a dental hygienist is a member of the school staff, he or she often has a variety of duties, including acting as a resource person for classroom teachers regarding dental health, making topical applications of sodium fluoride, cleaning children's teeth, and administering limited dental inspections.

NATURE. A difference of opinion exists on whether or not schools should provide dental examinations for pupils. Those in favor of such a practice point to its value as a motivating device to encourage parents and children to visit the dentist. Furthermore, they say it helps children in the low-income classes and focuses attention on the dental needs of children. Those not in favor of such a practice argue that as a result of school examinations children and parents visit their dentist less often and in some cases even substitute this examination for regular dental care. They further point out that it is the responsibility of everyone to make provisions for his or her own dental care and that the school is not the agency responsible for providing such a service. The question of the school's responsibility should be decided in each local community through conferences with dentists, educators, parents, and others interested in the problem. It can then be resolved in a manner that will best meet the needs of the children.

SCOPE. The scope of the school dental program usually concerns itself with the dental inspections and prophylaxis or cleaning. There are a few schools, however, that treat emergency cases and provide other dental care for children of parents who cannot afford such services. Dental inspection may be used to determine dental needs, to help communities meet the needs, and for purposes of evaluating the dental health program.

DENTAL PROBLEMS. The problems concerned with dental health are dental caries, or decayed teeth; malocclusion, a condition in which the teeth do not uniformly fit together when the jaws are closed; and periodontal diseases in which the tissues surrounding the teeth become infected, such as gingivitis (inflammation of the gums) or Vincent's infection (trench mouth). Although

dental caries is the most common problem, the others should receive due consideration.

Dental caries can best be prevented and controlled through good dental hygiene that includes frequent brushing, especially after eating; reducing sugar intake; topical fluoride applications; and fluoridation of water supplies, which experiments have shown reduces dental caries from 40% to 65%.

EDUCATIONAL IMPLICATIONS. The educational implications of dental health services are far reaching. Pupils and parents can be motivated to practice good oral hygiene and to visit their dentist regularly. The proper attitudes can be developed, resulting in good dental habits.

Screening for vision and hearing defects

Vision. Screening for vision requires a consideration of many factors.

VISION HEALTH SERVICES. The vision health services program in the school is concerned with the examinations given by physicians and appraisal of visual acuity. The appraisal of visual acuity is accomplished through continuous observations by the teacher and screening examinations. Both are necessary for the continual and satisfactory appraisal of the vision of school children.

FREQUENCY OF SCREENING TESTS. Tests of visual acuity should be given annually. The optimal time for such screening is immediately after the opening of school in the fall. They can be given to children in the early grades, as soon as they are old enough to cooperate satisfactorily. If possible, there should be a complete eye examination before the child enters school. A screening test for color acuity should be given during the early school years so that guidance can be given in regard to vocational opportunities.

ADMINISTRATION OF SCREENING TESTS. The teacher, after proper instruction and training, is qualified to administer various screening devices for vision. These devices, however, are only for purposes of detecting those individuals who need special care in respect to their vision. Their use is not a diagnostic technique.

SELECTION OF SCREENING DEVICES. The particular device that is utilized for checking visual acuity, together with the plans for appraisal, should be selected and arranged through conferences of school administrators, teachers, nurses, physicians, ophthalmologists, and optometrists.

It has been found that with young children, the Snellen E chart seems effective. For older children, the Snellen and Massachusetts Vision Tests have received wide recommendation. These devices should be administered according to prescribed instructions and pupils should be properly prepared for the examinations.

If needed, there are techniques for determining color acuity, such as the Holmgren test, and for determining muscle balance, such as the "cover test."

REFERRALS. The results of the screening examinations should be recorded and studied. In the light of these results and the teacher's observations, children with difficulties should be referred to the proper place for an eye examination. According to the Joint Committee of the National Education Association and the American Medical Association, "parents should be urged to secure eye examinations for children who are in the following categories: (1) those who consistently exhibit symptoms of visual disturbance, regardless of the results of the Snellen test, (2) older children (eight years and older) who have a visual acuity of 20/30 or less in either eye, with or without symptoms, and (3) younger children (seven years of age or less) who have a visual acuity of 20/40 or less in either eye, with or without symptoms."*

TEACHER'S OBSERVATIONS. The teacher as well as the parent should be alert to visual difficulties and problems among children. By being aware of certain actions and manifestations of the child from day to day under varying situations, it is possible to detect many eye difficulties that should be referred for examination. Many of these eye difficulties might go unnoticed unless the alert teacher or parent is aware of certain characteristics that indicate vision problems.

The Joint Committee has listed certain manifestations of visual difficulty in children before they begin to read and after reading activities have begun:

Before the child begins to read:
   Attempts to brush away blur
   Blinking more than usual
   Frequent rubbing of the eyes
   Squinting when looking at distant objects
   Frequent or continuous frowning
   Stumbling over small objects
   Undue sensitivity to light
   Red, encrusted, or swollen eyelids
   Recurring styes
   Inflamed or watery eyes
   Crossed eyes, "wall" eye, or "wandering" eye (regardless of degree)
After reading activities have begun:
   Holding a book too far away from or too close to the face when reading
   Inattention during reading periods, chalkboard, chart or map work
   Difficulty in reading or in other work requiring close use of the eyes
   Inability, or lack of desire, to participate in games requiring distance vision
   Poor alignment in written work
   Tilting head to one side or thrusting head forward when looking at near or distant objects
   Irritability when doing close work
   Shutting or covering one eye when reading*

Hearing. Following are administrative guides for conduct of health services in regard to hearing.

SCOPE. The main responsibility of the schools in respect to auditory health services is to detect those pupils with hearing difficulties as early as possible. This can be accomplished through such means as teacher observations and screening tests. A counseling and followthrough program that aims at remedying the defect should also be a part of the total plan.

FREQUENCY. Continuous observations should be a part of the school routine. Annual screening tests during the elementary years and one every 2 years at the secondary level are recommended. There should be a minimum of three tests during the first 8 years of school. It is also recommended that a preschool test of auditory acuity should be given wherever possible.

TECHNIQUE. The pure-tone audiometer is recommended as one of the most effective techniques for pupils of all school ages. This is a reliable instrument and allows for checking of either or both ears.

---

*Joint Committee of American Medical Association and National Education Association, op. cit., pp. 81-82.

*Joint Committee of American Medical Association and National Education Association, op. cit., p. 76.

REFERRALS. Students with a hearing loss in one or both ears should be rechecked to determine the accuracy of screening. If results are consistent, parents should be informed and encouraged to follow through with more complete examination.

Teachers who observe mouth breathing, ear discharge, or other abnormalities or characteristics that might arouse suspicion of hearing loss should refer the case to the proper authorities.

TEACHER'S OBSERVATIONS. The teacher can play an important part in continually observing the child for indications of hearing loss. He or she is also a key person in administering screening techniques. He or she should be watchful for such mannerisms as speech difficulties, requests for repetition of questions, turning of head to better hear what is said, and inattention, together with such noticeable characteristics as discharging ears, earaches, and other departures from the normal makeup of the child. Through such observations the teacher will detect individuals who need to be referred for more careful study and examination. All teachers should be alert for such manifestations.

PERSONNEL. Teachers, nurses, or technicians may be utilized in administering the various screening devices. All should be well trained in the use and purpose of such instruments. They should recognize that these are screening instruments and not diagnostic devices. There should be a careful check to determine that the instruments are in good working order and yield accurate results.

Teachers' observations. Teachers' observations are of great importance in detecting the health needs of school children. Furthermore, they increase in importance in the absence of nurses and doctors. Although this subject has been discussed previously, it is of such great importance that it is considered again here in more detail. Teachers, through observations of the appearance and behavior of pupils from day to day, become very well acquainted with each individual child. Any deviations from normal in appearance and in action will be detected very quickly by the alert teacher. For many of the health needs this provides the only means of discovering problems. Very often they would not be detected through medical examinations

and other health services. Therefore, the teacher's role in health services, through his or her continual association and observation of children, is a major one.

Such observations, after careful examination by nurses and physicians, may disclose various deficiencies. They may show that some children are maladjusted socially and emotionally, are undernourished, are in the early stages of a communicable or other disease, have some neurologic difficulties or other physical defects, or have developed poor health habits. Along with referral to nurses and physicians, the parents should also be informed of such discoveries. It should be reemphasized that in no case does the teacher diagnose. Instead, he or she refers the matter to the nurse, physician, and parent for further action.

There are many physical, social, and behavioral conditions that the teacher should be alert to in the classroom and the gymnasium. Some of these conditions are noted in the following paragraphs.

General physical condition. The teacher should take notice of such conditions as malnutrition, distended abdomen, excessive obesity or underweight, paleness, drawn look, tiredness or apathy, and rapid loss or gain of weight.

Eyes. Any of the following eye conditions should be noted and referred to proper medical supervision: tearing, styes, crusted eyelids, inflammation, squinting, protusion, excessive blinking or rubbing, squinting, and twitching eyelids.

Ears. Notice and medical referral should take place if any of the following conditions exist: inattention, difficulty hearing teacher or other students, earache or discharge from ear, excessive noisiness, or ear picking.

Nose and throat. Any of the following conditions require medical attention: mouth breathing, persistent coughing, sore throat, recurrent cold, nose bleeds, and nasal speech pattern.

Teeth and mouth. Dental supervision may be needed in the following conditions: visible or painful cavities, gum inflammation, bleeding gums, lack of cleanliness, mouth odor, tooth irregularities, and habits such as thumb sucking or nail biting.

Skin and scalp. Special attention should be

paid to any of the following conditions: hair infestation, skin rashes, excessive dandruff or other scalp condition, and general cleanliness.

Heart and glands. Any swelling of neck glands or thyroid should be referred to medical treatment. Indications of possible heart defects include excessive tiredness or listlessness, blue lip coloring, pallor, and breathlessness.

Behavioral problems. Any of the following conditions should be referred to school or private counseling services: withdrawal, overaggressive behavior, inability to adapt to group situations, rapid change of moods, uncontrollable behavior patterns, lack of self-confidence, chronic lying, stealing, constant antagonism, or problems of a sexual nature.

HS-29
4-60-20M

COLUMBUS PUBLIC SCHOOLS

Elementary Immunization Record Card (K-6)

Name.. School........................... Teacher..............

Room..............

This section pertains to pupils in **ALL GRADES.**

SMALLPOX VACCINATION
☐ Requirement met by a written statement of parent or physician, or by a scar

This section pertains to pupils in **ALL GRADES.**

POLIOMYELITIS — 3 injections
☐ School records show immunization completed
☐ Completed by written statement of parent or physician
☐ Received 1st injection.............. Date
☐ Received 2nd injection (1-month interval)........ Date
☐ Received 3rd injection (7-month interval)....... Date

This section pertains to all pupils in **GRADES K-2.**
DIPHTHERIA, WHOOPING COUGH, TETANUS — 3 injections + 1 Booster
☐ School records show immunization completed
☐ Completed by written statement of parent or physician
☐ Received 1st injection.............. Date
☐ Received 2nd injection (1-month interval)....... Date
☐ Received 3rd injection (1-month interval)....... Date
☐ Received booster injection (1-year interval)....... Date

This section pertains only to pupils in **GRADES 3-6** who did not receive injections for diphtheria and tetanus in grades K-2.
DIPHTHERIA, TETANUS — 2 injections + 1 Booster
☐ Completed by written statement of parent or physician
☐ Received 1st injection.............. Date
☐ Received 2nd injection (1-month interval)....... Date
☐ Received booster injection (1-year interval)....... Date

☐ **Parental objection (written)**

COLUMBUS PUBLIC SCHOOLS

Secondary Immunization Record Card (7-12)

Name.. School........................... Teacher..............

Room..............

All **THREE** sections of this card pertain to **ALL PUPILS.**

(1) SMALLPOX VACCINATION
☐ Requirement met by a written statement of parent or physician, or by a scar

(2) POLIOMYELITIS — 3 injections
☐ School records show immunization completed
☐ Completed by written statement of parent or physician
☐ Received 1st injection.............. Date
☐ Received 2nd injection (1-month interval)....... Date
☐ Received 3rd injection (7-month interval)....... Date

(3) TETANUS — 2 injections plus 1 Booster
☐ School records show immunization completed
☐ Completed by written statement of parent or physician
☐ Received 1st injection.............. Date
☐ Received 2nd injection (1-month interval)....... Date
☐ Received booster injection (1-year interval)....... Date

☐ **Parental objection (written)**

Health records. Following are some administrative guides in connection with health records:

1. As part of the overall school or college record, there should be a health record that contains a complete appraisal of the student's health. This should include such items as health history, vision and hearing data, teacher's observations, results of various medical, psychologic, dental, and other examinations given, reports of all conferences held with student, health defects that have been corrected, and any other information that has a bearing on the health of the student.

2. The health record should follow the student wherever he or she goes—when he or she moves from one community to another or when he or she is transferred from one school to another.

3. The records should be cumulative in nature, pointing out the complete health history of the student, together with a continuous appraisal of his or her health.

4. The health record should be made available to school or college medical and other personnel who are concerned with and who work toward the maintenance and improvement of a student's health. Professional ethics should govern the handling of such information.

5. The health record, if kept up to date and accurate, will prove a useful and effective device in furthering the health of all students.

Health histories

1. The history of the student's health should be in recorded form as an aid to teachers, nurses, physicians, and others in order to better understand the total picture of the student's health.

2. This record should be kept on a prepared form and should contain a complete history of communicable diseases, operations, accidents, immunizations, dental history, emotional maladjustments, physical abnormalities, nutritional problems, athletic injuries, menstruation, and any other factors that would be of help in better interpreting the total health picture.

3. The health history should be brought up to date before the medical examination is given so that the examining physician may use it as an aid.

Height-weight records. Following are administrative guides in connection with height-weight records:

1. The teacher, or students under supervision, should measure and record the height and weight of pupils at least three times a year. It is recommended that this be done at the beginning, middle, and toward the end of the year.

2. Height-weight records should not be utilized as a device to diagnose such elements as nutritional status. Instead, they should be used as indications that some health problems may exist if, for example, a child's weight does not increase during any 3-month period. They are best utilized not when compared against the height and weight of other children but when used as a comparison and history of a child's own growth from time to time.

3. Height-weight records provide an interesting and worthwhile phase of health education since students are interested in observing their growth and become curious about some of the reasons that encourage or deter growth.

*Accident records.** Accident records, as a means of health appraisal, provide information as to reasons for physical abnormalities and emotional maladjustment that may occur in children. They should be carefully kept and contain complete information.

Health counseling

In the light of the findings gathered through appraisal techniques, health matters are discussed with students and parents. Such problems as the need for medical and dental treatment, better health practices, diagnostic examinations, special services, and analysis of behavior problems are discussed. Through such counseling procedures a better understanding of the health of children and youth is achieved.

Health counseling is an important phase of the total health services program. As health needs and problems are revealed through medical examinations and other techniques, it is essential that defects be corrected, advice given, and a planned procedure established to provide for these needs and eliminate the problems.

---

*For further discussion of accident records see Chapter 18 on Legal Liability and Insurance Management.

Health counseling by qualified persons can help in achieving these goals.

Purposes. One general objective of health counseling is to provide students and parents with a better understanding of their health needs and the procedures that should be followed in order to satisfy these needs. Also, health counseling serves as a device for health education. Through conferences and discussion regarding health problems it is possible to develop sound health attitudes. Facts are presented that indicate the need for following acceptable health practices. The parent and student are motivated to alter their behavior in accordance with acceptable health standards. In addition, health counseling can help to develop a feeling of responsibility in pupils and parents for the correction of health defects and for promoting school and community health programs.

The objectives of health counseling have been well stated by the Joint Committee on Health Problems in Education of the National Education Association and the American Medical Association:

1. To give students as much information about their health status, as revealed by appraisal, as they can use to good advantage.
2. To interpret to parents the significance of health conditions and to encourage them to obtain needed care for their children.
3. To motivate students and their parents so that they will want and accept needed treatment and to accept desirable modifications of their school programs.
4. To promote each student's acceptance of responsibility for his own health, in keeping with his stage of maturity.
5. To encourage students and their parents to utilize available resources for medical and dental care to best possible advantage.
6. To encourage, if necessary, the establishment or enlargement of treatment facilities for students from needy families.
7. To contribute to the health education of students and parents.
8. To obtain for exceptional students educational programs adapted to their individual needs and abilities.*

In utilizing counseling as part of the health services program, it should be clearly recog-

*Reprinted with permission of the Joint Committee on Health Problems in Education of National Education Association, and American Medical Association, School health services, Chicago, 1964, National Education Association and American Medical Association, pp. 111-112.

nized that it has limitations. Counselors cannot always change individuals. This has been true, for example, of some handicapped individuals who may be subjected to pity or ridicule. Counselors can only help individuals to understand themselves, realize their potentialities, and live out their natural lives in a happy and productive manner. In some individuals, however, the social and physical environments have left their stamp so indelibly that counseling can do only a limited amount of good.

The counselor. The classroom teacher, school principal, physician, nurse, psychologist, physical education teacher, social worker, recreation leader, guidance person, and others have potentialities as counselors in the field of health. All have relationships with students that place them in a position to offer helpful advice and guidance. Whether or not they carry out such responsibilities effectively will depend on certain basic requirements.

Basic requirements for the counselors are concerned with their interest in people, personality, and competency in counseling skills.

To be effective, a counselor must be interested in people from the standpoint of service. The desire to help others live a happy and successful life and to help eliminate those problems that handicap the achievement of such goals must predominate in the counselor's mind.

A second basic requirement is the counselor's personality. Counseling procedure involves divulging personal problems and other matters that are brought out only when there is good rapport between the counselor and student or parent. Personality is a key to the establishment of a warm and cooperative counselor-client rapport. The counselor's personality must reflect such essentials as friendliness, interest in others' problems, and the desire to help. He or she must be a good listener and respect the views of others. A good counselor does not talk down to the pupil but confers with the student in an atmosphere of mutual understanding and respect.

A third requirement is competency in counseling skills. As in all specialized services, there are certain competencies that are essential to doing a good job. Studies have shown that the person who has developed competency in counseling gets more effective results and does a better job than the unskilled individual. Skills are necessary in establishing rapport with clients, understanding the implications of behavior patterns, communicating with students, analyzing pupil problems, conducting group discussions, administering conference procedures, and preparing records.

Conference method. The conference method of counseling that brings about a face-to-face relationship between the counselor, the pupil, and the parent is the best method for achieving desirable results. The use of written notices and standard forms is not recommended because of the possibility of misinterpretation and the lack of a clear understanding of the problems involved.

The success of the conference method will depend on the skill and the degree to which the counselor has planned for the conference. It is essential that the counselor have all the necessary records at hand, together with a complete understanding of the community, home, and problems surrounding the pupil in question.

The counselor must establish the proper relationship among the individuals who are present. A friendly and understanding atmosphere is necessary for the achievement of the desired results. The discussion of health matters must be carried on effectively and in a sound manner so that the pupil and parent will recognize the problems that exist and endorse the action that must be taken. No school person engaged in health counseling should attempt to diagnose diseases or select a physician or dentist for a pupil.

When the conference comes to an end there should be a common understanding among the counselor, pupil, and parent as to the next steps to be taken in the elimination of the health problems.

Correction of remediable defects

Two phases of school health services have been discussed. The student's health must first be appraised. Second, there must be a counseling procedure whereby the student and the parents are informed of health needs and problems so that the necessary action can be taken. After health appraisal and health counseling have been accomplished, the job is not completed. Next there must be a followthrough to see that remediable defects are corrected.

Students have many health defects that can be corrected. Dental caries is an example. It has been estimated that about 50% of 2-year-old children have one or more teeth that are carious. When they start school the number has risen to three and the number increases as the child progresses in school. In regard to vision defects it has been pointed out that eye problems increase from about 15% at 6 years of age to about 32% at 14 years of age.[*] Laxity in the correction of remediable defects seems to be especially prevalent in respect to teeth and eyes. There are also many other defects that can be corrected in the areas of malnutrition, hearing, speech, postural defects, diseased tonsils and adenoids, and emotional disorders.

The school has the responsibility for not only detecting such defects, whenever possible, but also putting forth every effort to see that they are corrected. The school's responsibility is to help every child attain optimal health; to encourage the removal of physical handicaps, defects, or anomalies that might constitute an obstacle to growth through correction or other helpful adjustment; and to guide parents, school staff, children, and others involved to a greater understanding of the factors related to better total health.

Community philosophy. The philosophy in respect to the methods that will be used to correct remediable defects will depend upon the community and the public at large. Although it is generally believed that the school should be concerned with educating parents and the public about the importance of correcting such defects, rather than with becoming a treatment agency, this belief and practice do not exist in all communities. Basically, the schools should not treat. They are not equipped with the personnel, facilities and other necessities for such a purpose. However, it is a community prerogative to decide such an issue. As a result, in some communities the school provides for the correction of dental, nutritional, postural, and other defects. In other communities this is considered a parental responsibility, and the school takes over only when indigent parents cannot afford such services. In many communities the school

---

[*]Joint Committee of American Medical Association and National Education Association, op. cit., p. 72.

does not treat in any way. The community must decide which method is most effective for the correction of defects.

Getting results. To obtain the best results in the correction of remediable defects, there must be planning, conferences, and accurate record keeping.

The teacher, nurse, health counselor, principal, and school physician should play active roles in planning such a program. A written plan should be developed and distributed so that all will be acquainted with the procedure that is to be followed. The responsibility for record keeping, home visitation, periodic checkups to see if defects have been corrected, and all other essential phases of the plan should be clearly designated. Good results will not be obtained if planning is a "hit-and-miss" affair. It will be effective only if it is done in advance of the detection of defects. If necessary, it should also be reviewed and amended periodically.

A second requisite for getting results is home and school conferences. As previously pointed out, written notices are cold and formal and do not achieve the desired results, as do personal conferences. If possible, the parents should come to the school for such purposes. However, where parents are reluctant to come to school, there should be visits to the home, preferably by the nurse. This also affords an opportunity to observe home conditions that affect the health of the child. At these conferences or visitations every attempt should be made to interest the pupil and the parent in the correction of the defects.

Two of the main reasons why health defects are not corrected are lack of money to provide the necessary service and indifference on the part of both pupil and parent. Conferences should aim at eliminating the indifference and attempting to provide the ways and means when financial problems exist. In most communities there are charitable organizations, civic groups, or others who will be happy to defray such expenses.

A third requirement for getting good results is accurate record keeping. As a part of health appraisal the defects should be properly recorded. It is essential to keep a record of all conferences and home visitations. Progress that has been made should be noted. Accurate and complete records will make it possible to know the current status of each pupil.

Community resources. Community resources should be tapped for aid in the correction of remediable defects. Public clinics, welfare agencies, and voluntary organizations should be utilized to give aid to indigent families where financial status prevents such treatment. A list of the hospitals, specialists, and clinics for various types of treatment could be provided when parents want additional information. In most cases it is better to suggest the names of several specialists rather than just one.

The school should work cooperatively with the various community agencies interested in this work. In some cases, time during the school day might be provided for students who must have treatment. Literature and other information prepared by various community agencies might be distributed. Meetings between leaders in the school and community agencies might be held to plan a program. A community health council is an ideal place for discussing and formulating plans for the correction of remediable defects. By mobilizing and utilizing community resources, remediable defects will be corrected.

Care and education of exceptional students*

The term *exceptional* refers to those students who are handicapped mentally, physically, socially, or emotionally and also to those who are gifted intellectually or in other ways.

A democratic society rests on the premise that all individuals should have equal opportunities to develop the various talents that they possess. This means that all children and youth in the schools should be granted the right to have an education adapted to their particular physical, mental, social, and emotional endowments. Therefore, whether an individual is gifted, normal, or handicapped, he or she should have the right to pursue the educational program that is best adapted to his or her particular needs and that enables him or her to achieve potentialities as a human being.

In any discussion of the care and education of

---

*See also Chapter 8 on The Adapted Program.

the exceptional child, it is important to consider (1) identifying the exceptional student, (2) discovering the exceptional child, (3) adapting the educational program, and (4) discussing the personnel that should be concerned with the care and education of the exceptional student.

Who are the exceptional students? Exceptional children include those students with superior intellectual capacity, those with learning disabilities, the mentally retarded, those with handicaps derived from physical defects or disease, and those who are emotionally disturbed or socially maladjusted.

According to one source,* out of every 1,000 students about 59 will have some physical handicap that requires special attention. These 59 can be broken down as follows: partially seeing and blind, 2; hard of hearing and deaf, 15; speech defective, 15; crippled, 10; lowered vitality, 15; and epileptic, 2. In the same group of 1,000 students, about 40 will deviate markedly in respect to mental ability.

The prevalence of exceptional school children is evident in every community. These children should be identified and referred for special services, and the educational program should be adapted to their needs and abilities.

Discovering the exceptional student. It is very important that each school develop a planned procedure for determining those pupils who are exceptional. It is very simple to identify some cases, such as those that are crippled, defective in their speech, or socially maladjusted. However, in others, where cardiac defects or tuberculosis causes the handicap, it is not as easy.

The exceptional child may be identified through the various phases of health appraisal that are conducted as part of the health services program. Through a thorough medical examination, the cardiac-handicapped student, for example, will be identified; through a psychologic examination the mentally or emotionally maladjusted pupil will be singled out; and through screening procedures, those with vision and hearing handicaps will be known.

The health history that should be a part of

every student's health record is another source for information leading to the identification of exceptional characteristics. A health history that lists all the significant diseases, accidents, and other aspects of the health history of a child should also list any exceptional characteristics that exist.

Teachers' observations also play a very important part. Through continuous observations on the part of a teacher, deviations from normal behavior will be identified. The individual who is listless might require further examination, a child who displays exceptional talent might be a genius in the class, or a child who finds it difficult to keep up with other boys his age in physical education activities should have further attention. Many of the children who fall into the exceptional group will have to be identified by teachers who work with them every day if they are to be singled out for special help.

Conferences with parents, teacher conferences with the school nurse, certain classroom tests, and reports from family physicians will help to identify exceptional individuals.

All of these methods should be carefully considered as potential media for identifying the many exceptional children who are regularly attending the public schools.

Adapting the educational program to the exceptional student. Some administrative guides for adapting the educational program and caring for the exceptional child are suggested here:

1. The school, as a general rule, should not undertake the treatment of handicapped students. However, it should do everything within its power to see that the necessary medical care is provided those who need such service. Through its referral service the school can carry out this responsibility.

2. Exceptional pupils should be treated as individuals rather than dealt with as groups of children with similar characteristics. Consideration should be given to each student.

3. Whether or not the exceptional individual is part of the regular group in the school situation, a part of a separate group, or in a separate school will depend upon the individual. The decision should be based on the question of which situation will allow the greatest possibil-

---

*Joint Committee of American Medical Association and National Education Association, op. cit., p. 129.

ity for improvement of the child's condition and for his or her total growth and development.

4. Special classes will aid certain individuals such as students who are hard of hearing, have speech and visual defects, and are severely crippled, homebound, or mentally retarded.

5. There is a need for an adequate supervisory program in connection with special classes for exceptional children. Good supervision will ensure periodic examinations to determine the status of the individual in respect to his or her exception, make sure that the program is as much like a regular school program as possible, and see that the child is returned to the regular class with normal children as soon as possible.

6. There are many different courses of action

for the education and care of exceptional students. A few methods for making provisions for the various classifications are listed. This listing, however, is in no way complete, and special resources should be consulted for a more complete description of the school's responsibility.

The *deaf*, when so classified by a competent specialist, are those that have a hearing loss of 70 decibels or more. Generally, they should be placed in special schools.

The education and care of the *hard of hearing* will vary with hearing loss (slight—loss of 20 to 30 decibels; mild to moderate—loss of 30 to 40 decibels; moderate to severe—loss of 40 to 70 decibels; and severe—loss of more than 70 decibels). Provisions can be made, such as

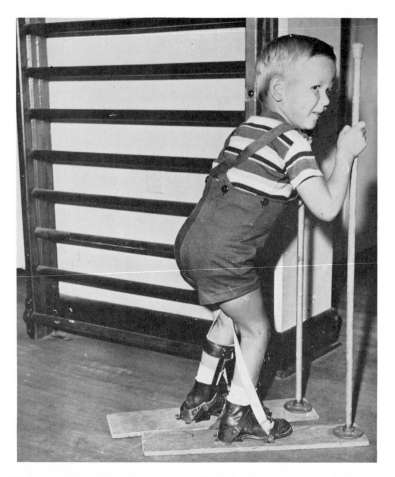

The school should do everything within its power to help obtain the necessary medical care for the orthopedically handicapped child. (United States Office of Education, Department of Health, Education and Welfare.)

special arrangements for seating and instruction, hearing aids, speech and lipreading, special classes, and special schools.

The *blind* (20/200 in better eye with glasses) may be provided for either by a special school or by special classes where braille is used.

The *partially sighted* (between 20/70 and 20/200 with glasses) can be provided for by proper fitting of correct glasses, sight-saving classes, provision within regular classroom, proper seating, advantageous scheduling of classes, and special materials, such as typewriters.

The *orthopedically handicapped* child should be cared for in regular classes whenever it is possible. Special provisions for children handicapped in this group include: "(1) transportation in school buses with an attendant, (2) physical and occupational therapy, (3) speech therapy, if needed, and (4) general health supervision by the teacher under the general direction of the school medical adviser and nurse, if such are available."*

The speech defective student's first need is a complete examination with medical and surgical care, if necessary, to remove the cause of the speech defect. Speech defects such as stuttering, stammering, and phonetic difficulties can be aided through work with a speech therapist, especially in the case of young children. Special classes are usually not needed; the student can attend regular classes and get the necessary treatment at a speech clinic or other place.

Malnourished and *undervitalized* children will usually be cared for on both an individual and a community basis. Health education aimed at raising the nutritional status of the home, a careful perusal of health histories to identify the causes, adjustment of the school program, and in some cases provision for special rest rooms will contribute to the solution of the defects.

The *mentally retarded* child (50 to 70 intelligence quotient, or I.Q.) should have a program that stresses, according to his or her individual abilities, proper health, safety, and social habits; information and skills essential to constructive community living, such as care of children,

proper maintenance of the home, and the community health resources that are available; and skills for creative and leisure-time activities that will lead to cultural development.*

The *mentally gifted* child (I.Q. of approximately 140 or over) has been helped in at least four ways: (1) an accelerated program adapted according to his or her ability to achieve higher standards, (2) enrichment of the curriculum so that it is adapted more to the child's abilities, (3) attendance in special classes, and (4) addition of elective courses.†

Cardiac-handicapped children should be provided for after complete examination by competent medical personnel. A few will require special classes, others will require modified programs, and some will need instruction to help them understand and live within certain restrictions.

The *tubercular-handicapped* child, if he or she has a case of active tuberculosis, should not be in school. The school programs for children who have had the disease should be adapted to their needs. This should be done in consultation with the appropriate medical person. This may mean only part-time attendance at school, provision for rest periods, limited physical activity, and special transportation.

Emotionally atypical students should be provided for in relation to their maladjustments. Some will need the help of a qualified psychologist or psychiatrist. Others will be helped by the guidance counselor or teacher. In most cases the teacher can play a key role in providing an emotional atmosphere where the child reacts favorably to the group.

The *socially exceptional* should also be provided for in relation to the extent of their maladjustments. Children with the most severe cases will need confinement to institutions; the rest will need rehabilitation, care, or developmental opportunities to restore them to normalcy.

There are many other methods of making special provisions for handicapped students. These methods include:

Desks, chairs, lamps, and equipment should be specially constructed for the orthopedically disabled child.

---

*Joint Committee of American Medical Association and National Education Association, op. cit., p. 136.

*Ibid., p. 143.
†Ibid., p. 145.

Children with visual or hearing problems should be seated close to the front of the room.

Hearing aids should be provided according to medical advice.

Screening tests for learning disabilities should be provided.

Rest periods and comportable rest areas should be provided for cardiac and other chronic disease patients.

All classes should be scheduled on one floor if at all possible.

Permission should be granted for partial daily attendance and adapted classes in physical education.

Students should receive individualized attention whenever possible.

Bus service should be offered to coincide with the schedule of handicapped students.

Such provisions enable many handicapped pupils to attend regular classes.

The child with learning disabilities is discussed here separately because although this condition is not new, the rapidly growing movement by parents, schools, and state and federal governments is new. There are several dimensions of learning disability problems, and one definition is very difficult for all persons involved to agree upon. The official definition of learning disabilities was created by the United States Congress in the Specific Learning Disabilities Act of 1969. The definition is as follows:

Children with specific learning disabilities exhibit a disorder in one or more of the basic psychological processes involved in understanding or in using spoken or written language. These may be manifested in disorders of listening, thinking, talking, reading, writing, spelling, or arithmetic. They include conditions which have been referred to as perceptual handicaps, brain injury, minimal brain dysfunction, dyslexia, developmental aphasia, etc. They do not include learning problems which are due primarily to visual, hearing, or motor handicaps, to mental retardation, emotional disturbance or to environmental disadvantage.

There are varying estimates of the numbers of children with learning disabilities. A study conducted at Northwestern University screened 2,800 school-age children and found 7 to 8% as having learning disabilities.* Other studies have estimated that 1 to 3% of school population may be identified as having learning disabilities.

Early identification of these children is essential, and kindergarten teachers should be especially observant in recognizing symptoms.

The school doctor and nurse can also perform specific tests to indicate possible impairment. These tests include such factors as coordinating right-left, discriminating muscle tone, and speech and language articulation and comprehension.

Personnel. The teachers who work with exceptional children should be well trained for their duties. Whether or not the child is able to adjust satisfactorily to the group, improve, and be educated and cared for in a desirable manner will depend to a great degree upon the teacher.

Teachers should be well prepared for the particular grade or subject to which they are assigned. In addition, they should be trained to work with exceptional children with specific disabilities. The nature or type of disability will determine the training needed. The teacher should be emotionally stable and have the temperament suitable for working with abnormal children. The size of classes for exceptional children should be smaller than for regular classes. If progress is to be achieved, the individual approach must be applied as much as possible.

In addition to the teacher, there are other individuals in the school and community who can render contributions to this phase of the health service program. Where they are part of the school staff, the nurse, guidance director, school physician, psychologist, social worker, and director of special education should work closely with the teacher and school administrator in planning the program. Other individuals, such as ophthalmologists, psychiatrists, orthopedists, speech correctionists, otologists, directors of agencies dealing with the handicapped, and members of state departments of health and education, should be utilized for advice, planning, referrals, inservice education, and other contributions to this phase of the health service program.

Communicable disease control

Whenever students congregate there is the possibility of spreading disease. The school, as a place for children and youth to congregate, is unique in that the law requires attendance. Therefore, if it is compulsory to go to school, there should also be certain protective measures and precautions taken to ensure that everything

---

*Lerner, J. W.: Learning disabilities: a school health problem, The Journal of School Health **42:**320, 1972.

is done to guard the health of the child. This includes the necessary procedures for controlling communicable disease. Although students are not required to go to college, higher educational institutions also have the responsibility for communicable disease control.

The problem of communicable disease control can be discussed under two main headings, first, responsibility, and second, the various measures that should be applied in the school situation.

Responsibility. The legal responsibility for communicable disease control rests with state and local departments of health. This means that public health officials have control over school and college personnel in this matter. In most cases, however, this is a case of cooperation rather than compulsion. School and college officials should work closely with public health officials so that cases of communicable disease are reported and proper measures taken to prevent other children from contracting the disease.

The responsibility for communicable disease control falls upon many individuals. These include public health personnel, school and college administrative personnel, nurse, school physician, teacher, custodian, and the parent. The teacher, parent, and nurse must be continually vigilant to notice symptoms of various communicable diseases, isolate such individuals immediately, and refer these cases to the school, college, or family physician. There must be close cooperation among these three since all play key roles in the control of communicable diseases. If the parent plays his or her role effectively and the child is isolated immediately, the exposure of other individuals to disease will be considerably lessened. If the child is in school, the alert teacher and nurse will take the necessary precautions.

The superintendent, principal, university physician, and other administrative officers have the responsibility for establishing policy, working cooperatively with public health officials, providing encouragement and inservice training for teachers, and developing among parents and the public in general an understanding that will be most conducive to communicable disease control.

The custodian, through his or her control over the sanitation of the equipment and facilities, can perform his or her responsibilities so effectively that a healthful environment is always in evidence and thus the spread of disease is decreased.

The school or college physician should advise the teacher, nurse, administrative officers, and others who are closely related to the whole problem of communicable disease control as to the necessary measures that should be provided. Through specialized knowledge, he or she can contribute much toward the establishment of an effective and workable plan.

Control measures. There are many control measures that every school or college should follow to prevent the spread of disease. Some of the more important of these measures are discussed here.

*Healthful environment.** Some of the provisions for a healthful environment that are necessary for the control of communicable disease include sufficient space to avoid undue crowding, adequate toilet and washroom facilities, proper ventilation and heating, safe running water, properly installed drinking fountains, use of pasteurized milk, a system of exclusions and control of admissions for students who may have communicable disease, and policies toward student and teacher absences that do not require teachers to be in school when they may be ill and capable of spreading communicable disease germs.

Isolation of students. The student who is a "suspect" in regard to some communicable disease should immediately be isolated from the group. Isolating a student does not constitute diagnosis. The details and procedures followed in each school or college regarding isolation should be in writing and clearly understood by all concerned. The adopted plan should have the approval of the health service staff.

The teacher should be continually on the lookout for "suspects." Some indications of communicable disease that should be recognized by the teacher are the following:

Unusual pallor or flushed face
Unusual listlessness or quietness
Red or watery eyes
Eyes sensitive to light
Skin rash
Cough

---

*See also Chapter 14.

Need for frequent use of toilet
Nausea or vomiting
Running nose or sniffles
Excessive irritability
Jaundice*

After the teacher isolates the ''suspect'' from the group, the student should not be left alone. Furthermore, the nurse or school or college physician should be notified. In the event neither of these individuals is available, the teacher and school administrator must decide on exclusion. The best solution is to arrange for the student to return home or to be sent to the infirmary, where the services of a physician should be procured as soon as possible. Furthermore, the case should be reported to the local health authorities.

Readmitting students to school or college. After having a communicable disease a student should not be readmitted to school or college until it is certain that his or her return is in the best interests of the health of both the student concerned and also the other students with whom he or she will come in contact. There should be strict conformance to the law that governs communicable diseases. In addition, there should be approval for such readmission

---

*Joint Committee of American Medical Association and National Education Association, op. cit., p. 210.

indicated in writing by a qualified physician or the local health department. In minor cases a note from the parent or the decision of the nurse or other staff member may suffice.

Immunization. Every student should receive immunization against preventable diseases. Most of this should be done in the preschool years when danger from such diseases is prevalent. Every child should be immunized against tetanus, poliomyelitis, diphtheria, smallpox, and whooping cough. The school can play an important part in the health education of parents to see that children are immunized against these diseases before starting school. The children who come to school and have not received the benefit of such services need special attention. It is a public health and medical problem and should be dealt with through members of these professions. If the community decides that the school is the best place for immunization, the school should cooperate fully and keep complete records on initial immunizations and booster doses. Written permission should be secured from parents concerned.

Attendance. There should not be an overemphasis on perfect attendance for school children. This often results in children coming to school regardless of the condition of their health and the danger to others. Furthermore, state aid

---

SAN FRANCISCO DEPARTMENT OF PUBLIC HEALTH
IMMUNIZATION AND TEST CONSENT

Date_____

Name_____ Address_____ Phone No._____

School_____ Grade_____ Room_____ Phy. Ed. Period_____ P. E. Teacher_____ Birth-date_____

In looking over your child's health record, it is recommended that the following immunizations and/or tests be given. Please sign your name opposite the recommended procedure if you wish your child to have the benefit of the test or immunization.

If your child has had a positive Tuberculin Test in the past, it will probably remain positive and should not be repeated. If your child's test was ever positive, please indicate when or approximately when

Negative Tuberculin Tests may be repeated yearly.

F 1515 1-56

Immunizations and Tests	Recommended	Parent's Signature
Smallpox Vaccination		
Diphtheria ⎫ Pertussis ⎬ D.P.T. Tetanus ⎭		
Polio Vaccination		
Tuberculin Test		

PLEASE RETURN TO PUBLIC HEALTH NURSE

should be based on some method other than attendance.

Epidemics. The viewpoint on closing schools and colleges during epidemics has changed somewhat in recent years. Formerly, it was generally believed that schools should be closed. Today, it is felt that under many circumstances they should remain open. The deciding factor is whether or not the school provides regular inspections, observations, adequate staff, and facilities to screen out those who indicate signs of having the disease. If this service can be performed and if the closing of schools will result in many contacts on playgrounds and other places where children congregate, then, according to the latest thinking, the schools should remain open. This is particularly true in urban areas. Many times in rural areas, where children will not come in contact with each other if schools are closed, it may be advisable to have schools closed.

If an epidemic occurs during a vacation period it is often wise to postpone the opening of school, since such opening might result in increased contact with the disease.

Emergency care

Elementary and secondary schools are responsible for providing each student with the necessary protection and care. The school acts in loco parentis (in place of the parent), and it is assumed that the child will receive the same care and protection during the hours of school that he or she would receive at home. Children often become sick or injured during school hours. Therefore, the school must provide the necessary attention until this can be undertaken by the parents.

According to the Joint Committee on Health Problems, the school has four responsibilities in respect to emergency care procedures. These are ''(1) giving immediate care, (2) notifying

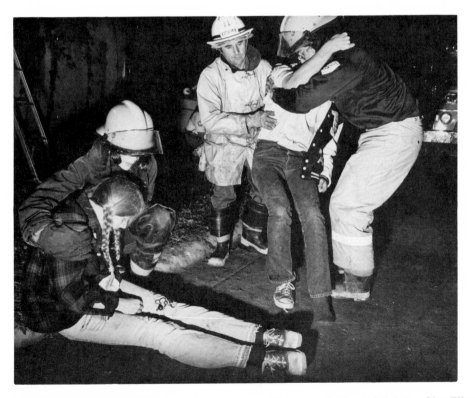

Schools and colleges have responsibility for emergency care. Students at College of DuPage, Glen Ellyn, Ill., participate in local emergency drill.

the pupil's parents, (3) arranging for the pupil to get home, and, (4) guiding parents, when necessary, to sources of treatment."*

Some administrative guides for emergency care are as follows:

1. Every school and college should have a written plan for emergency care. It should be carefully prepared by the school administration with the help of the school or college physician, parents, medical and dental professions, hospitals, nurse, teachers, and others interested and responsible in this area. The time to plan and decide on procedure is before an accident occurs. This should be one of the first administrative responsibilities that is accomplished.

The written plan should contain such essentials as first-aid instructions; procedures for getting medical help, transportation, and notifying parents; staff responsibilities, supplies, equipment, and facilities available; and any other information that will help clarify exactly what is to be done in time of emergency.

The plan should be reviewed periodically and revised so that it is continually up to date. It should be posted in conspicuous places and discussed periodically with school staff and community groups, whenever necessary.

2. As many staff members as possible should be trained in first-aid procedures. There is a need for special knowledge and training in respect to emergency care that might entail first aid for broken bones, use of artificial respiration, control of hemorrhage, and proper care of patients suffering from shock. The more staff members that are trained in these specific first-aid procedures, the better coverage there is for accidents that may occur at any time when school activities are in progress.

Some schools have the American Red Cross give inservice courses in first-aid procedures. Such inservice training will help to ensure that the staff is competent along this line.

When a nurse is on duty it would usually be expected that his or her responsibility includes seeing that proper first-aid procedures are carried out.

Professional preparation institutions should give due consideration to instruction in first-aid and emergency care procedures as part of the training of all teachers and school and college personnel.

3. A health room for first aid and emergency care should be available.* It should possess the necessary equipment and supplies; have good lighting; be clean, of adequate size, and always available for emergency cases.

In addition to furniture and routine equipment, the health room should also have available as a minimum the following:

Stethoscope	Tuning fork for hearing
Thermometer, clinical	tests
Sphygmomanometer	Mouth mirror
Electric ophthalmoscope	Probes, dental
Electric otoscope	Forceps
Reflex hammer	Syringes
Tape measure	Needles
Platform scale (not a spring	Eye droppers
model)	Graduated medicine
Illuminated eye test charts	glasses

The staff responsible for the health room should be fixed and such responsibility should include training and competency in first-aid procedures.

4. Proper emergency equipment and supplies, in addition to being located in the health room, should also be available in strategic school or college locations that are accident-prone because of activity courses and in places remote from the health room. Such locations might include gymnasium, laboratories, shops, school buses, annexes, and buildings housing school activities apart from the central unit.

5. School and college records should contain complete information on each student. This might include such information as his or her address; parent's name, address, and phone number; business address of parent and phone number; family physician, address, and phone number; family dentist, address, and phone number; parent instruction in case of emergency; choice of hospital; and any other pertinent information.

6. There should be a complete record of every accident, including first aid given and emergency care administered in the event of

---

*Joint Committee of American Medical Association and National Education Association, op. cit., pp. 222-223.

*See description in Chapter 15.

first aid chart for athletic injuries

FIRST AID, the immediate and temporary care offered to the stricken athlete until the services of a physician can be obtained, minimizes the aggravation of injury and enhances the earliest possible return of the athlete to peak performance. To this end, it is strongly recommended that:

ALL ATHLETIC PROGRAMS include prearranged procedures for obtaining emergency first aid, transportation, and medical care.

ALL COACHES AND TRAINERS be competent in first aid techniques and procedures.

ALL ATHLETES be properly immunized as medically recommended, especially against tetanus and polio.

Committee on the
Medical Aspects of Sports
AMERICAN MEDICAL ASSOCIATION

to protect the athlete at time of injury,
FOLLOW THESE FIRST STEPS FOR FIRST AID

STOP play immediately at first indication of possible injury or illness.

LOOK for obvious deformity or other deviation from the athlete's normal structure or motion.

LISTEN to the athlete's description of his complaint and how the injury occurred.

ACT, but move the athlete *only* after serious injury is ruled out.

BONES AND JOINTS

fracture Never move athlete if fracture of back, neck, or skull is suspected. If athlete *can* be moved, carefully splint any possible fracture. Obtain medical care at once.

dislocation Support joint. Apply ice bag or cold cloths to reduce swelling, and refer to physician at once.

bone bruise Apply ice bag or cold cloths and protect from further injury. If severe, refer to physician.

broken nose Apply cold cloths and refer to physician.

HEAT ILLNESSES

heat stroke Collapse—with dry warm skin—indicates sweating mechanism failure and rising body temperature.
THIS IS AN EMERGENCY; DELAY COULD BE FATAL. Immediately cool athlete by the most expedient means (immersion in cool water is best method). Obtain medical care at once.

heat exhaustion Weakness—with profuse sweating—indicates state of shock due to depletion of salt and water. Place in shade with head level or lower than body. Give sips of dilute salt water. Obtain medical care at once.

sunburn If severe, apply sterile gauze dressing and refer to physician.

IMPACT BLOWS

head If any period of dizziness, headache, incoordination or unconsciousness occurs, disallow any further activity and obtain medical care at once. Keep athlete lying down; if unconscious, give nothing by mouth.

teeth Save teeth, if completely removed from socket. If loosened, do not disturb; cover with sterile gauze and refer to dentist at once.

solar plexus Rest athlete on back and moisten face with cool water. Loosen clothing around waist and chest. Do nothing else except obtain medical care if needed.

testicle Rest athlete on back and apply ice bag or cold cloths. Obtain medical care if pain persists.

eye If vision is impaired, refer to physician at once. With soft tissue injury, apply ice bag or cold cloths to reduce swelling.

MUSCLES AND LIGAMENTS

bruise Apply ice bag or cold cloths and rest injured muscle. Protect from further aggravation. If severe, refer to physician.

cramp Have opposite muscles contracted forcefully, using firm hand pressure on cramped muscle. If during hot day, give sips of dilute salt water. If recurring, refer to physician.

strain and sprain Elevate injured part and apply ice bag or cold cloths. Apply pressure bandage to reduce swelling. Avoid weight bearing and obtain medical care.

OPEN WOUNDS

heavy bleeding Apply sterile pressure bandage using hand pressure if necessary. Refer to physician at once.

cut and abrasion Hold briefly under cold water. Then cleanse with mild soap and water. Apply sterile pad firmly until bleeding stops, then protect with more loosely applied sterile bandage. If extensive, refer to physician.

puncture wound Handle same as cuts; refer to physician.

nosebleed Keep athlete sitting or standing; cover nose with cold cloths. If bleeding is heavy, pinch nose and place *small* cotton pack in nostrils. If bleeding continues, refer to physician.

OTHER CONCERNS

blisters Keep clean with mild soap and water and protect from aggravation. If already broken, trim ragged edges with sterilized equipment. If extensive or infected, refer to physician.

foreign body in eye Do not rub. Gently touch particle with point of clean, moist cloth and wash with cold water. If unsuccessful or if pain persists, refer to physician.

lime burns Wash thoroughly with water. Apply sterile gauze dressing and refer to physician.

EMERGENCY PHONE NUMBERS

Physician		Phone:	
Physician		Phone:	
Hospital		Ambulance	
Police	Fire		Other

illness. Such information preserves for future reference the procedures followed in each case. This record is very important in the event questions arise in the future. Time results in forgetfulness, misinterpretation, misunderstanding, and inaccurate conclusions being drawn. Records can also be used to disclose hazards that should be eliminated and weak spots in procedures for emergency care that should be improved. Finally, such records aid in impressing upon students, staff, parents, and other individuals who are concerned the importance of good procedures for safe and healthful living.

7. The legal aspects of problems involved in regard to emergency care should be discussed and understood by the entire school or college staff. Such discussion will make for a better understanding of the laws of a particular state or locality and show the importance of avoiding negligence in duty.

8. Insurance plans for staff, athletes, and students should be made clear. They should be in writing and well publicized so that each individual will know the extent to which expenses, claims, and other items will be paid in event of accident, or the extent to which he or she can or should procure additional coverage.

9. Disasters in the form of fires, floods, tornadoes, and air raids can occur at any time. In order to provide proper emergency care under such circumstances, there must be advance planning. Schools and colleges should recognize their responsibility along this line. Adequate insurance coverage should be maintained. Supplies for emergency care should be on hand. Responsibilities should be fixed in key positions. Plans should be laid for taking children to safest place possible. Drills should be conducted. Close cooperation should exist between the schools and such organizations as Civil Defense or the Red Cross.

Environmental sanitation

Another health service responsibility of schools and colleges is that of ensuring a sanitary environment. Since many aspects of this topic are covered in Chapter 14, as well as earlier in this chapter, it will be discussed only briefly here. Some aspects of environmental sanitation that need particular attention are the

school's or college's responsibility for ensuring a safe water supply; sanitary sewage disposal; and sanitary cafeterias, kitchens, locker rooms, showers, and swimming pools.

If desirable environmental sanitation standards are adhered to, it will not only help to reduce the incidence of the spread of disease but also will be conducive to a more comfortable, pleasant environment that will contribute to optimal learning.

Health of school and college personnel

Educational organizations need to give attention to the health of school and college personnel in order to ensure efficiency of teachers, administrators, and other members of the staff; to provide examples for children and young people that are worth emulating; and to promote the most healthful and pleasant environment possible. Boards of education, boards of trustees, and other persons who are involved in making pertinent decisions, therefore, need to concern themselves with such matters as sick leave, health insurance, sabbatical leaves, retirement provisions, maternity leaves, medical examinations, exclusion from school or college of teachers with health conditions that have implications for students' health and well-being, and other matters that concern the health of all employees of the school district or college. The health of school and college personnel is as important a consideration as health of school and college students.

Questions and exercises

1. What are the component parts of a school or college health service program? What is the importance to the student of each part?
2. What is the relationship between health services and other phases of the school or college health program?
3. Discuss the most important factors involved in providing medical services to athletes. How can athletic injuries be prevented?
4. What should be the relationship between the public health department and the school or college health department in relation to school health services?
5. Discuss the responsibilities of athletic trainers. If your school employs athletic trainers, interview one to determine his or her background and functions.
6. Outline what you consider to be a sound health appraisal program for an elementary school.
7. Describe the nature and scope of the school medical

examination. Relate how it can be an educational experience for boys and girls.

8. Prepare a list of arguments to be presented to the board of education to justify the addition of a psychologist to the school staff.

9. What part do the teacher's observations play in a health services program? What are his or her responsibilities in the matter?

10. Identify pure-tone audiometer, whisper test, Massachusetts Vision Test, caries, Snellen E Chart, follow-through, exceptional child, and child with learning disabilities.

11. What are the essential health records that should be maintained to conduct a desirable health services program?

12. Prepare a mock health counseling conference with a child and his mother after a medical examination that has revealed several defects that need correction.

13. What recommendations could you make in order to ensure the greatest possible correction of remediable health defects?

14. Take one type of exceptional child, do considerable research on the type of educational program that is best suited to this particular individual, make recommendations to the class.

15. After careful study of all factors involved, outline a program for a particular community as to how the public health department and school health education division can most effectively work together for communicable disease control.

16. Prepare a written plan for emergency care of injuries for your school or college, which will then be submitted to the class for approval and then presented to the school health services division of your institution for comment.

Reading assignment in *Administrative Dimensions of Health and Physical Education Programs, Including Athletics:* Chapter 10, Selections 55 to 58.

Selected references

Committee on the Medical Aspects of Sports of the American Medical Association: The team physician, The Journal of School Health **37:**497, 1967.

Corliss, L. M.: Multiple handicapped children—their placement in the school education program, The Journal of School Health **37:**113, 1967.

Day, H. P.: University administration views the health service, American College Health Association Journal **15:**140, 1966.

Delforge, G., and Klein, R.: High school athletic trainers internship, Journal of Health, Physical Education, and Recreation **44:**42, 1973.

Forbes, O.: The role and functions of the school nurse as perceived by 115 public school teachers from three selected counties, The Journal of School Health **37:**101, 1967.

Hutton, L., and Silkin, J.: Needed: women athletic trainers, Journal of Health, Physical Education, and Recreation **43:**77, 1972.

Joint Committee on Health Problems in Education of National Education Association and American Medical Association: Health appraisal of school children, Washington, D. C., 1969, National Education Association.

Joint Committee on Health Problems in Education of National Education Association and American Medical Association: Health education, Washington, D. C., 1961, National Education Association.

Joint Committee on Health Problems in Education of National Education Association and American Medical Association: School health services, ed. 2, Washington, D. C., 1964, Nation Education Association.

Lerner, J. W.: Learning disabilities: a school health problem, The Journal of School Health **42:**320, 1972.

National Committee on School Health Policies: Suggested school health policies, ed. 3, Chicago, 1962, American Medical Association.

Neilson, E. A.: Health education and the school physician, The Journal of School Health **39:**377, 1969.

Oyeda, F.: The detection of learning disabilities in the early school age child, The Journal of School Health **42:**214, 1972.

Rolnick, M.: Health supervision of intercollegiate sports in junior and community colleges, JUCO Review **24:**20, 1972.

Ryan, A. J.: Prevention of sports injury: a problem solving approach, Journal of Health, Physical Education, and Recreation **42:**24, 1971.

Ryan, A. J.: Providing medical services for athletes, School Activities, November, 1967.

Schneeweiss, S. M., and Locke, A.: New horizons in school health services: the computer, The Journal of School Health **37:**349, 1967.

Schwank, W. C., and Miller, S. S.: New dimensions for the athletic training profession, Journal of Health, Physical Education, and Recreation, **42:**41, 1971.

Tower, B., and Fay, P.: Can contracted school health services work? The Journal of School Health **38:**339, 1968.

Wetzel, N. C.: New dimensions in the simultaneous screening and assessment of school children, Journal of Health, Physical Education, and Recreation **37:** January, 1966.

Wilson, H., and Albohn, M.: Women athletic trainers, Journal of Health, Physical Education, and Recreation **44:**57, 1973.

14

Providing
a healthful
environment
for students

A healthful school or college environment must take the individual into consideration. He or she must be given a safe, healthful, pleasant, and emotionally secure environment. The environment also includes the out-of-doors where everything possible should be done to control land, water, and air pollution. In addition, the total environment must also be healthy and pleasant for the teachers and other school staff members. The contentment of the staff is directly related to the students' well-being. This chapter will explore the physical and psychologic environment essential to good physical, mental, and social health.

THE PHYSICAL ENVIRONMENT

The general health features of the physical environment will be discussed here under the following headings: site, building, lighting, heating and ventilation, furniture, plant sanitation, and acoustics.

Site

There are many aspects to consider in the selection of a suitable site. These considerations will differ, depending on the community. Whether it is a rural or an urban community will have a bearing on the location of the site.

In an urban community it is desirable to have the school situated near transportation facilities, but at the same time located away from industrial concerns, railroads, noise, heavy traffic, fumes, and smoke. Consideration should be given to the trends in population movements and future development of the area in which the buildings are planned. Adequate space for play and recreation should be provided. Some standards recommend 5 acres of land for elementary schools, 10 to 12 acres for junior high schools, and 20 acres for senior high schools. The play area should consist of a minimum of 100 square feet for every child. The National Council on Schoolhouse Construction* has suggested that, although larger sites may be used, standards that provide a minimum of 5 acres plus an additional acre for each 100 pupils of projected enrollment for elementary schools and a minimum of 10 acres plus an additional acre for each 100 pupils of projected enrollment for junior and senior high schools should be followed. Thus an elementary school of 200 pupils would have a site of 7 acres, for example, and a high school of 500 pupils a site of 15 acres.

Attention should be given to the esthetic features of a site because of its effect on the physical and emotional well-being of students

---

*National Council of Schoolhouse Construction, East Lansing, Michigan.

and staff. The surroundings should be well landscaped, attractive, and free from disturbing noises or odors.

The American Association of School Administrators and the National Council on Schoolhouse Construction can supply detailed information on the selection of a site.

Building

Some trends in modern building construction have already been discussed and consideration of some of the special areas is still to come. The trend is toward one-story construction at the precollege educational level, where possible, with stress on planning from a functional rather than an ornamental point of view. The building should be constructed from the standpoint of use. As much natural lighting as possible should be utilized. The materials used should make the building attractive and safe. According to the National Safety Council, a high percentage of children's accidents occur in school buildings. Every precaution should be taken to protect against accidents from fire, slippery floors, and other dangers. The walls should be painted with light colors and treated acoustically. Doors should open outward. Space for clothing should be provided.

These are only a few of the considerations in planning a school building. It is important that an architect plan such facilities with special regard to the educational needs of those who utilize it. Educators should formulate a plan and use it in discussions with the architect.

Lighting *

Proper lighting is important to conserve vision, prevent fatigue, and improve morale. There should be proper lighting including both quality and quantity. In the past it had been recommended that natural light should come into the room from the left and that artificial light should be provided as needed. There is a trend now toward allowing natural light from more than one direction. Artificial light, moreover, should come from many sources rather than one in order to prevent too much concentration of light in one place. Switches for artificial light should be located in many parts of the room.

Light intensity in most classrooms, according to expert opinion, usually varies from 15 to 100 footcandles.† Most authorities suggest between 30 and 70 footcandles for reading and close work. In gymnasiums and swimming pools it is recommended that intensity range from 10 to 50 footcandles. Glare is undesirable and should be eliminated. Fluorescent lights should be properly installed and adjusted for

---

*A good source of information for acceptable standards on lighting is the Illuminating Engineering Society, New York, N. Y.

†A footcandle is the unit by which light is measured in intensity at a given point.

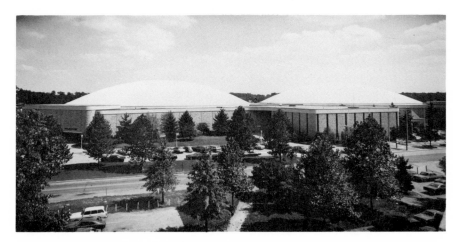

The University of Notre Dame's Athletic and Convocation Center provides a healthful environment for part of its athletic program. (Courtesy University of Notre Dame.)

best results. Strong contrasts of color such as light walls and dark floors should be avoided.

Windows, according to most experts, should extend as far up toward the ceiling as possible and should consume space equal to about one-fourth to one-fifth of the floor area.

Window shades aid in controlling light. They should be durable, of light color, and located in the middle of the window so that they may be adjusted either up or down.

Heating and ventilation*

Efficiency in the classroom, gymnasium, special activities rooms, and other places is determined to some extent by thermal comfort. Thermal comfort is determined in the main by heating and ventilation.

The purpose of heating and ventilation are many. Some of the more common are to remove excess heat, unpleasant odors, and, in some cases, gases, vapors, fumes, and dust from the room; to prevent rapid temperature fluctuations; to diffuse the heat within a room; and to supply heat to counteract loss from the human body through radiation and otherwise.

Heating standards vary according to the activities engaged in, the clothing worn by the participants, and section of the country. The following represents an approximate average of various suggested standards for temperatures:†

1. Classrooms, offices, and cafeterias—68° to 76° F. (30 inches above floor)
2. Kitchens, closed corridors, shops, and laboratories—65° to 68° F. (60 inches above floor)
3. Gymnasiums and activity rooms—55° to 65° F. (60 inches above floor)
4. Locker and shower rooms—70° to 78° F. (60 inches above floor)
5. Swimming pools—80° to 85° F. (60 inches above the deck)

In respect to ventilation, the range of recommendations is from 8 to 21 cubic feet of fresh air per minute per occupant. Adequate venti-

lating systems are especially needed in dressing, shower, and locker rooms, toilet rooms, gymnasiums, and swimming pools. The recommended humidity ranges from 35% to 60%. The type and amount of ventilation will vary with the specific needs of the particular area to be served.

Furniture

The furniture that students use most is desks and chairs. Seats and desks that are adjustable and movable are recommended by most educators. There are many different kinds of seats and desks that are available in both wood and metal. The desk should be of proper height and fit the pupil comfortably and properly. Desks should be arranged to provide the best light for the students.

Plant sanitation

Various items concerned with plant sanitation should not be overlooked. Sanitation facilities should be well provided and well maintained. The water supply should be safe and adequate. If any question exists, the local or state health department should be consulted. In regard to water supply, one authority suggests that at least 20 gallons per pupil per day is needed, for all purposes.

Drinking fountains of various heights should be recessed in corridor walls and should be of material that is easily cleaned. Approximately one drinking fountain should be provided for every 75 students. A stream of water should flow from the fountain in such a manner that it is not necessary for the mouth of the drinker to get too near the drain bowl.

Water closets, urinals, lavatories, and washroom equipment such as soap dispensers, toilet paper holders, waste containers, mirrors, bookshelves, and hand-drying facilities should be provided as needed.

Waste disposal should be adequately cared for. There should be provision for cleanup and removal of paper and other materials that make the grounds and buildings a health and safety hazard as well as unsightly. Proper sewage disposal and prompt garbage disposal should also be provided.

---

*A good source for ventilating and heating information is the American Society of Heating, Refrigerating, and Air-Conditioning Engineers, New York, N. Y.

†Because of the energy crisis, temperatures should be set lower than these standards wherever possible.

Acoustics

Concentration is necessary in many kinds of school, college, and recreational work. Noise distracts attention, causes nervous strain, and results in the loss of many of the activity's benefits. Therefore, noise should be eliminated as effectively as possible. This can be achieved by acoustical treatment of such important places as corridors, gymnasiums, swimming pools, shops, music rooms, and libraries.

Acoustical materials include plasters, fibers, boards, tiles, and various types of fabrics. Some areas should be given special attention. Floor covering that reduces noise can be used in corridors, and acoustical material can be used in walls. In classrooms, special attention should be given to materials that absorb sound in the upper walls and to tight floor coverings. In cafeterias there should be sound-absorption materials on floors, tables, counter tops, ceilings, and walls. Furthermore, the kitchen with its noises should be separated from the dining room. The music room and shop areas should be isolated as much as possible in addition to having acoustically treated walls. Swimming pools and gymnasiums need special treatment to control the various noises associated with joyous and enthusiastic play participation. Ceiling and wall acoustical treatment will help control noises in the gymnasium, while the use of mineral acoustical material, which will not be affected by high humidity, will be found helpful in the swimming pool.

Special considerations for a healthful environment for physical education

Physical educators including teachers, coaches, and others should contribute to a healthful environment by providing safe and sanitary conditions for their program and the construction and maintenance of safe facilities.

Outdoor physical education facilities. Playing fields and playgrounds should have good turf and be clear of rocks, holes, and uneven surfaces. A dirty, dusty surface, for example, can aggravate such conditions as emphysema, chronic bronchitis, and allergies. Artificial turf is now being used more and more. However, it needs improvement in several areas in order to reduce injuries and other problems associated with the type of surfacing. Safety precautions should also be provided in terms of well-lined areas, regularly inspected equipment, and fenced-in playfields and playgrounds, particularly where there is heavy traffic adjoining these facilities. Rubber asphalt, synthetic materials, and other substances that require little maintenance and help to free an area from cinders, gravel, stones, and dust are being used more and more on outdoor surfaces. In some sections of the country limited shelters are also being used to provide protection from the rain, wind, and sun. All outdoor areas should provide for sanitary drinking fountains and toilet facilities as needed.

Indoor physical education facilities. Just as safe and properly constructed equipment should be a part of outdoor facilities, so should they be a part of indoor physical education facilities. There should be adequate space provided for all the activity phases of the program whether they are in the gymnasium, swimming pool, or auxiliary areas. Mats should be used as a protective measure on walls and other areas where participants may be injured. Drinking fountains should be recessed and doors should open away from the playing floor. Proper flooring should be used—tile-cement floors are sometimes undesirable where activity takes place. Space should be provided for the adapted physical education program where students in wheelchairs and on crutches can be accommodated.

Clothing and equipment. Clothing and equipment used in physical education activities should meet health standards. If not, odors and germs will thrive, causing an unpleasant environment that may help to spread disease. Gymnasium mats, for example, should be kept clean. Regular physical education clothing, not street clothes, should be worn in most classes. Social dancing or similar activities, of course, would be exceptions. Clean clothing, including all types of athletic costumes, should be required. Footwear should be fitted properly. Socks should be clean. Many schools provide facilities for laundering physical education clothing.

Shower and locker facilities. Special attention should be paid to shower facilities. The shower room should be kept clean and plenty

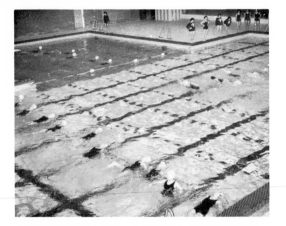

Richwoods Community High School, Peoria Heights, Ill.

of soap and warm water should be available. Proper heating and ventilation should be provided; a nonslip floor surface should be installed; and ceilings should be constructed to prevent condensation. The drying area should be washed daily to prevent athlete's foot and other contaminations. A towel service should be initiated if it doesn't already exist. Adequate time for showering should be allowed in the schedule.

Locker rooms should provide dressing as well as storage lockers for all students starting with the upper-grade elementary school. Adequate space should be provided so that dressing is not done in cramped quarters. Occasional locker inspections are considered to be necessary.

Swimming pools. Swimming pools need special attention whether they are of the indoor or outdoor variety. First, the pool should be properly constructed to provide for adequate filtration, circulation, and chlorination. There should be a daily diary kept of such things as temperature of water, hydrogen ion concentration, residual chlorine, and other important matters. Regulations should be established and students acquainted with them in regard to pool use. A list of pool regulations advocated by the National Education Association and the American Medical Association include:

1. Everyone using the pool should have an overall bath, in the nude, with soap and water, washing carefully the armpits, the genital and rectal areas, and the feet.

2. Before taking a shower, the bladder should be emptied. Pupils needing to urinate during the swimming period should be excused to go to the toilet.
3. Anyone leaving the pool to go to the toilet must take another cleansing bath with soap and water before returning.
4. Pupils should expectorate only in the overflow trough.
5. Boys and men should swim in the nude or wear sanitized trunks. Girls and women should wear sanitized tank suits.
6. Girls and boys with long hair should wear rubber bathing caps. Caps keep hair, dandruff, and hair oil from contaminating the water. They also keep hair out of the eyes.
7. Each pupil should be inspected by the instructor or the pool guard before he enters the pool. Pupils with evidence of skin infection, eye infection, respiratory disease, open cuts or sores, or bandages should be excluded.
8. There must be no rough or boisterous play and no running or playing tag in or around the pool area.
9. Pupils should wear ear plugs or nose clips if these have been recommended by their physicians. Some pupils, on medical recommendation, may need to be excused, at least temporarily, from participation in the aquatic program.
10. A qualified person, either the instructor or other person qualified as a lifeguard, should be on duty whenever the pool is in use. No pupil should enter the pool unless a guard is present. All doors leading to the pool should be locked when the pool is not in use and a guard on duty.
11. Since dirt from shoes may be tracked into the pool and contaminate the water, spectators should be prohibited from entering the pool deck.*

Environmental health. Environmental health also includes air pollution, which is an important factor for athletes and physical educators alike. The dangers from air pollution are great; thousands of persons die annually from bronchitis and emphysema. Clean air is essential to health, and polluted air is dangerous for everyone, especially athletes who participate in outdoor activities. In some areas of this country, children cannot play outside during times when the air is heavily polluted.

It is the responsibility of the physical and health educator to expose students and community members to the facts concerning air pollution. Students and faculty can conduct

---

*Joint Committee on Health Problems in Education of the National Education Association and the American Medical Association: Healthful school environment, Washington, D. C., 1969, The Association, pp. 234-235.

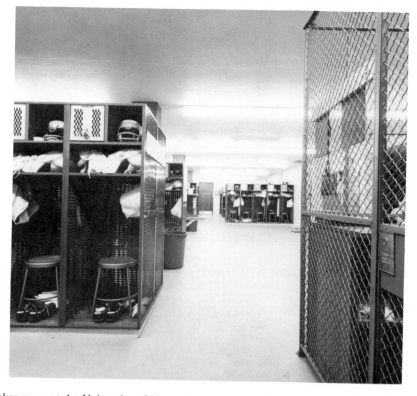

Locker room at the University of Notre Dame accents a healthy environment for athletes.

programs to educate the community in this area. Sources of pollution in the school and community should be stopped and clean-air methods introduced. Information concerning air pollution can be obtained through the federal or state Environmental Protection Agency.

Athletics. All the suggestions previously stated for a healthful environment refer to athletics as a phase of the total physical education program. In addition, athletes need some special considerations. All athletes should have medical examinations and medical supervision. The coach should be concerned about the health of the athlete at all times. This responsibility ranges from not putting undue pressure on an athlete to win to providing proper competition with teams of comparable ability. The coach also has great influence on the health habits of the athlete and as such should use it in a way that will reduce the amount of cigarette smoking, use of drugs, undue weight reduction brought about by crash diets, and improper nutrition.

The Joint Committee on Health Problems of the National Education Association and the American Medical Association has set forth a set of guidelines for safeguarding the health of the athlete. These can be found in Chapter 13.

THE PSYCHOLOGIC ENVIRONMENT

The World Health Organization defines health as follows: "Health is a state of complete physical, mental, and social well-being, and not merely the absence of disease or infirmity." In order to have a mentally healthful and educational environment, therefore, one should not be concerned merely with providing the proper physical facilities. It is necessary also to take into consideration the administrative practices that play such an important part in providing for the total health of the student. It has been estimated that one of every ten school children is emotionally disturbed. This fact shows the necessity for coming to grips with this problem in every way possible. Health and physical educators should be especially concerned with mental and emotional health because of their close relationship with physical health and illness. During the last few years the psychosomatic aspects of illness have increasingly been given more attention.

Mental health implies a state of mind that allows the individual to adjust in a satisfactory manner to whatever life has to offer. Good mental health cannot be thought of as a subject included in the school curriculum. Instead, it must permeate the total life of the educational institution. It means that programs are flexible and geared to individual needs, a permissive climate prevails, children are allowed considerable freedom, and students become self-reliant and responsible for their own actions. It means that the child is recognized and has a satisfying educational experience. The National Association for Mental Health points out that the well-adjusted person is the one who has the right attitudes and feelings toward himself or herself, other people, and the demands that life places upon him or her.

School and college programs offer an excellent laboratory for developing good human relations, democratic methods, responsibility, self-reliance, and other essentials to happy and purposeful living. The degree to which this laboratory is utilized for such purposes depends upon administrative officers, teachers, custodians, and other staff members. Such important considerations as the administrative policies established, teachers' personalities, program, human relations, and professional help that is given will determine to what extent educational programs justify their existence in human betterment. Some of the important implications for a healthful and educational environment are discussed in more detail.

Administrative practices

A few of the administrative practices that have a bearing upon the mental and emotional health of the students and participants deal with organization of the school day, student achievement, play and recreation, homework, attendance, personnel policies, administrative emphasis, and discipline.

Organization of the school day. The organization of the school day will have a bearing upon whether a healthful environment is provided for the child. The length of the school day must be in conformance with the age of the child. Classes should be scheduled in a manner that does not result in excessive fatigue. Subjects that require considerable concentration should be scheduled when the individual is more mentally efficient. Usually this is during the early part of the day. Boredom and tension will arise from scheduling similar classes close together, without any breaks. The program should be flexible to allow for variety, new developments, and satisfying children's interests. Adequate periods of rest and play should be provided, not only as a change from the more arduous routine of close concentration but also as a necessity for utilizing the big muscles of the body. "Big-muscle" activity is essential during the growing years. The length of classes should be adequate for instructional purpose but not so excessively long that the law of diminishing returns sets in.

Recent studies indicate that individuals have their own biologic clocks. In other words, different people have higher or lower activity periods at different times during the day. Research is currently being conducted to determine the feasibility of grouping students in physical education programs according to their individual performance on tests geared to determine the times of the day when one is at a peak performance level. This type of research has numerous implications for organizing the school day with the individual in mind. Computer utilization would also be a factor in this type of scheduling.

Student achievement. Success is an experience essential to the development of self-confidence and an integrated person. One who experiences success will be better stimulated to do good work than one who consistently fails. The child or youth who consistently fails is likely to have behavior disorders. In view of this, it is important that educational programs recognize their responsibility for developing each individual. Experiences should be provided that are adapted to the individual, allow for student involvement, and are planned so that each person will have a series of successful experiences.

Individual differences. It is important to

recognize that individuals differ. They differ in respect to intellect, physique, skill, personality, and many other qualities. In a fifth-grade class, for example, although the average chronologic age may be 11 years, the mental age could range from 6 to 16 years. Similar differences abound in other characteristics.

It is very important for administrators, teachers, and leaders to recognize that these differences do exist and that programs must be planned accordingly. The same goals cannot be established for all. If goals are standardized, some individuals will become frustrated because it is impossible for them to achieve the standards, and others will become very bored because there is no challenge. Goals that are within reach for everyone should be established. Administrators and teachers sometimes become so engrossed in the idea of setting high standards that they forget to consider the individual.

Grades. Excessive emphasis should not be placed on marks. Too often the individual is interested more in the mark received than in the knowledge, attitudes, and self-improvement inherent in the activity. It seems that, if marks must be given, as broad a category as possible should be used. These could be stated in terms such as "passed" and "did not pass' or "satisfactory" and "unsatisfactory." Whenever possible, descriptive statements of the student's progress should be given without any marks whatsoever. Parent-teacher conferences are probably the best way to evaluate a student's progress in the most effective manner. These procedures are being followed in some elementary schools with excellent results. In many physical education programs, students and teachers consult with each other in grade determination.

Tests and examinations. It is generally agreed that some method is needed to check on the progress that has been made in the acquisition of knowledge, skills, or attitudes. Harmful effects of such tests and examinations result when they are used by teachers and leaders to instill fear in the individual. Frequently, individuals harm themselves physically, mentally, and emotionally when they become worked up over an approaching examination. They stay up all night cramming, cannot sleep, are tense, and generally find it a very trying experience.

This is especially true at the college level. Students should understand that examinations are a means by which greater help can be given to them. Such help is not possible unless information is gained about what the person knows at certain points along the way. In physical education programs, tests are often determined on the basis of completion of certain performance objectives outlined by both student and teachers.

Intelligence ratings. Intelligence ratings can be of some value in the hands of a trained person. It is important to recognize, however, that such measuring devices are not definite, exact, and accurate in indicating the mental capacity of an individual. Furthermore, intelligence is only one factor that makes for success of an individual. In fact, it has been shown through Terman's study of gifted children, where all received high intelligence ratings, that intelligence does not necessarily ensure the achievement of prominent position in life.

Furthermore, intelligence ratings are often in error. One test should never be used as the criterion. Instead, several tests should be given before definite conclusions are drawn. Even then, as the work of Allison Davis and others at the University of Chicago has shown, intelligence tests measure a person's environment and the cultural experiences open to him to a greater extent than they do his native intelligence.

Play and recreation. The impression that achievement in so-called academic subjects is the only criterion necessary to ensure successful living is erroneous. In addition, there should be achievement in the areas of human relations, personality development, physical development, acquisition of skills for leisure hours, and other areas even more vital to the success of the individual than so-called scholastic achievement.

Dr. William Menninger and other experts in the field of psychiatry have pointed to the contributions of play and recreation to mental health. Furthermore, to achieve success in the competitive society of today, a person needs a sound body that possesses stamina and endurance and that will support long hours of work. Also, the skills in physical activities, music, industrial arts, and allied areas that are learned

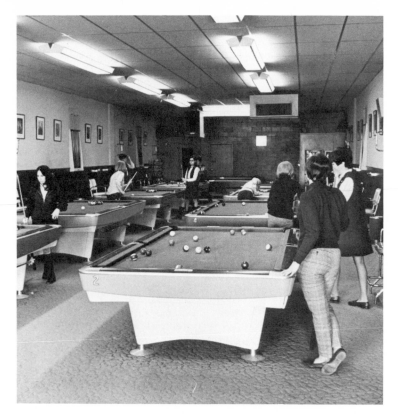

Play and recreation are important aspects of a healthy regimen for students. Students at Florissant Valley Community College in St. Louis have opportunities for recreation at the pool table. (Photograph by LeMoyne Coates.)

during the early years of an individual's life will determine to a great degree his or her hobbies or leisure-time pursuits during adult years.

For these and other reasons, it is important that physical education and other subjects falling into this category be recognized for the contribution they can make to the total growth of the individual.

Homework. Educators are increasingly recognizing that homework should be assigned in a manner that is in the best interest of the whole child. If it is given for the purpose of busywork, to keep someone occupied during hours after dinner at night, or solely for enabling a person to surpass his or her classmates, it cannot be justified. Children as well as adults need time for play and recreation. They are entitled to time after school for such purposes. For young children in elementary school, homework assignments should take into con-

sideration that young bodies need great amounts of physical activity. Ample exercise is necessary for body organs and muscles that are developing and gaining strength for future years. In junior high school, the homework assigned should be reasonable in nature. In high school it should not be given in such large amounts that it requires late hours of work. Instead, it should promote achievement and allow the student opportunity for independent work and help to promote the development of the whole individual.

Attendance. In many states financial aid is based upon school attendance. In some cases this has resulted in harmful effects to the health of children. Administrators have been known to stress attendance to the point where students come to school with colds and other illnesses when they should be home in bed. This not only endangers their own health, but at the same time it exposes many healthy children to harmful germs.

It is important to have regular attendance at school. However, if the student is ill and in need of rest or parental and medical care, it is much better that he or she stay home. In order not to abuse this privilege, administrators, teachers, and others should try to educate the parents on what constitutes good reasons for absences from school.

Furthermore, if the student is well enough to attend school, then it would seem that he or she should attend all classes. Too often a student is dismissed from a physical education class because of some minor disorder. If the program is adapted to the needs of the individual, special consideration can be given to such cases. It is just as important that regular attendance prevail in physical education as in social studies, mathematics, or any other subject.

Personnel policies. The administration's personnel policies in regard to teachers and other staff members will determine in some measure whether or not a healthful environment is created. A teacher who is required to punch a clock when he or she comes to work in the morning and leaves at night, is never greeted with a smile, never experiences an enjoyable conversation with the principal, is held responsible for many unnecessary details, is required to be at work regardless of how he or she feels, receives no administrative support when subject to community prejudices, and finds that the administrative policies that are established do not result in happiness, security, and confidence in doing the job, cannot help but reflect such policies in his or her dealings with students and colleagues.

Administrators should try to establish the best possible working conditions for all members of a staff. Only if they feel happy and well adjusted in their jobs will a healthful environment exist.

Differentiated staffing can be a great aid in providing for the teacher's work load and psychologic adjustment. Paraprofessionals and teacher-aides can help to alleviate the tremendous amount of paper work with which the teacher is frequently burdened. In addition,

more staff members allow for the teacher to be involved with the activities that he or she excels in and enjoys teaching.

Administrative emphasis. The administrative emphasis should be on the students and on those experiences that will help them to grow and develop into healthy and educated human beings. Administrative policies should be established that reflect human beings as the centers of the program, allow for flexibility, encourage initiative on the part of the students and teachers, are adapted to the needs and interests of the participants, and provide in every way for a healthful physical and nonphysical environment.

Discipline. The school and college should be a place where individuals receive joy and satisfaction from their experiences. A spirit of cooperation should exist among the administration, staff, and members of the organization. The emphasis in student discipline should be on self-government. As much freedom as possible should be given. The individual who is surrounded on all sides by restrictions and who is not trusted will rebel. As many educators have discovered, abrupt use of authority invites resistance. There should be a permissive attitude toward individual variations from acceptable behavior, coupled with a firm but kind insistence on higher standards of conduct. Responsibility should go along with freedom. A climate of opinion should be established that allows as much freedom as possible without encroaching on the rights of others. A strong student government can be one of the best educational devices for self-discipline.

Regulations should not be accepted just because they are regulations. Rather, they should be accepted because they are essential to securing the rights of everyone so that all can enjoy and benefit from the programs that are offered.

If antisocial behavior develops, it is important to look into the reasons for such behavior and work to eliminate the causes, rather than to abruptly and harshly discipline some person. Unless this is done, such antisocial behavior will continue to show itself. Furthermore, in time it may become so obstreperous that isolation of the individual from society will be re-

Table 14-1. Analysis of 193 student discipline provisions in negotiation agreements *

Clause	Agreements with clause	
	Number	Percent
Joint committee established to study disciplinary policy	11	5.7
Board disciplinary policy or public law tied into agreement by contract language	22	11.4
General statement of teacher board disciplinary philosophy	156	80.8
Reasons for disciplinary action		
Disruptive behavior	52	26.9
Persistent misbehavior	40	20.7
Gross offenses	39	20.2
Physical violence (assault, fighting)	18	9.3
Gambling, drugs, alcohol, tobacco, pornography, weapons	14	7.3
Disrespect or insubordination	10	5.2
Vandalism, arson, theft, extortion	9	4.7
False bomb reports, inciting violence	6	3.1
Abusive language	5	2.6
Threatening or belligerent manner	4	2.1
Truancy/skipping	3	1.6
Health/physical appearance	3	1.6
Procedures for initial identification and handling of disciplinary problems		
Reasonable force for protection and restraint	19	9.8
Child sent to office or principal notified	6	3.1
Teacher reports punishable offenses and points out emotional or disciplinary problem students to principal	47	24.4
Parents called to conference	28	14.5
Punishment for offenses		
Temporary exclusions from class		
By teacher	56	29.0
By principal	1	9.5
Detention	6	3.1
Corporal punishment	14	7.3
Transfer to another class (before suspension)	13	6.7
Suspension	32	16.6
Expulsion	4	2.1
Limitation on punishment	6	3.1
Special consideration given to teachers with one or more children who have emotional or behavior problems		
Reduced class size only	1	0.5
More or longer relief periods and/or reduced class size	2	1.0
Equal distribution of problem children among teachers	1	0.5
General statement	1	0.5
Need for help from specialists recognized		
Psychiatrists, psychologists, physicians, counselors	103	53.4
Law enforcement personnel	80	41.5
Special classes or services for emotional and behavior problem children		
Special classes exist	6	3.1
Expansion of special education	2	1.0
Board to prepare program	1	0.5
Removal from classroom of those who cannot adjust	6	3.1
Record of disciplinary cases kept	4	2.1
Miscellaneous clauses	7	3.6

*From NEA Research Bulletin **47**:59, 1969.

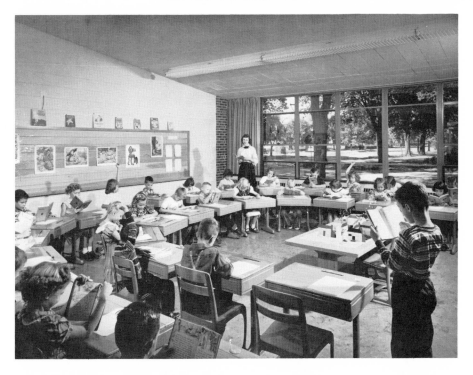

The school should be a place for student learning experiences in a healthful environment as shown here at the Washington Irving Elementary School, Waverly, Iowa. (Courtesy Burnett and Logan, Chicago, Ill.)

quired. If a constructive approach is taken, such measures may be avoided.

The teacher

Good mental health in a school program is closely tied to the teacher. The manner in which the teacher and student interact with one another is very important. It is important for the teacher to think of youngsters as living, feeling, and developing human beings who pursue different and varied courses on their ways to maturity. They are not inanimate objects or receptacles into which the instructor pours knowledge.

One of the main responsibilities of any teacher in health or physical education should be student counseling. Quite frequently specialists in these areas are the ones to whom the child goes in search of information. Anyone who is to perform such an important job as counseling should be well adjusted, understand himself or herself, and get along well with others.

The teacher must be in good physical condition in order to do a good job. A teacher may come to a job in excellent physical condition, but if large classes are assigned, the salary is insufficient, and outside work is necessary, physical harm may result. Furthermore, if there is no provision for sick leave and as a result the teacher must be on the job even when sick or ill, his or her physical condition will suffer. When this happens, the students also suffer.

The teacher's personality has important implications for the mental and emotional health of those with whom he or she comes in contact. The teacher who is happy, wears a smile, is kind, considerate, and likes people in general will impart these qualities to the students. It is bound to "rub off" in the daily interaction that takes place. Conversely, the teacher or leader who is sarcastic, depressed, prejudiced, and intolerant will also impart these qualities to the children with whom he or she associates. The leader's personality is also reflected in the appearance of the classroom and the teaching methods employed.

Administrators should be cognizant of the factors that result in maladjusted personalities for members of their staffs. A few years ago the National Educational Association found that many faculty members were plagued by personal and working conditions that influenced their mental outlooks. Some of these were as follows: financial difficulties, serious illness of relatives or friends, unsatisfactory progress of pupils, matters of personal health, being unmarried and without normal family relationships, disciplinary problems, an official rating by a superior, possible loss of position, work on a college course, being unhappily married, and religious problems. Many of these frustrating factors could have been eliminated.

All teachers should have satisfactory working conditions. They should receive an adequate salary to eliminate financial worries, be encouraged to develop out-of-school interests in the community, have hobbies in which they can engage after school hours and during vacation periods, and have adequate provisions for sick and sabbatical leaves and leaves of absence so that proper rest and adequate educational standards may be assured. Furthermore, there should be ample opportunities provided for affiliation with professional groups and the development of cultural and other interests conducive to better leadership qualifications. By providing such essentials teachers and leaders will be made happier and have better mental and emotional health. In turn, this will be reflected in the total health of the children with whom they come in contact.

Human relationships

Human relationships are a most important consideration if one is to grow into a happy, successful, and well-adjusted individual. Of all

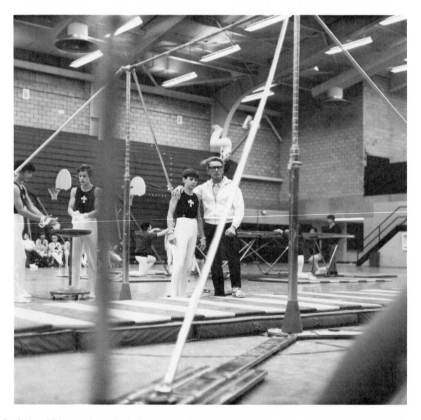

Each individual should be made to feel that he or she belongs to the group and has something to contribute, as symbolized here in Thornwood High School, South Holland, Ill.

the traits that should be developed in health and physical education, human relationships rank toward the top of the list. Through counseling, participation in group games and activities under good leadership, and other phases of the programs, the potentialities are great for developing in students good human relationships.

Each individual should be made to feel that he or she belongs to the group and has something to contribute in its behalf. There must never be an attempt to make a member of the group feel insignificant and unimportant. More praise should be dispensed than criticism. Every attempt should be made to help each person maintain his or her self-respect. The atmosphere that pervades the classroom, gymnasium, or recreation center should be relaxed and friendly. The emotional needs of every individual should be taken into consideration in the class or group activities that are held.

The teacher should have good relationships with his or her colleagues. Any faculty or staff that is infested with cliques, jealousies, and strife communicates these attitudes to the students.

There must be good human relationships among the students themselves. They are dependent upon the feeling of the group toward them and whether or not they are accepted. It is important to have status among one's associates. The teacher can play an important part in helping to see that everyone gains recognition. This is especially important with such individuals as the dull child in the classroom, the awkward, uncoordinated youngster on the playfield, and the intellectually gifted student in a recreation setting.

The teacher should be careful not to accentuate any characteristic that makes a child markedly different from the rest of the group. This applies to the whole realm of deviations, including scholastic, physical, mental, social, and economic.

Professional services

The factors discussed thus far in respect to the nonphysical environment have been largely preventive in nature. They have attempted to show the importance of providing an environment where the individual has freedom, self-respect, and security and experiences satisfaction in his or her activities. However, despite emphasis upon preventive measures, there will always be some individuals who become behavior problems and will need professional help.

The teacher can play an important part by identifying those individuals who need help. He or she can also render guidance and such other aid as is possible in the school or college situation. The teacher can often do a great deal of good by evaluating the student thoroughly in respect to his or her school, home, and community environment. Through such a study and by working closely with parents, many minor maladjustments can be eliminated. If further help is needed, the student should be referred to the proper professional persons.

In some schools there are counselors who have had preparation that goes beyond that of the ordinary teacher or leader. Their special knowledge of guidance and mental hygiene should be utilized in dealing with problem cases.

With the increasing emphasis on mental health, many schools and colleges are utilizing the services of social workers, psychologists, and psychiatrists. The more serious cases should be referred to such professional people. They are trained in dealing with such problems and can render a great deal of personal help as well as promote a more healthful environment.

Recently, there has been a marked growth of child guidance clinics across the country. These are sponsored by various organizations interested in securing professional guidance for individuals with behavior problems. These clinics guide parents and community groups in good mental hygiene practices and needs, aid children who have various mental maladjustments, and seek support and understanding within the community to help promote better mental hygiene. They have trained people on their staffs who are competent to assist in preventing and solving problems that involve psychology.

CHECKLIST FOR ADMINISTRATIVE PRACTICES FOR A HEALTHFUL ENVIRONMENT

Organization of the school day

Length of the school day   *Yes*   *No*

1. The length of the school day should be adapted to the age of the child, starting with one-half day in kindergarten.
2. Play and rest periods are provided in accordance with pupil needs.

Scheduling

1. Subjects demanding diligent application are scheduled early in the day.
2. Subjects requiring more mental concentration and academic effort are interspersed with those requiring less mental effort.
3. The amount of time devoted to a specific task is assigned with regard to the age, readiness, and needs of the child.
4. There is ample time between classes to ensure student promptness without excessive haste.
5. A leisurely lunch break is provided for each pupil.
6. The educational program is a flexible one, so that it is possible to schedule special programs or activities without hindering the regular program.

Student achievement

Individual differences

1. There is provision in the school program for individual differences among children in respect to physical handicaps, readiness to learn, academic ability, and environmental background.
2. Consideration is given to the physical and mental growth of each child.
3. The abilities of each child are recognized and instruction is adjusted to individual ability.

Grades

1. Provision is made for clerical and special assistance in helping the teacher to spend more time with teaching responsibilities.
2. The program is planned so that each child experiences a series of educational successes.
3. Goals are adjusted to fit each pupil, and marks are used to indicate progress toward stated goals.
4. Provision is made for a descriptive evaluation along with the grade.

Reporting pupil progress

1. The means used to report pupil progress include personal conferences, checklists, graphs, letters, progress reports, and report cards.
2. Problems, weaknesses, and potential of child are items for teacher-parent conferences.

Tests and examinations

1. Examinations are used as a means of helping pupil and teacher discover the progress that has been made in the acquisition of knowledge.
2. Tests help the learner attain satisfaction and a sense of achievement when he is doing as well as he should.
3. Tests help the teacher judge how effective his teaching methods are.
4. Tests assist in making administrative judgments in respect to grouping and other procedures.
5. Tests provide emphasis on diagnosis rather than on rating of overall merit, upon individual improvement rather than comparison with others, and are used more as guides than as final measures.

CHECKLIST FOR ADMINISTRATIVE PRACTICES FOR A HEALTHFUL ENVIRONMENT—cont'd

	Yes	No

Intelligence ratings

1. Intelligence tests are selected and administered by a trained person.
2. Tests are used with a view to how the children can profit with suitable instruction.

Physical education and recreation

1. Physical education class size ranges from thirty to forty pupils.
2. Physical education is offered daily and stresses basic skills and movement experiences.
3. The physical education program is concerned with the social, mental, and emotional aspects of the child, as well as the physical.
4. Recreational activities are based on pupil interests.

Homework

1. Homework is assigned in accordance with the age, interest, ability, and needs of the child.

Pupil attendance

1. The school nurse determines whether the child should attend school and when he should be sent home.
2. The child does not return to school after sickness until he is able to attend all classes.
3. The nurse and attendance officer play a major role in communication with the parent regarding proper health practices.

Discipline

1. Behavior is evaluated with the knowledge that misconduct is a sign of maladjustment and an attempt is made to find the cause.
2. The staff upholds the same general standards of behavior.
3. All pupil abilities are recognized and an effort is made to maintain the self-respect of the child through the use of praise.
4. Fear is not used as a technique of control.
5. Children are encouraged to assist in developing standards of behavior and to assist in their enforcement.

Student grouping

1. Grouping is flexible so that administration and organization exist only to expedite the process of learning.
2. Differences in learners and subject matter are considered in grouping.
3. Promotion practices are flexible.
4. Grouping is such that children do not bear labels, for example, "fast group" or "slow learner."

Teacher-pupil relationships

1. There is cooperative thinking and effort between teachers and pupils rather than emphasis upon the sole direction and authority of the teacher.
2. The teacher sets a good example for the pupil.
3. A primary teacher responsibility is that of pupil counseling.
4. The pupil is made to feel that he is part of the group and contributes to it.
5. The atmosphere of the classroom is relaxed and friendly.
6. The teacher shows interest in each pupil.
7. The teacher recognizes the various environmental factors that compose pupil personality and behavior.
8. The teacher has good relationships with his colleagues.
9. The teacher has an enthusiastic and confident attitude.

Continued.

CHECKLIST FOR ADMINISTRATIVE PRACTICES FOR A HEALTHFUL ENVIRONMENT—cont'd

	Yes	No

Teacher-pupil relationships—cont'd

10. The teacher enjoys his work and takes pride in it.
11. The teacher is secure in his job.

Professional services

1. The administration provides for guidance, psychologist, psychiatrist, and social worker services.
2. Specialists in ''1'' work closely with the home in providing necessary help for the child.

Personnel policies

1. Relationships between administrators and teachers are harmonious.
2. The administration promotes good social and professional relations among members of the staff.
3. Administrators help educate the public to its true responsibilities to the schools and seek the support and assistance of the public in the promotion of educational goals.

The teacher

Qualities

1. The teacher likes children.
2. The teacher is well adjusted and mentally healthy.
3. The teacher understands the growth and development of children.
4. The teacher is able to identify children with serious problems and knows how and when to refer them for help.
5. The teacher helps pupils meet their basic emotional needs.
6. The teacher has a pleasing appearance and manner and is physically healthy, patient, and impartial.
7. The teacher respects the child's personality, understands his limitations and creates an overall atmosphere of security.

Working conditions

1. The physical conditions of the job are good (salary, sick leave, class load).
2. Administration is aware of factors that might affect the mental health of the teacher and helps to eliminate such problems.

Improving instruction

1. Administration utilizes opportunities to commend teacher achievement and effort.
2. The beginning teacher is helped over the rough spots and is also assisted in obtaining a broad professional orientation.

Questions and exercises

1. Define what is meant by the ''physical'' and ''nonphysical'' environments. What are the implications of each for total health?
2. Prepare a research report on administrative practices for a healthful and educational environment as they relate to a school with which you are very familiar.
3. Prepare a list of administrative practices in health, physical education, or recreation that are nationally in evidence and should be eliminated in order to provide greater total health.
4. What part does each of the following play in mental health of school children: (a) organization of the school day, (b) achievement, (c) marks, (d) play and recreation, (e) homework, (f) attendance, and (g) discipline?
5. How does the mental and emotional health of a teacher affect the mental and emotional health of school children?

6. Discuss environmental health in relation to school health programs.
7. To what degree are the physical features of a school related to mental and emotional health?
8. Why is it so important to have good human relationships within the school?
9. How can the school and community coordinate their efforts to further better physical, mental, emotional, and social health for all residents?
10. What is the role of professional services in the school program?

Reading assignment in *Administrative Dimensions of Health and Physical Education Programs, Including Athletics:* Chapter 11, Selections 59 to 62.

Selected references

American Association for Health, Physical Education, and Recreation: School safety policies with emphasis on physical education, athletics, and recreation, Washington, D. C. 1964, The Association.

American Medical Association, Committee on Medical Aspects of Sports: Proceedings of the National Conference on the Medical Aspects of Sports—I through IX, Chicago, 1960-1967, The Association.

American Medical Association, Committee on Medical Aspects of Sports: Tips on athletic training—I through IX, Chicago, 1960-1967, The Association.

Brennan, A. J. J.: Environmental health: a look at the cost of air pollution, The Journal of School Health **43**:300, 1973.

Castetter, W. B.: The personnel function in educational administration, New York, 1971, The Macmillan Co.

Daniels, A. S., and Davies, E. A.: Adapted physical education, ed. 2, New York, 1965, Harper & Row, Publishers.

Engelhardt, N. L.: Complete guide for planning new schools, West Nyack, New York, 1970, Parker Publishing Co.

Fitch, K., and others: Life science and man, New York, 1973, Holt, Rinehart and Winston, Inc.

Goldstein, J.: Environmental education for teachers, Journal of Health, Physical Education, and Recreation **44**:38, 1973.

Grout, R. E.: Health teaching in schools, Philadelphia, 1968, W. B. Saunders Co.

Illinois Office of Public Instruction: Guidelines for evaluating programs in physical education, Springfield, Ill., Office of Public Instruction.

Jefcoat, A.: Health and human values: an ecological approach, New York, 1972, John Wiley and Sons, Inc.

Johns, E.: Health for effective living, New York, 1973, McGraw-Hill Book Co., Inc.

Joint Committee on Health Problems in Education of National Education Association and American Medical Association: School health services, Washington, D. C., 1964, National Education Association.

Joint Committee on Health Problems in Education of National Education Association and American Medical Association: Healthful school living, Washington, D. C., 1957, National Education Association.

Joint Commitee on Health Problems in Education of National Education Association and American Medical Association: Health education, Washington, D. C., 1961, National Education Association.

Kirk, R., and others: Personal health in ecological perspective, St. Louis, 1972, The C. V. Mosby Co.

Konopa, V., and Zimering, S.: Noise—the challenge of the future, The Journal of School Health **42**:172, 1972.

Phillips, J.: Environmental health, Dubuque, Iowa, 1970, William C. Brown Co.

Waldbott, G. L.: Health effects of environmental pollutants, St. Louis, 1973, The C. V. Mosby Co.

PART FOUR

Administrative functions

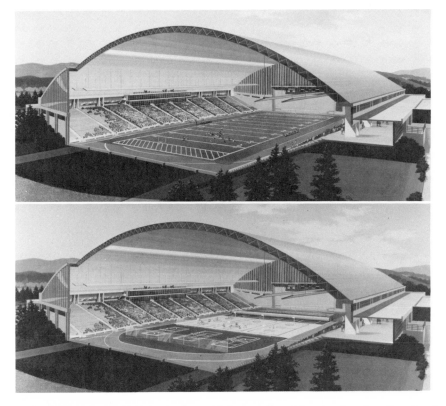

Architect drawings of New Idaho Stadium with its portable gridiron in place (top picture) and portable gridiron partly rolled up (bottom picture) over permanent synthetic floor marked for basketball, tennis, volleyball, badminton, and track. (Courtesy Scholastic Coach.)

The physical plant

The physical considerations of any school or college physical education and health complex are essential for the safety and education of the students. Physical plants require careful planning, and specialists in this area of architecture must be consulted. Administrators, physical educators, and other personnel should participate in the planning of new facilities and be knowledgeable about their structure and functions. Trends and innovative structural concepts should be thoroughly examined in order to provide a healthful and efficient physical plant.

The physical plant is a major consideration in most health, physical education, and athletic programs. New architectural ideas are being introduced and new concepts developed in order to have a more economical and functional plant. Some building concepts include *convertibility*, for example: rearranging interiors by using elements such as movable walls and partitions and utilizing such areas as the gymnasium and amphitheater for a variety of activities such as basketball, ice skating, and baseball. Such versatility is needed in order to accommodate a number of different activities so that small and large group instruction and independent study spaces may be provided. This flexibility also ensures such important functions

as team teaching and proper installation and use of electronic aids.

Another concept that is being developed involves obtaining air-rights over some locations in cities so that schools may be constructed over railroad yards, water, or highways. An example is New York City's Northeast Bronx School, which is constructed above the Hutchinson River Parkway.

Educational parks represent another new concept; these result in a cluster of schools of several educational levels from elementary school through college located in the same geographic place. East Orange, New Jersey, for example, is planning such an educational park.

An important inner-city innovation is Storefront Schools that are developed to serve such segments of the population as unemployed young people, school drop-outs, and other innercity youth. Youth receive a form of education with which they can identify and which is adapted to their needs and interest. The education takes place in their own neighborhoods.

In the following paragraphs are listed a few schools and colleges throughout the nation where new concepts have been put to good use in the physical plants:

Oak Grove High School, San Jose, California. This school has a movable interior partitioning system with adjustable lighting, acoustics, and air conditioning that can accommodate different types of activities on short notice.

Nova High School, Fort Lauderdale, Florida. This school spent 10% of the school's total cost on teaching aids so that all types of audiovisual materials could be utilized or piped into most classrooms and teaching stations in the school.

Poway High School, Poway, California. Teachers' offices are located adjacent to resource centers in the school with the result that they are easily accessible to students.

Aspen Senior High School, Aspen, Colorado. This high school provides for an open-walled concept, which has space that can be used for multiple purposes.

Andrews Senior High School, Andrews, Texas. Here the open court has a windowless exterior and faces inward to a concourse and a domed rotunda. Along the concourse there are a swimming pool and gymnasium and under the rotunda there is an assembly area for students.

Holland High School, Holland, Michigan. This school built its plant on the compass plan with four small schools. Physical education facilities are shared by all schools.

John Marshall High School, Portland, Oregon. Here facilities were adapted to the flexible modular programs, thus accommodating team teaching, independent study, large and small group instruction, open laboratories, and resource centers.

New Haven, Connecticut Public Schools. This city adapted its facilities to the community school concept with each school including community facilities involving the city's social and welfare agencies where such problems as health, family relations, and unemployment are a major concern.

Portland State University, Oregon. Here the roof of the physical education building was covered with artificial surfacing to provide tennis courts and a general sports area.

Brooklyn Polytech in New York City. A bubble was erected on top of the Physics Building for a gymnasium.

University of Texas at El Paso. This university covered its outdoor swimming pool with prefabricated material in order to have an all-weather, year-round facility.

LaVerne College, California. Here what some persons call a "super tent," involving a cable-supported fabric roof structure made of fiberglass and Teflon, houses theater, gymnasium, cafeteria, bookstore, and health clinic.

The University of Minnesota. Administrators are considering placing a dome over the football

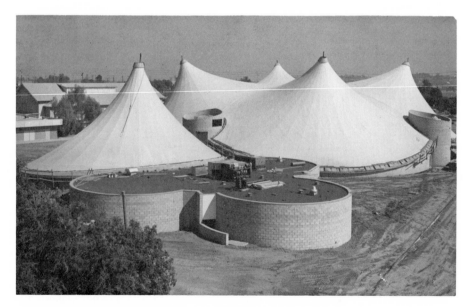

"Super tent" at LaVerne College, Calif.

field in order to provide additional activity space.

Cuyahoga Falls, Ohio. Here a roof was installed over the swimming pool so that it could be used during the winter as well as the summer months. In the summer months the roof is removed.

Thomas Jefferson Junior High School, Arlington, Virginia. This school has implemented the shared facilities concept by housing together performing arts, recreation, and physical education.

Harvard University, Massachusetts. Here the largest air supported structure for a new track facility has been erected; it is 250 feet wide, 300 feet long, and 60 feet high.

Lewis and Clark Elementary School in St. Louis, Missouri. A physical education partial shelter has been erected with the sides of the open structure protected by banks of shrubbery.

Boston College, Massachusetts. A roof design of hyperbolic parabaloids is utilized. This very efficient structure spans a large area— 42,000 square feet of floor space.

BASIC CONSIDERATIONS IN PLANNING

At the outset, two principles should be very much in the minds of health and physical educators in relation to facility management: (1) facilities emanate as a result of program needs and (2) cooperative planning is essential to avoid common mistakes. The objectives, activities, teaching methods and materials, administrative policies, and equipment and supplies represent program considerations regarding facilities. The educational and recreational needs of both the school and community, the thinking of both school administrators and health and physical educators, and the advice of both architects and lay persons are other considerations if facilities are to be planned wisely.

Another set of principles basic to facility planning relate particularly to the optimal promotion of a healthful environment for the students. Included in this set of principles is the provision for facilities that take into account physiologic needs of the student, including proper temperature control, lighting, water supply, and noise level. A second principle

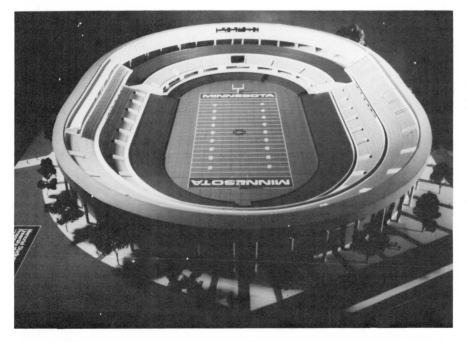

Model, University of Minnesota, stadium encapsulation. (Courtesy Gassner Nathan Browne, Architects Planners Inc., 265 Court Avenue, Memphis, Tenn. Otto Baitz, Photography of Architecture, Cliffwood, N. J.)

would be the provision of facilities that provide protection against accidents. The facilities would be planned so that the danger of fire, the possibility of mechanical accidents, and the hazards involved in student traffic would be eliminated or kept to a minimum. A third principle would concern itself with protection against disease. This would mean attention to such items as proper sewage disposal, sanitation procedures, and water supply. Finally, a fourth principle is the need to provide a healthful psychologic environment. This would have implications for space, location of activities, color schemes, and elimination of distractions through such means as soundproof construction.

A third set of principles has been developed by Bookwalter.* These may be used as guides for the planning, construction, and utilization of facilities for school health and physical education programs:

1. *Validity.* Standards for space, structure, and fixtures must be compatible with the rules

---

*Bookwalter, K. W.: Physical education in the secondary schools, Washington, D. C., 1964, The Center for Applied Research in Education, Inc. (The Library of Education), pp. 84-86.

essential for the effective conduct of the program. According to the New York State Department of Education, the number of teaching stations needed for a school will depend upon school enrollment, physical education class size, periods of physical education scheduled each week for a teaching station, the number of periods of physical education each week for which a pupil is scheduled, activities offered, and pupils in and out of class programs.

2. *Utility.* Facilities should be adaptable for different activities and programs without affecting such items as safety and effective instruction.

3. *Accessibility.* Facilities should be readily and directly accessible for the individuals who will be using them.

4. *Isolation.* Facilities should be planned to reduce to a minimum distractions, offensive odors, noise, and undesirable activities and groups.

5. *Departmentalization.* Functionally related services and activity areas should be continuous or adjacent for greatest economy and efficiency.

6. *Safety, hygiene, and sanitation.* The maintenance of proper health standards should

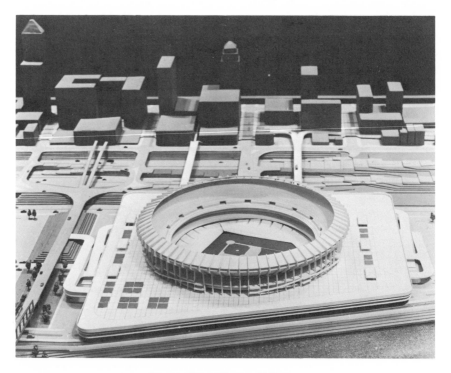

Home of the Cincinnati Reds.

be a major consideration in all facility planning.

7. *Supervision.* Facilities should take into consideration the need for proper teacher supervision of activities under his or her jurisdiction. Therefore, visibility and accessibility are essential considerations.

8. *Durability and maintenance.* Facilities should be easy and economical to maintain and should be durable.

9. *Beauty.* Facilities should be attractive and esthetically pleasing with the utilization of good color dynamics and design.

10. *Flexibility and expansibility.* Changes in enrollments, program, and other considerations for future expansion should be considered. Modern thinking has stressed the principle of flexibility in regard to physical education facilities. Flexibility should provide for immediate change through folding partitions, such as doors that separate gymnasiums, for overnight change with very little effort in cases in which partitions cannot be removed immediately, and for

greater change that can be made within a period of 1 or 2 months, such as during the summer vacation.

11. *Economy.* The best use of funds, space, time, energy, and other essential factors should be considered as they relate to facility planning.

A summary of some of the important guidelines and principles for facility planning for school and college health and physical education programs includes the following:

1. All planning should be based on goals that recognize that the total physical and nonphysical environments must be safe, attractive, comfortable, clean, practical, and adapted to the needs of the individual.

2. The planning should include a consideration of the total school or college health and physical education facilities and the recreational facilities of the community. The programs and facilities of these areas are essential to any community. Since they are closely allied, they should be planned coordinately and based on the

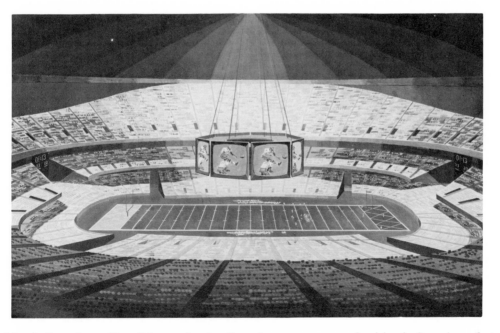

Louisiana's Superdome, New Orleans, showing Superdome superscreens. Louisiana's Superdome features a closed-circuit, full-color television system (six screens, each 56 feet wide and 36 feet high), attached to a gondola suspended from the stadium ceiling. The TV system, which is adjustable for height, provides close-up showings of in-stadium events (sports, entertainment, conventions) as they happen as well as "instant replay" from your seat in the stadium. The giant screens have a multiplicity of uses, including commercial advertising, attractiveness to conventions and trade shows, and closed-circuit showings of out of stadium events such as prize fights, collegiate football, and so forth.

needs of the community. Each should be a part of the overall community pattern.

3. Facilities should be geared to health standards. They play an important part in protecting the health of individuals and in determining the educational outcomes.

4. Facilities play a part in disease control. The extent to which schools and colleges provide for play areas, ample space, sanitary considerations, proper ventilation, heating, and cleanliness will to some extent determine how effectively disease is controlled.

5. Administrators must make plans for facilities long before an architect is consulted. Technical information can be procured in the forms of standards and guides from various sources, such as state departments of education, professional literature, building score cards, and various manuals. Information may also be secured from such important groups as the American Association of School Administrators, National Council on Schoolhouse Construction, and American Institute of Architects.

6. Standards should be utilized as guides and as a starting point. They will prove very helpful. However, it is important to keep in mind that standards cannot always be used entirely as developed. They usually have to be modified in the light of local needs, conditions, and resources.

7. Building and sanitary codes administered by the local and state departments of public health and the technical advice and consultation services available through these sources should be known and utilized by administrators in the planning and construction of facilities. Information concerned with acceptable building materials, specifications, minimum standards of sanitation, and other details may be procured from these informed sources.

8. Health, physical education, and recreation personnel should play important roles in the planning and operation of facilities. The specialized knowledge that such individuals have is very important. Provisions should be made so that their expert opinion will be utilized in the promotion of a healthful and proper environment.

9. Facilities should be planned with an eye to the future. Too often, facilities are constructed and outgrown within a very short time. Units should be sufficiently large to accommodate peak-load participation in the various activities. The peak-load estimates should be made with future growth in mind.

10. Planning should provide for adequate allotment of space to the activity and program areas. They should receive priority in space allotment. The administrative offices and service units, although important, should not be planned and developed in a spacious and luxurious manner that goes beyond efficiency and necessity.

11. Geographic and climatic conditions should be taken into consideration in planning facilities. By doing this, the full potentialities for conducting activities outdoors as well as indoors can be realized.

12. Architects do not always pay as much attention as they should to the educational and health features when planning buildings and facilities. Therefore, it is important that they be briefed on certain requirements that educators feel are essential in order that the health and welfare of children, youth, and adults may be provided for. Such a procedure is usually welcomed by the architect and will aid him in rendering a greater service to the community.

13. Facilities should take into consideration all the necessary safety features so essential in programs of health, physical education, and recreation. Health service substations near the gymnasium and other play areas, proper surfacing of activity areas, adequate space, and proper lighting are a few of these considerations.

14. It should be kept in mind that the construction of school or college health, physical education, and recreational facilities often tends to set a pattern that will influence parents, civic leaders, and others. This in turn will promote a healthful and safe environment for the entire community.

COMMON ERRORS OF HEALTH AND PHYSICAL EDUCATION PERSONNEL IN FACILITY MANAGEMENT

Some common mistakes made by health and physical educators in facility management include the following:

1. Failure to adequately project enrollments and program needs into the future (Facilities are difficult to expand or change, so this is a significant error.)
2. Failure to provide for multiple use of facilities
3. Failure to provide for adequate accessibility for students in health and physical education classes and also for community groups for recreation purposes
4. Failure to observe basic health factors in planning facilities in regard to lighting, safety, and ventilation
5. Failure to provide adequate space for the conduct of a comprehensive program of physical education activities
6. Failure to provide appropriate accommodations for spectators
7. Failure to soundproof areas of the building where noise will interfere with educational functions
8. Failure to meet with the architect to present views on program needs
9. Failure to provide adequate staff offices
10. Failure to provide adequate storage space
11. Failure to provide adequate space and privacy for medical examinations
12. Failure to provide large enough entrances to transport equipment
13. Failure to observe desirable current professional standards
14. Failure to provide for adequate study of cost in terms of durability, time, money, and effective instruction
15. Failure to properly locate teaching stations with service facilities

THE PLANNING TEAM

Planning for meaningful facilities is a team effort. It includes such persons as members of the board of education or board of trustees, representatives of the administration, students, custodians, curriculum specialists, educational consultants, members of the community, and selected teachers and department heads.

WORKING WITH THE ARCHITECT

The architect is the specialist in facility planning and the leader in the designing of school and college buildings. As such, he or she

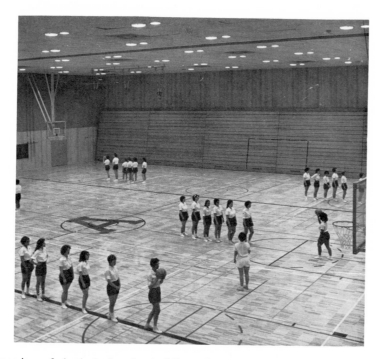

Gymnasium of physical education building. (University of Alaska, College, Alaska.)

is an important consideration for all persons engaged in health and physical education work. The architect, through his or her training and experience, is a specialist who is competent to give advisory service in all aspects of facility management.

The qualifications of the architect include:

1. The architect should be legally qualified to practice in the state and should be in good standing in the profession. He or she must have unquestioned professional character and integrity and must possess high ethical standards.

2. The architect should have had previous successful experience in designing buildings that demonstrate competence in architectural work. The buildings previously designed by the architect should also reflect a careful study of the peculiar needs of each client.

3. The architect should possess the vision and imagination to translate the educational aims and program specified by the educator into functional buildings. There should be an avoidance of stereotypes. The architect should not possess set, preconceived ideas that are hard to change. He or she must be able and willing to mold design to fit needs.

4. The architect must have a record of working cooperatively and harmoniously with clients, educational advisors, and contractors.

5. The architect must have an adequate staff of trained personnel to carry out the building program without undue delay. The architect should either have qualified engineering services available in his or her own organization or should specify qualified engineering specialists who will work with him or her.

6. The architect should keep abreast of recent research and study concerning materials and mechanical equipment used in school buildings.

7. The architect should show such economy in the use of space and materials as is consistent with educational needs.

8. The architect should be competent in the field of site planning and the utilization of space for educational and recreational purposes.

9. The architect must give adequate supervision to his or her buildings. This is a very important part of the architect's services.

10. The architect should be informed concerning state and municipal building regulations and codes and must show care in complying with them.

11. The architect must demonstrate sound business judgment, proper business procedures, and good record keeping on the job.*

Physical educators should carefully think through their own ideas and plans for their special facilities and submit them in writing to

*From Leu, D. J.: Planning education facilities, New York, 1965, The Center for Applied Research in Education, Inc. (The Library of Education), p. 50.

the architect during the early stages of school and college planning. There should also be several conferences in which the architect and physical education specialist exchange views in regard to the educational and architectural possibilities to be considered.

Many architects know little about programs of health and physical education and therefore welcome the advice of specialists in these fields. The architect might be furnished with such information as the names of school or college plants where excellent facilities exist, kinds of activities that will constitute the program, space requirements for various activities, storage and equipment areas needed, temperature requirements, relation of dressing, showering, and toilet facilities to program, teaching stations needed, best construction materials for activities, and lighting requirements. The physical educator may not have all this information readily available, including some of the latest trends and standards recommended for his or her field. However, such information can be obtained through professional organizations, other schools where excellent facilities have been developed, and facility books developed by experts in the area.

Mr. William Haroldson, Director of Health and Physical Education for the Seattle, Washington, Public Schools, has developed a procedural outline in cooperation with three architectural firms, in which are listed some essential considerations for health and physical educators in their relationships and cooperative planning with architects. Some of the main points stressed in this outline are discussed.

Educational specifications

Adequate educational specifications provide the basis for good planning by the architect:

1. General description of the program, such as the number of teaching stations necessary to service the health and physical education programs for a total student body of approximately _____ boys and _____ girls.

2. Basic criteria that pertain to the gymnasium: the number of teaching periods per day, capacities, number and size of courts, lockers, and projected total uses contemplated for the facility.

a. Availability to the community
b. Proximity to parks
c. Parking
d. Size of groups that will use gymnasium after school hours
e. Whether locker rooms will or will not be made available to public use

3. Specific description of aspects of the health and physical education programs that are of concern to the architects.

a. Class size and scheduling, both present and possible future; number of instructors, present and future
b. Preferred method of handling students, for example, flow of traffic in classrooms, locker rooms, shower rooms, and going to outside play area (This item has a direct bearing on the design of this area.)
c. Storage requirements and preferred method of handling all permanent equipment and supplies (Here, unless a standard has been established, requirements should be specific—for example, request should state number and size of each item rather than "ample storage.")
d. Team and other extracurricular use of facilities (It is of assistance to the architect if the educational specifications can describe a typical week's use of the proposed facility, which would include a broad daily program, afterschool use, and potential community use.)

Meeting with the architect

At this point, it is advisable to meet with the architect to discuss specifications in order to ensure complete understanding and to allow the architect to point out certain restrictions or limitations that may be anticipated even before the first preliminary plan is made.

Design

The factors to be considered in the design of the facility and discussed with the architect should include the following:

1. *Budget.* An adequate budget should be allowed. Gymnasiums are subject to extremely hard usage, and durability should not be sacrificed for economy.

2. *Acoustics.* Utilize the service of acoustical consultants.
3. *Public address system.* How is it to be used—for instruction, athletic events, general communication?
4. *Color and design.* Harmonize with surrounding neighborhood if it is a new school or match other areas if it is an addition to an old school.
5. *Fenestration* (window treatment). Consider light control, potential window breakage, vision panel; gymnasium areas should have safety glass (preferred) or wire protectors.
6. *Ventilation.* The area should be zoned for flexibility of usage. This means greater ventilation when a larger number of spectators are present, or a reduction for single class groups, or isolated areas, such as locker rooms. Special attention must be given to proper ventilation of uniform drying rooms. gymnasium storage areas, locker and shower areas. (Current and off-season uniform storage areas require constant ventilation when plant is shut down.) Ventilation equipment should have a low noise level.
7. *Supplementary equipment in the gymnasium.* Such equipment should be held to a minimum. Supplementary equipment, such as fire boxes, should be recessed.
8. *Compactness and integration.* Keep volume compact—large, barnlike spaces are unpleasant, costly to heat and maintain. Integrate as far as budget permits.
9. *Mechanical or electrical features.* Special attention should be given to location of panel boards, chalk boards, fire alarm, folding doors, and so on.

Further critique with the architect

1. The architect begins the development of plans from an understanding of the initial requirements that he or she has considered in relation to the design factors listed.
2. When it becomes evident that the basic plan is set, the architect will usually call in consulting engineers to discuss the structural and mechanical systems prior to approval of the plan by the school district. These systems

will have been given previous attention by the architect but cannot be discussed with the consultants other than in generalities before the plan is in approximate final form.

3. A further series of meetings are then held with school personnel regarding approval of preliminary plans and proposed structural and mechanical systems and the use of materials after the incorporation in the preliminary plans.

4. If supplementary financing by governmental agencies other than the school district is involved, the drawing or set of drawings will have been submitted to those agencies with a project outline or specifications as soon as the plan has been sufficiently developed to establish the area. If the other agency approves the application as submitted by the architect, the final preliminary working drawings are started.

Final processing

It is advisable that all matters that can be settled are decided during preliminary planning in order to save time. If this method is used, greater clarity is assured and less changing or misunderstanding results. Preliminary plans are drawn with the intent of illustrating the plan for the school district; working drawings are technical in nature and often difficult to interpret. However, should school personnel wish to check the working drawings before their completion, they should be welcome to do so.

GENERAL TRENDS IN FACILITY CONSTRUCTION

In respect to educational buildings in general, there has been considerable change. Traditionally rectangular in shape, buildings of all shapes and sizes have appeared in recent years, including round, semicircular, quadrangular, hexangular, oval, and pentangular buildings. New types of rooms have also been introduced, including large rooms for team teaching and large lecture groups; classrooms of various shapes and sizes; special rooms including those for dramatics, science, band, choral groups, business machines, and television broadcasting; and more office and conference rooms for such people as counselors and health program and administrative assistants. Furthermore, with the greater use of overhead lighting, there has been a trend to more windowless rooms. In fact, some buildings have no windows whatsoever.

School sites are becoming larger and located away from busy industrial centers. More space is also being provided for parking.

The designs of school buildings and other facilities concerned with health and physical education programs and recreation today stress two factors: the educational needs of the children and others who pursue programs in such areas and the need for economy at a time when construction costs are so high.

The trend is to do away with many of the so-called frills in order to achieve economy but at the same time not to compromise educational standards. Educational leaders advocate taking greater advantage of labor-, material-, and space-saving devices. For example, they suggest that the ceilings in regular classrooms be cut down from the traditional 12 feet to 8 feet. They maintain that good lighting can be gained under most conditions with only 8-foot ceilings. Also, multipurpose halls can be constructed to double as exhibit and social areas, and gymnasiums can be used for physical education and community purposes rather than merely for spectator entertainment.

It has further been pointed out that several practices are not economical in some of the construction going on today. An example of this is the application of Gothic and Colonial architecture merely to enhance appearance. Buildings should be planned with emphasis on the functional, inside aspects, rather than on the outside ornamentation. Also, it is not economical to have a large auditorium constructed that will be only half filled except on commencement day.

These features have received the support of the American Association of School Administrators. Bright plastic floor covering, improved lighting, and colorful painted walls are important. Classrooms should be large, with movable furniture, work alcoves, and conference rooms. Large, well-planned play areas are important features in the selection of a school site, with 10 to 20 acres of land frequently used for such sites. On both the elementary and secondary levels, one-story buildings are becoming increasingly common. Single-story construction is safer, more economical, and decreases noise. Walls are being constructed with special attention to acoustical treatment to reduce noise. Ceilings that slope are increasingly utilized in order to improve light distribution and to reduce the space to be heated. Many rooms and facilities are being located to facilitate community use. Finally, there is evidence of the practicability of single-loaded corridors, which run along the outer walls of the building. In this way classrooms open onto the hall from only one side.

Flexibility of design is an important trend in facility management today, with the inclusion of folding partitions and multiple use of facilities for different types of activities.

Some new materials that are being used are:

1. *Structural steel.* One of the most versatile of building materials, used in various shapes, sizes, and strengths, providing for greater stability, flexibility, and adaptability
2. *Structural pine.* Used for such purposes as laminated beams to form roof structures and uprights of buildings and other purposes, providing economy of design, beauty, safety, and ease of maintenance
3. *Concrete block.* Increasingly being used to enclose framework and as interior walls; economical and easily removed from non–load-bearing walls to develop flexibility
4. *Stone.* Used to a great extent for attractive exteriors on schools and for permanence
5. *Corrugated steel.* Provides an economical method of long-span roofing
6. *Carpeting of classrooms.* Helps eliminate noise and is easy to clean and requires less man hours to maintain

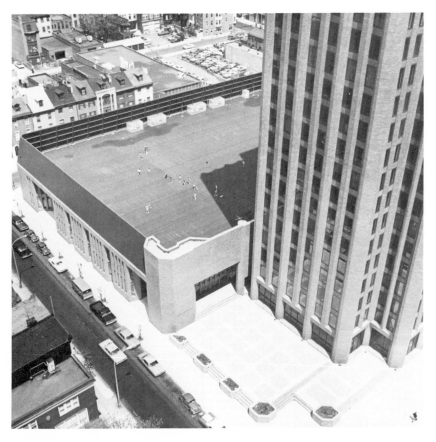

Friends Select School, Philadelphia, with rooftop playing fields utilizing AstroTurf surfacing. The synthetic surface has a ⅝ inch absorbing pad. (Courtesy Mirick Pearson Ilvonen Batcheler Architects, Philadelphia.)

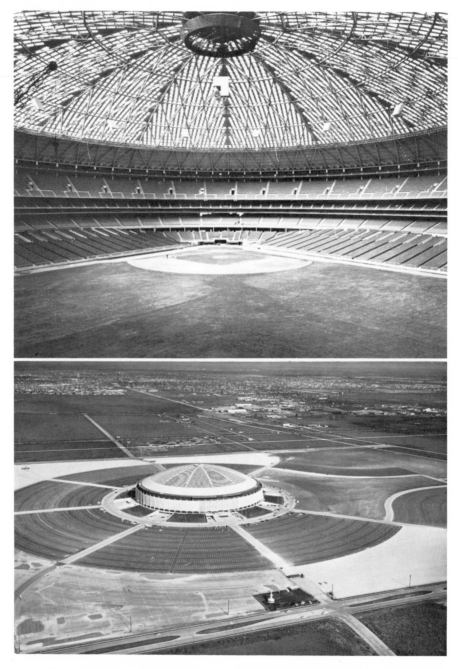

Houston's Astrodome. (Courtesy Houston Sports Association, Inc., Houston, Tex.)

NEW FEATURES IN THE CONSTRUCTION OF PHYSICAL EDUCATION FACILITIES

There are many new trends in facilities and materials for physical education programs. New paving materials, new types of equipment, improved landscapes, new construction materials, new shapes for swimming pools, partial shelters, and synthetic grass are just a few of the many new developments. Combination indoor-outdoor pools, physical fitness equipment for outdoor use, all-weather tennis courts, and lines that now come in multicolors for various games and activities are other new developments.

In gymnasium construction some of the new features include the utilization of modern engineering techniques and materials. This has resulted in welded steel and laminated wood modular frames; arched and gabled roofs; domes that provide areas completely free from internal supports; exterior surfaces of aluminum, steel, fiberglass, and plastics; different window patterns and styles; several kinds of floor surfaces of nonslip material; prefabricated wall surfaces; better lighting systems with improved quality and quantity and less glare. Facilities are moving from use of regular glass to either plastic and fiberglass panel or to an overhead skydome. Lightweight fiberglass, sandwich panels, or fabricated sheets of translucent fiberglass laminated over an aluminum framework are proving popular. They require no painting, the cost of labor and materials is lower, there is no need for shades or blinds to eliminate glare and the breakage problem is reduced or eliminated.

Locker rooms and service areas are including built-in locks that involve combination locks with built-in combination changers that permit the staff to change combinations when needed. There is more extensive use of ceramic tile

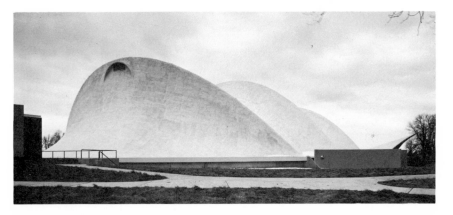

Graceland Fieldhouse, Lamoni, Iowa. (Courtesy Shaver & Co., Salina, Kan.)

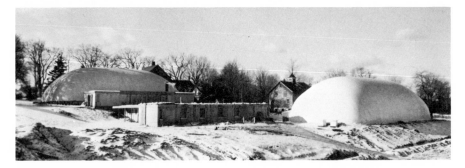

Forman School, Litchfield, Conn. (Courtesy Educational Facilities Laboratories, New York, N. Y.)

because of its durability and low-cost maintenance. Wall-hung toilet compartment features permit easier maintenance and sanitation with no chance for rust to start from the floor. Odor control is being effectively handled by new dispensers. New thin-profile heating, ventilating, and air-conditioning fan coil units are now being used.

The health suite is being modernized by making it more attractive and serviceable. There is also a trend toward better ventilation, heating, and lighting and more easily cleaned materials on walls and floors to guarantee improved sanitation.

New developments in regard to indoor swimming pools include automatic control boards, where one person can have direct control over all filters, chlorinators, chemical pumps, and level controllers; much larger deck space area constructed of nonslip ceramic tile; greater use of diatomaceous earth rather than sand filters to filter out small particles of matter including some bacteria; underwater lighting; water-level deck pools (where the overflow gutters are placed in the deck surrounding the pool instead of in the pool's side walls and provision is made for grating that is designed so that the water that overflows is drained to a trench under the deck without the possibility of debris returning to the pool); air-supported roofs that can serve as removable tops in a combination indoor-outdoor pool; and movable bulkheads.

New developments in regard to outdoor swimming pools involve new shapes—including oval, wedge, kidney, figure eight, cloverleaf, and bean shaped—as well as modern accessories, including gas heaters, automatic water levelers, and retractable roofs and sides. More supplemental recreational facilities, such as shuffleboard courts, volleyball, and horseshoes, and more deck equipment including guard rails, slides, and pool covers, are being included around larger pools.

Selected physical education facilities

The features discussed in this section should be of special interest to administrators, physical educators, and recreation specialists because of their adaptability to school and college physical education programs.

Limited shelters for physical education. The shelter or limited shelter provides protection from extremes of climate, uses the desirable elements of the natural environment, and creates an interesting background for physical

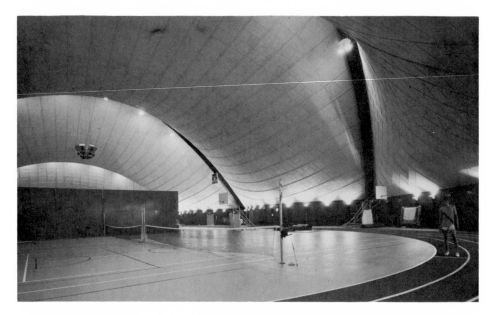

Graceland Fieldhouse, Lamoni, Iowa. (Courtesy Shaver & Co., Salina, Kan.)

education activities. See diagrams on p. 404 for utilization of limited shelters.

The actual design of the shelter is determined by climate, use, and the activity program. Methods of controlling air movement may be developed by using natural elements (trees and plantings), architectural elements (wall, roofs, and screens), and mechanical devices (fan, moving walls, and screens). Solar radiation may be controlled with natural shading and moving walls.

Limited shelters are presently being used in schools throughout the country. The Oneonta School System, Oneonta, Alabama has in use a 4,500 square foot, hard surfaced floor without walls. In the Cobb County public schools,

Marietta, Georgia, a 6,000 square foot all-weather surface is attached to the main building. Such shelters may be designed for elementary school students in view of the type of activities in the program and the shorter periods. These shelters cost about half as much as the traditional gymnasium.

Air-supported structures. This innovation consists of a large plastic bubble that is inflated and supported by continuous air pressure. It is the least expensive building that one can erect, costing from one-fifth to one-half of what a solid structure would cost. These facilities have served for housing military equipment, theaters, factories, swimming pools, tennis courts, and gymnasiums.

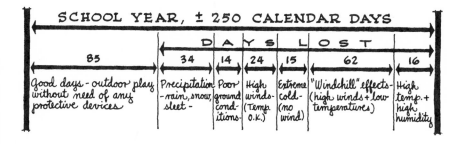

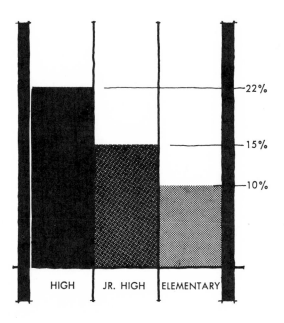

BUILDING SPACE DEVOTED TO PHYSICAL ACTIVITIES

Charts showing amount of space devoted to physical activities in schools, the implications of weather conditions for the physical education program, and some ideas for partial shelters for physical education programs. (From Shelter for physical education: a study of the feasibility of the use of limited shelters for physical education, College Station, Texas, Texas Engineering Experiment Station, Texas A & M University.)

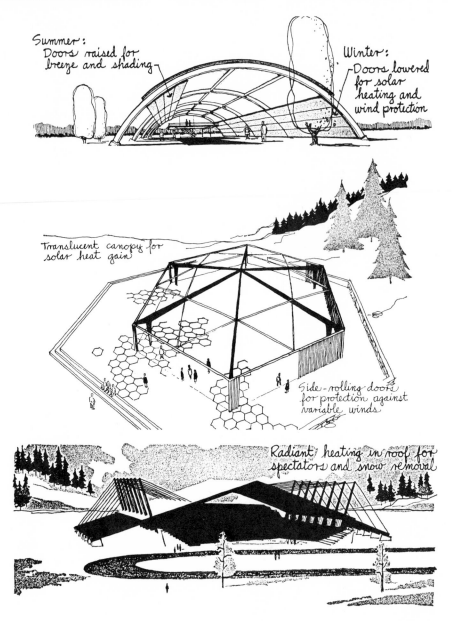

Summer:
Doors raised for
breeze and shading

Winter:
Doors lowered
for solar
heating and
wind protection

Translucent canopy for
solar heat gain

Side-rolling doors
for protection against
variable winds

Radiant heating in roof for
spectators and snow removal

Partial shelters for physical education.

The outside construction is usually made of vinyl-coated or Dacron polyester, which is lightweight, strong, and flexible. The fabric is flame-retardant, waterproof, tear-resistant, and mildew- and sunlight-resistant. Installation is simple and may be completed in a few hours by a minimum crew. The installation process includes placement of vinyl envelope and inflation. The bubble is supported by a blower that provides a constant flow of air pressure. The bubble may be easily dismantled by stopping the blower, opening the door, unhitching the attachments, and folding the bubble compactly. These structures will last a minimum of 5 to 7 years with continuous usage. They can be reconditioned at half the original price and will last longer if used less frequently.

Mini-gyms and fitness corners. Children,

especially young children, like to be active most of the time. However, most school children must confine their physical activities to the physical education class that may not meet every day. Even in gym classes, students are often required to participate amidst an atmosphere of formality when time is taken up in attendance lineups, exercises, testing and other planned activities. How can this be changed?

The answer may be found in the mini-gyms that would become a part of the daily school experience. The mini-gyms would be operated in the halls and alcoves of the school building. They might consist of climbing, pulling, and hanging apparatus that the students could use between classes, at study hours, lunch, and recess. This idea is to actually distribute the gymnasium throughout the school. Some other suggestions may include mats, chinningbars, inclines, walls to throw balls against, and carpeted corridors for stunts and tumbling.

In addition, classrooms too can be turned into mini-gyms with fitness corners for exercise and equipment such as stationary bicycles, rowing machines, and stand-up desks to promote activity.

This approach to exercise is inexpensive, a valuable aid to physical and emotional health, and an inducement to learning.

Artificial turf has been developed and successfully tried. Although there are some disadvantages to this type of surfacing, the initial reaction of students and teachers is that the turf provides excellent traction and helps the acoustics. It is easily cleaned with a vacuum.

Rubber-cushioned tennis courts are being used in some places. They consist of tough durable material about 4 inches thick, with the individual advantages of clay, turf, and composition courts being combined into one type of surfacing.

Other new developments in health and physical education facilities that have come into use in schools across the country are numerous. Sculptured play apparatus has been produced by a number of firms. It is designed to be more conducive to imaginative movements and creativity than conventional equipment. Hard-surfaced, rubberized, all-weather running tracks, radiant heating of decks on swimming pools, floating roofs with the elimination of non–load-bearing walls, interior climate control, better indoor and outdoor lighting, rubber padding for use under apparatus, park-school concept with land being used for school and recreational purposes, outdoor skating rinks, translucent plastic materials for swimming pool canopies and other uses, electrically operated machinery to move equipment and partitions and bleachers, and auxiliary gymnasiums used for both activity and classroom use are a few more of the new developments in facilities for health and physical education programs.

Park-school facilities

The park-school complex is another innovation that should be mentioned. In this type of setup the school is erected near a park, and the park facilities are used by both the school and the community. This has implications particularly for physical education and recreation programs, since the school usually uses the park facilities during school hours and the recreation department uses them after school hours, on weekends, and during vacation periods.

The T. Wendall Williams Community Education Center in Flint, Michigan is situated on a two-block site that adjoins a 72 acre park. The area consists of thirty classrooms, a lower elementary group activity area, a large sunken learning resources center, five team-teaching rooms, and a large gymnasium. The recreation area is located on park property and administered by the Flint Recreation and Park Department. Baseball, softball, soccer, football, basketball, and picnicking are provided for. There are swimming areas, tennis courts, and small-child activity areas. In the winter the pool is covered for all-year swimming, and the tennis courts are converted into a large artificial ice-skating rink. The park also provides natural areas for learning and recreation for all.

Utilizing community resources

Schools should take community resources into consideration in order to augment their facilities. Such facilities as parks, bowling alleys, swimming pools, ski slopes, and skating arenas, to name only a few, can extend the school physical education program and related sports activities. Most community facilities can be utilized during off-hours and after school, and the charge is frequently nominal.

TEACHING STATIONS

The teaching station concept should be taken into consideration when scheduling physical education classes. A teaching station is the space or setting where one teacher or staff member can carry on physical education activities for one group of students. The number and size of teaching stations available together with the number of teachers on the staff, the size of the group, the number of times the group meets, the number of periods in the school or college day, and the program of activities are important items to consider in planning.

According to the participants in the National Facilities Conference,* the following formulas are listed for determining the number of teaching stations needed.

Secondary schools and colleges

The formula for computing the number of teaching stations needed for physical education

---

*Participants in National Facilities Conference: Planning areas and facilities for health, physical education, and recreation, Washington, D. C., 1965, American Association for Health, Physical Education, and Recreation, p. 83.

in colleges and secondary schools is as follows:

$$\text{Minimum number of teaching stations} = \frac{\text{Number of students}}{\text{Average number of students per instructor}} \times$$

$$\frac{\text{Number of periods class meets each week}}{\text{Total number of class periods in school work}}$$

For example, if a school system projects its enrollment to 700 students and plans six class periods a day with an average class size of thirty students, and physical education is required daily, the formula is as follows:

$$\text{Minimum number of teaching stations} = \frac{700 \text{ students}}{30 \text{ per class}} \times$$

$$\frac{5 \text{ periods per week}}{30 \text{ periods per week}} = \frac{3,500}{900} = 3.9$$

Colleges could substitute pertinent facts into the same formula to determine the number of teaching stations they would need.

Elementary schools

The formula for computing the number of teaching stations needed for physical education in the elementary schools is:

$$\text{Minimum number of teaching stations} = \frac{\text{Number of classrooms of students}}{} \times$$

$$\frac{\text{Number of physical education periods per week per class}}{\text{Total periods in school week}}$$

For example, in an elementary school with six grades, with three classes at each level (approximately 450 to 540 students), ten 30-

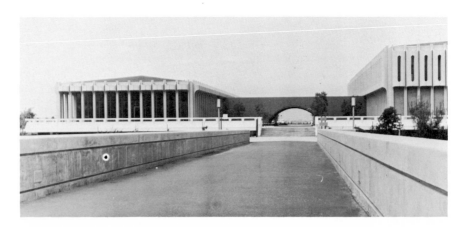

Overpass to athletic facilities. A unique feature of overall campus planning permits access to facilities from parking lots and academic buildings without the necessity of crossing a main thoroughfare. (University of California at Irvine.)

minute physical education periods per day, and physical education conducted on a daily basis, the teaching station needs are calculated as follows:

$$\text{Minimum number of teaching stations} = 18 \text{ classroom units} \times$$

$$\frac{5 \text{ periods per week}}{50 \text{ periods per week}} = \frac{90}{50} = 1.8$$

INDOOR FACILITIES

Several special areas and facilities are needed by programs of health, physical education, and recreation. A few of the indoor areas that are important and prominent in the conduct of these specialized programs are briefly discussed in this section.

Administrative and staff offices*

It is important, as far as practical and possible, for professional persons working in health, physical education, and recreation to have a section of a building set aside for administrative and staff offices. As a minimum there should be a large central office with a waiting room. The central office provides a

*See also Chapter 21 on Office Management.

place where the secretarial and clerical work can be performed, space for keeping records and files, and storage closets for office supplies. The waiting room can serve as a reception point where students and visitors can wait until staff members are ready to see them.

Separate offices for the staff members should be provided, if possible. This allows for a place where conferences can be held in private and without interruption. This is a very important consideration for health counseling and for discussing scholastic, family, recreational, and other problems. If separate offices are not practical, a desk should be provided for each staff member. In this event, there should be a private room available to staff members for conferences.

Other facilities that make for a more efficient and enjoyable administrative and staff setup are staff dressing rooms, departmental library, conference room, and toilet and lavatory facilities.

Locker, shower, and drying rooms

Health, physical education, and recreation activities require facilities for storage of clothes, showering, and drying. These are essential to good health and for a well-organized program.

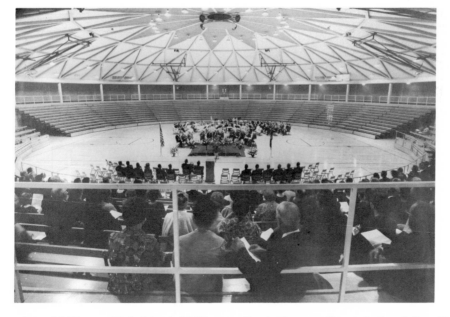

Gymnasium. (McPherson High School, McPherson, Kan.) (Courtesy Shaver & Co., Salina, Kan.)

ROOMS	FLOORS — Asphalt, Rubber, Linoleum Tile	Cement, Abrasive and Non-absorbent	Maple, hard	Terrazo Abrasive	Tile, ceramic	Brick	Brick, glazed	Cinder Block	Concrete	Plaster	LOWER WALLS — Tile, ceramic	Wood Panel	Moisture-proof	Brick	Brick, glazed	Cinder Block	Plaster	UPPER WALLS — Acoustic	Moisture-resistant	Concrete or Structure Tile	Plaster	CEILINGS — Tile, acoustic	Moisture-resistant
Apparatus Storage Room	1	2			1		2	1		C													
Classrooms	2	1	1		2		2	1	1		2				2	2	1			C	1	1	
Clubroom	2	1	1		2		2	1	1		2				2	1	1			C	1	1	
Corrective Room	1	1		2	1		2				2			2	1	2	2				1	1	
Custodial Supply Room			1	2																			
Dance Studio	2	1	1		2		1													C	1	1	
Drying Room (equip.)	1		2	2	1	1	1					1	1		1		*			C	*	1	
Gymnasium		1	1	2	1		2	1	1		2	2	2	2	1	2	1			C	1	1	
Health-Service Unit	1	1			2		2	1			C				2	1	1				1	1	
Laundry Room	2		1	2	1		2	2	1	1	C	*	1		1		*	*			*	*	
Locker Rooms	3		2	1	2	1	2	2	3	1		*	1		1	2			1	C	1	1	
Natatorium			1	2	1	3	2	2	1	1	1	*	2	2	1		*	*	1	C	*	*	
Offices	2	1			2		2	1	1		1		2		2	1	1			C	1	1	
Recreation Room	2	1		2	1		2	1	1		1	*	2		1	2	1	*		C	1	1	
Shower Rooms	3		2	1	1		1		2	1	1	*	2	1	2	2		*	1		1	*	
Special-activity Room	2	1	1		2		2	1	1		1		1		1	1	1			C	1	1	
Team Room	3		2	1	2	1	2	2	3	1		*	1		1	2			1	C	1	1	
Toilet Rooms	3		2	1	1		2	2	2	1		*	1		1	1	1		2	C	1	1	
Toweling-Drying Room (bath)	3		2	1	1		2	2	2	1		*	2		2	2	1	*			1	*	

Note: The numbers in the Table indicate first, second, and third choices. "C" indicates the material as being contrary to good practice. An * indicates desirable quality.

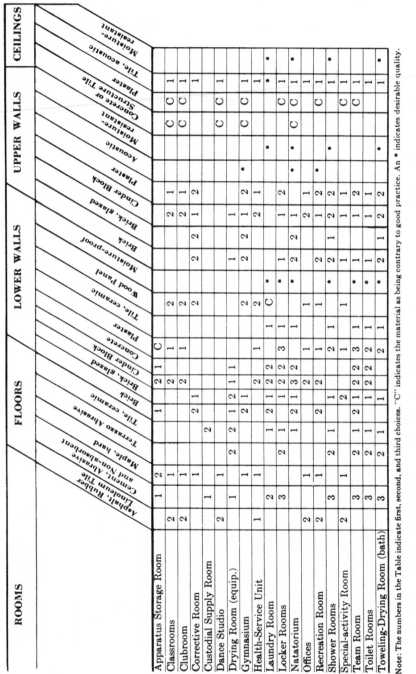

Suggested indoor surface materials. (From Participants in National Facilities Conference: Planning areas and facilities for health, physical education, and recreation, revised, Chicago, 1965, The Athletic Institute.)

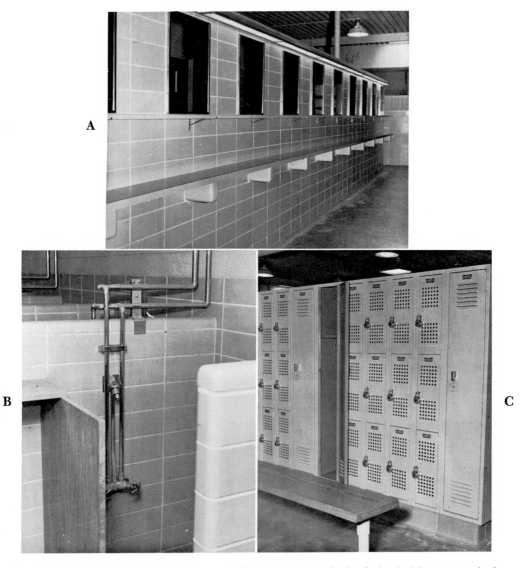

A, Dual-shelf system in the girls' dressing room. Books, purses, and other in-hand objects go on the lower shelf. Bobby pins, combs, compacts, and lipstick, of course, need to be at hand on the smaller upper shelf. **B,** A girl's shower stall. Picture taken from an upper angle. **C,** Locker arrangement utilized in both girls' and boys' locker rooms. The perforated storage lockers are 9 inches wide, 20 inches high, and 15 inches deep. Hook hangers provide a place to hang gymnasium wear. Each student has his own personal lock rented from the school. Shelves in the dressing lockers were lowered from 12 inches to 16 inches to make room for the large folios that many students carry. The dressing lockers are 8 inches high, 12 inches wide, and 15 inches deep. There is room for books, shoes, and clothes. (Courtesy Spring Branch Independent School District, Houston, Tex.)

The reason such facilities are often not fully utilized is that poor planning makes them inadequate and uncomfortable.

Locker and shower rooms should be readily accessible to activity areas. Locker rooms should not be congested places that students want to get out of as soon as possible. Instead, they should provide ample room, both storage and dressing type lockers, stationary benches, mirrors, recessed lighting fixtures, and drinking fountains.

An average of 14 square feet per individual at peak load, exclusive of the space utilized by the lockers, is required to provide proper space.

Storage lockers should be provided for each individual in the school or recreational program. An additional 10% should be installed for purposes of expanded enrollments or membership. These are lockers for the permanent use of each individual and can be utilized to hold essential clothing and other supplies. They can be smaller than the dressing lockers and some recommended sizes are these: 7½ by 12 by 24 inches, 6 by 12 by 36 inches, and 7½ by 12 by 18 inches. The basket type lockers are not looked upon with favor by many experts, because of the hygiene factor, the fact that an attendant is required for good administration of this system, and the necessity of carting the baskets from place to place.

Dressing lockers are utilized by participants only when actually engaging in activity. They are large in size, usually 12 by 12 by 54 inches or 12 by 12 by 48 inches in elementary schools and 12 by 12 by 72 inches for secondary schools and colleges and for community recreation programs.

Shower rooms should be provided that have both group and cubicle type showers. Some facility planners recommend that girls have a number of shower heads equal to 40% of the enrollment at peak load and the boys, 30% of the enrollment at peak load. Another recommendation is one shower head for four boys and one for three girls at peak load. These should be 4 feet apart. If showers are installed where a graded change of water temperature is provided and where the individual progresses through such a gradation, the number of shower heads can be reduced. The shower rooms should

also be equipped with liquid soap dispensers, good ventilation and heating, floors constructed of nonslip material, and recessed plumbing. The ceiling should be dome-shaped so that it will more readily shed water.

The drying room adjacent to the shower room is an essential. This should be equipped with proper drainage, good ventilation, towel bar, and a ledge that can be used to place a foot upon while drying.

A report of a conference on the planning of facilities for health, physical education, and recreation lists the following common errors in service facilities:

Failure to provide adequate locker and dressing space
Failure to plan dressing and shower area so as to reduce foot traffic to a minimum and establish clean, dry aisles for bare feet
Failure to provide a nonskid surface on dressing, shower, and toweling room floors
Failure to properly relate teaching stations with service facilities
Inadequate provision for drinking fountains
Failure to provide acoustical treatment where needed
Failure to provide and properly locate toilet facilities to serve all participants and spectators
Failure to provide doorways, hallways, or ramps so that equipment may be moved easily
Failure to design equipment rooms for convenient and quick check-in and check-out
Failure to provide mirrors and shelving for boys' and girls' dressing facilities
Failure to plan locker and dressing rooms with correct traffic pattern to swimming pool
Failure to construct shower, toilet, and dressing rooms with sufficient floor slope and properly located drains
Failure to place shower heads low enough and in such a position that the spray is kept within the shower room
Failure to provide shelves in the toilet room*

Gymnasiums

The type and number of gymnasiums that should be part of a school or recreational plant will depend on the number of individuals who will be participating, the variety of activities that will be conducted in this area, and the school level concerned.

General construction features to which most individuals will agree include smooth walls, hardwood floors (maple preferred—laid length-

---

*Planning facilities for health, physical education, and recreation, revised edition, Chicago, 1956, The Athletic Institute, Inc., p. 70.

This unit provides:

Two teaching stations

One standard inter-school basketball court

Two court areas for instruction and intra-mural basketball

Two court areas for volleyball, newcomb, etc.

Four court areas for badminton, paddle tennis, etc.

Two circle areas for instruction, dodge ball, and circle games

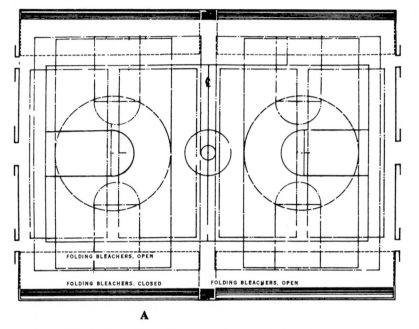

A

This unit provides:

Two teaching stations

One standard inter-school basketball court

Two court areas for in-struction and intra-mural basketball

Three court areas for volleyball, new-comb, etc.

Six court areas for badminton, paddle tennis, etc.

Four circle areas for instruction, dodge ball, and circle games

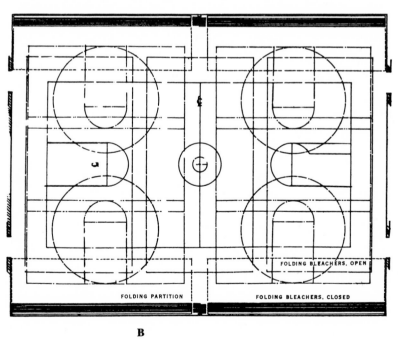

B

A, Illustrative plan of two teaching stations for junior high school gymnasium. **B,** Illustrative plan of two teaching stations for senior high school gymnasium. (From Participants in National Facilities Conference: Planning areas and facilities for health, physical education, and recreation, revised, Chicago, 1965, The Athletic Institute.)

wise), recessed lights, recessed radiators, adequate and well-screened windows, and storage space for the apparatus and other equipment utilized. It is also generally agreed that in schools it is best to have the gymnasium located in a separate wing of the building to isolate the noise and also as a convenient location for community groups that will be anxious to use such facilities.

The American Alliance for Health, Physical Education, and Recreation has listed several important factors to keep in mind when planning the gymnasium:

1. Hard maple flooring which is resilient and non-slippery.
2. Smooth interior walls to a height of 10 or 12 feet.
3. Upper walls need not be smooth.
4. The ceiling should reflect light and absorb sound, and there should be at least 22 to 24 feet from the floor to exposed beams.
5. Windows should be ten to twelve feet above floor and placed on long side of room.
6. Heating should be thermostatically controlled, radiators recessed with protecting grill or grate if placed at floor level.
7. Sub-flooring should be moisture- and termite-resistant and well ventilated.
8. Prior consideration must be given concerning the suspension of apparatus from the ceiling and the erection of wall-type apparatus.
9. Mechanical ventilation may be necessary.
10. Proper illumination meeting approved standards and selectively controlled for various activities must be designed.
11. Floor plates for standards and apparatus must be planned, as well as such items as blackboards, electric clocks and scoreboards, public address system, and provisions for press and radio.
12. Floor markings for various games should be placed after prime coat of seal has been applied and prior to application of the finishing coats.*

Many gymnasiums have folding doors that divide them into halves, thirds, or fourths and allow for activities to be conducted simultaneously on each side. This has proved satisfactory where separate gymnasiums could not be provided.

In elementary schools that need only one teaching station, a minimum floor space of 36 feet by 52 feet is required. Where two teaching stations are desired, floor space of 52 feet by 72 feet may be divided by a folding partition. In junior and senior high schools where only one teaching station is desired, a minimum floor space of 48 feet by 66 feet is necessary. If two teaching stations are necessary, an area 66 feet by 96 feet of floor space, exclusive of bleachers, will provide these teaching stations of minimum size. The folding partition that provides the two teaching stations should be motor driven. Where seating capacity is desired, additional space will be needed. If more than two teaching stations are desired, the gymnasium area may be extended to provide an additional station or activity rooms may be added. Of course, the addition of a swimming pool also provides an additional teaching station.

Other considerations for gymnasiums should include provisions for basketball backboards, mountings for various apparatus that will be used, recessed drinking fountains, places for hanging mats, outlets for various electric appliances and cleaning devices, proper line markings for activities, bulletin boards, and other essentials to a well-rounded program.

Common errors in construction of gymnasiums are:

Provision for spectator space at the sacrifice of instructional space.

Failure to mark floor for possible court games such as badminton, basketball, and volleyball.

Construction of a combination auditorium-gymnasium when separate facilities could be provided.

Installation of permanent bleachers instead of folding bleachers, resulting in loss of maximum use of floor space.

Failure to provide ventilated space below a built-up gymnasium floor.

Natural lighting construction permitting leakage and glare problems.*

Guidelines in gymnasium planning. The following guidelines are valid for administrators, architects, board members, and other persons involved in gymnasium planning. Many

*American Association for Health, Physical Education, and Recreation: Administrative problems in health education, physical education, and recreation, Washington, D. C., 1953, The Association, p. 83.

*Planning facilities for health, physical education, and recreation; revised edition, Chicago, 1956, The Athletic Institute; Inc., p. 63.

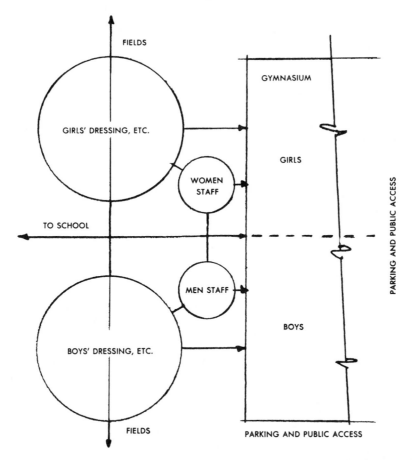

Orientation of gymnasium to related areas. (From Participants in National Facilities Conference: Planning areas and facilities for health, physical education, and recreation, revised, Chicago, 1965, The Athletic Institute.)

of these guidelines are overlooked by those responsible for gymnasium construction.

The roof. If the roof is not properly designed before construction, costly changes in equipment installation may occur at a later time. Ceiling support beams are also essential for the physical educator to make maximal use of the facility. The design of the roof should allow for support beams sufficient in strength to absorb the stress placed upon them in various activities. Support beams should be placed in such a manner that maximal flexibility in the location of apparatus is allowed for. The design should also consider the placement of gymnastic apparatus so that students are saved from obstructions in the event of falls.

The floor. The floor is a vital part of the gymnasium and should be constructed from hardwood, not tile. Although expensive, hardwood is safer, does not become slick, and is better for athletic performance. Plates for floor apparatus such as the highbar should be designed with safety and flexibility in mind.

The walls. Electrical outlets should be provided for throughout the gymnasium so that audiovisual areas can be used at each activity station. Walls behind baskets should be recessed and padded. This is safer than hanging pads near glazed tile walls. It is a good idea to provide a wall for students to practice their tennis skills. A line should be painted along the wall to indicate the height of the tennis net. The wall can also be used for hardball and other ball skills.

Lighting. Adequate durable lighting with recessed fixtures is essential. This type of fixture helps to prevent bulb breakage from ball activities.

Acoustics. Noise control should be a primary consideration in any gymnasium construction. Acoustic treatment of ceilings and walls can help to reduce or eliminate noise.

Special activity areas. Although gymnasiums are large and take up considerable space, there should still be additional areas for activities essential to school programs of health, physical education, and recreation.

Wherever possible, additional activity areas should be provided for remedial or adapted activities, apparatus, handball, squash, weight lifting, dancing, rhythms, fencing, and dramatics and for various recreational activities such as arts and crafts, lounging and resting, and bowling. The activities to be provided will depend on interests of participants and type of program. The recommended size of such auxiliary gymnasiums is 30 by 50 by 24 feet, or preferably 40 by 60 by 24 feet.

Another special room especially desirable in the elementary school is the all-purpose room that could be used for such activities as games, music, dramatics, and social events.

In reference to special activity areas, it should also be pointed out that regulation classrooms can be converted into these special rooms. This may be feasible where the actual construction of such costly facilities may not be practical.

The remedial or adapted activities room should be equipped with items such as horizontal ladders, mirrors, mats, climbing ropes, stall bars and benches, pulley weights, dumbbells, Indian clubs, shoulder wheels, and other such equipment suited for the particular needs of the individuals participating.

Auxiliary rooms. The main types of auxiliary areas found in connection with school and college health and physical education and recreation facilities are supply, checkout, custodial, and laundry rooms.

Supply rooms should be easily accessible from the gymnasium and other activity areas. In these rooms are stored balls, nets, standards, and other equipment needed for the programs that are offered. The size of these rooms varies according to the number of activities offered and the number of participants.

Checkout rooms should be provided on a seasonal basis. They house the equipment and supplies used in various seasonal activities.

Custodial rooms provide a place for storing equipment and supplies utilized in the maintenance of these specialized facilities.

Laundries should be adequate in size to accommodate the laundering of such essential items as towels, uniforms, and swimming suits.

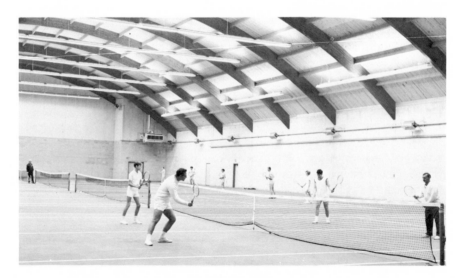

Special tennis structure. (Brigham Young University, Provo, Utah.)

Swimming pools

In the year 1900 there were very few indoor swimming pools in the public schools in the United States. Today, however, there are approximately 2,500 swimming pools in public schools.

According the Gabrielsen,* schools should have swimming pools for many reasons. Swimming is the number one recreational activity in America, and it is often listed by elementary and secondary school students as their favorite activity. Teaching all children how to swim could reduce the more than 8,000 deaths by drowning that occur in the United States each year. Knowing how to swim leads to many other excellent aquatic activities such as surfing, sailing, canoeing, fishing, scuba diving, and water skiing.

Gabrielsen in his report cited the major de-

sign decisions that must be made if a school or college decides to construct a pool. These include such items as the nature of the program to be conducted in a pool, type of overflow system to be used, dimensions and shape of pool, depth of the water, type of finish, type of filters and water treatment system, construction material to be used, amount of deck area, climate control, illumination, and number of spectators to be accommodated.

Some mistakes that Gabrielsen says should be avoided in the construction of a pool include entrances to the pool from the locker rooms opening onto the deep rather than the shallow end of the pool, pool base finished with slippery material such as glazed tile, insufficient depth of water for diving, improper placement of ladders, insufficient rate of recirculation of water to accommodate peak bathing loads, inadequate storage space, failure to use acoustic material on ceiling and walls, insufficient illumination, slippery tile on decks, and an inadequate overflow system at the ends of the pool.

Finally, in this report are listed some trends

---

*Professor M. A. Gabrielsen, New York University. From a speech given at the Conference on Planning, Constructing, Utilizing Physical Education, Recreation, and Athletic Facilities, sponsored by the Ohio Department of Education, Columbus, Ohio, December 10, 1969.

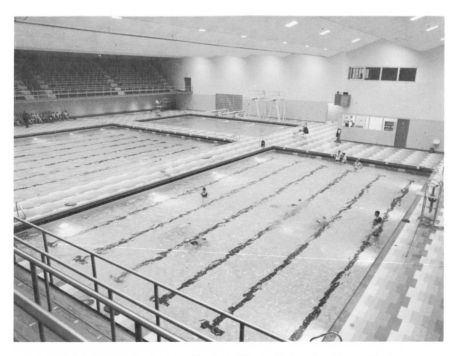

Swimming pool complex. (Brigham Young University, Provo, Utah.)

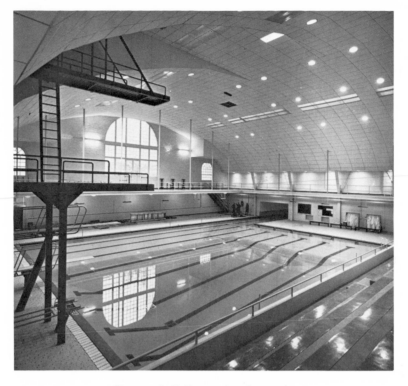

Dartmouth College swimming pool.

and innovations in pool design and operation. These include: the Rim-Flow Overflow System, inflatable roof structure, the skydome design, pool tent cover, floating swimming pool complex, prefabrication of pool tanks, automation of pool recirculating and filter systems, regenerative cycle filter system, adjustable height diving platform, variable depth bottoms, fluorescent underwater lights, automatic cleaning systems, and wave making machines.

Present types of swimming pools have in the main two objectives, one to provide instructional and competitive programs and the other for recreation.

The swimming pool should be located on or above the ground level, have southern exposure, be isolated from other units in the building, and be easily accessible from the central dressing and locker rooms. Materials that have been found most adaptive to swimming pools are smooth, glazed, light-colored tile or brick.

The standard indoor pool is 75 feet in length. The width should be a multiple of 7 feet, with a minimum of 35 feet. Depths vary from 2 feet

6 inches at the shallow end to 4 feet 6 inches at the outer limits of the shallow area. The shallow or instructional area should comprise about two-thirds of the pool. The deeper areas taper to 9 to 12 feet in depth. An added but important factor is a movable bulkhead that can be used to divide the pool into various instructional areas.

The deck space around the pool should be constructed of a nonslip material and provide ample space for land drills and demonstrations. The area above the water should be unobstructed. The ceiling should be at least 25 feet above the water if a 3-meter diving board will be used. The walls and the ceiling of the pool should be acoustically treated.

The swimming pool should be constructed to receive as much natural light as possible, with the windows located on the sides rather than on the ends. Artificial lighting should be recessed in the ceilings. Good lighting is especially important in the areas where the diving boards are located. Underwater lighting is beautiful but not an essential.

There should be an efficient system for ade-

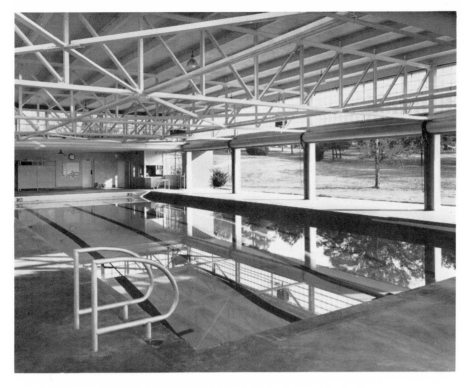

Swimming pool. (Alabama College, Montevallo, Ala.)

quately heating and circulating the water. The temperature of the water should range from 75° to 80° F.

If spectators are to be provided for, it is recommended that a gallery separate from the pool room proper be erected along the length of the pool.

An office adjacent to the pool where records and first-aid supplies can be kept is advisable. Such an office should be equipped with windows that overlook the entire length of the pool. Also, there should be lavatory and toilet facilities available.

The swimming pool is a costly operation. Therefore, it is essential that it be planned with the help of the best advice obtainable. Specialists who are well acquainted with such facilities and who conduct swimming activities should be brought into conferences with the architect, a representative from the public health department, and experts in such essentials as lighting, heating, construction, and acoustics.

Innovations in swimming pool complexes are a current trend. The Art Linkletter Natatorium at Springfield College, Springfield, Massachusetts measures 44 feet by 169 feet. One wall can be positioned anywhere along the length of the pool, thus forming two areas of any chosen size. Beneath the water level in the pool are picture windows that look into classrooms where swimming techniques can be studied.

Another innovative design in swimming pools is the aquatic center at Princeton University. This complex was designed to meet the needs of swimming as a spectator sport. Seating is provided for 3,500 persons, and the 50-meter pool features a submersible deck that can be lowered to divide the pool into varsity and teaching areas. The diving decks are hydraulically operated for height adjustments, and sidewall windows have been eliminated because of the possible danger of mistaking window glare for the pool surface.

HEALTH SCIENCE INSTRUCTION FACILITIES

The health science instruction program should have facilities especially designed to meet the needs of educating students in respect to health matters. The National Facilities Conference stresses the following standards:

1. Space for 35 square feet per pupil, maximum of 30 pupils
2. Flexible teacher location
3. Provision for various teaching methods, including laboratory demonstration
4. Flexibility of seating
5. Hot and cold running water and gas outlet
6. Educational exhibit space
7. Storage space
8. Provision for using audio-visual devices (electrical outlets, window shades, screens)
9. Access to health service unit
10. Exemplary environmental features
11. Adequate handwashing facilities, drinking fountains, and toilets
12. Air-conditioning
13. Accessible to and usable by the disabled
14. Planned jointly for community use *

*Participants in National Facilities Conference: Planning areas and facilities for health, physical education, and recreation, Washington, D. C., 1965, American Association for Health, Physical Education, and Recreation, p. 209.

The recommended sizes in square feet for a floor plan for a health instruction laboratory are given in Table 15-1.

Classrooms

Classrooms utilized for health instruction should include the requirements discussed in relation to seating, lighting, color of walls and ceilings, heating and ventilation, acoustics, and sanitation. All classrooms should be healthful, comfortable, and adaptable, regardless of whether they are being used for health instruction or some other subject.

There is one feature, however, that should receive consideration if there is not a special room set aside for such a purpose. This is the use of audiovisual equipment. There are ample resources for audiovisual material that can be utilized very effectively in any health instruction program. There should be available projection and sound equipment including an opaque projector, slide projector, filmstrip projector, motion picture projector, and turntables.

Table 15-1. Recommended sizes in square feet of health service facilities for schools of various sizes *

| | Enrollment | | | | | |
	200 to 300	301 to 500	501 to 700	701 to 900	901 to 1,100	1,101 to 1,300
Waiting room	80	80	100	100	100	120
Examining room†	200	200	200	240	240	240
Rest room (total area for boys and girls)‡	100	180	220	260	300§	240§
Toilets (48 square feet total area—provide one for girls and one for boys)						

Optional areas

Dental clinic	100 square feet for all schools
Office space	80 square feet for each office provided
Eye examination	120 square feet minimum for all schools

*From Participants in National Facilities Conference: Planning areas and facilities for health, physical education, and recreation, Chicago, 1965, The Athletic Institute, p. 211. Based on data from State Department of Education: School planning manual, School Service Section, vol. 37, 1954, Richmond, Va.

†Examining room areas include 6 square feet for clothes closet and 24 square feet for storage closets.

‡For determining the number of cots, allow one cot per 100 pupils up to 400 pupils, and one cot per 200 pupils above 400. Round out fractions to nearest whole number. Allow 50 square feet of floor space for each of the first two cots and 40 square feet for each additional cot.

§In schools enrolling 901 to 1,100, a three-cot rest room is suggested for boys and a four-cot rest room for girls, and in 1,101-pupil to 1,300-pupil schools, a three-cot rest room is suggested for boys and a five-cot rest room for girls.

Note: For larger schools, add multiples of the above areas to obtain total needs.

There should also be outlets for electrical connections. Projection equipment should be installed in the rear of the room and audio equipment outlets in the front. There should be shades or other facilities for darkening the room. Finally, a screen should be available.

Another consideration in any health instruction room is a large display board that can be used to illustrate the material that is presented.

Health service facilities

The health services are a very important part of the health program and require adequate facilities to carry out the responsibilities assigned to this health area. DeWeese and Moore * made an extensive study of the health service facilities and concluded that at least 720 square feet of floor surface should be provided and include the following:

1. Administrative office
2. Library for health science instruction material

---

*DeWeese, A. O., and Moore, V. M.: The organization of a school health service comprising from 500 to 1000 pupils from kindergarten through high school, Journal of School Health **34:**415, 1964.

3. Rest rooms
4. Examination room
5. Conference facilities
6. Space for first-aid care and treatment
7. Space for scientific and educational displays
8. Storage and toilet facilities

Health service suite. To have a practical health service setup that can accommodate examination work, a suite is needed rather than just one room. Experts recommend at least four rooms, which include examining, waiting, and rest rooms for boys and for girls. In addition there should be toilet facilities for each sex. Several exits from the examining room are recommended as a means of expediting the conduct of health services and eliminating confusion.

The health service suite may also become the nurse's headquarters. In this case, there should be room for various items such as health records, desk, and files.

The color and furnishings of the waiting room should provide an attractive and cheerful atmosphere. A desk for clerical help can also be provided. There should be screens, if necessary, to give privacy to the examining and rest rooms

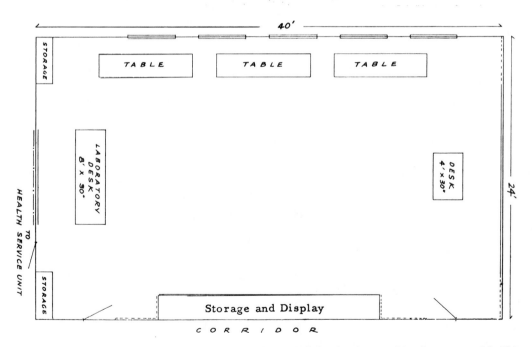

Health instruction laboratory. (From Participants in National Facilities Conference: Planning areas and facilities for health, physical education, and recreation, revised, Chicago, 1965, The Athletic Institute.)

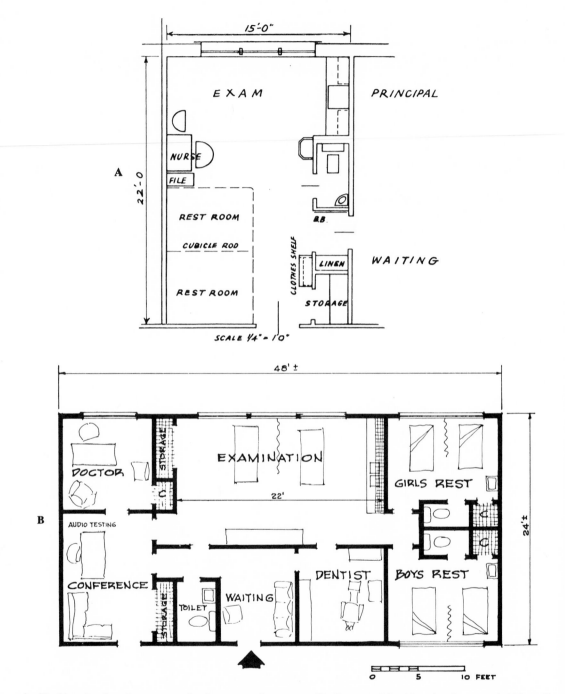

A, Health suite for elementary school—seven classrooms. **B,** Suggested health suite for over 1,100-pupil school. **C,** Suggested health suite for up to 700-pupil school. (From Participants in National Facilities Conference: Planning areas and facilities for health, physical education, and recreation, revised, Chicago, 1965, The Athletic Institute.)

that are part of the health suite and attached to the waiting room.

The examining room should be large enough to accommodate all the necessary equipment, supplies, and measuring devices. Provisions for eye testing, weighing, first aid, examining procedures, parent interviews, and other essentials should be kept in mind.

The rest rooms should be large enough to hold necessary cots, tables, and other items. They should also be equipped with subdued lighting, walls and ceilings that keep noise to a minimum, and other conveniences that contribute to rest.

A Committee on School Health Service Facilities of the American School Health Association conducted an extensive study of health service units throughout the country. This committee, recognizing that there could be no standard health unit that would meet the needs of schools everywhere, did, however, indicate what an average health unit might be, on the basis of statistical information gathered from their survey. According to this committee, the elementary school health service unit consisting of approximately 400 square feet would probably contain the following:

Examination room
Cot-room
Toilet room
Storage spaces
Testing and
    dressing room

Waiting room
Dental examination
    room, in some
    cases

Health service units for secondary schools would require approximately 600 to 700 square feet of floor space and consist of the following:

Examination room
Two cot rooms
Two toilet rooms

Storage spaces
Waiting room
Testing room

The following general statements help describe some essential considerations for a health service unit:

1. Future expansion should be considered.
2. The unit should be located near the administrative area, for ease of supervision, and away from noisy areas such as the shops, gymnasiums and music rooms.
3. Finishes should be of a type that can be easily maintained.
4. Attractive colors are important.
5. Service facilities such as sinks, lavatories, counters, and toilets should be of appropriate size for the pupils to be served.
6. Telephones are a necessity.

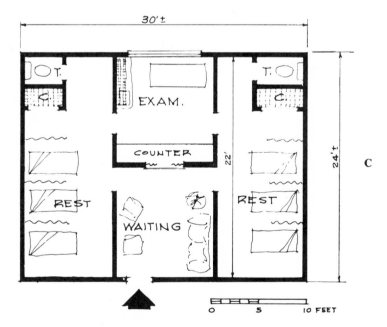

For legend see opposite page.

Cafeteria

The school lunch is a vital factor in the general health of any child and is an important part of his or her educational experiences. Furthermore, the cafeteria in any school or college recreational or other building is an important consideration and concern of individuals engaged in health, physical education, and recreation work.

The cafeteria should be easily accessible from anywhere within the building, as well as the service driveway. The size depends on the number of individuals to be served. In general, from 10 to 12 square feet per person is required to peak load for the dining area.

The size of the kitchen area depends on the number of meals to be prepared. The kitchen should contain all the equipment and supplies essential to the preparation and serving of good meals. Such equipment as ranges, ovens, sinks, dish-washing machines, refrigerators, tables, service trucks, counters, and kitchen machines such as mixers, peelers, and slicers should be provided.

The dining-room part of the cafeteria should be equipped with the necessary tables and chairs, serving counter, refrigerated counters, silver, napkins, plates, trays, drinking fountain, and other essentials.

The physical appearance of the cafeteria should be attractive, with adequate lighting, light colors, and floors that are easy to clean. The cafeteria should be quiet and conducive to enjoyable and satisfactory eating conditions.

OUTDOOR FACILITIES

The outdoor facilities that will be discussed in this section are (1) play areas, (2) game areas, (3) outdoor swimming pools, and (4) camps.

Play areas

Many factors must be taken into consideration when planning outdoor facilities for schools and colleges. The location, topography, soil drainage, water supply, size, shape, and natural features are a few important considerations before a site is selected. The outdoor facilities should be as near the gymnasium and locker rooms as possible and yet far enough from the classrooms so that the noise will not be a disturbing factor.

The play areas should serve the needs and interests of the students for the entire school year and at the same time should provide a setting for activities during vacation periods. The needs and interests of the citizens of the community must also be taken into consideration, since the play areas can be used for part of the community recreation program. This is especially important in some communities where such facilities can be planned as education and recreation centers. Since the community uses the areas after the school day is over, the plan is feasible.

The size of the playground area should be determined on the basis of activities offered in the program and the number of individuals who will be using the facilities at peak load. Possibilities for expansion should also be kept in mind.

Playground and recreation areas will be discussed under the three headings of elementary, junior high, and senior high school.

Elementary school. The activities program in the elementary school suggests what facilities should be available. Children of the primary grades engage in big muscle activity involving adaptations of climbing, jumping, skipping, kicking, throwing, leaping, and catching. The children in the intermediate and upper elementary grades utilize not only these activities but also others as games of low organization, team games, and fundamental skills used in playing these games.

The playground area for an elementary school should be located near the building and should be easily accessible from the elementary classrooms. The kindergarten children should have a section of the playground for their exclusive use. This should be at least 5,000 square feet in size and separated from the rest of the playground. It should consist of a surfaced area, a grass area, and a place for sand and digging. The sand area should be enclosed to prevent the sand from being scattered. It is also wise to have a shaded area where storytelling and similar activities may be conducted. Some essential equipment would include swings, slides, seesaws, climbing structures, tables, and seats.

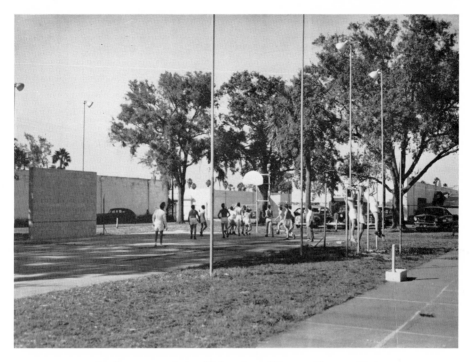

Outdoor gymnasium. (University of Tampa, Tampa, Fla.)

The children older than kindergarten age in the elementary school should have play space that includes turf, apparatus, shaded, multiple-use paved, and recreation areas.

The turf area provides space for many field and team games. Provisions for speed ball, soccer, field hockey, softball, and field ball could be included.

The apparatus area should provide such equipment as climbing bars in the form of a Jungle Jim, horizontal bars, and Giant Strides. There should be ample space to provide for the safety of the participants.

The shaded area may provide space for such activities as marbles, hopscotch, or ring toss and also storytelling.

The multiple-use paved area may serve for a variety of purposes and activities on a year-round basis by both school and community. It can house basketball, tennis, and handball courts, games of minimum organization, and other activities. This area should be paved with material that takes into consideration resiliency, safety, and durability. Rapid and efficient drainage is essential. Lines may be painted on the area for the various types of games. Schools should allow additional space adjacent to this area for possible future expansion.

Other recreation areas that have important implications for the community are a landscaped, parklike area, a place for quiet activites such as dramatics and informal gatherings, a wading pool, a place for older adults to congregate, and a place for children to have gardening opportunities.

Junior high school. The junior high school play and recreation area, planned and developed for the children who attend the school and also for the adults in the community, should be located on a larger site than that for the elementary school. Some suggestions have been made that it consist of from 10 to 25 or more acres. Local conditions will play a part in deciding the amount of area available.

Many of the facilities of the elementary school will be a part of the junior high school. In many cases, however, the various areas should be increased in size. There should be a place for small children, apparatus, quiet games, and a wading pool, as in the elementary schools. The multiple-use paved area or turf area for games should be increased in size.

The program for junior high school girls should stress a broad base in fundamentals for participation in such activities as archery, volleyball, tennis, and hockey.

The boys' program may include soccer, touch football, baseball, speed ball, softball, and golf. A track should also be included. Therefore, the necessary facilities should provide for those activities that will be part of the regular physical education class as well as the intramural program.

A landscaped, parklike area should be provided for the various recreational activities in which people in the community like to engage, such as walking, picnicking, skating, and fly casting.

Senior high school. The senior high school physical education program is characterized to a more pronounced degree by a team game program in various activities. This emphasis, together with the fact that facilities are needed for the recreational use of the community, requires an even larger area than those for the two previous educational levels. Estimates range from 10 to 40 acres for such a site.

Most of the areas that have been listed in discussing the elementary and junior high schools should again be included at the senior high school. This means there would be facilities for young children, such as apparatus, pool, and a place for quiet activities. Where there was an increase in size of many areas at the junior high over the elementary level, there should again be an increase in size at the high school level over the junior high.

There should be considerably more space for the various field games so that not only can physical education class instruction take place but also at the same time fullsized official fields will be available for such activities as softball, field hockey, soccer, speed ball, lacrosse, football, and baseball. This would be on an intramural as well as an interscholastic basis. Also, the community recreation program could make use of these facilities.

Football and track can be provided for in an area of approximately 4 acres, with the football field being placed within the track oval. A baseball field is questionable in such an area, because track and baseball are both spring sports. Baseball needs an area of about 350 feet by 350 feet. This allows for a minimum of 50 feet from home plate to the backstop and also allows for adequate space outside the first and third base lines.

Game areas

The recommended dimensions for game areas for school physical education programs have been outlined by a group of experts as shown in Table 15-2. An area of about 1 acre will accommodate four tennis courts, four handball courts, three badminton courts, and two volleyball courts.

There should be a separate area for high school girls with a minimum area of 320 feet by 280 feet, which is approximately 2 acres in size. Such an area will permit basic physical education instructional classes to be held and also provide fields for softball, field hockey, soccer, speedball, lacrosse, and other activities.

High school boys should also be adequately provided for in addition to the many courts areas that include basketball, softball, and other activities. There should be proper space for track if desired, an oval one-fourth mile in length or at least a straightaway of 380 feet and 15 to 20 feet in width. Of course, there is also the need for the interschool athletic area, which usually includes football, track, baseball, and soccer.

Not to be forgotten should be the winter activities. With such activities gaining increased popularity, provision should be made for skiing, sleds, skating, and other winter activities.

The New York State Department of Education* recommends that the outdoor facilities for the basic needs of a physical education and recreation program, from kindergarten to grade twelve, should consist of a minimum of 12 acres of land. This area should be divided into an elementary area of 3 acres; courts area of 1 acre; high school girls' area of 2 acres, a high school boys' intramural area of 3 acres, and an interschool athletic area of 3 acres. With the trend

*New York State Department of Education: Planning the outdoor physical education facilities, Albany, 1964, The Department.

Table 15-2. Recommended dimensions for game areas * †

	Elementary	Upper grades	High school (adults)	Area size (sq. ft.)
Basketball	40' × 60'	42' × 74'	50' × 84'	5,000
Volleyball	25' × 50'	25' × 50'	30' × 60'	2,800
Badminton			20' × 44'	1,800
Paddle tennis			20' × 44'	1,800
Deck tennis			18' × 40'	1,800
Tennis		36' × 78'	36' × 78'	7,200
Ice hockey			85' × 200'	17,000
Field hockey			180' × 300'	54,000
Horseshoes		10' × 40'	10' × 50'	1,000
Shuffleboard			6' × 52'	648
Lawn bowling			14' × 110'	7,800
Tetherball	10' circle	12' circle	12' circle	
Croquet	38' × 60'	38' × 60'	38' × 60'	2,275
Handball	18' × 26'	18' × 26'	20' × 34'	1,280
Baseball			350' × 350'	122,500
Archery		50' × 150'	50' × 300'	20,000
Softball (12'' ball)‡	150' × 150'	200' × 200'	250' × 250'	62,500
Football—with 440-yard track—220-yard straightaway			300' × 600'	180,000
Touch football		120' × 300'	160' × 360'	68,400
6-man football			120' × 300'	49,500
Soccer			165' × 300'	57.600

*From Planning facilities for health, physical education, and recreation, revised edition, Chicago, 1956, The Athletic Institute, Inc., p. 26.
†Table covers a single unit; many of above can be combined.
‡Dimensions vary with size of ball used.

toward more coeducational activities, the boys' and girls' areas might be combined. The interschool athletic area would be used for baseball in the spring and summer and football or soccer in the fall. A quartermile track could also be added, but in this case the interschool athletic program should have 7 acres of land. The recommendation further points out that if archery, golf, natural theater, picnic area, skiing, and tobogganing area are desired, additional land will be necessary.

A new concept in play areas is the multi-purpose sports court. This small, self-contained, fenced in court provides for a variety of activities in a small area. The average sport court is 12 feet by 24 feet by 10½ feet and is completely enclosed (including top) with a weather-proofed steel-tube and link fence that rests like a box on the floor of the court. Low-cost lighting and canvas covering can be used for evening and colder weather activities. The floor is frequently a raised wooden deck that allows for quick drainage and a weather-resistant playing surface. However, pads of other playing surfaces can be laid over the wooden deck. The court can be used for basketball, volleyball, paddle tennis, handball, and other activities. This type of court is excellent for crowded urban areas, industrial recreation programs, schools, apartments, and individual homes.

Outdoor swimming pools

The outdoor swimming pool is a popular and important facility in many communities. To a great degree climatic conditions will determine the advisability of such a facility.

Outdoor pools are built in various shapes, including oval, circular, T-shaped, and rectangular. Rectangular pools are most popular because of easier construction and because they lend themselves better to competitive swimming events.

The size of pools varies, depending upon the

number of persons they are to serve. One recommendation has been made that 12 square feet of water space per swimmer be allotted for swimming purposes, or, if the deck is taken into consideration, 20 square feet of space for swimming and walking area per swimmer.

The decks for outdoor pools should be larger than those for indoor pools. This larger space will serve to accommodate more people and also provide space for sunbathing.

Shower facilities should be provided to ensure that every swimmer takes a soapy shower in the nude before entering the water. A basket system for storing clothes has been found practical instead of the locker type of system that is used inside. In cases where the pool is located adjacent to the school, it sometimes is practical to use the locker and shower facilities of the school. However, it is strongly advised that wherever possible separate shower and basket facilities be provided. Toilets should also be provided for the convenience of the swimmers.

Since swimming is popular at night as well as in the daytime, lights should be provided in order that a great percentage of the population may participate in this healthful and enjoyable activity.

Diving boards generally are of wood or metal, but in recent years glass and plastic ones have proved popular. The standard heights of boards are 1 and 3 meters. The 1-meter board should be over water 9 to 10 feet in depth and the 3-meter board over 10 to 12 feet in depth. The board or any diving takeoff area should have a nonskid covering. The boards should be securely fastened to the ground or foundation.

The rules and regulations concerning diving equipment should be clearly posted near the diving areas. Roping off and patrolling the area are good safety precautions.

The checklist at the end of the chapter provides further information on swimming pool standards. *

Camps †

Since camping is becoming an increasingly popular activity in both school and recreational programs, it should receive consideration.

Camps should be located within easy reach of the school and community. They should be in locations that are desirable from the standpoints of scenic beauty, safety, accessibility, water, and natural resources pertinent

*For more information on swimming pools, see pp. 415-417.
†See Chapter 25.

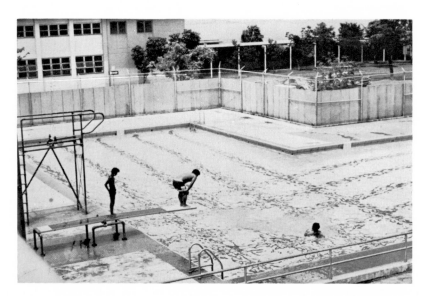

Swimming pool. (Wallace Rider Farrington High School, Honolulu, Hawaii.)

to the program offered. Activities usually offered include fishing, hiking, swimming, campcraft, boating, nature study, and appropriate winter sports. The natural terrain and other resources can contribute much toward such a program.

There should be adequate housing, eating, sanitary, waterfront, and other facilities essential to camp life. These do not have to be as elaborate as those in the home or school but instead can be very simple. Adequate facilities for protection against the elements are essential, however. Facilities should also meet acceptable standards of health and sanitation. In general, camp structures should be adapted to the climatic conditions of the particular area in which the camp is located. It is wise to consult public health authorities when selecting a camp site. Sometimes existing facilities can be converted to camp use. The camp site should be purchased outright or a long-term lease acquired.

CHECKLIST FOR FACILITY PLANNERS *

General

	Yes	No
1. A clear-cut statement has been prepared on the nature and scope of the program, and the special requirements for space, equipment, fixtures, and facilities dictated by the activities to be conducted.		
2. The facility has been planned to meet the total requirements of the program as well as the special needs of those who are to be served.		
3. The plans and specifications have been checked by all governmental agencies (city, county, and state) whose approval is required by law.		
4. Plans for areas and facilities conform to state and local regulations and to accepted standards and practices.		
5. The areas and facilities planned make possible the programs which serve the interests and needs of all the people.		
6. Every available source of property or funds has been explored, evaluated, and utilized whenever appropriate.		
7. All interested persons and organizations concerned with the facility have had an opportunity to share in its planning (professional educators, users, consultants, administrators, engineers, architects, program specialists, building managers, and builder—a team approach).		
8. The facility and its appurtenances will fulfill the maximum demands of the program. The program has not been curtailed to fit the facility.		
9. The facility has been functionally planned to meet the present and anticipated needs of specific programs, situations, and publics.		
10. Future additions are included in present plans to permit economy of construction.		
11. Lecture classrooms are isolated from distracting noises.		
12. Storage areas for indoor and outdoor equipment are adequately sized. They are located adjacent to the gymnasia.		
13. Shelves in storage rooms are slanted toward the wall.		
14. All passageways are free of obstructions; fixtures are recessed.		
15. Facilities for health services, health testing, health instruction, and the first-aid and emergency-isolation rooms are suitably interrelated.		
16. Buildings, specific areas, and facilities are clearly identified.		
17. Locker rooms are arranged for ease of supervision.		
18. Offices, teaching stations, and service facilities are properly interrelated.		
19. Special needs of the physically handicapped are met, including a ramp into the building at a major entrance.		

* Adapted from Participants in National Facilities Conference: Planning areas and facilities for health, physical education, and recreation, Washington, D. C., 1965, American Association for Health, Physical Education, and Recreation, pp. 256-260.

Continued.

CHECKLIST FOR FACILITY PLANNERS—cont'd

General—cont'd

	Yes	No
20. All "dead space" is used.		
21. The building is compatible in design and comparable in quality and accommodation to other campus structures.		
22. Storage rooms are accessible to the play area.		
23. Workrooms, conference rooms, and staff and administrative offices are interrelated.		
24. Shower and dressing facilities are provided for professional staff members and are conveniently located.		
25. Thought and attention have been given to making facilities and equipment as durable and vandalproof as possible.		
26. Low-cost maintenance features have been adequately considered.		
27. This facility is a part of a well-integrated master plan.		
28. All areas, courts, facilities, equipment, climate control, security, etc. conform rigidly to detailed standards and specifications.		
29. Shelves are recessed and mirrors are supplied in appropriate places in rest rooms and dressing rooms. Mirrors are not placed above lavatories.		
30. Dressing space between locker rows is adjusted to the size and age level of students.		
31. Drinking fountains are conveniently placed in locker-room areas or immediately adjacent thereto.		
32. Special attention is given to provision for the locking of service windows and counters, supply bins, carts, shelves, and racks.		
33. Provision is made for the repair, maintenance, replacement, and off-season storage of equipment and uniforms.		
34. A well-defined program for laundering and cleaning of towels, uniforms, and equipment is included in the plan.		
35. Noncorrosive metal is used in dressing, drying, and shower areas except for enameled lockers.		
36. Antipanic hardware is used where required by fire regulations.		
37. Properly placed hose bibbs and drains are sufficient in size and quantity to permit flushing the entire area with a water hose.		
38. A water-resistant, coved base is used under the locker base and floor mat, and where floor and wall join.		
39. Chalkboards and/or tackboards with map tracks are located in appropriate places in dressing rooms, hallways, and classrooms.		
40. Book shelves are provided in toilet areas.		
41. Space and equipment are planned in accordance with the types and number of enrollees.		
42. Basement rooms, being undesirable for dressing, drying, and showering, are not planned for those purposes.		
43. Spectator seating (permanent) in areas which are basically instructional is kept at a minimum. Roll-away bleachers are used primarily. Balcony seating is considered as a possibility.		
44. Well-lighted and effectively displayed trophy cases enhance the interest and beauty of the lobby.		
45. The space under the stairs is used for storage.		
46. Department heads' offices are located near the central administrative office, which includes a well-planned conference room.		
47. Workrooms are located near the central office and serve as a repository for departmental materials and records.		
48. The conference area includes a cloak room, lavatory, and toilet.		
49. In addition to regular secretarial offices established in the central and department chairmen's offices, a special room to house a secretarial pool for staff members is provided.		
50. Staff dressing facilities are provided. These facilities may also serve game officials.		

CHECKLIST FOR FACILITY PLANNERS—cont'd

General—cont'd

	Yes	No
51. The community and/or neighborhood has a ''round table''—planning round table.		
52. All those (persons and agencies) who should be a party to planning and development are invited and actively engaged in the planning process.		
53. Space and area relationships are important. They have been carefully considered.		
54. Both long-range plans and immediate plans have been made.		
55. The body comfort of the child, a major factor in securing maximum learning, has been considered in the plans.		
56. Plans for quiet areas have been made.		
57. In the planning, consideration has been given to the need for adequate recreation areas and facilities, both near and distant from the homes of people.		
58. Plans recognize the primary function of recreation as being enrichment of learning through creative self-expression, self-enhancement, and the achievement of self-potential.		
59. Every effort has been exercised to eliminate hazards.		
60. The installation of low-hanging door closers, light fixtures, signs, and other objects in traffic areas has been avoided.		
61. Warning signals—both visible and audible—are included in the plans.		
62. Ramps have a slope equal to or greater than a 1-foot rise in 12 feet.		
63. Minimum landings for ramps are 5 feet × 5 feet, they extend at least 1 foot beyond the swinging arc of a door, have at least a 6-foot clearance at the bottom, and have level platforms at 30-foot intervals on every turn.		
64. Adequate locker and dressing spaces are provided.		
65. The design of dressing, drying, and shower areas reduces foot traffic to a minimum and establishes clean, dry aisles for bare feet.		
66. Teaching stations are properly related to service facilities.		
67. Toilet facilities are adequate in number. They are located to serve all groups for which provisions are made.		
68. Mail services, outgoing and incoming, are included in the plans.		
69. Hallways, ramps, doorways, and elevators are designed to permit equipment to be moved easily and quickly.		
70. A keying design suited to administrative and instructional needs is planned.		
71. Toilets used by large groups have circulating (in and out) entrances and exists.		

Climate control

	Yes	No
1. Provision is made throughout the building for climate control—heating, ventilating, and refrigerated cooling.		
2. Special ventilation is provided for locker, dressing, shower, drying, and toilet rooms.		
3. Heating plans permit both area and individual room control.		
4. Research areas where small animals are kept and where chemicals are used have been provided with special ventilating equipment.		
5. The heating and ventilating of the wrestling gymnasium have been given special attention.		

Electrical

	Yes	No
1. Shielded, vaporproof lights are used in moisture-prevalent areas.		
2. Lights in strategic areas are key controlled.		
3. Lighting intensity conforms to approved standards.		
4. An adequate number of electrical outlets are strategically placed.		
5. Gymnasium and auditorium lights are controlled by dimmer units.		
6. Locker-room lights are mounted above the space between lockers.		
7. Natural light is controlled properly for purposes of visual aids and other avoidance of glare.		

Continued.

CHECKLIST FOR FACILITY PLANNERS—cont'd

Electrical—cont'd

	Yes	No
8. Electrical outlet plates are installed 3 feet above the floor unless special use dictates other locations.		
9. Controls for light switches and projection equipment are suitably located and inter-related.		
10. All lights are shielded. Special protection is provided in gymnasia, court areas, and shower rooms.		
11. Lights are placed to shine between rows of lockers.		

Walls

1. Movable and folding partitions are power-operated and controlled by keyed switches.		
2. Wall places are located where needed and are firmly attached.		
3. Hooks and rings for nets are placed (and recessed in walls) according to court locations and net heights.		
4. Materials that clean easily and are impervious to moisture are used where moisture is prevalent.		
5. Shower heads are placed at different heights—4 feet (elementary) to 7 feet (university) —for each school level.		
6. Protective matting is placed permanently on the walls in the wrestling room, at the ends of basketball courts, and in other areas where such protection is needed.		
7. An adequate number of drinking fountains is provided. They are properly placed (recessed in wall).		
8. One wall (at least) of the dance studio has full-length mirrors.		
9. All corners in locker rooms are rounded.		

Ceilings

1. Overhead-supported apparatus is secured to beams engineered to withstand stress.		
2. The ceiling height is adequate for the activities to be housed.		
3. Acoustical materials impervious to moisture are used in moisture-prevalent areas.		
4. Skylights, being impractical, are seldom used because of problems in waterproofing roofs and the controlling of sun rays (gyms).		
5. All ceilings except those in storage areas are acoustically treated with sound-absorbent materials.		

Floors

1. Floor plates are placed where needed and are flush-mounted.		
2. Floor design and materials conform to recommended standards and specifications.		
3. Lines and markings are painted on floors before sealing is completed (when synthetic tape is not used).		
4. A coved base (around lockers and where wall and floor meet) of the same water-resistant material used on floors is found in all dressing and shower rooms.		
5. Abrasive, nonskid, slip-resistant flooring that is impervious to moisture is provided on all areas where water is used—laundry, swimming pool, shower, dressing and drying rooms.		
6. Floor drains are properly located and the slope of the floor is adequate for rapid drainage.		

Gymnasiums and special rooms

1. Gymnasiums are planned so as to provide for safety zones (between courts, end lines, and walls) and for best utilization of space.		
2. One gymnasium wall is free of obstructions and is finished with a smooth, hard surface for ball-rebounding activities.		

CHECKLIST FOR FACILITY PLANNERS—cont'd

Gymnasiums and special rooms—cont'd

	Yes	No
3. The elementary school gymnasium has one wall free of obstructions; a minimum ceiling height of 18 feet; a minimum of 4,000 square feet of teaching area; and a recessed area for housing a piano.		
4. Secondary school gymnasiums have a minimum ceiling height of 22 feet; a scoreboard; electrical outlets placed to fit with bleacher installation; wall attachments for apparatus and nets; and a power-operated, sound-insulated, and movable partition with a small pass-through door at one end.		
5. A small spectator alcove adjoins the wrestling room and contains a drinking fountain (recessed in the walls).		
6. Cabinets, storage closets, supply windows, and service areas have locks.		
7. Provisions have been made for the cleaning, storing, and issuing of physical education and athletic uniforms.		
8. Shower heads are placed at varying heights in the shower rooms on each school level.		
9. Equipment is provided for the use of the physically handicapped.		
10. Special provision has been made for audio and visual aids, including intercommunication systems, radio, and television.		
11. Team dressing rooms have provisions for:		
a. Hosing down room		
b. Floors pitched to drain easily		
c. Hot- and cold-water hose bibbs		
d. Windows located above locker heights		
e. Chalk, tack, and bulletin boards, and movie projection		
f. Lockers for each team member		
g. Drying facility for uniforms		
12. The indoor rifle range includes:		
a. Targets located 54 inches apart and 50 feet from the firing line		
b. 3 feet to 8 feet of space behind targets		
c. 12 feet of space behind firing line		
d. Ceilings 8 feet high		
e. Width adjusted to number of firing lines needed (1 line for each 3 students)		
f. A pulley device for target placement and return		
g. Storage and repair space		
13. Dance facilities include:		
a. 100 square feet per student		
b. A minimum length of 60 linear feet for modern dance		
c. Full-height viewing mirrors on one wall (at least) of 30 feet; also a 20-foot mirror on an additional wall if possible		
d. Acoustical drapery to cover mirrors when not used and for protection if other activities are permitted		
e. Dispersed microphone jacks and speaker installation for music and instruction		
f. Built-in cabinets for record players, microphones, and amplifiers, with space for equipment carts		
g. Electrical outlets and microphone connections around perimeter of room		
h. An exercise bar (34 inches to 42 inches above floor) on one wall		
i. Drapes, surface colors, floors (maple preferred), and other room appointments to enhance the room's attractiveness		
j. Location near dressing rooms and outside entrances		
14. Training rooms include:		
a. Rooms large enough to administer adequately proper health services		
b. Sanitary storage cabinets for medical supplies		
c. Installation of drains for whirlpool, tubs, etc.		
d. Installation of electrical outlets with proper capacities and voltage		
e. High stools for use of equipment such as whirlpool, ice tubs, etc.		

Continued.

CHECKLIST FOR FACILITY PLANNERS—cont'd

Gymnasiums and special rooms—cont'd

	Yes	*No*
f. Water closet, hand labatory, and shower	___	___
g. Extra hand lavatory in the trainer's room proper	___	___
h. Adjoining dressing rooms	___	___
i. Installation and use of hydrotherapy and diathermy equipment in separate areas	___	___
j. Space for the trainer, the physician, and the various services of this function	___	___
k. Corrective-exercise laboratories located conveniently and adapted to the needs of the handicapped	___	___
15. Coaches' rooms should provide:		
a. A sufficient number of dressing lockers for coaching staff and officials	___	___
b. A security closet or cabinet for athletic equipment such as timing devices	___	___
c. A sufficient number of showers and toilet facilities	___	___
d. Drains and faucets for hosing down the rooms where this method of cleaning is desirable and possible	___	___
e. A small chalkboard and tackboard	___	___
f. A small movie screen and projection table for use of coaches to review films	___	___

Handicapped and disabled

Have you included those considerations that would make the facility accessible to, and usable by, the disabled? These considerations include:

1. The knowledge that the disabled will be participants in almost all activities, not merely spectators, if the facility is properly planned.	___	___
2. Ground-level entrance(s) or stair-free entrance(s) using inclined walk(s) or inclined ramp(s).	___	___
3. Uninterrupted walk surface; no abrupt changes in levels leading to the facility.	___	___
4. Approach walks and connecting walks no less than 4 feet in width.	___	___
5. Walks with a gradient no greater than 5%.	___	___
6. A ramp, when used, with rise no greater than 1 foot in 12 feet.	___	___
7. Flat or level surface inside and outside of all exterior doors, extending 5 feet from the door in the direction that the door swings, and extending 1 foot to each side of the door.	___	___
8. Flush thresholds at all doors.	___	___
9. Appropriate door widths, heights, and mechanical features.	___	___
10. At least 6 feet between vestibule doors in series, i.e., inside and outside doors.	___	___
11. Access and proximity to parking areas.	___	___
12. No obstructions by curbs at crosswalks, parking areas, etc.	___	___
13. Proper precautions (handrails, etc.) at basement-window areaways, open stairways, porches, ledges, and platforms.	___	___
14. Handrails on all steps and ramps.	___	___
15. Precautions against the placement of manholes in principal or major sidewalks.	___	___
16. Corridors that are at least 60 inches wide and without abrupt pillars or protrusions.	___	___
17. Floors which are nonskid and have no abrupt changes or interruptions in level.	___	___
18. Proper design of steps.	___	___
19. Access to rest rooms, water coolers, telephones, food-service areas, lounges, dressing rooms, play areas, and auxiliary services and areas.	___	___
20. Elevators in multiple-story buildings.	___	___
21. Appropriate placement of controls to permit and to prohibit use as desired.	___	___
22. Sound signals for the blind, and visual signals for the deaf as counterparts to regular sound and sight signals.	___	___
23. Proper placement concealment, or insulation of radiators, heat pipes, hotwater pipes, drain pipes, etc.	___	___

CHECKLIST FOR FACILITY PLANNERS—cont'd

Swimming pools   *Yes*   *No*

1. Has a clear-cut statement been prepared on the nature and scope of the design program and the special requirements for space, equipment, and facilities dictated by the activities to be conducted?

2. Has the swimming pool been planned to meet the total requirements of the program to be conducted as well as any special needs of the clientele to be serviced?

3. Have all plans and specifications been checked and approved by the local board of health?

4. Is the pool the proper depth to accommodate the various age groups and types of activities it is intended to serve?

5. Does the design of the pool incorporate the most current knowledge and best experience available regarding swimming pools?

6. If a local architect or engineer who is inexperienced in pool construction is employed, has an experienced pool consultant, architect, or engineer been called in to advise on design and equipment?

7. Is there adequate deep water for diving (minimum of 9 feet for 1-meter boards, 12 feet for 3-meter boards, and 15 feet for 10-meter towers)?

8. Have the requirements for competitive swimming been met (7-foot lanes; 12-inch black or brown lines on the bottom; pool 1 inch longer than official measurement; depth and distance markings)?

9. Is there adequate deck space around the pool? Has more space been provided than that indicated by the minimum recommended deck/pool ratio?

10. Does the swimming instructor's office face the pool? And is that a window through which the instructor may view all the pool area? Is there a toilet-shower-dressing area next to the office for instructors?

11. Are recessed steps or removable ladders located on the walls so as not to interfere with competitive swimming turns?

12. Does a properly constructed overflow gutter extend around the pool perimeter?

13. Where skimmers are used, have they been properly located so that they are not on walls where competitive swimming is to be conducted?

14. Have separate storage spaces been allocated for maintenance and instructional equipment?

15. Has the area for spectators been properly separated from the pool area?

16. Have all diving standards and lifeguard chairs been properly anchored?

17. Does the pool layout provide the most efficient control of swimmers from showers and locker rooms to the pool? Are toilet facilities provided for wet swimmers separate from the dry area?

18. Is the recirculation pump located below the water level?

19. Is there easy vertical access to the filter room for both people and material (stairway if required)?

20. Has the proper pitch to drains been allowed in the pool, on the pool deck, in the overflow gutter, and on the floor of shower and dressing rooms?

21. Has adequate space been allowed between diving boards and between the diving boards and sidewalls?

22. Is there adequate provision for lifesaving equipment? Pool-cleaning equipment?

23. Are inlets and outlets adequate in number and located so as to ensure effective circulation of water in the pool?

24. Has consideration been given to underwater lights, underwater observation windows, and underwater speakers?

25. Is there a coping around the edge of the pool?

26. Has a pool heater been considered in northern climates in order to raise the temperature of the water?

27. Have underwater lights in end racing walls been located deep enough and directly below surface lane anchors, and are they on a separate circuit?

Continued.

CHECKLIST FOR FACILITY PLANNERS—cont'd

Swimming pools—cont'd

	Yes	No
28. Has the plan been considered from the standpoint of handicapped persons (e.g., is there a gate adjacent to the turnstiles)?		
29. Is seating for swimmers provided on the deck?		
30. Has the recirculation-filtration system been designed to meet the anticipated future bathing load?		
31. Has the gas chlorinator (if used) been placed in a separate room accessible from and vented to the outside?		
32. Has the gutter waste water been valved to return to the filters, and also for direct waste?		

Indoor pools

1. Is there proper mechanical ventilation?
2. Is there adequate acoustical treatment of walls and ceilings?
3. Is there adequate overhead clearance for diving (15 feet above low springboards, 15 feet for 3-meter boards, and 10 feet for 10-meter platforms)?
4. Is there adequate lighting (50 footcandles minimum)?
5. Has reflection of light from the outside been kept to the minimum by proper location of windows or skylights (windows on side walls are not desirable)?
6. Are all wall bases coved to facilitate cleaning?
7. Is there provision for proper temperature control in the pool room for both water and air?
8. Can the humidity of the pool room be controlled?
9. Is the wall and ceiling insulation adequate to prevent "sweating"?
10. Are all metal fittings of noncorrosive material?
11. Is there a tunnel around the outside of the pool, or a trench on the deck which permits ready access to pipes?

Outdoor pools

1. Is the site for the pool in the best possible location (away from railroad tracks, heavy industry, trees, and open fields which are dusty)?
2. Have sand and grass been kept the proper distance away from the pool to prevent them from being transmitted to the pool?
3. Has a fence been placed around the pool to assure safety when not in use?
4. Has proper subsurface drainage been provided?
5. Is there adequate deck space for sunbathing?
6. Are the outdoor lights placed far enough from the pool to prevent insects from dropping into the pool?
7. Is the deck of nonslip material?
8. Is there an area set aside for eating, separated from the pool deck?
9. Is the bathhouse properly located, with the entrance to the pool leading to the shallow end?
10. If the pool shell contains a concrete finish, has the length of the pool been increased by 3 inches over the "official" size in order to permit eventaul tiling of the basin without making the pool "too short"?
11. Are there other recreational facilities nearby for the convenience and enjoyment of swimmers?
12. Do diving boards or platforms face north or east?
13. Are lifeguard stands provided and properly located?
14. Has adequate parking space been provided and properly located?
15. Is the pool oriented correctly in relation to the sun?
16. Have windshields been provided in situations where heavy winds prevail?

Questions and exercises

1. Discuss some of the new concepts utilized in physical plant construction. Are any of these concepts used in your school? If so, explain in what way they are used.
2. Prepare a sketch of what you consider to be an ideal physical education plant. In your plans consider both outdoor and indoor facilities.
3. Plan a health suite that you consider to be ideal.
4. What are ten basic considerations in planning facilities?
5. Discuss the following statement: the trend in school-house construction is away from the so-called frills.
6. Develop a list of standards for outdoor play areas and locker, shower, and drying room facilities in the following areas: (a) lighting, (b) heating and ventilation, (c) plant sanitation, (d) furniture.
7. What are some of the essential factors to keep in mind when planning the gymnasium?
8. What should be provided in the school in the way of special activity areas?
9. What are some of the essential factors to keep in mind when planning the swimming pool?
10. What considerations should be made in school facilities for recreation?
11. Draw up a list of references for obtaining authoritative information on various aspects of facility construction and maintenance.

Reading assignment in *Administrative Dimensions of Health and Physical Education Programs, Including Athletics:* Chapter 12, Selections 63 to 69.

Selected references

American Association for Health, Physical Education, and Recreation: Planning areas and facilities for health, physical education, and recreation, Washington, D. C., 1965, The Association.

Architectural Research Group: Shelter for physical education, College Station, Texas, 1961, Publications Department, Texas Engineering Experiment Station, A & M College of Texas.

Athletic Institute and American Association for Health, Physical Education, and Recreation: Equipment and supplies for athletics: athletics, physical education, and recreation, Chicago, 1960, The Institute.

Bingham, J. H.: A multipurpose court for all seasons, Parks and Recreation Trends, May, 1973.

California State Department of Education: Brief statement of principles involving the construction of school unit, State Health Committee Bulletin, Sacramento, The Department.

California State Joint Committee on School Health: Guide and check list for healthful and safe school environment, Sacramento, The Committee.

DeWeese, A. O., and Moore, V. M.: The organization of a school health service comprising from 500 to 1000 pupils from kindergarten through high school, Journal of School Health **34:**415, 1964.

Dickey, D. D.: Athletic lockers for schools and colleges, Minneapolis, Minnesota, Post Office Box 6630, 1967.

Educational Facilities Laboratories, Inc.: Air structures for school sports, New York, 1964, The Laboratories.

Englehardt, N. L.: Complete guide for planning new schools, West Nyack, New York, 1970, Parker Publishing Co.

Environmental education facility resources: A report from the Educational Facilities Laboratory, New York, 1972, The Laboratories.

Ezersky E., and Theibert, R.: City schools without gyms, Journal of Health, Physical Education, and Recreation **41:** April, 1970.

Ezersky, E. M.: Mini-gyms and fitness courts, Journal of Health, Physical Education, and Recreation **43:**38, 1972.

Gabrielsen, M. A.: Swimming pool planning and utilization, Speech delivered at the Conference on Planning, Constructing, Utilizing Physical Education, Recreation, and Athletic Facilities, Columbus, Ohio, December 10, 1969.

Grieve, A.: Legal considerations of equipment and facilities, The Athletic Journal **47:**38, 1967.

Joint Committee on Health Problems in Education of National Education Association and American Medical Association: Healthful school environment, Washington, D. C., 1969, The Association.

Kelsey, L., Kolflat, F., and Schaefer, R.: New generation gyms, Nation's Schools, December, 1969.

Let's look at new sports arenas: American School and University, August, 1968.

Leu, D. J.: Planning educational facilities, New York, 1965, The Center for Applied Research, Inc. (The Library of Education).

New York State Department of Education: Planning the indoor physical education facilities, Albany, 1962, The State Department of Education.

Pettine, A. M.: Planning a gymnasium, Journal of Health, Physical Education, and Recreation **44:**58, 1972.

Puckett, J.: Two promising innovations in physical education facilities, Journal of Health, Physical Education, and Recreation **43:**40, 1972.

Theibert, P. R.: On facilities for lifetime sports, American School & University, November, 1971.

The State Education Department, The University of the State of New York: Planning the outdoor physical education facilities for central schools, Albany, 1964, The Department.

Wetzel, C. H.: Planning gym seating for long-range needs, Scholastic Coach **30:**48, 1961.

Woods, H. W.: Vinyl flooring, the surface of the future, Athletic Journal **43:** December, 1972.

Annuals and periodicals

Professional architectural and educational magazines devote considerable space to the planning, designing, constructing, equipping, and managing of school facilities. The school facilities articles appearing in the annuals and periodicals listed below are usually concerned with specific school plants of recent construction and are illustrated with drawings and photographs. Some of these periodicals issue special editions that are devoted entirely to school facilities.

Architectural

Architectural Forum, Time, Inc., 9 Rockefeller Plaza, New York, N. Y. 10020

Architectural Record, F. W. Dodge Corp., 119 W. 49th St., New York, N. Y. 10018

Progressive Architecture, Reinhold Publishing Corp., 430 Park Ave., New York, N. Y. 10022

Educational

American School and University, Buttenheim Publishing Corp., 470 Park Ave. South, New York, N. Y. 10016 (annual).

American School Board Journal, Bruce Publishing Co., Milwaukee, Wis.

Nation's Schools, Modern Hospital Publishing Co., Inc., 1050 Merchandise Mart, Chicago, Ill. 60654

Overview, Buttenheim Publishing Corp., 470 Park Ave. South, New York, N. Y. 10016

School Management, School Management, Inc., 22 W. Putman Ave., Greenwich, Conn.

School Planning, School Planning, Inc., 75 E. Wacker Dr., Chicago, Ill. 60601

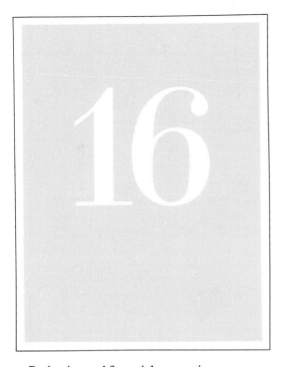

Budget preparation and financial accounting

Budgeting and financial accounting are essential administrative functions that provide for efficient money management in schools and colleges. In recent years, traditional fiscal management in many cases has been replaced by the PPB System or similar systems that analyze financial needs in terms of program objectives. The PP Budgeting System will be discussed in detail in this chapter.

The administrator must thoroughly understand the needs and objectives of all the departments under his or her supervision. Budgeting must take all department requests into consideration on equal terms without being influenced in a prejudicial manner. Within departments students must also be given equitable treatment in matters of funding. Women should have facilities, materials, equipment, transportation, and uniforms equal to those of men. The fiscal management of an institution is a difficult, challenging job, and the manner in which it is handled is reflected in the efficiency or lack of it in the institution and its personnel.

IMPORTANCE OF FISCAL MANAGEMENT

The services that a school system provides, whether personal help, facilities, instructional materials, or other items, usually involve the disbursement of money. This money must be secured from proper sources, be expended for educational purposes, and be accounted for item by item. The budget, the master financial plan for the entire school or college system or any subdivision, is constructed with this purpose in mind.

There must be well thought through policies for the raising and spending of school or college money. Educators should know the procedures for handling such funds with integrity, the basic purposes for which the educational program exists, the school laws, and the codes and regulations concerning fiscal management. Education is big business and is rapidly occupying a major role in the fiscal planning of national, state, and local units of government. Only as the funds are used wisely and in the best interests of the students and all people concerned can the large outlay of monies be justified.

PLACE OF FINANCIAL MANAGEMENT IN HEALTH AND PHYSICAL EDUCATION PROGRAMS

Of all the subject matter areas in elementary, secondary, or college and university educational systems, health and physical education require one of the largest outlays of funds in order that the educational programs may be conducted effectively. The cost of personnel, health services, facilities, and supplies and equipment are only a few of the items that amount to large sums of money. As much as 25% of many school and college plants are devoted to these programs. There are probably 200,000 physical educators and coaches getting collectively paid millions of dollars annually in salaries. More than 60 million children and young people are the focus of attention in health and physical education.

Gymnasiums, swimming pools, health suites, playgrounds, and other facilities are being constructed at the cost of astronomical sums to taxpayers.

With such a great outlay of funds for health and physical education programs, there must be sound financial management to see that the monies are utilized in the best way possible. This is one of the most important responsibilities that educators, and particularly administrators, have.

Purposes of financial management

Some of the principal purposes for which financial management exists in health and physical education programs are as follows:

1. To prevent misuse and waste of funds that have been allocated to these special fields.
2. To help coordinate and relate the objectives of health and physical education programs with the money appropriated for achieving such outcomes.
3. To ensure that monies allocated to health and physical education will be based upon research, study, and a careful analysis of the pertinent conditions that influence such a process.
4. To involve the entire staff in formulating policies and procedures and in preparing budgetary items that will help ensure that the right program directions are taken.
5. To utilize funds in a manner that will develop the best programs of health and physical education possible.
6. To exercise control over the process of fiscal management in order to guarantee that the entire financial process has integrity and purpose.
7. To make the greatest use of personnel, facilities, supplies, equipment, and other factors involved in accomplishing educational objectives.

Responsibility

The responsibility for fiscal management, although falling largely upon the shoulders of the administration, involves every person who is a member of the school staff, as well as the pupils themselves.

Formulation and preparation of the budget, for example, is a cooperative enterprise in many respects. It is based on information and reports that have been forwarded by faculty and staff through the various departments and subdivisions of the organization. These reports must contain information on programs, projects, obligations that exist, funds that have been spent, and monies that have been received from various sources. Staff members help in this process. Administrators must have an overall picture of the entire enterprise at their fingertips. They must be cognizant of the work being done throughout the establishment, functions that should be carried out, needs of every facet of the organization, and other items that must be considered in the preparation of the budget. The larger the organization, the larger should be the budget organization under the administrator. The efficiency of the enterprise depends upon expert judgment in fiscal matters. Students themselves play a part in many school and college systems. For example, through general organizations, budgets are prepared and outlays of funds relating to many activities, such as plays and athletics, are either approved, amended, or rejected. Fiscal management involves many people, but the job of leadership and direction falls upon the administration.

PPBS—PLANNING, PROGRAMMING, BUDGETING SYSTEM

PPBS has already been introduced in Chapter 1; however, its great importance to budgeting and fiscal accounting demands a more complete discussion in this chapter. PPBS came about as a solution to problems of fiscal accountability and optimal utilization of limited resources.

PPBS—a history

The PPBS started in 1949 when the Hoover Commission report, on the organization of the Executive Branch, recommended that the government adopt a budget based on function, activities, and objectives. In 1954 the Rand Corporation developed a performance budget for use in military spending. Planning-Programming-Budgeting System—PPBS was the title given to this system. The Du Pont Corporation and the Ford Motor Company were among the first to use the PPB System. In the early 1960s Robert McNamara introduced the system to the Defense Department. The results of the system were so impressive that President Johnson ordered all federal departments and agencies to adopt PPBS by August 1965. Presently, many schools and colleges are using this system and many more are researching the feasibility of using it in their particular cases.

Definition of PPBS

A PPB System may be defined as a long-range plan for the accomplishment of an organization's objectives, utilizing continual feedback and updating of information to allow for greater efficiency of the decision-making process. The three basic elements of PPBS are explained by writer Edward L. Katzenbach, as follows:

1. Planning—establishing objectives
2. Programming—combining activities and events to produce distinguishable results
3. Budgeting—allocating resources, the financial plan for meeting program needs*

First, the objectives of the organization must be clearly defined. All those activities that contribute to the same objective, regardless of placement in the organization, are grouped together. A financial plan designed to reach these objectives is formulated for a particular time period. An analysis document discusses long-range needs and an evaluation of the adequacy and effectiveness, costs, benefits, and difficulties inherent in the proposed program. Under the PPB System, funds must be utilized with definitive goals in mind. In this way accountability for expenditures is stressed. In using the PPB System, each activity and educational program is taken into consideration, not only by itself but also in respect to other educational programs that comprise the whole system. In this way the needs of the entire school system rather than just one part are taken into consideration.

The PPBS cycle

The steps necessary to the utilization of a PPBS program are as follows:

1. *Goals and objectives must be determined.* Goals and objectives should be stated in terms of behavior and performance. The deserved results of the program should also be determined in relation to knowledges, skills, and attitudes.

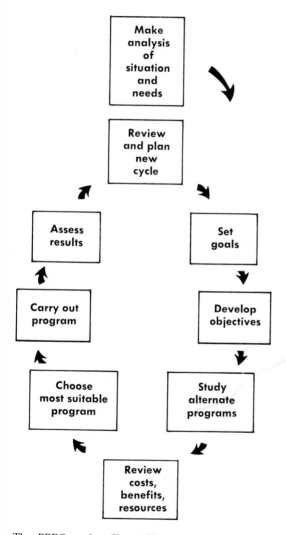

The PPBS cycle. (From Clegg. A. A., Jr.: The teacher and manager of the curriculum, Educational Leadership, January, 1973, p. 308.)

*Katzenbach, E.: Planning, Programming Budgeting Systems: PPBS and Education, Cambridge, Massachusetts, 1968, New England School Development Council.

2. *Statement of needs and problems.* Needs and problems of the particular organization must be adequately defined.

3. *A determination of expected satisfaction of needs is essential.* Numbers of persons and skills must also be determined.

4. *Constraints and feasibility.* Both of these items must be evaluated to determine whether the system can overcome certain limitations (personnel, materials, facilities, etc.). The system may need modification in terms of needs or objectives in order to overcome the existing limitations.

5. *Alternative programs.* These programs outline the different ways that the organization can reach its goals. Alternative programs should be evaluated in terms of needs, goals, and constraints of the system.

6. *Resource requirements must be estimated.* The resource needs of each alternative must be computed. The easiest way to do this is to derive the faculty teaching cost per student credit hour and then add department costs, counseling, administration, equipment, and clerical costs.

7. *Estimate benefits to be gained from each alternative.* The benefits of the program must be determined in relationship to student accomplishment presently and in the future.

8. *Develop an operating plan.* From the data collected, all alternatives should be weighed against such fixed criteria as: cost of implementation and risk involved, estimated benefits, and future budget allocations.

9. *Pilot implementation of best alternative.* A pilot program should be conducted at a level where it could be modified or changed without involved or costly effort.

10. *Evaluation.* The data from the pilot program should be used in determining whether it is meeting the objectives of the organization. It should be modified accordingly.

11. *Feedback and further modification.*

Once the PPB System is in process, it should be continually reevaluated and modified to ensure that the goals and objectives agreed upon are being met.

Advantages and disadvantages of PPBS

Before implementing a PPB System into his or her institution, the administrator must be thoroughly familiar with the advantages and disadvantages of such a system. Each situation differs and careful analysis prior to implementation is essential.

Some of the advantages of PPBS are:

1. The system aids in formulating goals, objectives, and skills.

2. Curriculum can be designed to meet the objectives formulated.

3. Staff can be provided with prior planning and resource material.

4. Alternative plans can be more systematically analyzed.

5. Costs and accomplishments may be compared.

6. Teachers and other staff members are more involved in decision-making.

7. Instructural costs may be easily identified.

8. Innovation can be promoted in teaching and programs.

9. Evaluating criteria is continually applied to system.

10. Public awareness and understanding are increased.

The disadvantages of such a system can be seen in the following points:

1. Staff time is limited and staff members with sufficient technical skills in these areas are also limited.

2. Implementation may lead to conflict and resistance from community members.

3. Cost-benefit analysis is a difficult example to quantitate; some benefits from education are not easily measurable.

4. Communication among staff may be limited as a result of centralization of system planning.

5. PPBS is a method of indicating the best use of funds; however, in doing so, funds are also expended and limited budgets

may not be able to implement such a system.

6. The vocabulary is vague to those who are not directly involved in using such a system.
7. PPBS may be mistakenly seen as a substitute for management rather than a tool of management.
8. Alternatives with great potential are passed up because of their high chance of failure according to PPBS criteria.
9. Some educators may feel that they are answerable to the "system" for their instructional program; however, the "system" should be an aid to the educator not a deterrent.

Utilization of PPBS

Recent surveys indicate that there were between 800 and 1000 schools in the United States developing PPBS type budgets in the 1972-73 school year. Twenty states, during this time, were also in the process of mandating some form of PPBS. Some examples of PPBS utilization are given in the following paragraphs.

The Michigan program. Michigan has adopted a PPB System in its 42 publicly funded institutions of higher learning. Although the system will cost more money, it will also enable administrators to have greater information for decision-making and will give tax payers a better indication of where their money is being spent.

California program. Under the direction of the Advisory Commission on School District Budgeting and Accounting, fifteen pilot school districts are utilizing PPBS. They have simplified the plan so that it is readily understandable to voters in the hope that the public's understanding will aid in the passage of school bond issues. In two of the pilot districts, El Monte and Hillsborough, positive results can already be seen. In El Monte, the health services program had been harshly criticized. When explained in terms of objectives and expected accomplishment, the voters supported the budget. In Hillsborough, students were found to be doing poorly on science achievement tests. When it was determined through PPBS that the science budget was not as high as it should be,

a remedial program was initiated and successful results were obtained.

It is obvious from these examples that PPBS is a total process that can help to best utilize available funds, point up problem areas, and improve curriculum defects. In addition, the public is given clear and understandable data to aid in deciding on budgets.

How can PPBS be applied to physical education?

Physical education has much to gain through the implementation of PPBS. If this system is used, physical education programs and budget requests cannot be arbitrarily dropped or refused because of inadequate funding. Each segment of the curriculum must be given equal emphasis according to objectives and benefits derived from meeting these objectives.

Physical education budgets prior to PPBS were considered in terms of bats and balls rather than total program needs and benefits. PPBS is now used by physical education departments in order to present in a comprehensive manner needed information required by administrators. PPBS provides administrators with a detailed list of goals and objectives, an analysis of problems, alternatives, solutions, and recommendations. The most important accomplishment of PPBS is the way it relates program costs to expected accomplishments.

COST ANALYSIS

Cost analysis of materials consumed or used in a program is a derivative of cost accounting. The need for cost analysis is to aid the administrator to evaluate present operations as well as to project future planning. Cost analysis is limited to the types of accounting systems being used as well as designating the unit to be compared. For example, some schools operate on grades one to eight, kindergarten to grade twelve, or some other educational pattern. Naturally, there would be a great difference in expenditures per pupil in the various patterns or organization.

Various units are used in cost analysis for the general education fund. The number of pupils in attendance, the census, average daily attendance, and average daily membership are some of those that are used. There are advantages and disadvantages to each of the various units.

Knezevich and Fowlkes* found several years ago in their study a practice that is still true today in most school systems, namely that the most common raw per capita unit used in cost analysis is per pupil in average daily attendance. In other words, educational costs are figured on a per pupil basis, and the total number of pupils involved is computed by determining what the average daily pupil attendance is in a school or educational system. This figure is arrived at by adding the aggregated days of attendance of all pupils and then dividing by the number of days school was in session. The number of pupils in average daily attendance is then divided into the total of the educational costs in order to obtain the cost per pupil in average daily attendance. It should be recognized, however, there is no universally accepted definition of average daily attendance. Whereas some states would permit all pupils to be counted in attendance when teachers are attending a state teachers meeting, others would not.

Knezevich and Fowlkes also pointed out that as a raw measure of educational burden, the average daily membership is a better measure than the average daily attendance. Teachers' salaries must be paid whether pupils are in 90% or 100% attendance, and desks and school books must be available whether pupils are in attendance or not. With respect to raw per capita units, the average daily membership is a better unit to measure the educational burden than the more commonly used average daily attendance unit. Tradition, however, has favored the average daily attendance unit over that of average daily membership.†

Cost analysis as it relates to equipment and supplies for health and physical education may be simply handled by allowing a certain number of dollars per pupil enrolled in the district or on the various levels in the school system. The New York State Education Department, for example, publishes an analysis of the monies spent on different budget categories on a pupil basis, depending on the type and size of the school.* This is very helpful and offers the business administrator a guide to the problem of budget allocation.

Good business administration should allow a space on the budget sheet for personnel in all departments to list any needs over the specified allocations and a place to state reasons for the listing. One of the drawbacks of using cost analysis sheets is that it is physically impossible for the data to be current.

Some experts in fiscal management feel that a per capita expenditure allocation for health and physical education represents a good foundation program. However, they recommend, in addition, (1) an extra percentage allocation for program enrichment, (2) an extra percentage allocation for variation in enrollment, and (3) a reference to a commodity index (current prices of equipment and supplies) that may indicate need for changes in the per capita expenditure because of current increase or decrease in the value of the items being purchased.

Cost analysis in practice in physical education programs

In order to provide the reader with an understanding of the amount of money allocated to physical education programs throughout the United States and how it is determined, a survey of selected school systems was accomplished. The following paragraphs are cited examples of money allocation in several cities.

California. A large city system in California reports that physical education supplies are included in each school's allocation for instructional supplies, with the amount being based upon the number of pupils enrolled—elementary schools, $3.25 per pupil; junior high schools, $2.44 per pupil; and senior high schools, $2.15 per pupil.

Physical education equipment was included in the budget for the year at a figure of $32,000. The maintenance of physical education equip-

*Knezevich, S. J., and Fowlkes, J. G.: Business management of local school systems, New York, 1960, Harper & Row, Publishers, p. 157.

†Knezevich, S. J., and Fowlkes, J. G., op. cit., p. 15.

*Bureau of Statistical Services: Expenditures per pupil in average daily attendance, Division of Educational Management Services, State Education Department, The University of the State of New York, Albany, N. Y.

ment was provided for, as needed, by the board of education. The board of education also provided the towels and laundry service. In regard to the athletic program, the board of education provided extra pay for coaches and intramural directors, all the necessary athletic uniforms, the cleaning and repair of these uniforms and equipment, officials, and accident insurance for all boys and girls participating in the extramural and interschool athletic programs.

In another large school district in California, there was an allocation of $1.35 per pupil (boys) in junior and senior high schools for physical education programs. Girls were allocated the amount of $1.05 per pupil at the same educational level for the same period. The amount varied from year to year based upon need and prior experience. If the total amount allocated was not used during the school year, an amount not to exceed 20% of the total year's allocation could be carried over. The school district provided the expenses of transportation and instruction for the athletic program. Supplies needed in connection with the athletic program were provided through student body funds derived from student fees, sales at student stores, and admissions to athletic activities.

Florida. As reported to the author, Florida as a general policy does not favor ear-marked funds for any single program in the schools. The procedure recommended is that county school districts receive what is called a teacher-unit allocation from the state for each twenty-seven students in average daily attendance. Each unit carries with it a certain amount of money for expendable supplies. The local school district holds a percentage of this money for general district-wide use and reallocates the remaining amount to individual schools based on formulas such as pupil enrollment. Each individual school is encouraged to involve its faculty in determining the priority of needs for the coming year. Therefore, health and physical education could have a high priority one year and a low one another year. As a general rule, health and physical education appear to receive the same consideration as other phases of the curriculum. In a few instances, physical education needs are met through such fund-raising activities as dances and PTA drives.

Illinois. A high school in Illinois reported that no set figure or set formula was used to arrive at the allocation for health or physical education programs. The board of education subsidized the program of physical education beyond the gate receipts. At the time of the survey there was an equipment budget of $1,000 and a supplies budget of $1,300. The board of education reviews the anticipated budget each year for approval. The Director of Health and Physical Education submits a list of anticipated expenditures for such items as equipment, supplies, transportation, and officials. Gate receipts are also estimated. The difference between the two figures is the amount the board must approve or adjust before approval.

Indiana. One medium-sized school system in Indiana reported that each school (elementary, junior high, senior high, and so on) is allocated so much money for each student enrolled, and then the principal assigns the amount for each phase of the school program.

A county school corporation in Indiana budgets 10 cents per pupil for elementary schools in two accounts—one for instructional supplies and one for repair and replacement. Junior high and senior high schools are budgeted 35 cents per pupil in both accounts. In addition to the above-mentioned accounts, each junior and senior high school principal is budgeted 35 cents per pupil per school as additional money that can be used where he or she feels the greatest need exists.

A large city school system in Indiana does not have a formula for determining the amount of money allocated for physical education. Budget requests are prepared by the high school department heads for grades nine to twelve and by the supervisor of health and physical education for grades one to eight. The amount requested is based on inventory, program needs of individual schools, and requirements for supplying new schools and additions to present plants.

Another Indiana school system finances the entire interscholastic athletic program from gate receipts. Extra pay for coaches and maintenance of athletic facilities is financed through the general fund. In respect to the physical education program, each department is given an allocation of funds based on the number of students served.

New Jersey. One large school system in New Jersey reported an allocation of 50 cents per student for physical education supplies, and a smaller school system reported an allocation of $3,000 to $6,000 for supplies and coaches' salaries for athletics. Most school districts in New Jersey, it was reported, do not seem to have difficulty in getting reasonable physical education supplies based on needs. For athletics, most schools in New Jersey are subsidized in whole or part by board of education funds.

New York. Twenty-five New York State schools were surveyed to determine the amount of money allocated to their physical education programs. The amounts allocated were then changed into a per pupil allotment in order to provide a means of comparison. The items for which the money was allocated included athletic and gymnasium supplies and equipment, various athletic fees, officials, transportation, police, reconditioning of equipment, supplies and equipment needed in physical education classes, and intramurals and extramurals for both men and women. In those schools in which the administrative pattern grouped grades seven to twelve, the highest allocation per pupil was $33.86 and the lowest was $10.07. In those schools in which budgets were figured on a kindergarten to grade twelve school administrative pattern, the highest per capita allocation was $13.22 and the lowest was $5.30. In those schools in which the administrative pattern included grades nine to twelve, the highest per capita allocation was $35.24 and the lowest was $13.68.

Each school surveyed was asked how the amount that was allocated per student was determined. The general practice was that the Director of Health and Physical Education submitted and substantiated the following:

1. Needs—for the coming school year
2. Increased expenditures—a sound estimate of projected increases in regard to pupil program participation based on increased enrollments, pupil interest, program changes, and the anticipated cost of equipment and supplies to be used
3. Inventory—present equipment and supplies on hand and the condition of these items
4. Previous year's budget—amounts allocated in previous year or years

These four items represent the basis on which most allocations of funds to programs of health and physical education were determined.

Directors of health and physical education programs surveyed felt that where they were granted increases in per capita allocations it was the result of such factors as increase in the number of participants, a careful evaluation of the number of participants and the time they spent using the equipment and supplies, the cost per hour (for example, it was determined in one community that it cost less than 50 cents per hour per child to participate in football), and an excellent working rapport with the board of education.

The survey also disclosed that most schools have a contingency fund to meet emergency needs, that many schools used the money that was saved when the proposed budget allocation was in excess of the actual bid price on certain supplies and equipment, that some schools used part of the money received from gate receipts, and that some other schools used part of the money from the sale of general organization tickets.

Oklahoma. A city school system in Oklahoma reported that budget allocations for health and physical education programs for boys and girls vary according to pupil enrollment. The superintendent of schools and the board of education decide the amount that will be allocated to each of the special programs. Athletics are self-supporting and the board of education does not allocate money directly to them.

Texas. An independent school district in Texas pointed out that it does not have a formula for physical education or health education. The board of education and school administration decide the total budget.

BUDGETING

Budgeting is the formulation of a financial plan in terms of work to be accomplished and services to be performed. See previous discussion of PPBS. All expenditures should be closely related to the objectives that the organization

SCHOOL DISTRICT — TAX BUDGET.

Assessed Valuation		$59,681,265.00
Rate per $1,000.00		32.34
Amount of Budget to be Raised by Taxation		1,930,067.00

GENERAL CONTROL:

2/2	Board of Education—Legal, Auditing	$	1,225.00
2/3	Board of Education—Supplies, Travel, etc.		5,700.00
2/7	Central Office—Salaries		66,680.00
2/8	Central Office—Supplies, Travel, etc.		4,600.00
2/10	Attendance & Census Service—Salaries		450.00
2/11	Attendance & Census Service—Supplies		165.00
	Total General Control	$	78,820.00

INSTRUCTIONAL SERVICE:

3/3	Salaries of Principals	$	87,225.00
3/4	Salaries of Clerical & Other Help		36,405.00
3/6	Other Expenses of Supervision—Supplies, Travel, etc.		8,850.00
3/9	Salaries of Teachers		1,277,015.00
3/10	Textbooks		18,800.00
3/11	Supplies Used in Instruction		38,250.00
3/13	Tuition to Other Districts		12,600.00
3/14	Other Expenses of Instruction		10,100.00
	Total, Instructional Service (Day Schools)	$	1,489,245.00

OPERATION OF SCHOOL PLANT:

4/1	Wages—Building Service Employees	$	110,575.00
4/2	Fuel Oil		20,900.00
4/3	Water		3,875.00
4/4	Light & Power		21,800.00
4/5	Custodial Supplies		5,600.00
4/7	Services Other Than Personal (Telephone, Laundry, Piano Tuning)		7,100.00
	Total, Operation of School Plant	$	169,850.00

MAINTENANCE OF SCHOOL PLANT:

5/1	Upkeep of Grounds	$	8,175.00
5/2	Repair of Buildings		57,160.00
5/3	Repair & Replacement of Heating, Lighting & Plumbing Equipment		20,400.00
5/4	Repair & Replacement of Instructional Equipment		14,182.00
5/5	Repair & Replacement of Furniture		9,920.00
5/6	Repair & Replacement—Other Equipment		5,457.00
5/11	Other Expenses of Maintenance		1,985.00
	Total, Maintenance of School Plant	$	117,279

FIXED CHARGES:

6/1	Pensions—State Teachers' Ret. System	$	226,000.00
6/2	Pensions—Other Employees		35,525.00
6/3	Insurance		37,410.00
6/4	Taxes		3,200.00
6/5	Membership—State School Boards Assn.		400.00
6/6	Employers Contrib. to F.I.C.A. (Soc. Sec.)		37,500.00
	Total, Fixed Charges	$	340,035.00

DEBT SERVICE:

7/1	Payment of Bonds	$	175,000.00
7/4	Payment of Interest on Bonds		56,555.00
7/7	Refunds		—
7/8	Other Expenses of Debt Service		225.00
	Total, Debt Service	$	231,780.00

CAPITAL OUTLAY:

8/2	Improvement of Grounds	$	800.00
8/3	Architect & Engineer Fees		2,500.00
8/4	New Buildings & Bldg. Equipment		—
8/9	Alteration of Bldgs. (Not Repairs)		1,920.00
8/11	Instructional Equip. & Furniture		19,157.00
8/12	Other Equipment		1,971.00
8/15	New Library Books		5,700.00
8/14	Gift Fund		—
	Total, Capital Outlay	$	32,048.00

AUXILIARY AGENCIES AND OTHER SUNDRY ACTIVITIES:

9/1	Library Salaries	$	20,800.00
9/2	Library—Repair & Repl. of Books		3,500.00
9/3	Library—Other Expenses		1,350.00
9/4	Health Service—Med. Inspection		5,100.00
9/5	Health Service—Nurses' Salaries		32,800.00
9/6	Health Service—Dental Hyg. Salary		500.00
9/7	Health Service—Other Expenses		1,400.00
9/8	Transportation Services		19,000.00
			22,500.00
9/10	Cafeteria		8,400.00
9/12	Recreation & Sports		4,135.00
9/13	Other Expenses		50.00
9/14	Psychological Services		11,175.00
	Total, Auxiliary Agencies	$	130,710.00
	Grand Total of Budget	$	2,596,067.00
	Amount of State Aid (Estimated)		550,000.00
	Miscellaneous Receipts (Estimated)		53,000.00
		$	1,930,067.00
	Reduction of Contingent Fund		63,000.00
	Amount to be Raised by Taxes	$	1,930,067.00
	Assessed Valuation		$59,681,265.00
	Tax Rate per $1,000.00 (Estimated)	$	32.34

Certified to be a true and correct copy

Sgd:

Sgd: District Clerk

Sample budget summary for a school system.

is trying to achieve. In this aspect the administration plays a very important part in the budgeting process.

Budgets should be planned and prepared with a thought to the future. They are an important part of the administration's 3-, 5-, or 7-year plan and the program of accomplishment that has been outlined for a fiscal period. Projects of any size should be integrated progressively over many years. Thus the outlay of monies to realize such aims requires long-term planning.

According to the strict interpretation of the word, a budget is merely a record of receipts and expenditures. As used here, however, it reflects the long-term planning of the organization, pointing up the needs with their estimated costs, and then ensuring that a realistic program is planned that will fit into the estimated income.

The budget forecasts revenues and expenses for a period of 1 year, known as the fiscal year, which is not always synonymous with the school or college year.

Purposes of budgets

The purposes of budgets are as follows:

1. They express the plan and program for the departments of health and physical education. They determine such things as (a) size of classes, (b) supplies, equipment, and facilities, (c) methods used, (d) results and educational values sought, and (e) personnel available.

2. They reflect the school's or college's educational philosophy and policies and those of the professional fields of health and physical education. They provide an overview of these specialized areas.

THE ROLE OF THE ADMINISTRATOR IN BUDGETING *

A. Preliminary considerations in preparing the budget
   1. Program additions or deletions
   2. Staff changes
   3. Inventory of equipment on hand

B. Budget preparation: additional considerations
   1. Athletic gate receipts and expenditures—Athletic Association fund
   2. Board of education budget—allocations for physical education, including athletics
   3. Coaches requests and requests of teachers and department heads
   4. Comparison of requests with inventories
   5. Itemizing and coding requests
   6. Budget conferences with administration
   7. Justification of requests

C. Athletic association funds: considerations
   1. Estimated income
      a. Gate receipts
      b. Student activities tickets
      c. Tournament receipts
   2. Estimated expenditures
      a. Awards
      b. Tournament fees
      c. Films
      d. Miscellaneous
      e. Surplus

D. General budget: considerations
   1. Breakdown
      a. By sport or activity
      b. Transportation
      c. Salaries of personnel
      d. Insurance
      e. Reconditioning of equipment
      f. Supervision
      g. General and miscellaneous
      h. Equipment
      i. Officials
   2. Codes
      a. Advertising
      b. Travel
      c. Conferences
      d. Others

E. Postbudget procedures
   1. Selection of equipment and supplies
   2. Preparation of list of dealers to bid
   3. Request for price quotations
   4. Requisitions
   5. Care of equipment
   6. Notification of teachers and coaches of amounts approved

F. Ordering procedures
   1. Study the quality of varius products
   2. Accept no substitutes for items ordered
   3. Submit request for price quotations
   4. Select low quotes or justify higher quotes
   5. Submit purchase orders
   6. Check and count all shipments
   7. Record items received on inventory cards
   8. Provide for equipment and supply accountability

* Adapted from recommendations of Director's Workshop, New York University, 1968.

THE ROLE OF THE ADMINISTRATOR IN BUDGETING—cont'd

G. Relationships with administration
  1. Consultation—program plans with building principal and/or superintendent
  2. Make budget recommendations to administration
  3. Advise business manager of procedures followed
  4. Discuss items approved and deleted with business manager
  5. Advise teachers and coaches of amounts available and adjust requests

H. Suggestions for prospective directors of physical education programs

  1. Develop a philosophy and approach to budgeting
  2. Consult with staff for their suggestions
  3. Select quality merchandise
  4. Provide proper care and maintenance of equipment and supplies
  5. Provide for all programs on an equitable basis
  6. Budget adequately but not elaborately
  7. Provide a sound well-rounded program of physical education
  8. Emphasize equality for girls and boys
  9. Provide for basic instructional, adapted, intramural and extramural, and interscholastic parts of the program
  10. Conduct a year-round public relations program
  11. Try to overcome these possible shortcomings:
      a. Board of education not oriented to needs of physical education
      b. Program not achieving established goals
      c. Staff not adequately informed and involved in administrative process

---

3. They determine what phases of the program are to be emphasized. They aid in an analysis of all aspects of health and physical education programs.

4. They interpret to the principal, superintendent of schools, board of education (or trustees), dean, and the public in general the needs of health and physical education.

5. They assist, together with the budgets of other educational subdivisions, in determining the tax levy for the school district.

6. They make it possible, upon approval by the recognized officials, to authorize expenditures for the program of health and physical education.

7. They make it possible to administer the health and physical education program economically by improving accounting procedures.

Types of budgets

There are short-term and long-term budgets. The short-term is usually the annual budget that runs for a 12-month period. The long-term budget represents long-term fiscal planning, possibly for a 10-year period. Most health and physical education personnel will be concerned with short-term or annual budgets whereby they plan their financial needs for a period covering the school year.

Responsibility for budgets

The responsibility for the preparation of the overall school or college budget may vary from one locality to another. In most systems the superintendent of schools is responsible. In colleges it is the responsibility of the president and the dean. Where these situations exist, it is often possible for principals, department heads, teachers, and professors to participate in preparation of the budget by submitting various requests for budget items. In other situations the budget may be first prepared in nearly all its details and then submitted to the subdivisions for consideration.

In some large school systems the superintendent of schools frequently delegates much of the budget responsibility to a business manager, a clerk, or an assistant or associate superintendent.

The final official school authority in respect to school budgets is the board of education. This body can approve, reject, or amend. But even beyond the board of education rests the authority of the people, who in most communities have the right to approve or reject the budget.

In colleges the budget may be handled in the dean's office, or the director or chairman of the physical education department may have the responsibility. In some cases the director of athletics is responsible for the athletic budget.

Within school departments of health and physical education the chairman, supervisor, or director is the person responsible for the budget. However, he or she will usually consult with members of the department and receive their suggestions.

Criteria for a good budget

A budget for health and physical education should meet the following criteria:

1. The budget will clearly present the financial needs of the entire program in relation to the objectives sought.

2. Key persons in the organization have been consulted.

3. The budget will provide a realistic estimate of income to balance the expenditures that are anticipated.

4. The budget should reflect equitable allocations to boys' and girls' athletic programs.

5. The possibility of emergencies is recognized through flexibility in the financial plan.

6. The budget will be prepared well in advance of the fiscal year in order to leave ample time for analysis, thought, criticism, and review.

7. Budget requests are realistic, not padded.

8. The budget meets the essential requirements of students, faculty, and administrators.

Budget preparation and planning

Four general steps for procedure in budget planning that health and physical education personnel might consider are as follows:

1. Actual preparation of the budget by the chairman of the department with his or her staff, listing the various estimated receipts, expenditures, and any other information that needs to be included.

2. Presentation of the budget to the principal, superintendent, dean, board of education, or other person or group that represents the proper authority and has the responsibility for reviewing it.

3. After formal approval of the budget, its use as a guide for the financial management and administration of the department or organization.

4. Critical evaluation of the budget periodically to determine its effectiveness in meeting educational needs, with notations being made for the next year's budget.

The preparation of the budget, representing the first step, is a long-term endeavor that cannot be accomplished in a day or two. The budget is something that can be well prepared only after a careful review of program effectiveness and appraisal over an extended period of time. However, the actual finalization of the budget usually is accomplished in the early spring after a detailed inventory of program needs has been taken. The director of health and/or physical education, after close consultation with staff members and the principal, dean, superintendent of schools, or other responsible administrative officer, should formulate the budget.

In preparing the budget many records and reports will be of value. The inventory of equipment and supplies on hand will be useful, and copies of inventories and budgets from previous years will provide good references. Comparison of budgetary items with those in schools and colleges of similar size may be of help. Accounting records will be valuable.

The preparation of the budget should be accomplished in such a way that it is flexible and will allow for readjustments to be made, if necessary. It is difficult to accurately and specifically list each detail in the way that it will be needed and executed.

The budget should represent a schedule that can be justified. This means that each budgetary item must satisfy the most meaningful educational needs and interests of all concerned. Furthermore, each item that constitutes an expenditure should be reflected in budget specifications.

Richard G. Mitchell, writing on "administrative planning," lists these five important considerations in budget preparation:

1. What was planned last year? This constitutes the tying together of the proposed budget with the one approved last year to check on long-term planning goals.
2. What was accomplished last year? This step relates last

year's accomplishments to the achievement of the department's long-term objectives.

3. What can realistically be accomplished this year? In light of past years, future trends, and the master plan, what can be accomplished this year?

4. What needs to be done? This constitutes the minimum essentials that must be accomplished this year. These items have priority.

5. How is it to be done? Such items as staff, equipment, supplies, and other requirements for accomplishment and meeting of needs would be outlined.*

Budget organization

Budgets can be organized in many ways. One pattern that consists of four sections or divisions and that might prove useful for a health or physical education administrator is described here:

1. An introductory message enables the administration to present the financial proposals in terms that a board of education or person outside the specialized fields might readily understand. This section offers to persons who have specialized in these areas an opportunity to discuss some aspects of the program in lay terms and some of the directions that need to be taken in order to provide for the health and physical fitness of the students.

2. The second section presents an overall view of the budget, with expenditures and anticipated revenues arranged in a clear and systematic fashion so that any person can compare the two.

3. A third section, with an estimate of receipts and expenditures in much more detail, should enable a principal, superintendent of schools and/or board of education, or other interested person or group to understand the budget specifically and to follow up any item of cost.

4. A fourth section might include supporting schedules to provide additional evidence for the requests outlined in the budget. Many times a budget will have a better chance of approval if there is sufficient documentation to support some items. For example, extra pay for coaching may be thought to be desirable. Salary schedules for coaches in other school systems could be included to support such a proposition.

Another type of budget organization might be

one that consists of the following three parts: (1) an introductory statement of the objectives, policies, and program of the health and physical education department; (2) a résumé of the objectives, policies, and program interpreted in terms of proposed expenditures; and (3) a financial plan for meeting the educational needs during the fiscal period.

Not all budgets are broken down into these four or three divisions. All budgets do, however, give an itemized account of receipts and expenditures.

In a physical education budget common inclusions are items concerning instruction, such as extra compensation for coaches; matters of capital outlay, such as a new swimming pool or handball court; the replacement of expendable equipment, such as basketballs and baseball bats; and provision for maintenance and repair, such as refurbishing football uniforms or doing some grading on the playground. It is difficult to estimate many of these items without making a careful inventory and analysis of the condition of the facilities and equipment.

Sources of income

The sources of income for most school and college health and physical education programs include the general school or college fund, gate receipts, health, general organization, and activity fees, and some other revenues.

General school or college fund. At the elementary and secondary levels the health program would be supported, usually entirely, through general school funds, and the physical education program would be financed in the same way, to a large extent. At the college and university level the general fund of the institution would also represent a major source of income.

Gate receipts. Gate receipts play an important part in some schools in the financing of at least part of the physical education program. Although there is usually less stress on gate receipts at lower educational levels, colleges and universities sometimes finance their entire athletic, intramural, and physical education programs through such a method. At a few high schools throughout the country, gate receipts have been abolished because of the feeling that

---

*Mitchell, R. G.: Administrative planning—its effective use, Recreation **44:**426, 1961.

if athletics represent an important part of the education program, they should be paid for in the same way that science and mathematics programs, for example, are financed.

Health, general organization, and activity fees. Some high schools either require or make available to students separate health, general organization, or activity fees and tickets or some other inducement that enables them to attend the athletic, dramatic, and musical events that are offered. In colleges and universities a similar plan is generally used, thus providing students with reduced rates to the various out-of-class activities offered by the institution. A

Table 16-1. General organization athletic account—financial report (September-December)

Expenses		
Football		
Officials (four home games)	$ 240.00	
Equipment and supplies	1,182.01	
Transportation	87.50	
Supervision (police, ticket sellers and takers)	476.00	
Reconditioning and cleaning equipment	656.60	
Medical supplies	62.70	
Scouting	30.00	
Film	15.68	
Guarantees	260.00	
Football dinner	115.50	
Miscellaneous (printing tickets, meetings)	86.00	
Total football expense		$3,211.99
Cross country		
State and county entry fees	$ 5.00	
Transportation	32.00	
Total cross country expense		$ 37.00
Basketball		
Supervision (three games)	$ 18.00	
Custodian (three games)	13.00	
Police (one game)	6.00	
Total basketball expense		$ 37.00
Cheerleaders		
Transportation	$ 26.10	
Sixteen sweaters	160.00	
Cleaning sweaters	48.00	
Total cheerleader expense		$ 234.10
Total expenses		$3,520.09
Receipts		
Football		
Newburgh game	$ 655.85	
Norwalk game	909.80	
Yonkers game	564.75	
Bridgeport game	550.00	
Guarantee (New Haven)	60.00	
Total receipts		$2,740.40

health fee also is quite common at higher education levels. Table 16-1 shows a general organization financial statement.

Other sources of income. Some other sources of income, not so common to all educational levels, are (1) *special foundation, governmental, or individual grants or gifts* intended to promote physical fitness, athletics, or some phase of health and physical education programs; (2) the sale of *radio and television rights* at the college level, especially for those institutions that have nationally ranking teams and where the athletic contests have great public appeal; (3) *concessions* at athletic contests and other activity events; and (4) *special fund-raising events* such as a faculty-varsity basketball game or a gymnastic circus.

Some steps that might be followed for estimating receipts in the general school budget and that also have application to the health and physical education budget include:

1. Gathering and analyzing all pertinent data, including past and current information
2. Estimating all income based on comprehensive view of income sources
3. Organizing and classifying receipts in appropriate categories
4. Estimating revenue from all gathered data
5. Comparing estimates with previous years and drawing up final draft of receipts

Expenditures

In health and physical education budgets, typical examples of expenditures are items of *capital outlay,* such as a dental chair or swimming pool; *expendable equipment,* such as tongue depressors or basketballs; and a *maintenance and repair provision,* such as towel and laundry service and the repair of pure-tone audiometers or refurbishing of football uniforms. See Table 16-2 for a sample list of expenditures for athletics.

Some expenditures are very easy to estimate but others are more difficult, requiring the keeping of accurate inventories, examination of past records, and careful analysis of the condition of the equipment. Some items and services will need to be figured by averaging costs over a period of years, such as cleaning and mending athletic equipment. Other examples of items that require careful consideration in order to list

expenditures accurately are awards, new equipment needed, guarantees to visiting teams, and medical services for emergencies.

Some sound procedures to follow in estimating expenditures include:

1. Determine objectives and goals of program.
2. Analyze expenditures in terms of program objectives.
3. Prepare a budgetary calendar that states what accomplishments are expected and by what date.
4. Estimate expenditures by also considering past, present, and future needs.
5. Compare estimates with expenditures for previous years.
6. Estimates should be thoroughly evaluated prior to preparing final draft.

Budget presentation and adoption

Budgets in health and physical education, after being prepared, should usually be submitted to the superintendent through the principal's office. The principal represents the person in charge of his or her particular building and, therefore, subdivision budgets should be presented to him or her for approval. Good administration would mean, furthermore, that the budgetary items would have been reviewed with the principal during their preparation so that approval is usually a routine matter.

In the case of college and university, the proper channels should be followed. This might mean clearance through a dean or other administrative officer. Each person, of course, who is responsible for budget preparation and presentation should be very familiar with the proper working channels.

For successful presentation and adoption, the budget should be prepared in final form only after careful consideration so that little change will be needed. Requests for funds should be justifiable, and ample preliminary discussion of the budget with persons and groups most directly concerned should be held so that needless difficulty will be avoided.

Budget administration

After the presentation and approval of the budget, the next step is to see that it is administered properly. This means that it should be

Table 16-2. A sample list of expenditures for athletics

	Baseball	Basketball	Football	Cross country	Girls' sports	Golf	Hockey	Soccer	Swimming	Tennis	Track	Total
Equipment and supplies	$369.55	$116.70	$278.68	$45.80	$41.60	$36.10	$251.65	$70.40	$80.05	$27.20	$231.77	$1,549.50
Transportation	208.50	248.70	39.60	83.20	84.98	48.40	495.00	63.70	108.80	8.80	120.90	1,510.48
Officials	122.00	391.35	50.00					52.00				615.35
Cleaning	65.70	30.95	129.40				95.60	57.20			141.10	519.95
Supervision		66.00										66.00
Custodian		37.00										37.00
Additional coaching			350.00					100.00				450.00
Entry fees						7.00			17.21	4.00	22.50	50.75
Rental, boys' club pool									250.00			250.00
Totals	$765.75	$890.70	$847.68	$129.00	$126.58	$91.50	$842.25	$343.20	$456.10	$40.00	$516.27	$5,049.03

followed as closely as possible with periodic checks on expenditures to see that they fall within the budget appropriations that have been provided. The budget should function as a good guide for economical and efficient administration.

Budget appraisal

Periodic appraisal calls for an audit of the accounts and an evaluation of the school program resulting from the administration of the current budget. Such appraisal should be done in all honesty and with a view to eliminating weaknesses in current budgets and strengthening future ones. It should also be remembered that the budget will be only as good as the administration makes it and that the budget will improve only as the administration improves.

FINANCIAL ACCOUNTING

The great amount of money involved in health and physical education programs means that strict accountability must be observed. This means the maintenance of accurate records, proper distribution of materials, and adequate appraisal and evaluation of procedures. Financial accounting should provide:

1. A record of receipts and expenditures for all departmental transactions
2. A permanent record of all financial transactions for future reference
3. A pattern for expenditures that is closely related to the approved budget
4. A tangible documentation of compliance with mandates and requests either imposed by law or by administrative action
5. Some procedure for evaluating, to ensure that funds are dealt with honestly, and proper management in respect to control, analysis of costs, and reporting

Most of the state departments of education publish manuals on school accounting. Each chairperson of health and physical education should have a copy of his or her own state's school accounting procedure and should read and follow it carefully.

Reasons for financial accounting

Some reasons why financial accounting is needed in health and physical education include the following:

1. To provide a method of authorizing expenditures for items that have been included and approved in the budget. This means proper accounting records are being used.

2. To provide authorized procedures for making purchases of equipment, supplies, and other materials and to let contracts for various services.

3. To provide authorized procedures for paying the proper amounts (a) for purchases of equipment, supplies, and other materials, which have been checked upon receipt, (b) for labor that actually has taken place, and (c) for other services that have been rendered.

4. To provide a record of each payment that has been made, including the date, to whom, for what purpose, and other pertinent material.

5. To provide authorized procedures for handling various receipts and sources of income.

6. To provide the detailed information that is essential for proper auditing of accounts, such as confirmation that money has been spent for accurately specified items.

7. To provide material and information for the preparation of future budgets.

8. To provide a tangible base for the development of future policies relating to financial planning.

Administrative principles and policies for financial accounting

The Athletic Institute* has prepared some excellent material on accountability, in which it brings out such important principles and policies as the following:

1. The administrative head has the final responsibility for accountability for all equipment and supplies in his or her organization.

2. Departments should establish and enforce policies covering loss, damage, theft, misappropriation, or destruction of equipment and supplies or other materials.

3. A system of accurate record keeping should be established and be uniform throughout the department.

4. Accountability should demonstrate the close relationship that exists between equipment and supplies and the program objectives.

*The Athletic Institute: Equipment and supplies for athletics, physical education and recreation. Chicago, 1960, The Institute, chap. 5.

Table 16-3. Sample sports program, general organization, and board of education report of expenditures and receipts

Sports	Board of education	General organization	Total
Total expenditures			
Baseball	$ 765.75		$ 765.75
Basketball	890.70	$ 106.34	997.04
Football	847.68	3,943.09	4,340.77
Cross country	129.00	37.00	166.00
Girls' sports and cheerleaders	126.58	249.10	375.68
Golf	91.50		91.50
Hockey	842.25	48.95	891.20
Soccer	343.20		343.20
Swimming	456.10	41.10	497.20
Tennis	40.00	4.00	44.00
Track	516.27	15.03	531.30
Total	$5,049.03	$3,994.61	$9,043.64
Total general organization receipts			
Football		$2,740.40	
Basketball		381.30	
Total			$3,121.70

5. A system of policies should be developed that will guarantee the proper use and protection of all equipment and supplies within the department.

6. The person to whom equipment and supplies are issued should be held accountable for these materials.

7. Accurate inventories are essential to proper financial accounting.

8. A system of marking equipment and supplies as proof of ownership should be instituted.

9. A meaningful procedure should be established for the proper distribution of all equipment and supplies.

10. The discarding of equipment and supplies should take place only in accordance with established procedures and by authorized persons.

Accounting for receipts and expenditures

A centralized accounting system is very advantageous, with all funds being deposited with the school treasurer or business manager. Purchase orders and other procedures are usually then countersigned or certified by the school treasurer, thus better guaranteeing integrity in the use of funds. A system of bookkeeping wherein books are housed in the central office by the finance officer helps to ensure better control of finances by the school and allows for all subdivisions or departments in an educational system to be financially controlled in the same manner. Such a procedure also provides for better and more centralized record keeping. The central accounting system fund accounts, in which are located the physical education and health funds, should be audited annually by qualified persons not associated with the school funds. Finally, an annual financial report should be made and publicized to indicate receipts, expenditures, and other pertinent data associated with the enterprise.

All receipts and expenditures should be recorded in the ledger in the proper manner, providing such important information as the fund in which it has been deposited, or from which it was withdrawn, and the money received from such sources as athletics and dues to school organizations should be shown with sufficient cross references and detailed information. Supporting vouchers should also be at hand. Tickets to athletic and other events should be numbered consecutively and checked to get an accurate record of ticket sales. Students should not be permitted to handle funds except under the supervision of some member of the administrative staff or faculty. All accounts should be properly audited at appropriate intervals.

Purchase orders on regular authorized forms issued by the school should be used, so that accurate records may be kept. To order verbally is a questionable policy. By preparing written purchase orders, on regular forms and according to good accountability procedure, legality of contract is better ensured, together with prompt delivery and payment. For more information see Chapter 17 on the purchase and care of supplies and equipment.

CHECKLIST FOR BUDGETING AND FINANCIAL ACCOUNTING

	Yes	No
1. Has a complete inventory been taken and itemized on proper forms as a guide in estimating equipment needs?		
2. Does the equipment inventory include a detailed account of the number of items on hand, size and quantity, type, condition, etc.?		
3. Is the inventory complete, current, and up-to-date?		
4. Are budgetary estimates as accurate and realistic as possible without padding?		
5. Are provisions made in the budget for increases expected in enrollments, increased pupil participation, and changes in the cost of equipment and supplies?		
6. Have supply house and the school business administrator been consulted on the cost of new equipment?		
7. Has the Director of Health and Physical Education consulted with his staff on various budget items?		

CHECKLIST FOR BUDGETING AND FINANCIAL ACCOUNTING—cont'd

	Yes	No

8. Has the Director of Health and Physical Education consulted with the school business administrator in respect to the total budget for his department?

9. Are new equipment and supply needs for health and physical education determined and budgeted at least one year in advance?

10. Was the budget prepared according to the standards desired by the chief school administrator?

11. Are statistics and information for previous years indicated as a means of comparison?

12. Is there a summary of receipts and expenditures listed concisely on one page so that the total budget can be quickly seen?

13. If receipts from athletics or other funds are to be added to the budget, is this shown?

14. Are there alternate program plans with budgetary changes in the event the budget is not approved?

15. Has a statement of objectives of the program been included that reflects the overall educational philosophy and program of the total school and community?

16. Has the budget been prepared so that the major aspects may be viewed readily by those persons desiring a quick review and also in more detail for those persons desiring a further delineation of the budgetary items?

17. Is the period of time for which the budget has been prepared clearly indicated?

18. Is the health and physical education budget based on an educational plan developed to attain the goals and purposes agreed upon by the director and his staff within the framework of the total school's philosophy?

19. Is the health and physical education plan a comprehensive one reflecting health science instruction, health services, and a healthful environment, physical education class, adapted, intramural and extramural, and interscholastic program?

20. Does the plan include a statement of the objectives of the health and physical education programs and are these reflected in the budget?

21. Are both long-range and short-range plans for achieving the purposes of the program provided?

22. Have provisions been made in the budget for emergencies?

23. Are accurate records kept on such activities involving expenditures of money as transportation, insurance, officials, laundry and dry cleaning, awards, guarantees, repairs, new equipment, medical expenses, and publicity?

24. Are accurate records kept on the receipt of monies from such sources as gate receipts and advertising revenue?

25. Once the budget has been approved, is there a specific plan provided for authorizing expenditures?

26. Are specific forms used for recording purchase transactions?

27. Are purchases on all major items based on competitive bidding?

28. Are requisitions used in obtaining supplies and equipment?

29. Are requisitions numbered and do they include such information as the name of the person originating the requisition, when the item to be purchased will be needed, where to ship the item, the description and/or code number, quantity, unit price, and amount?

30. With the exception of petty cash accounts, is a central purchasing system in effect?

31. Is the policy of quantity purchasing followed wherever possible and desirable in the interests of economy?

32. If quantity purchasing is used, is advanced thought and planning given to storage and maintenance facilities and procedures?

33. Are performance tests made of items purchased? Are state, regional, or national testing bureaus or laboratories utilized where feasible?

34. Are receipts of equipment and supplies checked carefully?

35. Is an audit made of all expenditures?

36. Are specific procedures in effect to safeguard money, property, and employees?

37. Is there a check to determine that established standards, policies, and procedures have been followed?

Continued.

CHECKLIST FOR BUDGETING AND FINANCIAL ACCOUNTING—cont'd

	Yes	No
38. Are procedures in operation to check condition and use of equipment and supplies?	____	____
39. Is a financial report made periodically?	____	____
40. Are there proper procedures for the care and maintenance and accountability of all equipment and supplies?	____	____
41. Are accurate records kept on all equipment and supplies including condition, site, and age?	____	____
42. Have established procedures been developed and are they followed in regard to the issuance, use, and return of equipment?	____	____
43. Have provisions been made for making regular notations of future needs?	____	____

Questions and exercises

1. Write a detailed essay discussing the history, definition, utilization, advantages, and disadvantages of the PPB System.
2. Does your school or individual department utilize PPBS in budget planning? If so, briefly discuss the use of this system. If it is not used, write a brief PPBS plan for your department, gathering data from key individuals in this area.
3. Prepare a budget for a high school or college department of physical education.
4. What are five reasons for fiscal management in health and physical education?
5. Collect budgets from five school systems or colleges and critically evaluate them.
6. Where does the responsibility fall for budget preparation?
7. Outline the procedure you would follow in the preparation of a budget if you were the chairperson of the department of health and physical education for a city educational system.
8. What are the criteria for a good budget?
9. What are the most common sources of receipts and expenditures in a health and/or physical education department?
10. Formulate ten policies to ensure good financial accounting.

Reading assignment in *Administrative Dimensions of Health and Physical Education Programs, Including Athletics:* Chapter 13, Selections 70 to 76.

Selected references

Andrew, L., and Robertson, L.: PPBS in higher education: a case study, Educational Record **54**:61, 1973.

Athletic Institute: Equipment and supplies for athletics, physical education, and recreation, Chicago, 1960, The Institute.

Avedisian, C.: Planning, programming, budgeting systems, Journal of Health, Pysical Education, and Recreation **43**:37, 1972.

Boston, R. E.: Management by objectives: A management system for education, Educational Technology **12**:49, 1972.

Casey, L. M.: School business administration, New York, 1964, The Center for Applied Research in Education, Inc. (The Library of Education).

Cosgrove, J. N., editor: Budgeting-experts say it's wise planning, not pinching pennies, The National Underwriter **50**:42, 1967.

Fleischmann, M., chairman: Report of the New York State Commission on the quality, cost and financing of elementary and secondary education, vol. 1., Albany, New York, 1972, New York State Commission on the quality, cost and financing of elementary and secondary education.

Hartley, H. J.: Educational planning-programming-budgeting, a systems approach, Englewood Cliffs, New Jersey, 1968, Prentice-Hall Inc.

Hartley, H. J.: PPBS: A status report with operational suggestions, Educational Technology **12**:21, 1972.

Jenkins, W. A., and Lehman, G. O.: Nine pitfalls of PPBS, School Management **16**:2, 1972.

Johns, R. L., and Morphet, E. L.: The economics and financing of education, a systems approach, Englewood Cliffs, New Jersey, 1969, Prentice-Hall Inc.

Johns, R. L., and others: Planning to finance education, vol. 3, Gainsville, Florida, 1970, The National Education Finance Project.

Knezevich, S. J., and Fowlkes, J. G.: Business management of local school systems, New York, 1960, Harper & Row, Publishers.

Ranney, D. C.: The determinants of fiscal support for large city educational systems, Administrators Notebook **15**: December, 1966.

Sisson, R. L., and others: An introduction to the educational planning, programming, budgeting system, Educational Technology **12**:54, 1972.

Weathersby, G. B.: PPBS: purpose, persuasion, backbone, and spunk, Liberal Education **57**:211, 1971.

Wilsey, C. F.: Budget for equipment replacement, School Board Journal, p. 10, May, 1967.

The purchase and care of supplies and equipment including audiovisual materials

Educational technology is no longer a new concept in school and college physical education programs. Videotapes and instant play-back machines are being used for such diverse functions as tennis skill instruction and teacher behavior observation. Cable television has numerous educational uses that enable administrators and teachers to participate in program development. These and other audiovisual breakthroughs will be explored in this chapter along with the essentials of purchase and care of equipment and supplies.

Health and physical education programs utilize many supplies and equipment that cost thousands of dollars. *Supplies* are those materials that are expendable and that need to be replaced at frequent intervals, such as shuttlecocks and adhesive tape. *Equipment* is the term used for those items that are not considered expendable but are utilized over a period of years, such as parallel bars and audiometers.

Since so much money is expended upon supplies and equipment and since such materials are vital to school and college health and safety, to good playing conditions, and to values derived from the programs, it is important that this administrative phase of the specialized fields of

health and physical education be considered carefully. The purchase of supplies and equipment should also be related to the achievement of objectives as designated by the PPB System. It is important that administrators and physical educators express their need for equipment and other materials in terms of the educational goals that these aids represent.

Many different sources for purchasing equipment exist, many grades and qualities of materials are available, and many methods of storing and maintaining such merchandise are prevalent. Some of these sources, grades, and methods are good and some are questionable. In order to obtain the greatest values for the amount of money spent, basic principles of selecting, purchasing, and maintaining need to be known and understood. This chapter includes a brief discussion of these matters and also a discussion of audiovisual materials.

SUPPLY AND EQUIPMENT NEEDS VARY

Supplies and equipment needed in a school or college system will vary according to certain influencing factors. These include, first, the programs themselves and the activities that are to be offered. The geographic location of the school will help to determine the activities scheduled, as will such other elements as the interests of students and their physiologic, psychologic, and sociologic needs. Another factor would be the other facilities and the health rooms and playing space available. Some schools and a few colleges do not have a health suite and have only limited physical education facilities. Under such conditions the supplies and equipment needed will differ from those required in settings where spacious accommodations exist. Other factors that will need to be taken into consideration are the nature of the clientele (in regard to age, sex, and number of students), the money available, the length of playing seasons, and provisions for the health and safety of participants. Those persons responsible for purchasing supplies and equipment should carefully study their own particular situations and estimate their own needs in an objective and realistic manner.

As pointed out previously, the types of equipment and supplies will vary with the program. In the health education area such articles as microscopes, mannequins, test materials, laboratory equipment, and audiovisual equipment will be needed. In the health service area there will be a need for such items as equipment for screening vision and hearing, first-aid supplies, scales, examining table, dental equipment and supplies, beds, towels, and sheets. In the physical education area, of course, all types of balls, apparatus, uniforms, timers, and racks will be needed if individual, team, formal, aquatic, dance, and other activities are to be offered. Different types of materials will be required for the interschool and intercollegiate athletic programs, the intramural and extramural programs, the adapted programs, and the class programs. Many decisions in the purchasing of equipment and supplies will depend upon the objectives being sought by the administration.

In general, however, the administration is interested in:

1. Trying to standardize supplies and equipment as much as possible
2. Supervising the entire process of selection, purchase, storage, and maintenance

3. Maintaining a list of sources of materials
4. Preparing specifications for various items that are to be purchased
5. Securing bids for large purchases and those required by law
6. Deciding upon or recommending organizations where materials are to be purchased
7. Testing products to see that specifications are satisfactorily met
8. Checking supplies and equipment to determine if all that were ordered have been delivered
9. Expediting the delivery of purchases so that materials are available as needed
10. Continually seeking new products that meet the needs of the program
11. Providing overall supervision of purchase, care, and use of supplies and equipment

SELECTION OF SUPPLIES AND EQUIPMENT

A discussion of some of the principles that should be observed in the selection of supplies and equipment for school and college health and physical education programs, including athletics, follows.

Selection should be based upon local needs. Supplies and equipment should be selected because they are needed in a particular school or college situation and by a particular group of students. Items should be selected that represent materials needed to carry out the program as outlined in the course of study and that represent essentials to fulfilling program objectives.

Selection should be based upon quality. In the long run, the item of good quality is the cheapest and the safest. Bargains too often represent inferior materials that wear out much earlier. Only the best grade of football equipment should be purchased. The author did a study of football deaths that occurred during a 25-year period and found that many of these deaths had resulted from the use of inferior helmets and other poor equipment. What is true of football is also true of other activities.

Selection should be made by competent personnel. The persons carrying out the assignment of selecting the supplies and equipment

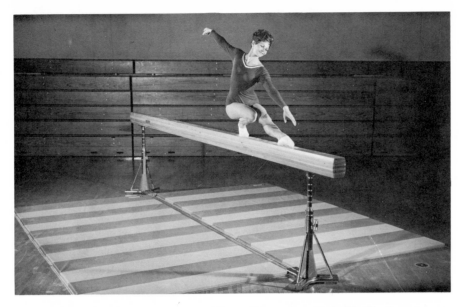

Gymnastic equipment. (Courtesy Nissen Corporation, Cedar Rapids, Iowa.)

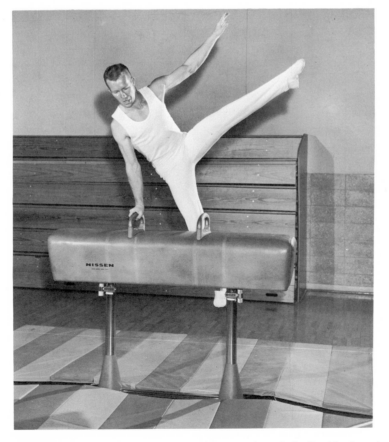

Gymnastic equipment. (Courtesy Nissen Corporation, Cedar Rapids, Iowa.)

KEY TO FIGURES

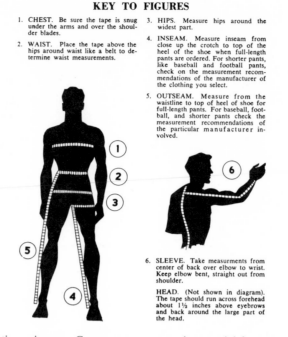

1. CHEST. Be sure the tape is snug under the arms and over the shoulder blades.

2. WAIST. Place the tape above the hips around waist like a belt to determine waist measurements.

3. HIPS. Measure hips around the widest part.

4. INSEAM. Measure inseam from close up the crotch to top of the heel of the shoe when full-length pants are ordered. For shorter pants, like baseball and football pants, check on the measurement recommendations of the manufacturer of the clothing you select.

5. OUTSEAM. Measure from the waistline to top of heel of shoe for full-length pants. For baseball, football, and shorter pants check the measurement recommendations of the particular manufacturer involved.

6. SLEEVE. Take measurments from center of back over elbow to wrist. Keep elbow bent, straight out from shoulder.

HEAD. (Not shown in diagram). The tape should run across forehead about 1½ inches above eyebrows and back around the large part of the head.

How to measure for athletic equipment. Correct measurement is essential for proper sizing of athletic equipment to ensure the comfort of the wearer, durability of equipment, proper protection, and appearance on the field. This illustration may be used as a measuring guide to ensure the proper fit of uniforms, jerseys, protective equipment, and warmup suits. This is a basic measuring guide for most types of athletic equipment. For a perfect fit it is also recommended that you state height, weight, and any special irregularities of build. (From How to budget, select, and order athletic equipment, Chicago, 1962, The Athletic Institute.)

needed in health and physical education programs should be competent to assume such a responsibility. To perform such a job efficiently means examining many types and makes of products, conducting experiments to determine such qualities as economy and durability, listing and weighing the advantages and disadvantages of different items, and knowing how each item is going to be used. The person selecting supplies and equipment should be interested in this responsibility, have the time to do the job, and possess those qualities needed to perform the function in an efficient manner. Some schools and colleges have purchasing agents who are specially trained in these matters. In small organizations the chairman, director, or coach frequently performs this responsibility. One other point is important: regardless of who the responsible person may be, the staff member who utilizes these supplies and equipment in his or her particular facet of the total program should have a great deal to say about the specific items

chosen. He or she is the one who understands the functional use of the merchandise.

Selection should be continuous. A product that ranks as the "best" available this year may not necessarily be the "best" next year. Manufacturers are constantly conducting research in order to come out with something better. There is keen competition among them. The administration, therefore, cannot be complacent and apathetic, thinking that because a certain product has served them so well in the past, it is the best buy for the future. Instead, there must be a continual search for the best product available.

Selection should take into consideration service and replacement needs. Items of supplies and equipment may be difficult to obtain in volume. Upon receipt of merchandise, sizes of uniforms may be wrong and colors may be mixed up. Additional materials may be needed on short notice. Such facts mean that in the selection process consideration should be given to selecting items that will be available in vol-

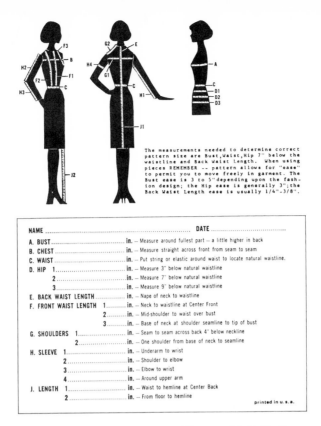

The measurements needed to determine correct pattern size are Bust, Waist, Hip 7" below the waistline and Back Waist Length. When using pieces REMEMBER -- pattern allows for "ease" to permit you to move freely in garment. The Bust ease is 3 to 5" depending upon the fashion design; the Hip ease is generally 3"; the Back Waist Length ease is usually 1/4"-3/8".

NAME		DATE	
A. BUST	in.	— Measure around fullest part — a little higher in back	
B. CHEST	in.	— Measure straight across front from seam to seam	
C. WAIST	in.	— Put string or elastic around waist to locate natural waistline.	
D. HIP 1	in.	— Measure 3" below natural waistline	
2	in.	— Measure 7" below natural waistline	
3	in.	— Measure 9" below natural waistline	
E. BACK WAIST LENGTH	in.	— Nape of neck to waistline	
F. FRONT WAIST LENGTH 1	in.	— Neck to waistline at Center Front	
2	in.	— Mid-shoulder to waist over bust	
3	in.	— Base of neck at shoulder seamline to tip of bust	
G. SHOULDERS 1	in.	— Seam to seam across back 4" below neckline	
2	in.	— One shoulder from base of neck to seamline	
H. SLEEVE 1	in.	— Underarm to wrist	
2	in.	— Shoulder to elbow	
3	in.	— Elbow to wrist	
4	in.	— Around upper arm	
J. LENGTH 1	in.	— Waist to hemline at Center Back	
2	in.	— From floor to hemline	

printed in u.s.a.

How to take a girl's measurements. (Courtesy McCall's Patterns.)

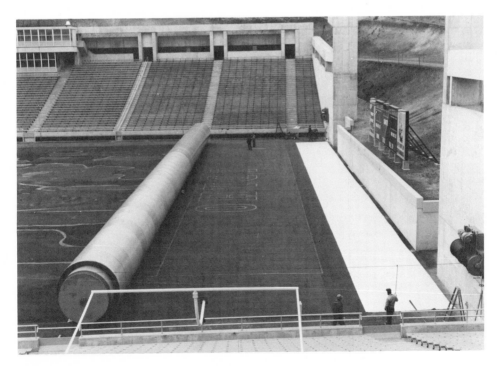

The University of Idaho purchased a new portable football field. The Tartan Turf is 200 by 370 feet and can be rolled up and stored on a 210 feet long steel drum. (Courtesy Scholastic Coach.)

ume, if needed, and that consideration should be given to dealing with a business firm that will service and replace materials and take care of emergencies without delay and controversy.

PURCHASING SUPPLIES AND EQUIPMENT

A discussion of several important considerations in making purchases of supplies and equipment follows.

Purchases should meet the requirements established by the educational system and have administrative approval

Each educational system has its own policy providing for the purchase of supplies and equipment. It is essential that the prescribed pattern be followed and that proper administrative approval be obtained. Requisition forms that contain such information as description of items, amounts, and costs; purchase orders that place the buying procedure on a written or contract basis; and voucher forms that show receipt of materials should all be utilized as prescribed by school or college regulations. The health and physical education administrator and staff should be familiar with and follow local purchasing policies.

Below are listed a series of steps that one school system uses in purchasing equipment:

1. *Initiation.* A request is made by the teacher for equipment to fulfill, augment, supplement, or improve the curriculum.

Purchase requisition.

2. *Review of request.* The building principal and central administration approve or disapprove request after careful consideration of need.

3. *Review of budget allocation.* A budget code number is assigned after availability of funds in that category has been determined.

4. *Preparation of specifications.* Specifications are prepared in detail, giving exact quality requirements, and made available to prospective contractors or vendors.

5. *Receipt of bids.* Contractors or vendors submit price quotations.

6. *Comparison of bids to specifications.* Careful evaluation is made to determine exact fulfillment of quality requirements.

7. *Recommendations to the board of education.* The business administrator prepares comparisons for the board of education, with specific recommendations for their approval.

8. *Purchase order to supplier.* After board of education approval, a purchase is made that fulfills the requirements at a competitive price.

Purchasing should be done in advance of need

The main and bulk purchases of supplies and equipment for programs of health and physical education should be completed well in advance of the time that the materials will be utilized. Late orders, rushed through at the last moment,

Purchase order.

may mean mistakes or substitutions on the part of the manufacturer. When purchase orders are placed early, manufacturers have more time to do their jobs and can carry out their responsibilities more efficiently. Goods that do not meet specifications can be returned and replaced, and many other advantages result. Items that are needed in the fall should be ordered not later than the preceding spring, and items desired for spring use should be ordered not later than the preceding fall.

Supplies and equipment should be standardized as far as possible and practical

Ease of ordering is accomplished and larger quantities of materials can be purchased at a saving when standardized items of supplies and equipment are used. Standardization means that certain colors, styles, and types of material are ordered consistently. This procedure can be followed after careful research to determine what is the best, most reliable, and most serviceable product for the money. However, standardization of supplies and equipment should never mean that further study and research to find the best materials in the light of program objectives are terminated.

Specifications should be clearly set forth when making purchases

The trademark, item number, catalogue number, type of material, and other important specifications should be clearly stated when purchasing material to avoid any misunderstanding of what is wanted and is being ordered. This procedure ensures that quality merchandise will be received when it is ordered. It also makes it possible to compare bids of competing business firms in a more meaningful manner.

Cost should be kept at the lowest figure possible without loss of quality

Quality of materials is a major consideration. However, among various manufacturers and business concerns, prices vary for products of equal quality. Since supplies and equipment are usually purchased in considerable volume, a few cents on each unit of purchase could represent a saving of many hundreds of dollars to taxpayers. Therefore, if quality can be maintained, materials should be purchased at the lowest cost figure.

Purchases should be made from reputable business firms

In some cases the decision concerning the firm from which supplies and equipment are to be purchased may be determined by the local board of education or college authorities. In the event of such a procedure, this principle is academic. However, where the business firm from which purchases will be made is determined by health and physical education personnel, it is wise to deal with established, reputable businesses that are known to have reasonable prices, reliable materials, and good service. In the long run this is the best and safest procedure to follow.

Local firms should be considered

The administration's main concern is to obtain good value for money expended. If local firms can offer equal values, render equal or better service for the same money, and are reliable, then preference should probably be given to local dealers. If such conditions cannot be met, however, a question can be raised about the wisdom of such a procedure. In some cases it is advantageous to use local dealers, since they are more readily accessible and can provide quicker and better service than firms located farther away.

Bids should be obtained

A good administrative procedure that helps to eliminate any accusation of favoritism and that assists also in obtaining the best price available is the use of competitive bidding. This procedure requires that special forms be distributed to many dealers who handle the supplies and equipment desired. In such cases, the specifics in regard to the kind, amount, and quality of articles desired should be clearly stated. After bids have been obtained, the choice can be made. Low bids do not have to be accepted. However, where they are not honored, proper justification should be set forth.

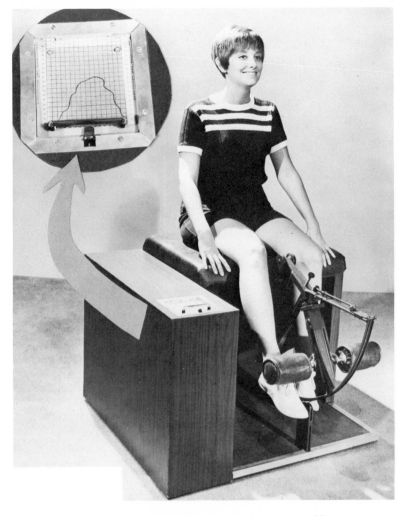

Mini-Gym. (Courtesy Mini-Gym, Independence, Mo.)

Gifts or favors should not be accepted from dealers

Some dealers and salesmen are happy to present an administrator or staff member with a new rifle, set of golf clubs, tennis racquet, or other gift if, in so doing, they believe it is possible to get a school or college on their account. It is poor policy to accept such gifts or favors. This places a person under obligation to an individual or firm and can only result in difficulties and harm to the program. An administrator or staff member should never profit personally from any materials that are purchased for use in his or her programs.

A complete inventory analysis is essential before purchasing

Before purchases are made such information should be available as the amount of supplies and equipment on hand and the condition of these items. This knowledge prevents overbuying and large stockpiles of materials that may be outdated when they become needed.

CHECKING, ISSUING, AND MAINTAINING SUPPLIES AND EQUIPMENT

Some guidelines for checking, issuing, and maintaining supplies and equipment are discussed in the following paragraphs.

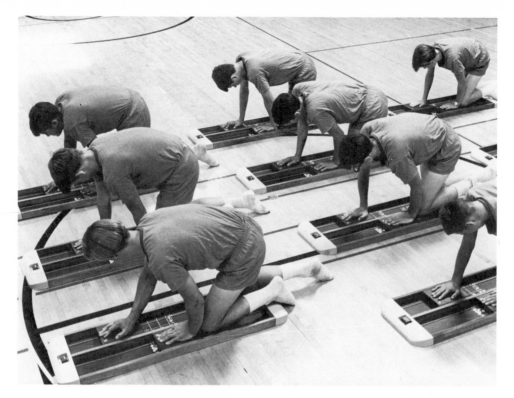

Exer-Cor. (Courtesy Health and Education Services, Bensenville, Ill.)

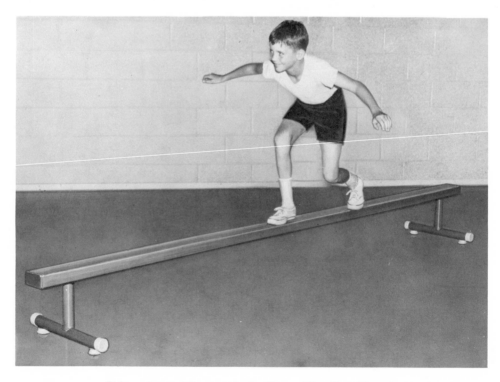

Balance beam. (Courtesy Jayfro Corp., Waterford, Conn.)

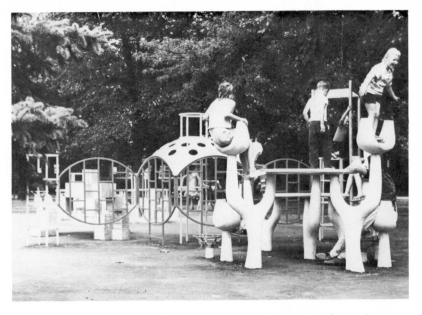

Playground equipment. (Courtesy Playground Corporation of America.)

All supplies and equipment should be carefully checked upon receipt

Equipment and supplies that have been ordered should not be paid for until they have been checked for amount, type, quality, size, and other specifications that were listed on the purchase order. If any discrepancies are noted, they should be corrected before payment is made. This is a very important procedure and responsibility and should be carefully followed. It represents good business practice in a matter requiring good business sense.

Supplies and equipment requiring organization identification should be labeled

Equipment and supplies are aften moved from location to location within the school plant and also are issued to students and to staff members on a temporary basis. It is a good procedure to stencil or stamp the school or college identification in some appropriate location in order to have a check on such material, to help trace missing articles, to discourage misappropriation of such items, and to know what is and what is not departmental property.

Procedures should be established for issuing and checking in supplies and equipment

There can be considerable loss of material if poor accounting procedures are followed. Procedures should be established so that items are issued in a prescribed manner, proper forms are completed, records are maintained, and at all times there is a clear understanding of where the material is located. Articles should be listed on the records according to various specifications of amount, size, or color, together with the name of the person to whom the item is issued. The individual's record should be classified according to name, street address, telephone, locker number, or other information important for identification purposes. In all cases the person or persons to whom the supplies and equipment are issued should be held accountable.

Equipment should be in a state of constant repair

Equipment should always be maintained in a serviceable condition. Procedures for caring for equipment should be routinized so that repairs are provided as needed. All used equipment should be checked and then repaired, replaced,

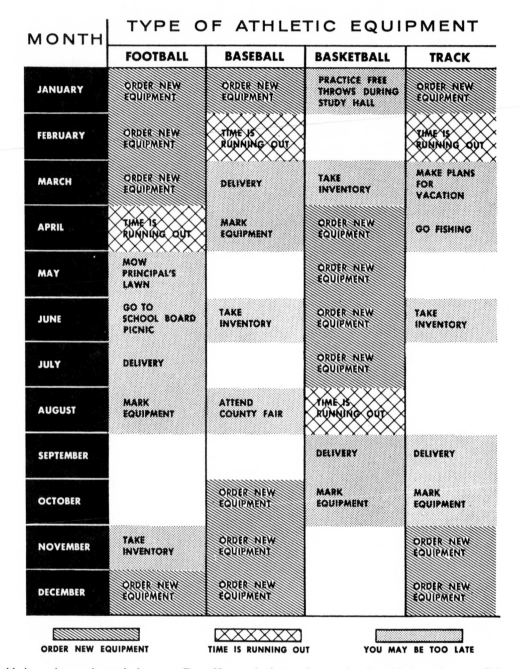

MONTH	TYPE OF ATHLETIC EQUIPMENT			
	FOOTBALL	**BASEBALL**	**BASKETBALL**	**TRACK**
JANUARY	ORDER NEW EQUIPMENT	ORDER NEW EQUIPMENT	PRACTICE FREE THROWS DURING STUDY HALL	ORDER NEW EQUIPMENT
FEBRUARY	ORDER NEW EQUIPMENT	TIME IS RUNNING OUT		TIME IS RUNNING OUT
MARCH	ORDER NEW EQUIPMENT	DELIVERY	TAKE INVENTORY	MAKE PLANS FOR VACATION
APRIL	TIME IS RUNNING OUT	MARK EQUIPMENT	ORDER NEW EQUIPMENT	GO FISHING
MAY	MOW PRINCIPAL'S LAWN		ORDER NEW EQUIPMENT	
JUNE	GO TO SCHOOL BOARD PICNIC	TAKE INVENTORY	ORDER NEW EQUIPMENT	TAKE INVENTORY
JULY	DELIVERY		ORDER NEW EQUIPMENT	
AUGUST	MARK EQUIPMENT	ATTEND COUNTY FAIR	TIME IS RUNNING OUT	
SEPTEMBER			DELIVERY	DELIVERY
OCTOBER		ORDER NEW EQUIPMENT	MARK EQUIPMENT	MARK EQUIPMENT
NOVEMBER	TAKE INVENTORY	ORDER NEW EQUIPMENT		ORDER NEW EQUIPMENT
DECEMBER	ORDER NEW EQUIPMENT	ORDER NEW EQUIPMENT		ORDER NEW EQUIPMENT

ORDER NEW EQUIPMENT   TIME IS RUNNING OUT   YOU MAY BE TOO LATE

Athletic equipment buyers' almanac. (From How to budget, select, and order athletic equipment, Chicago, 1962, The Athletic Institute.)

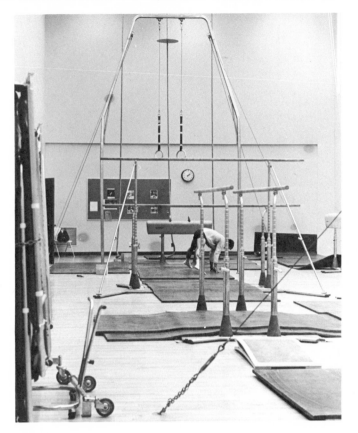

Gymnastic room with equipment. (University of California at Irvine.)

or serviced as needed. Repair can be justified, however, only when the cost for such is within reason. Supplies should be replaced when they have been expended.

Equipment and supplies should be stored properly

Supplies and equipment should be handled efficiently so that space has been properly organized for storing, a procedure has been established for ease of location, and proper safeguards have been taken against fire and theft. Proper shovels, bins, hangers, and other accessories should be available. Temperature, humidity, and ventilation are also important considerations. Items going into the storeroom should be properly checked for quality and quantity. An inventory should be constantly available on all items on hand in the storeroom. Every precaution should be taken to provide for

the adequate care of the material so that a wise investment has been made.

AUDIOVISUAL MATERIALS

Audiovisual aids and materials have become such an important part of health and physical education programs that space is provided for a discussion of the use, types, and guidelines for such supplies and equipment.

A recent survey among 100 schools and colleges found that more than one-half of them used some form of visual or audio aid in their programs. All of the persons surveyed felt that audiovisual media served as a valuable supplement to instruction in the learning of motor skills. The survey also found that videotaping is on the increase as an instructional tool. The audiovisual media used most frequently by those persons surveyed included cartridge films, loopfilms, 16- and 8-mm. films, wall charts, slide

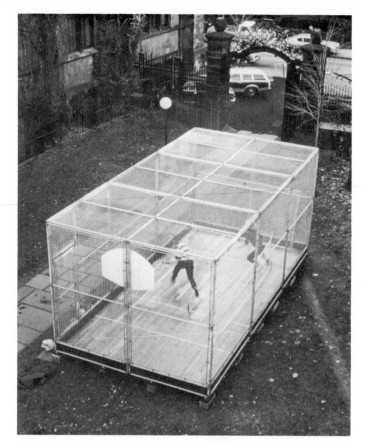

Sport Court, developed by Sportatron Company of America, Old Lyme, Conn., can provide much activity in a small amount of space.

films, film strips, and instructional television.

Reasons for increased use of audiovisual materials

There are several reasons why there is an increased use of audiovisual materials in health education and physical education programs. Some of these are:

1. *They enable the student to better understand concepts and the performance of a skill, events, and other experiences.* The old cliché, "One picture is worth a thousand words," has much truth. The use of a film, pictures, or other materials gives a clearer idea of the subject being taught, whether it is how a heart functions or how to perfect a golf swing.

2. *They help to provide a variety to teaching.*

There is increased motivation, the attention span of students is prolonged, and the subject matter of a course is much more exciting when audiovisual aids are used in addition to other teaching techniques.

3. *They increase motivation on the part of the student.* To see a game played, a skill performed, or an experiment conducted in clear, understandable, illustrated form helps to motivate the student to engage in a game, perform a skill more effectively, or want to know more about the relation of exercise to health. This is particularly true in video replay, for example, where a student can actually see how he performs a skill and then can compare his performance to what should be done.

4. *They provide for an extension of what can normally be taught in a classroom, gymnasium,*

The board of education of ___(legal name)___ School District

No. ___ of the Town(s) of _____ popularly known

as _____ , (in accordance with Section 103 of

Article 5-A of the General Municipal Law) hereby invites the sub-

mission of sealed bids on _____ for use in the

schools of the district. Bids will be received until _____ on the
                                                       (hour)

_____ day of _____ , 19 ___ , at _____
(date)   (month)   (place of bid

_____ , at which time and place all bids will be publicly opened.
opening)

Specifications and bid form may be obtained at the same office. The

board of education reserves the right to reject all bids. Any bid

submitted will be binding for _____ days subsequent to the date of

bid opening.

Board of Education

_____ School District No. ___

of the Town(s) of _____

County(ies) of _____

_____
(Address)

By _____
        (Purchasing Agent)

_____
(Date)

Note: The hour should indicate whether it is Eastern Standard or
      Eastern Daylight Saving Time.

Sample notice to bidders form. (From School Business Management Handbook Number 5, The University of the State of New York, Albany, N. Y.)

EQUIPMENT ISSUE

Date...

I .... have

accepted school property ....

.... (write in article and its number)

and agree to return it clean and in good condition or pay for said uniform.

Signed ....

H. R. #

Home Phone #   Home Address..................................

Equipment issue form. (From Bucher, C. A., and Koenig, C. R.: Methods and materials in secondary school physical education, ed. 4, St. Louis, 1974, The C. V. Mosby Co.)

EQUIPMENT CHECKOUT RECORD

Player_____ Home Room_____

Address_____ Phone_____

Class_____ Height_____ Weight_____ Age_____

Parents Waiver_____ Examination_____ Insurance_____

Football   Cross Country   Basketball   Swimming   Wrestling

Baseball   Track   Tennis   Golf

	Out	In	Game Equipment	Out	In
Blocking pads			White jersey		
Shoulder pads			Maroon jersey		
Hip pads			White pants		
Thigh pads			Maroon pants		
Knee pads			Warm-up pants		
Helmet			Warm-up jacket		
Shoes			Stockings		
Practice pants					
Practice jersey					

I hereby certify that I have received the above-listed athletic equipment and will return same not later than the day following the last game of the season for the sport checked.

Signature_____

Equipment checkout record. (From Bucher, C. A., and Koenig, C. R.: Methods and materials in secondary school physical education, ed. 4, St. Louis, 1974, The C. V. Mosby Co.)

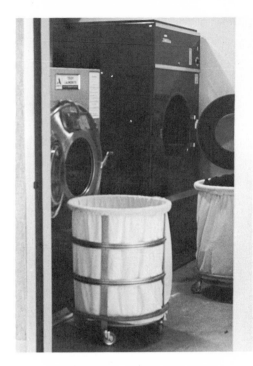

Laundry for washable supplies. (University of California at Irvine.)

or playground. Audiovisual aids enable the student to be taken to other countries, to experience sporting events that occur in other parts of the United States, and to witness events that are significant to world health. All of these are important to health and physical education programs and the instructional program for students.

5. *They provide a historical reference for the fields of health and physical education.* Outstanding events in sports, physical education, and health that have occurred in past years can be brought to life before students' eyes. In this way the student obtains a better understanding of these fields and the important role they play in our society and other cultures of the world.

Selected types of audiovisual aids

A partial list of audiovisual materials that are commonly used today by health and physical education teachers follows.

Visual aids (audiovisual in some cases)

Reading materials—books, magazines, encyclopedias, and almanacs

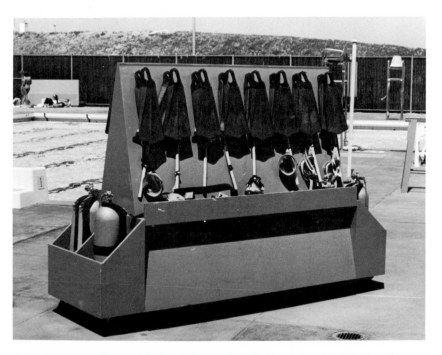

Rolling equipment cart, one of several designed for specific classes of the physical education program. These are stored in the equipment room and transported to activity areas by student helpers. (University of California at Irvine.)

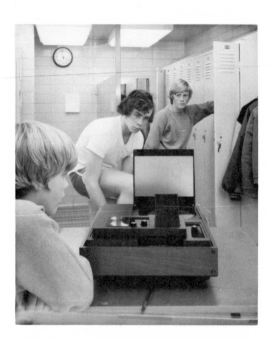

A visual teaching aid. (Courtesy Eastman Kodak Co.)

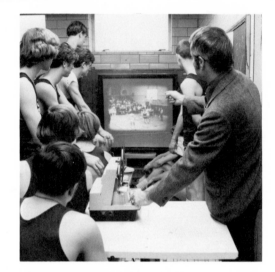

Courtesy Eastman Kodak Co.

ADMINISTRATOR'S CODE OF ETHICS FOR PERSONNEL INVOLVED IN PURCHASING *

1. To consider first the interests of the school district or college and the betterment of the educational program.

2. To be receptive to advice and suggestions of colleagues, both in the department and in the field of business administration, and others insofar as advice is compatible with legal and moral requirements.

3. To endeavor to obtain the greatest value for every dollar spent.

4. To strive to develop an expertise and knowledge of supplies and equipment that ensure recommendations for purchases of greatest value.

5. To insist on honesty in the sales representation of every product submitted for consideration for purchase.

6. To give all responsible bidders equal consideration in determining whether their product meets specifications and the educational needs of your program.

7. To discourage and to decline gifts that in any way might influence a purchase.

8. To provide a courteous reception for all persons who may call on legitimate business missions regarding supplies and equipment.

9. To counsel and help other educators involved in purchasing.

10. To cooperate with governmental or other organizations or persons and help in the development of sound business methods in the procurement of school and college equipment and supplies.

*Adapted from the New York State Association of School Business Officials: Code of ethics for school purchasing officials.

Chalkboards—for recording plays, thoughts, and ideas

Wall charts—of self-explanatory terms

Flat pictures, cartoons, posters, photographs

Graphs—bar, circle, line, and other types

Maps and globes

Bulletin boards—for posting materials pertaining to program

Models and specimens—the human body, skeleton, animals, insects, and others

Opaque projector—used to display on a screen an enlarged picture that is too small in the original for all students to readily see and understand its message

Overhead projector—a compact, lightweight machine that can be operated with ease and used to project materials on a screen. The material projected is in the form of a transparency, made of film that can either be purchased or made

Stereoscopes—machines that project a picture in three dimensions and thus give a better understanding of space relationships

Silent films

Slides—three types, generally speaking: 35-mm. individual slide encased in a cardboard holder; the larger lantern slide usually 3¼ by 4 inches, and the lantern slide that may be prepared for immediate use by a Polaroid transparency film

Filmstrips

Loop films—available in cartridges that can be inserted into a projector and shown with comparative ease. There are three types: a free 8-mm. loop film that can be shown in an 8-mm. projector; an 8-mm. cartridge film encased in a plastic cartridge that requires a special projector; and the super–8-mm. film encased in a plastic cartridge that requires a still different type of projection.

Motion pictures—usually in 8-, 16-, and 35-mm. sizes

Television—educational and closed circuit television and the kinescope recorder. Videotape recording that enables a student to actually see how he or she performs a particular skill, for example, has proved effective as an instructional medium.

Audio aids

Radio—educational and commercial programs

Records and transcriptions—of important events, speeches, musical productions, and music for dances

Tape recordings—special events are recorded and used to appraise student progress in conduct, skills, concepts, and appreciation and to cover current happenings pertinent to health and physical education

Administrative guidelines for the selection and use of audiovisual aids

1. *Audiovisual materials should be carefully selected and screened before using.* Such items as appropriateness for age and grade level of students, adequacy of subject matter, technical qualities, inclusion of current information, cost, and other factors are important to know when selecting audiovisual materials to be used.

2. *The presentation of materials should be carefully planned to provide continuity in the subject being taught.* Materials should be selected and used that amplify and illustrate some important part of the material being covered in a particular course. Furthermore, they should be used at a time that logically fits into the presentation of certain material and concepts.

3. *The materials should be carefully evaluated after they have been used.* Whether or not materials are used a second time should be determined on the basis of their worth the first time they were used. Therefore, a careful evaluation should take place after their use. Records of evaluation should be maintained.

4. *Slow-motion and stop-action projections are best when a pattern of coordination of movements in a skill is to be taught.* When teaching a skill, the teacher usually likes to analyze the various parts of the whole and also to stop and discuss various aspects of the skill with the students.

5. *Proper maintenance and preparation of equipment should be done.* Projectors, record players, television equipment, and other materials need to be kept in good operating condition and operated by qualified personnel in order to have an effective audiovisual program.

Innovations in educational technology

Educational technology, sometimes referred to as educational hardware, is an area devoted to facilitation of learning through the systematic development, organization, and utilization of a full range of learning resources. The basic thrust of educational technology is toward the following objectives: (1) the use of a broad range of learning resources, (2) emphasis on individualized and personalized learning, and (3) the use of the systems approach to learning. Some of these learning resources are discussed in the following paragraphs.

Individualized learning. Programmed learning through teaching machines is a major emphasis of individualized learning. Programmed learning functions with little intervention by the teacher as the student proceeds at his or her own rate. In any programmed system the selection of materials for use with the equipment is of utmost importance. Material must offer some degree of flexibility and lend itself to change. Frequent evaluation and modification of systems is essential to derive the best possible learning experience.

Dial access systems. The Dial Access Information Retrieval System provides immediate, automatic access to a wide variety of audiovisual materials. A coaxial television cable is connected to a centralized distribution center, school libraries, and selected classrooms. The teacher or student can consult a catalogue of available audiovisual materials and can request material, which is then directed through an electronic switching system to one of the television terminals in the school. The primary objective of the Dial Access program is to provide students and teachers individual access to all audiovisual materials.

Satellite TV. Satellite television has been considered in the state of Alaska to bring educational television to this large, remote state. In developing this type of program certain factors have to be considered: (1) adequate ground facilities that can send and transmit radio and television signals, (2) adequate teaching programs must be developed, (3) teachers must be trained in its use, and (4) scheduling of programs may be added by the use of videotape recorders to play back programs that were viewed at an earlier time.

Cable television. Cable television can be received by such institutors as libraries, schools, hospitals, and private homes. The possibilities for educational use are tremendous. Educators, administrators, and curriculum specialists can collaborate in the production of instructional programming. Students can also produce programs to be aired over cable television. For example, on Long Island, New York, an area educational service center known as SCOPE has worked with cable television to produce programs concerning school budgets, drug abuse, field trips, and a student film competition program.

Videotape systems. Videotape systems have already made a significant contribution to education and can make further contributions in many areas. This magnetic recording device makes it possible for film and sound programs to be recorded on tape and played back for immediate use (as used in sporting events) or stored for future presentation.

Videotaping can make a valuable contribution to physical education, as shown by the videotape laboratory at the State University of New York at Buffalo. The project was designed to complement laboratory experiences for physical education major students. A prototype videotape was produced to allow students to participate with motor skills shown on the tape. The tape was accompanied by a booklet that included immediate response questions and in-depth analyses that follow up the questions. The program was evaluated by students and teachers and found to be both interesting and educational.

Videotaping has also been suggested for use in improving teacher behavior. Videotapes of physical education teachers can be used for analyzing the teacher's behavior and the relationship of behavior to specific instructional objectives. This practice has great value in terms of teacher accountability and can be employed by school systems in teacher evaluation.

Other uses of videotaping include pretaping of instructional classes by the physical education teacher. This can be a great time saver for the teacher and provide a view at how he or she is teaching and whether modification of methods is necessary.

Computers

Computer use in education has shown dramatic increases in the past few years. One program used in school systems is computer-assisted instruction (CAI). CAI uses the computer as a teacher substitute; the student works with a computer through a typewriter or video aid. This type of instruction frees the teacher to spend more time with individual students. The computer-managed instruction (CMI) is a method of keeping a record of the child's learning experiences and needs. The data are used as an aid to instruction and individualized attention.

Computer-monitored physical education at Simmons Junior High, Aurora, Illinois allows students to progress at their own rate through self-directed activities with the computer keeping track of each student's progress. Students receive no grades and attend individual con-

CHECKLIST OF SELECTIVE ITEMS FOR THE PURCHASE AND CARE OF SUPPLIES AND EQUIPMENT

	Yes	No
1. Selection of equipment and supplies is related to the achievement of the goals of health and physical education.		
2. Equipment and supplies are selected in accordance with the needs and capacities of the participants including consideration for age, sex, skill and interest.		
3. A manual or written policies have been prepared regarding the procedure for purchasing and care of all supplies and equipment.		
4. Such mechanics of purchasing as the following are utilized: requisitions, specifications, bids and quotations, contracts and purchase orders, delivery date, receipt of merchandise, vendor invoices, and payment.		
5. The relationship of such functions as the following to purchasing is taken into consideration: programming, budgeting and financing, auditing and accounting, property maintenance, legal regulations, ethics, and philosophy of education.		
6. Such principles of purchasing as the following are adhered to: quality, quantity, storage, inventory, and salvage value.		
7. A close working relationship exists between department chairman and school or college business administrator.		
8. Both girls and boys have necessary equipment and supplies and have their own equipment and supplies when needed.		
9. Merchandise is purchased only from reputable manufacturers and distributors and consideration is also given to their replacement and the services provided.		
10. The greatest value is achieved for each dollar expended.		
11. Administration possesses current knowledge of equipment and supplies.		
12. Administration is receptive to advice and suggestions from colleagues who know, utilize, and purchase equipment and supplies.		
13. The coach of a sport is contacted when ordering merchandise for his or her activity, and specifications and other matters checked.		
14. The Director of Physical Education and/or Health Education consults with the business administration when equipment and supplies are needed and ordered.		
15. Local regulations for competitive purchasing are followed.		
16. Equipment and supply purchases are standardized wherever possible in order to make replacement easier.		
17. Administration is alert to improvements and advantages and disadvantages of various types of equipment and supplies.		
18. Specifications of brand, trademark, catalogue specifications, etc. are clearly defined in the purchase requisitions.		
19. Purchase orders are made on regular school forms.		
20. Functional quality of merchandise and the safety it affords are major considerations.		
21. The inventory is utilized when planning for replacements and additions.		
22. Complete and accurate records are kept on all merchandise purchased.		
23. New equipment and supply needs are determined well in advance.		
24. New materials and equipment are tested and evaluated before being purchased in quantity lots.		
25. Minimum safety requirements are utilized for equipment that is purchased.		
26. Honesty is expected in all sales representation.		
27. State contracts are utilized when they are available.		
28. Administration is prompt and courteous in receiving legitimate salesman and businessmen.		
29. All competitors who sell merchandise are given fair and equal consideration.		
30. Gifts or favors that are offered by salesmen or manufacturers are refused.		
31. Materials that are received are checked with respect to quality and quantity and whether they meet specifications that have been indicated in preschool requisitions.		
32. Prompt payment is assured on contracts that have been made.		

Continued.

CHECKLIST OF SELECTIVE ITEMS FOR THE PURCHASE AND CARE OF SUPPLIES AND EQUIPMENT—cont'd

	Yes	No
33. All orders are checked carefully for damaged merchandise, shortages, and errors in shipment.		
34. Policies have been established for designating procedure to be followed when there is theft, loss, or destruction of merchandise.		
35. People who are issued equipment and supplies are held accountable for them.		
36. Inventories are taken periodically to account for all materials.		
37. A uniform plan is established for marking equipment and supplies.		
38. A written procedure has been established for borrowing and returning equipment and supplies.		
39. A procedure has been established for holding students accountable for merchandise that is not returned.		
40. Proper storage facilities have been provided for the storing of merchandise used.		
41. Equipment is cleaned and repaired where necessary before it is stored.		

---

ferences with the teacher. A computer print-out aids in establishing the students' progress. Students use a variety of materials in achieving their specific cognitive and performance objectives. Each school year is a continuation of the previous year where students pick up at the specific skill level from the previous year.

Media centers

Media resource centers are being developed by various professional organizations as well as schools and colleges. These centers are concerned with the collection, storage, and dissemination of various audiovisual materials, such as videotapes to organizations and persons who desire them. For example, the National Center on Education Media and Material for the Handicapped is being developed by the Curriculum and Foundations Faculty in the College of Education at Ohio State University. Recently the Physical Education Division of the American Alliance for Health, Physical Education, and Recreation established a resource center on media in physical education where such functions are carried out as the duplication and dissemination of video- and audiotapes, collection of teachers' guides, and the storage of tapes of speeches and conference proceedings. This center is currently located at Wayne State University in Detroit, Michigan.

Questions and exercises

1. What factors need to be taken into consideration in relation to the purchase and care of supplies and equipment?
2. List and discuss five principles that should be followed in respect to the selection of supplies and equipment. Apply these principles in the procedure involved in selecting a diving board for a swimming pool.
3. List and discuss five principles that should be followed in respect to purchasing supplies and equipment. Apply these principles to the procedure involved in purchasing a trampoline for the gymnasium.
4. Prepare a report on the various types of audiovisual aids that could be used effectively in the teaching of tennis.
5. Prepare an administrative plan that you, as a chairman of a health and physical education department, would recommend for the checking, issuing, and maintenance of physical education supplies and equipment. Be specific, pointing out the steps that should be followed and procedure implemented to ensure sound property accountability.

Reading Assignment in *Administrative Dimensions of Health and Physical Education Programs, Including Athletics:* Chapter 13, Selections 73 to 76.

Selected references

American Association for Health, Physical Education, and Recreation: Equipment and supplies for athletics, physical education and recreation, Washington, D. C., The Association. (Published annually in the Journal of Health, Physical Education, and Recreation.)

Care of athletic equipment, River Grove, Ill., Wilson Sporting Goods Co.

Casey, L. M.: School business administration, New York, 1964, The Center for Applied Research in Education, Inc. (The Library of Education).

De Kieffer, R. E.: Audiovisual instruction, New York, 1965, The Center for Applied Research in Education, Inc. (The Library of Education).

Gibson, D. M.: Dial access systems, Today's Education **59:**35, 1970.

Greenberg, J. L.: How videotaping improves teaching behavior, Journal of Health, Physical Education, and Recreation **44:**36, 1973.

Hill, R. W.: Cable television, Today's Education **59:**39, 1970.

Hook, A. J., and others: Computer monitored physical education, Journal of Health, Physical Education, and Recreation **44:**24, 1973.

How to budget, select, and order athletic equipment. Available from Athletic Goods Manufacturers Association, Merchandise Mart, Chicago, Ill.; also through MacGregor & Rawlings Sporting Goods.

Irwin, A.: Put your equipment on wheels, Scholastic Coach **35:**10, 1966.

Koerner, J.: Educational technology, Saturday Review of Education **1:**43, 1973.

Participants in National Facilities Conference: Planning areas and facilities for health, physical education, and recreation, Chicago, 1965. The Athletic Institute, Inc.

Piscopo, J.: Videotape laborating: a programmed instructional sequence, Journal of Health, Physical Education, and Recreation **44:**32, 1973.

Selway, C. P.: Efficiency in the equipment and laundry rooms, Scholastic Coach **34:**30, 1965.

Studer, H.: Programmed learning systems, Today's Education **59:**34, 1970.

Suppes, P.: Computer confrontation, Saturday Review of Education **1:**48, 1973.

Tendow, M.: Computers, Today's Education **59:**40, 1970.

Van Houte, R.: Satellite Television, Today's Education, **57:**37, 1970.

Legal liability and insurance management

Legal liability and insurance management are crucial responsibilities of administrators and educators. Recent court cases have had to deal with such diverse situations as grooming regulations concerning athletes, eligibility requirements, the entrance of girls into interscholastic athletics, Little League teams, and general rulings concerning men and women engaging together in athletic competition. Legal liability and insurance management involve some very highly specialized areas, many of which will be discussed in this chapter.

According to Bouvier's *Law Dictionary,* liability is "the responsibility, the state of one who is bound in law and justice to do something which may be enforced by action." Another definition states: "Liability is the condition of affairs which gives rise to an obligation to do a particular thing to be enforced by court action."

Leaders in the fields of health and physical education should know how far they can go with various aspects of their programs and what precautions are necessary in order not to be held legally liable in the event of an accident. The fact that approximately 67% of all school jurisdiction accidents involving boys and 59% involving girls occur in physical education and recreation programs has implications for these specialized fields. Furthermore, the fact that an estimated 3 million boys and girls participate in interscholastic athletic programs alone indicates a further administrative concern for physical education programs. It is estimated that every year, one out of every 33 students attending school will be injured. It is alarming to note that physical educators are involved in more than 50% of the injuries sustained by students each year.*

The administration, which in the final analysis is responsible for the program, should clearly understand the implications of their work in this respect. Fear of personal liability can thwart an otherwise good educational program.

When an accident resulting in personal injury occurs on school property, the question often arises as to whether damages can be recovered. The National Commission on Safety Education points out that all school employees run the risk of suit by injured pupils on the basis of alleged negligence that causes bodily injury to pupils. Such injuries occur on playgrounds, on athletic fields, in science laboratories, in shop classes, or in any place where students congregate.

---

*Chambless, J. R. and Mangin, C.: Legal liability and the physical educator, Journal of Health, Physical Education, and Recreation **44:**42, 1973.

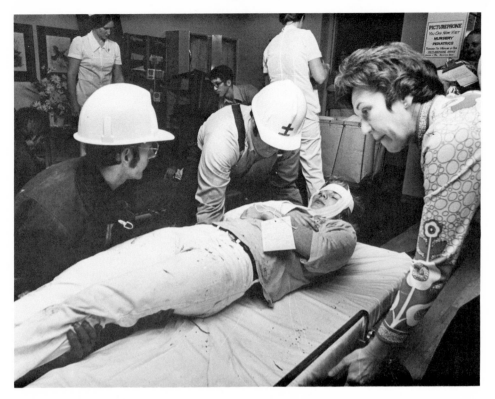

Liability may be involved when injuries occur. Students from College of DuPage, Glen Ellyn, Ill., are participating in a local emergency drill in order to be prepared in the event of emergency and injuries.

The legal rights of the individuals involved in such cases are worthy of study. Although the law varies from state to state, it is possible to discuss liability in a general way that has implications for all sections of the country. First, it is important to understand the legal basis for health, physical education, and allied areas.

THE LEGAL BASIS FOR HEALTH EDUCATION, PHYSICAL EDUCATION, AND ALLIED AREAS

Recent surveys concerning physical education requirements by law in the elementary grades and in junior and senior high schools indicated certain interesting trends. The surveys indicated an overall increase in required physical education programs in the years since a similar survey was taken (1964). The greatest increases in requirements seem to be at the elementary school level. Requirements at the secondary level increased in ten states and were reduced in three states.

The survey showed that all but five states have physical education requirements. Some degree of physical education instruction is required in grades 9 through 12 in 46 states. The range is from 1 to 4 years. Forty-four states had some degree of required programs in grades seven and eight. Forty-four states also required some type of physical education program at the elementary level. Physical education is required in all grades (one through twelve) to some degree in 14 states.*

Health education programs were found to be required to some degree in 36 states.† Grade

*Grieve, A.: State legal requirements for physical education, Journal of Health, Physical Education, and Recreation **42:** 19, 1971.

†Jensen, G. O.: State requirements in health and physical education, The Society of State Directors of Health, Physical Education, and Recreation, July 1973.

levels of requirements differed with 23 states requiring health instruction at the elementary, junior high school, and senior high levels.

LEGAL IMPLICATIONS FOR REQUIRING PHYSICAL EDUCATION

Shroyer* made a study of the legal implications of requiring pupils to enroll in physical education classes and found that the courts have handed down decisions from which the following conclusions may be drawn:

1. Students may be required to take physical education. However, there should be some flexibility to provide for those cases where an individual's constitutional rights might be violated if such activities are against his or her principles, for example, dancing.
2. Where reasonable parental demands for deviation from the physical education requirement are called for, every effort should be made to comply with the parent's wishes. However, unreasonable demands should not result in acquiescence.
3. Where rules and regulations may be questioned, the board of education should provide for a review of the rationale behind the rule or regulation and why the policy is needed.
4. A student may be denied the right to graduate and receive a diploma when a required course such as physical education is not taken.

LEGAL LIABILITY

Some years ago the courts recognized the hazards involved in the play activities that are a part of the educational program. An injury occurred to a boy while he was playing tag. The court recognized the possibility and risk of some injury in physical education programs and would not award damages. However, it pointed out that care must be taken by both the participant and the authorities in charge. It further implied that the benefits derived from participating in physical education activities

---

*Shroyer, G. F.: Legal implications of requiring pupils to enroll in physical education, Journal of Health, Physical Education, and Recreation **35**:51, 1964.

such as tag offset the occasional injury that might occur.

The cited decision regarding the benefits derived from participating in physical education programs was handed down at a time when the attitude of the law was that no government agency, which would include the school, could be held liable for the acts of its employees unless it so consented. Since that time a changing attitude in the courts has been in evidence. As more accidents occurred, the courts frequently decided in favor of the injured party when negligence could be shown. The immunity derived from the old common-law rule that a government agency cannot be sued without its consent is slowly changing in the eyes of the courts so that both federal government and state may be sued.

Those elements of a school curriculum that are compulsory, such as physical education, prompt courts to decide on the basis of what is in the best interests of the public. Instead of being merely a moral responsibility, safety has become a legal responsibility. Those who uphold the doctrine that a government agency should be immune from liability maintain that payments for injury to constituents is a misapplication of public funds. On the other hand, some persons feel it is wrong for the cost of injuries to fall on one or a few persons and, instead, should be shared by all. To further their case these persons cite the constitutional provision that compensation must be given for the taking or damaging of private property. They argue that it is inconsistent that the government cannot take or damage private property without just compensation on the one hand, yet on the other hand can injure or destroy the life of a person without liability for compensation. This view is being used more and more by the courts.

The rule of immunity (since school districts are instrumentalities of the state, and the state is immune from suit unless it consents, the state's immunity extends to the districts) is the law, with a few exceptions, in almost all the states. Some exceptions are California, Washington, and New York. However, as has been pointed out previously, the doctrine of immunity is starting to crumble. The case *Bingham v. Board of Education of Oregon City,* 223 P2d

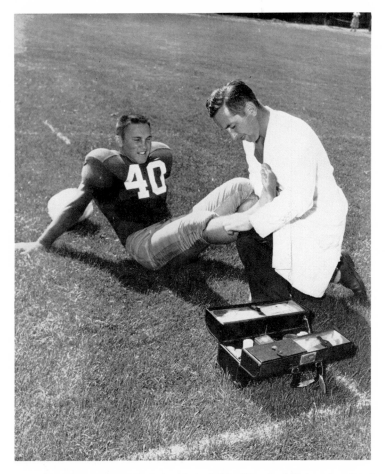

Many accidents occur on playgrounds and athletic fields. (Stanford University, Stanford, Calif.)

432, handed down by the Supreme Court in Utah in October, 1950, involved a 3-year-old child who, while riding her tricycle on the school grounds, fell into some burning embers left on the grounds and suffered severe burns. The school maintained an incinerator adjacent to the playground area in which rubbish was burned. From time to time embers and ashes were removed and scattered around the adjoining area. The parents sued to recover damages and the court held the district was not liable. Judge Latimer, who wrote the court's opinion, said: "While the law writers, editors, and judges have criticized and disapproved the foregoing doctrine of government immunity as illogical and unjust, the weight of precedent of decided cases supports the general rule and we prefer not to disregard a principle so well estab-

lished without statutory authority. We, therefore, adopt the rule of the majority and hold that school boards cannot be held liable for ordinary negligent acts."

The importance of this case lies in the fact that two judges dissented. The dissenting opinion pointed out: "I prefer to regard said principle for the purpose of overruling it. I would not wait for the dim distant future in never-never land when the legislature may act." It was also pointed out that the rule rests upon the "immortal and indefensible doctrine" that "the king (sovereign) can do no wrong" and that a state should not be allowed to use this as a shield.

There has been considerable court activity in regard to the principle of governmental immunity. In 1959 the Illinois Supreme Court (*Molitor* *v. Kaneland Community Unit,* District No. 302, 163 N. E. 2d 89) overruled the immunity doctrine. The supreme courts of Wisconsin, Arizona, and Minnesota legislature followed suit, but in 1963 the Minnesota legislature restored the rule but provided that where school districts had liability insurance they were responsible for damages up to the extent of the coverage. The principle of governmental immunity has also recently been put to the test in courts in such states as Colorado, Iowa, Kansas, Oregon, Pennsylvania, and Utah. However, the courts in these states are hesitant to depart from the precedent that has been set and furthermore insist that it is the legislature of the state rather than the courts that should waive the rule.*

In thirty-nine of fifty states school districts have governmental immunity, which means that as long as they are engaging in a governmental function they cannot be sued, even though negligence has been determined. In eleven states governmental immunity has been annulled either by legislation or judicial decision. In some states schools may legally purchase liability insurance (California requires and twenty-two other states expressly authorize school districts to carry liability insurance) protecting school districts that may become involved in lawsuits, although this does not necessarily mean that governmental immunity has been waived. Of course, in the absence of insurance and "save harmless" laws, which require that school districts assume the liability of the teacher, negligence, proved or not, any judgment rendered against a school district must be met out of personal funds. School districts in Connecticut, Massachusetts, New Jersey, and New York have "save harmless" laws. Wyoming permits school districts to idemnify employees.

School districts that still enjoy governmental immunity usually are either required or permitted to carry liability insurance that specifically covers the operation of school buses.

There is a strong feeling among educators and many in the legal profession that the doctrine of sovereign immunity should be abandoned. In fourteen states students injured as a result of negligence are assured recompense for damages directly or indirectly, either because governmental immunity has been abrogated or because school districts are legally required to indemnify school employees against financial loss. In eighteen other states, if liability insurance has been secured, there is a possibility that students may recover damages incurred.

Although school districts have been granted immunity in many states, teachers do not have such immunity. A decision of an Iowa court in 1938 provides some of the thinking in regard to the teacher's responsibility for his own actions (*Montanick v. McMillin,* 225 Iowa 442, 452-453, 458, 280 N. W. 608, 1938).

[The employee's liability] is not predicated upon any relationship growing out of his employment, but is based upon the fundamental and underlying law of torts, that he who does injury to the person or property of another is civilly liable in damages for the injuries inflicted. . . . The doctrine of *respondeat superior,* literally, "let the principle answer," is an extension of the fundamental principle of torts, and an added remedy to the injured party, under which a party injured by some act of misfeasance may hold both the servant and the master. The exemption of governmental bodies and their officers from liability under the doctrine of *respondeat superior* is a limitation of exception to the rule of *respondeat superior* and in no way affects the fundamental principle of torts that one who wrongfully inflicts injury upon another is liable to the injured person for damages. . . . An act of misfeasance is a positive wrong, and every employee, whether employed by a private person or a municipal corporation owes a duty not to injure another by a negligent act of commission. . . .

Tort

A tort is a legal wrong resulting in direct or indirect injury to another individual or to property. A tortious act is a wrongful act and damages can be collected through court action. Tort can be committed through an act of *omission* or *commission.* An act of omission results when the accident occurs during failure to perform a legal duty, such as when a teacher fails to obey a fire alarm after he or she has been informed of the procedure to be followed. An act of commission results when the accident occurs while an unlawful act is being performed, such as assault on a student.

The National Education Association points out that "A tort may arise out of the following acts: (a) an act which without lawful justification or excuse is intended by a person to cause harm

---

*Shapiro, F. S.: Your liability for student accidents, National Education Association Journal 54:46, 1965.

and does cause the harm complained of; (b) an act in itself contrary to law or an omission of specific legal duty, which causes harm not intended by the person so acting or omitting; (c) an act or omission causing harm which the person so acting or omitting did not intend to cause, but which might and should, with due diligence, have been foreseen and prevented."* The teacher, leader, or other individual not only has a legal responsibility as described by law but also is responsible for preventing injury. This means that in addition to complying with certain legal regulations, such as proper facilities, there must be compliance with the principle that children should be taught without injury to them and that prudent care, such as a parent would give, must be exercised. The term *legal duty* does not mean only those duties imposed by law but also the duty that is owed to society to prevent injury to others. A duty imposed by law would be one such as complying with housing regulations and traffic regulations. A duty that teachers owe to society in general consists of teaching children without injury to them. For example, it was stated in one case (*Hoose v. Drumm,* 281 N. Y. 54): "Teachers have watched over the play of their pupils time out of mind. At recess periods, not less than in the classroom, a teacher owes it to his charges to exercise such care of them as a parent of ordinary prudence would observe in comparable circumstances."

It is important to understand the legal meaning of the word *accident* in relation to the topic under discussion. According to Black's *Law Dictionary,* accident is defined as follows: "An accident is an unforeseen event occurring without the will or design of the person whose mere act causes it. In its proper use the term excludes negligence. It is an event which occurs without fault, carelessness, or want of proper circumspection for the person affected, or which could not have been avoided by the use of that kind and degree of care necessary to the exigency and in the circumstance in which he was placed." The case of *Lee v. Board of Education of City of New York* in 1941, for example, showed that

prudent care was not exercised, and the defendant was liable for negligence. A boy was hit by a car while playing football in the street as a part of the physical education program. The street had not been completely closed off to traffic. The board of education and the teacher were found negligent.

Negligence

Questions of liability and negligence occupy a very prominent position in connection with the actions of teachers and leaders in school health and physical education programs.

The law in America pertaining to negligence is based upon common law, previous judicial rulings, or established legal procedure. This type of law differs from that which has been written into the statutes by lawmaking bodies and is called statutory law.

Negligence implies that someone has not fulfilled his legal duty or has failed to do something that according to common-sense reasoning should have been done. Negligence can be avoided if there are common knowledge of basic legal principles and proper vigilance. One of the first things that must be determined in event of accident is whether there has been negligence.

Rosenfield* defines negligence as follows: "Negligence consists in the failure to act as a reasonably prudent and careful person would under the circumstances involved." The National Education Association's report elaborates further: "Negligence is any conduct which falls below the standard established by law for the protection of others against unreasonable risk of harm. In general, such conduct may be of two types: (a) an act which a reasonable man would have realized involved an unreasonable risk of injury to others, and (b) failure to do an act which is necessary for the protection or assistance of another and which one is under a duty to do.†

According to Garber, a school employee may be negligent because of the following reasons:

1. He did not take appropriate care

---

*National Education Research Division for the National Commission on Safety Education: Who is liable for pupil injuries? Washington, D. C., 1950, National Education Association, p. 5.

*Rosenfield, H. N.: Liability for school accident, New York, 1940, Harper & Row, Publishers.

†National Education Research Division for the National Commission on Safety Education, op. cit., p. 6.

2. Although he used due care, he acted in circumstances which created risks
3. His acts created an unreasonable risk of direct and immediate injury to others
4. He set in motion a force which was unreasonably hazardous to others
5. He created a situation in which third persons, such as pupils, or inanimate forces, such as shop machinery, may reasonably have been expected to injure others
6. He allowed pupils to use dangerous devices although they were incompetent to use them
7. He did not control a third person, such as an abnormal pupil, whom he knew to be likely to inflict intended injury on others because of some incapacity or abnormality
8. He did not give adequate warning
9. He did not look out for persons, such as pupils, who were in danger
10. He acted without sufficient skill
11. He did not make sufficient preparation to avoid an injury to pupils before beginning an activity where such preparation is reasonably necessary
12. He failed to inspect and repair mechanical devices to be used by pupils
13. He prevented someone, such as another teacher, from assisting a pupil who was endangered, although the pupil's peril was not caused by his negligence*

The National Education Association report includes the following additional comment:

> The law prohibits careless action; whatever is done must be done well and with reasonable caution. Failure to employ care not to harm others is a misfeasance. For example, an Oregon school bus driver who parked the bus across a driveway when he knew the pupils were coasting down the hill was held liable for injuries sustained by a pupil who coasted into the bus. (*Fahlstrom v. Denk,* 1933.)†

Negligence may be claimed when the plaintiff has suffered injury either to himself or to his property, when the defendant has not performed his legal duty and has been negligent, and when the plaintiff has constitutional rights and is not guilty of contributory negligence. The teacher or leader for children in such cases is regarded as *in loco parentis,* that is, acting in the place of the parent in relation to the child.

Since negligence implies failure to act as a reasonably prudent and careful person, necessary precautions should be taken, danger should be anticipated, and common sense should be

used. For example, if a teacher permits a group of very young children to go up a high slide alone and without supervision, he or she is not acting as a prudent person would act. If the teacher of health education, after giving a demonstration, leaves a deadly drug on the desk and it later results in the death of a child, he or she is not acting as a careful person should act. In the case previously cited of *Lee v. Board of Education of City of New York,* when the physical education class was held in a street where cars were also allowed to pass, negligence existed.

Four factors of negligence must be proved before a law suit can be won. First, there must be conformance to a standard of behavior that avoids subjecting a student to reasonable risk or injury. This factor is easy for the lawyer to prove since it is accepted by most persons that the teacher owes such a responsibility to his or her students. Secondly, a breach of duty must be shown. Thirdly, the breach of duty must be the cause of injury to the student. The final factor that must be proved is that injury did occur.

A verdict by the jury in a California district court points up negligence in the sport of football. Press dispatches indicated that the high school athlete who suffered a disabling football injury was brought into court on a stretcher. The award was $325,000 (against the school district) in a suit in which the parent charged that the coach ''was negligent in having the boy moved to the sidelines *too soon* after he was injured.'' The newspaper report seemed to infer that the negligence was involved not in the *method* of moving the boy from the field, but rather in the *time* at which he was moved.

An interesting case where the court ruled negligence occurred in New Jersey. In 1962 a student in the Chatham Junior High School was severely injured in an accident while participating in physical education. The testimony brought out that the physical education teacher was not present when the accident occurred but was treating another child for a rope burn. However, he had continually warned his class not to use the springboard at any time he was out of the room. (The student was trying to perform the exercise where he would dive from a springboard over an obstacle and finish with a forward

---

*Garber, L. O.: Law and the school business manager, Danville, Ill., 1957, Interstate Printers & Publishers, Inc., pp. 205-206.

†National Education Research Division for the National Commission on Safety Education, op. cit., p. 6.

roll.) The prosecution argued that the warning had not been stressed sufficiently and that the teacher's absence from the gymnasium, leaving student aides in charge, was an act of negligence. The court ruled negligence and in 1964 awarded the boy $1.2 million dollars for injuries. His parents were awarded $35,140. Upon an appeal, the award to the boy was reduced to $300,000, but the award to the parents remained the same. It is interesting to note that in this case the board of education felt there was no negligence on the part of the physical education teacher.

In respect to negligence, considerable weight is given in the law to the *foreseeability of danger*. One authority points out that "if a danger is obvious and a reasonably prudent person could have foreseen it and could have avoided the resulting harm by care and caution, the person who did not foresee or failed to prevent a foreseeable injury is liable for a tort on account of negligence."* If a teacher fails to take the needed precautions and care, negligence is constituted. However, it must be established upon the basis of facts in the case. It cannot be based upon mere conjecture.

Teachers and leaders must realize that children will behave in certain ways, that certain juvenile acts will cause injuries unless properly supervised, that hazards must be anticipated, reported, and eliminated. The question that will be raised by most courts of law is: "Should the teacher or leader have had prudence enough to foresee the possible dangers or occurrence of an act?"

Two court actions point up legal reasoning on negligence as interpreted in one state. In the case of *Lane v. City of Buffalo* in 1931, the board of education was found not liable. In this case a child fell from a piece of apparatus in the schoolyard. It was found that the apparatus was in good condition and that proper supervision was present. In the case of *Cambareri v. Board of Albany,* the defendant was found liable. The City of Buffalo owned a park that was supervised by the park department. While skating on the lake in the park a boy playing "crack the

whip" hit a 12-year-old boy who was also skating. Workers and a policeman had been assigned to supervise activity and had been instructed not to allow games that were rough or dangerous.

Although there are no absolute, factual standards for determining negligence, certain guides have been established that should be familiar to teachers and others engaged in the work under consideration in this book. Attorney Cymrot, in discussing negligence at a conference in New York City, suggested the following:

1. The teacher must be acting within the scope of his employment and in the discharge of his duties in order to obtain the benefits of the statute.
2. There must be a breach of a recognized duty owed to the child.
3. There must be a negligent breach of such duty.
4. The accident and resulting injuries must be the natural and foreseeable consequence of the teacher's negligence arising from a negligent breach of duty.
5. The child must be a participant in an activity under the control of the teacher or, put in another way, the accident must have occurred under circumstances where the teacher owes a duty of care to the pupil.
6. A child's contributory negligence, however modified, will bar his recovery for damages.
7. The plaintiff must establish the negligence of the teacher and his own freedom from contributory negligence by a fair preponderance of evidence. The burden of proof on both issues is on the plaintiff.
8. Generally speaking, the board of education alone is responsible for accidents caused by the faulty maintenance of plants (schools) and equipment.*

Some states have a "save harmless" law. For example in New Jersey the law reads:

Chapter 311, P. L. 1938. Boards assume liability of teachers. It shall be the duty of each board of education in any school district to save harmless and protect all teachers and members of supervisory and administrative staff from financial loss arising out of any claim, demand, suit or judgment by reason of alleged negligence or other act resulting in accidental bodily injury to any person within or without the school building; provided, such teacher or member of the supervisory or administrative staff at the time of the accident or injury was acting in the discharge of his duties within the scope of his employment and/or under the direction of said board of education; and said board of education may arrange for and maintain appropriate insurance with any company created by or under the laws of this state, or in any

---

*National Education Research Division for National Commission on Safety Education, op. cit., p. 6.

*Proceedings of the City Wide Conference with Principal's Representatives and Men and Women Chairmen of Health Education, City of New York Board of Education, Brooklyn, N. Y., 1953, Bureau of Health Education.

insurance company authorized by law to transact business in this state, or such board may elect to act as self-insurers to maintain the aforesaid protection.

Negligence concerning equipment and facilities. Defective or otherwise hazardous equipment or inadequate facilities are often the cause of injuries that lead to court action. If a teacher has noted that the equipment is defective, he or she should put this observation in writing for personal future protection. A letter should be written to the principal and superintendent of schools stating that danger does exist and the areas of such danger. The teacher should keep a copy for evidence in a possible lawsuit. In these cases the courts tend to agree with the student, even if dangerous conditions had been noted. Conditions cannot only be recognized but must also be corrected.

Negligence concerning instruction. Many cases result from situations concerning instruction in an activity. For example, if a child is injured from a fall from a trampoline, a case might ensue where the child and his or her parents may try to show that instruction had been inadequate. These cases are often found in favor of the student because of the inherent danger of the activity. Other students and their families have sued teachers because they did not follow a class syllabus that many states require of their teachers. Such a syllabus outlines the course content, and if injury occurs in an unlisted activity then a basis for suit is apparent.

Negligence in athletic participation. Many injuries are related to participation in athletics. Unequal competition is often the cause of athletic accidents. Teachers should consider sex, age, size, and skill of students in grouping players for an activity.

Defenses against negligence

Despite the fact that an individual is negligent, to collect damages one must show that the negligence resulted in or was closely connected with the injury. The legal question in such a case is whether or not the negligence was the "proximate cause" (legal cause) of the injury. Furthermore, even though it be determined that negligence is the "proximate cause" of the injury, there are still certain defenses upon which a defendant may base his case.

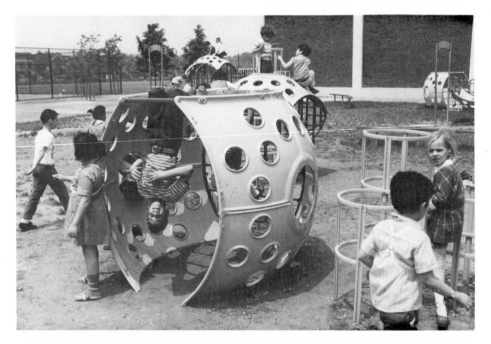

Equipment and supplies must be in good repair at all times in order to avoid negligence. Some playground equipment in the elementary school. (Courtesy Playground Corporation of America.)

Proximate cause. The negligence of the defendant may not have been the proximate cause of the plaintiff's injury.

Example: In the case of *Ohmon v. Board of Education of the City of New York,* 88 N.Y.S. 2d 273 (1949), it was declared that when a 13-year-old pupil in public school was struck in the eye by a pencil thrown in classroom by another pupil to a third pupil, who stepped aside, the proximate cause of injury was an unforeseen act of the pupil who threw the pencil and that absence of the teacher (who was stacking supplies in a closet nearby the classroom) was not proximate cause of injury so as to impose liability for the injury on the board of education.

Act of God. An act of God is a situation that exists because of certain conditions that are beyond the control of human beings. For example, a flash of lightning, a gust of wind, a cloudburst, and other such factors may result in injury. However, this assumption applies only in cases where injury would not have occurred had prudent action been taken.

Assumption of risk. This legal defense is especially pertinent to games, sports, and other phases of the program in health education and physical education. It is assumed that an individual takes a certain risk when engaging in various games and sports where bodies are coming in contact with each other and where balls and apparatus are used. Participation in such activity indicates that the person assumes a normal risk.

Example: In the case of *Scala v. City of New York,* 102 N.Y.S.2d 709, where the plaintiff when playing softball on a public playground was aware of the risks caused by curbing and concrete benches near the playing fields, it was decided that the plaintiff must be held to have voluntarily and fully assumed the dangers and, having done so, must abide by the consequences.

Example: In an action by Albert Maltz (*Maltz v. Board of Education of New York City,* 114 N.Y.S.2d 856, 1952) against the Board of Education of the City of New York for injuries, the court held that a 19-year-old boy who was injured when he collided with a doorjamb in a brick wall 2 feet from the backboard and basket in a public school basketball court and who

had played on that same court several times prior to the accident knew the basket and backboard were but 2 feet from the wall, had previously hit the wall or gone through the door without injury, was not a student at the school but a voluntary member of a team that engaged in basketball tournaments with other clubs, knew or should have known the danger, and thus assumed the risk of injury.

Contributory negligence. Another legal defense is contributory negligence. A person who does not act as would a normal individual of similar age and nature thereby contributes to the injury. In such cases negligence on the part of the defendant might be ruled out. Individuals are subject to contributory negligence if they expose themselves unnecessarily to dangers. The main consideration that seems to turn the tide in such cases is the age of the individual and the nature of the activity in which he engaged.

The National Education Association's report makes this statement in regard to contributory negligence:

> Contributory negligence is defined in law as conduct on the part of the injured person which falls below the standard to which he should conform for his own protection and which is legally contributing cause, cooperating with the negligence of the defendant in bringing about the plaintiff's harm. Reasonable self-protection is to be expected of all sane adults. With some few exceptions, contributory negligence bars recovery against the defendant whose negligent conduct would otherwise make him liable to the plaintiff for the harm sustained by him. Both parties being in fault, neither can recover from the other for resulting harm. When there is mutual wrong and negligence on both sides, the law will not attempt to apportion the wrong between them.
>
> Contributory negligence is usually a matter of defense, and the burden of proof is put upon the defendant to convince the jury of the plaintiff's fault and of its causal connection with the harm sustained. Minors are not held to the same degree of care as is demanded of adults.*

Contributory negligence has implications for a difference in the responsibility of elementary school teachers as contrasted with high school teachers. The elementary school teacher, because the children are immature, has to assume greater responsibility for the safety of the child. That is, accidents in which an elementary school

---

*National Education Research Division for the National Commission on Safety Education, op. cit., p. 9.

child is injured are not held in the same light from the standpoint of negligence as those involving high school students who are more mature. The courts might say that a high school student was mature enough to avoid doing the thing causing him to be injured, whereas if the same thing occurred with an elementary school child, the courts could say the child was too immature and that the teacher should have prevented or protected the child from doing the act from which he or she was injured.

Sudden emergency. This legal defense is pertinent in cases where the exigencies of the situation require immediate action on the part of a teacher and, as a result, an accident occurs. For example, an instructor in a swimming pool is suddenly alerted to the fact that a child is drowning in the water. The teacher's immediate objective is to save the child. He runs to the assistance of the drowning person and in doing so knocks down another student who is watching from the side of the pool. The student who is knocked down hits his head on the tile floor

and is injured. This would be a case of sudden emergency and, if legal action is taken, the defense could be based on this premise.

These are cases of sudden emergency, however, that can and are found against the instructor. For example in a recent case, a teacher left the gymnasium to take an injured student to the school nurse. In his absence, another student was hurt when he fell from a springboard that had been erected behind parallel bars. The teacher was sued by the student for failing to supervise a potentially dangerous activity. The court decided in favor of the student awarding him $300,000 in damages and $35,000 in medical bills. The court's decision in such cases is quite definite in expecting a teacher not to leave his or her class unsupervised under any circumstances.

Precautions

Certain precautions must be taken by the physical educator in order to avoid possible legal liability. Some of the precautions include:

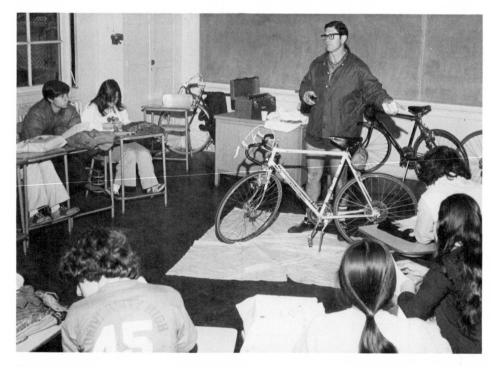

University High School of the Los Angeles Unified School District provides for proper understanding and care of equipment in order to prevent accidents from occurring. (Student Auxiliary Services Branch, Los Angeles Unified School District. Courtesy Gwen R. Waters.)

1. Be familiar with the health status of each student.
2. Take the individuals' skills into consideration in teaching new activities.
3. Group students together on equal competitive levels.
4. Be sure that both equipment and facilities are safe to use.
5. Organize and carefully supervise the class. Never leave the class unattended—even in emergencies. If an emergency occurs, get a replacement before leaving the room.
6. Administer only first aid—never prescribe or diagnose.
7. Utilize only qualified personnel to aid in classrooms.
8. Keep accurate accident records.
9. Provide adequate instruction especially in potentially dangerous activities.
10. Make sure that any injured student receives a medical examination.

Nuisance

Action can be instituted for nuisance when the circumstances surrounding the act are dangerous to life or health, result in offense to the senses, are in violation of the laws of decency, or cause an obstruction to the reasonable use of property.

An authentic source states in regard to a nuisance:

There are some conditions which are naturally dangerous and the danger is a continuing one. An inherent danger of this sort is called at law a "nuisance"; the one responsible is liable for maintaining a nuisance. His liability may be predicated upon negligence in permitting the continuing danger to exist, but even without a showing of negligence the mere fact that a nuisance does exist is usually sufficient to justify a determination of liability. For example, a junk pile in the corner of the grounds of a country school was considered a nuisance for which the district was liable when a pupil stumbled over a piece of junk and fell while playing at recess (*Popow v. Central School District No. 1, Towns of Hillsdale et al., New York*, 1938). Dangerous playground equipment available for use by pupils of all ages and degrees of skill has also been determined to be a nuisance (*Bush v. City of Norwalk, Connecticut*, 1937).

On the other hand, allegations that the district has maintained a nuisance have been denied in some cases; for example, when a small child fell into a natural ditch near the schoolyard not guarded by a fence, the ditch was held not to be a nuisance for which the district would be liable (*Whitfield v. East Baton Rouge Parish School Board,*

Louisiana, 1949). The court said this ditch did not constitute a nuisance; nor did the principle of *res ipsa loquitur* apply. Under this principle the thing which causes the injury is under the management of the defendant and the accident is such that in the ordinary course of events, it would not have happened if the defendant had used proper care.*

Mr. Cymrot, attorney at law, in addressing the Health Education Division of the New York City Schools had the following to say about an "attractive nuisance:"

Teachers need to be aware of decisions of the courts pertaining to "attractive nuisance," . . . an attractive contrivance which is maintained, alluring to children but inherently dangerous to them. This constitutes neglect. But it is not every contrivance or apparatus that a jury may treat as an "attractive nuisance." Before liability may be imposed, there must always be something in the evidence tending to show that the device was something of a new or uncommon nature with which children might be supposed to be unfamiliar or not know of its danger. Many courts have held, however, that for children above the age of 10 years the doctrine of "attractive nuisance" does not hold. Other children are expected to exercise such prudence as those of their age may be expected to possess.†

The following cases point up some court rulings in respect to "nuisance."

In the case of *Texas v. Reinhardt* in 1913, it was ruled that ball games with their noises and conduct were not a "nuisance" in the particular case in question and an injunction should not be issued stopping such activity.

In the case of *Iacono v. Fitzpatrick* in Rhode Island in 1938, a boy 17 years old, while playing touch football on a playground, received an injury that later resulted in his death. He was attempting to catch a pass and in so doing crashed into a piece of apparatus. The court held that the apparatus was in evidence and the deceased knew of its presence. It further stated the city had not created or maintained a nuisance.

In the case of *Schwarz v. City of Cincinnati, Ohio,* the city had permitted an organization to have fireworks in one of its public parks. Next day a 12-year-old boy was injured after lighting an unexploded bomb that he found. The court

*National Education Research Division for the National Commission on Safety Education, op. cit., p. 6.
†Proceedings of the City Wide Conference with Principals' Representatives and Men and Women Chairmen of Health Education, City of New York Board of Education, Brooklyn, N. Y., March, 1953, Bureau of Health Education.

ruled that the permit granted the association was ". . . not authority to create a nuisance . . . not authority to leave an unexploded bomb in the park." The city, which was the defendant in the case, was not held liable.

Governmental versus proprietary functions

The government in a legal sense is engaged in two types of activity: (1) governmental in nature and (2) proprietary in nature.

The *governmental function* refers to those particular activities that are of a sovereign nature. This theory dates back to the time when kings ruled under the divine right theory, were absolute in their power, and "could do no wrong." As such the sovereign was granted immunity and could not be sued without his consent for failing to exercise governmental powers or for negligence. Furthermore, a subordinate agency of the sovereign could not be sued. The municipality, according to this interpretation, acts as an agent of the state in a governmental capacity. The logic behind this reasoning is that the municipality is helping the state to govern the people who live within its geographic limits.

Many activities are classified under the *governmental function* interpretation. Such functions as education, police protection, and public health fall in this category.

In regard to public education, the courts hold that this is a governmental function and, therefore, entitled to state's immunity from liability for its own negligence. However, as has previously been pointed out, the attitude of the courts has changed and has taken on a broader social outlook that allows in some cases for the reimbursement of the injured.

Proprietary function pertains to government functions that are similar to those of a business enterprise. Such functions are for the benefit of the constituents within the corporate limits of the governmental agency. An example of this would be the manufacture, distribution, and sale of some product to the public. A cafeteria conducted for profit in a school is a proprietary function. In functions that are proprietary in nature a governmental agency is held liable in the same manner as an individual or a private corporation would be held liable.

In the case *Watson v. School District of Bay City,* 324 Mich. 1, 36 N.W.2d 195, a decision was handed down by the supreme court of Michigan in February, 1949. In this case a 15-year-old girl attended a high school night football game. In going to her car she was required to walk around a concrete wall. As she attempted to do this, she fell over the wall and onto a ramp. She suffered paralysis and died 8 months later. The parking area was very poorly lighted. The supreme court held that staging a high school football game was a governmental function and refused to impose liability upon the district.

From this discussion it can be seen that education, recreation, and health are governmental functions. While this distinction between governmental and proprietary functions precludes a recovery from the governmental agency if the function was governmental in nature, the federal government and some of the states by legislation have eliminated this distinction.

Fees

Most public recreation activities, facilities, and the like are offered free of charge to the public. However, there are certain activities that, because of the expenses involved, necessitate a fee in order that such activities may continue. For example, golf courses are expensive and charges are usually made so that they may be maintained. This is sometimes true also of such facilities as camps, bathing beaches, and swimming pools.

The fees charged have a bearing upon whether recreation is a governmental or a proprietary function. The courts in most states have upheld recreation as a governmental function, because of its contribution to public health and welfare and also because its devices are free to the public at large. When fees are charged, however, the whole picture takes on a different aspect.

The attitude of the courts has been that the amount of the fee and whether or not the activity was profit-making in nature are considerations in determining whether recreation is a governmental or a proprietary function. Incidental fees that are used in the conduct of the enterprise do not usually change the nature of the enterprise. However, if the enterprise is run for profit, the function changes from governmental to proprietary in nature.

Liability of the municipality

It has been previously pointed out that a municipality as a governmental agency performs both governmental and proprietary functions.

When the municipality is performing a governmental function, it is acting in the interests of the state, receives no profit or advantage, and is not liable for negligence on the part of its employees or for failure to perform these functions. However, this would not hold if there were a specific statute imposing liability for negligence. When the municipality is performing a proprietary function—some function for profit or advantage of the agency or people who comprise it—rather than the public in general, it is liable for negligence of those who are carrying out the function.

This discussion readily shows the importance of conducting recreation as a governmental function.

Liability of the school district

As a general rule the school district is not held liable for acts of negligence on the part of its officers or employees, provided a state statute does not exist to the contrary. The reasoning behind this is that the school district or district school board in maintaining public schools acts as an agent of the state. It performs a purely public or governmental duty imposed upon it by law for the benefit of the public and for the performance of which it receives no profit or advantage.

Some state laws, however, provide that the state may be sued in cases of negligence in the performance of certain duties, such as providing for a safe environment and competent leadership. Furthermore, the school district's immunity in many cases does not cover such acts as those that bring damage or injury through trespass of another's premises or where a nuisance exists on a school district's property, resulting in damage to other property.

Liability of school, park, and recreation board members

Generally speaking, members are not personally liable for any duties in their corporate capacities as board members that they perform negligently. Furthermore, they cannot be held personally liable for acts of employees of the district or organization over which they have jurisdiction on the theory of *respondeat superior* (let the master pay for the servant). Board members act in a corporate capacity and do not act for themselves. For example, in the state of Oregon the general rule as to the personal liability of members of district school boards is stated in 56C.J., page 348, section 223, as follows:

> School officers, or members of the board of education, or directors, trustees, or the like, of a school district or other local school organization are not personally liable for the negligence of persons rightfully employed by them in behalf of the district, and not under the direct personal supervision or control of such officer or member in doing the negligent act, since such employee is a servant of the district and not of the officer or board members, and the doctrine of *respondeat superior* accordingly has no application; and members of a district board are not personally liable for the negligence or other wrong of the board as such. A school officer or member of a district board is, however, personally liable for his own negligence or other tort, or that of an agent or employee of the district when acting directly under his supervision or by his direction.

However, a board member can be held liable for a *ministerial* act even though he cannot be held for the exercise of discretion as a member of the board. If the board acts in bad faith and with unworthy motives, and this can be shown, it can also be held liable.

Liability of teachers and leaders

The individual is responsible for negligence of his or her own acts. With the exception of certain specific immunity, the teacher or leader in programs of health, physical education, and recreation is responsible for what he or she does. The Supreme Court of the United States has reaffirmed this principle and all should recognize the important implications it has. Immunity of the governmental agency such as a state, school district, or board does not release the teacher or leader from liability for his or her own negligent acts.

In New York a physical education teacher was held personally liable when he sat in the bleachers while two strong boys, untrained in boxing, were permitted by the instructor to fight through nearly two rounds. The plaintiff was hit in the temple and suffered a cerebral hemorrhage. The court said: ''It is the duty of a teacher to exercise reasonable care to prevent injuries. Pupils should be warned before being permitted to engage in a dangerous and hazardous exercise. Skilled boxers at times are injured, and . . . these young men should have been taught the principles of defense if indeed it was a reasonable thing to permit a slugging match of the kind which the testimony shows this contest was. The testimony indicates that the teacher failed in his duties in this regard and that he was negligent, and the plaintiff is entitled to recover.'' (*LaValley v. Stanford,* 272 App. Div. 183, 70 N.Y.S. 2d 460.)

In New York (*Keesee v. Board of Education of City of New York,* 5 N.Y.S.2d 300, 1962) a junior high school girl was injured while playing line soccer. She was kicked by another player. The board of education syllabus listed line soccer as a game for boys and stated that ''after sufficient skill has been acquired two or more forwards may be selected from each team.'' The syllabus called for ten to twenty players on each team and required a space of 30 to 40 feet. The physical education teacher divided into two teams some forty to forty-five girls who had not had any experience in soccer. A witness who was an expert in such matters testified that in order to avoid accidents no more than two people should be on the ball at any time and criticized the board syllabus for permitting the use of more than two forwards. The expert also testified that pupils should have experience in kicking, dribbling, and passing before being permitted to play line soccer. The evidence showed that the teacher permitted six to eight inexperienced girls to be on the ball at one time. The court held that possible injury was at least reasonably foreseeable under such conditions and that the teacher had been negligent and that the teacher's negligence was the cause of the pupil being injured.*

Teachers and leaders are expected to conduct their various activities in a careful and prudent manner. If this is not done, they are exposing themselves to lawsuits for their own negligence. As respects administrators, the National Education Association's report has the following to say:

The fact that administrators (speaking mainly of principals and superintendents) are rarely made defendants in pupil-injury cases seems unjust to the teachers who are found negligent because of inadequate supervision, and unjust also to the school boards who are required to defend themselves in such suits. When the injury is caused by defective equipment, it is the building principal who should have actual or constructive notice of the defect; when the injury is caused by inadequate playground supervision, the inadequacy of the supervision frequently exists because of arrangements made by the building principal. For example, a teacher in charge of one playground was required to stay in the building to teach a make-up class; another teacher was required to supervise large grounds on which 150 pupils were playing; another teacher neglected the playground to answer the telephone. All of these inadequacies in playground supervision were morally chargeable to administrators; in none of these instances did the court action direct a charge of responsibility to the administrator. Whether the administrator in such cases would have been held liable, if charged with negligence, is problematical. The issue has not been decided, since the administrator's legal responsibility for pupil injuries has never been discussed by the courts to an extent that would make possible the elucidation of general principles; the administrator's moral responsibilities must be conceded.*

Accident-prone settings

Since many accidents occur on the playgrounds, during recess periods, in physical education classes, and at sports events, some very pertinent remarks are included here that have been stated in the National Education Association's report:

Playground and recess games

. . . [T]he unorganized games during recess and noon intermissions are more likely to result in pupil injuries than the organized games of physical education classes. Playground injuries may be pure accidents, such as when a pupil ran against the flagpole while playing (*Hough v. Orleans Elementary School District of Humboldt County, California,* 1943), or when a pupil was hit by a ball (*Graff v. Board of Education of New York City, New York,* 1940), or by a stone batted by another pupil (*Wilbur v. City of Binghamton, New York,* 1946). The courts have said in connection with this type of injury that every act of every pupil cannot be anticipated. However, the school district should make rules and regulations for pupils' conduct on playgrounds so as to minimize dangers. For example, it was held to be negligence to permit pupils to ride bicycles on the playground while other pupils were playing. (*Buzzard v. East Lake School District of Lake County, California,* 1939.)

Playgrounds should be supervised during unorganized

---

*School Law Series: The pupil's day in court: review of 1963, Washington, D. C., 1964, Research Division, National Education Association, p. 43.

*National Education Research Division for the National Commission on Safety Education, op. cit., p. 14.

play and such supervision should be adequate. One teacher cannot supervise a large playground with over a hundred pupils playing (*Charonnat v. San Francisco Unified School District, California,* 1943), and when the supervision is either lacking or inadequate districts which are not immune are liable for negligence in not providing adequate supervision (*Forgnone v. Salvadore Union Elementary School District, California,* 1940). Pupils are known to engage in fights and may be expected to be injured in fights; it is the responsibility of the school authorities to attempt to prevent such injuries. The misconduct of other pupils could be an intervening cause to break the chain of causation if the supervision is adequate; but when the supervision is not adequate, misconduct of other pupils is not an intervening superseding cause of the injury.

If a pupil wanders away from the group during playground games and is injured by a dangerous condition into which he places himself, the teacher in charge of the playground may be liable for negligence in pupil supervision (*Miller v. Board of Education, Union Free School District, New York,* 1943), although the district would not be liable in common-law state because of its immunity (*Whitfield v. East Baton Rouge Parish School Board, Louisiana,* 1949).

Supervision of unorganized play at recess or noon intermissions should be by competent personnel. A school janitor is not qualified to supervise play. (*Garber v. Central School District No. 1 of Town of Sharon, New York,* 1937.)

All injuries sustained by pupils on playground equipment are excluded in the Washington statute imposing liability for certain other kinds of accidents. Injuries may occur because playground equipment is in a defective condition. The New York courts have not been consistent in their rulings on this point. In one New York case the district was not liable for injury caused by a defect in a slide because there was no evidence that the defect had existed a sufficient length of time for the school authorities to have knowledge of it (*Handy v. Hadley-Luzerne Union Free School District No. 1, New York,* 1938), but another district in New York was held liable for a defect in a slide (*Howell v. Union Free School District No. 1, New York,* 1937).

Nor have the New York courts been consistent in fixing liability when the injury was sustained on playground equipment which was not defective but was dangerous for the individual pupil who played on it. One pupil who fell off a monkey bar was unable to collect damages because the court held specific supervision of each game and each piece of playground equipment would be an unreasonable requirement. The pupil merely met with an accident which was not the fault of the playground supervisor. (*Miller v. Board of Education of Union Free School District No. 1, Town of Oyster Bay, New York,* 1936.) However, another district was declared liable for injuries sustained by a pupil who fell from a ramp during recess, the court holding that liability rested upon the maintenance of a dangerous piece of playground equipment. This ramp had been constructed for the use of older boys and even they were to use it only under supervision; the injured pupil was a small child. (*Sullivan v. City of Binghamton, New York,* 1946.)

Where children of all ages share a playground extra precautions should be taken to prevent accidents, since some children are more adept in using equipment than others and some playground equipment is dangerous to the unskilled.

Physical education and sports events

Pupil injuries in this area occur when playground or gymnasium equipment is defective, when pupils attempt an exercise or sport for which they have not been sufficiently trained, when there is inadequate supervision of the exercise, when other pupils conduct themselves in a negligent manner, and even when the pupils are mere spectators at sports events.

It has been held that physical education teachers, or the school district in States where the district is subject to liability, are responsible for injuries caused by defective equipment. For example, there was liability for the injury to a pupil who was injured in a tumbling race when the mat, not firmly fixed, slipped on the slippery floor. (*Cambareri v. Board of Education of Albany, New York,* 1940.)

Defects in equipment should be known to the physical education instructor. There may be what is called actual or constructive notice of the defect. Actual knowledge is understandable; constructive notice means that the defect has existed for a sufficient time so that the instructor should have known of its existence, whether he did or not. Teachers of physical education should make periodic examination of all equipment at rather frequent intervals; otherwise they may be charged with negligence in not having corrected defects in equipment which have existed for a sufficient time that ignorance of the defect is a presumption of negligence.

Physical education teachers may be liable also for injuries which occur to pupils who attempt to do an exercise which is beyond their skills. A running-jump somersault is one such instance (*Govel v. Board of Education of Albany, New York,* 1944); boxing is another (*LaValley v. Stanford, New York,* 1947); and a headstand exercise is another (*Gardner v. State of New York, New York,* 1939). All of these exercises were found to be inherently dangerous by the courts, and the evidence showed that previous instruction had been inadequate and the pupils had not been warned of the dangers. However, where the previous instruction and the supervision during the exercise are both adequate, there is no liability so long as it cannot be proved that the teacher is generally incompetent (*Kolar v. Union Free School District No. 9, Town of Lenox, New York,* 1939). These cases suggest that teachers should not permit pupils to attempt exercises for which they have not been fully prepared by warnings of the dangers and preliminary exercises to develop the required skills.

As in other types of pupil injuries, the physical education teacher is not liable if the injury occurred without his negligence. If caused by the negligence of another pupil, the teacher will likely be relieved of liability if the other pupil's misconduct was not foreseeable. Pure accidents occur in sports also and if there is no negligence there is no liability (*Mauer v. Board of Education of New York City, New York,* 1945).

Sports events to which nonparticipating pupils and even the public are invited raise other problems of liability for the district or the physical education teacher in charge. If the locality is in a common-law State where the district is immune, the charge of an admission fee does not nullify the district's immunity or make the activity a proprietary function as an exception to the immunity rule (*Watson v. School District of Bay City, Michigan,* 1949). If the accident occurs in a State where the district is liable for at least certain kinds of injuries, such as California, the invitation to attend a sports event includes an invitation to use the nearby grounds and equipment, imposing liability for injury from hidden glass or other dangers (*Brown v. City of Oakland, California,* 1942). If a spectator is accidentally hit by a ball, however, there is no liability; even when a pupil was injured by being hit by a bottle at a game there was no liability because the misconduct of the other spectator was not foreseeable (*Weldy v. Oakland High School District of Alameda County, California,* 1937).*

Common areas of negligence

Common areas of negligence in health and physical education activities listed by Begley† in a New York University publication are situations involving poor selection of activities, failure to take protective procedures, hazardous conditions of buildings or grounds, faulty equipment, inadequate supervision, and poor selection of play area. Cases involving each of these common areas of negligence are as follows.

Poor selection of activities. The activity must be suitable to the child or youth. In *Rook v. New York,* 4 N.Y.S.2d 116 (1930), the court ruled that tossing a child in a blanket constituted a dangerous activity.

Failure to take protective measures. The element of "foreseeability" enters here and proper protective measures must be taken to provide a safe place for children and youth to play. In *Roth v. New York,* 262 App. Div. 370, 29 N.Y.S.2d 442 (1941), inadequate provisions were made to prevent bathers from stepping into deep water. When a bather drowned, the court held the state was liable.

Hazardous conditions of buildings or grounds. Buildings and grounds must be safe. Construction of facilities and their continual repair must have as one objective the elimination of hazards. In the case of *Novak et al. v. Borough of Ford City,* 141 Atl. 496 (Pa., 1928), unsafe conditions were caused by an electric wire over the play area. In the case of

Honaman v. City of Philadelphia, 185 Atl. 750 (Pa., 1936), unsafe conditions were caused by failure to erect a backstop.

Faulty equipment. All play and other equipment must be in good condition at all times. In the case of *Van Dyke v. Utica,* 203 App. Div. 26, 196 N.Y. Supp. 277 (1922), concerning a slide that fell over on a child and killed him, the court ruled that the slide was in a defective condition.

Inadequate supervision. There must be qualified supervision in charge of all play activities. In the case of *Garber v. Central School District No. 1, Town of Sharon, N.Y.,* 251 App. Div. 214, 295 N.Y. Supp. 850, the court held that a school janitor was not qualified to supervise school children playing in a gymnasium during the lunch hour.

Poor selection of play area. The setting for games and sports should be selected with a view to the safety of the participants. In the case *Morse v. New York,* 262 App. Div. 324, 29 N.Y.S.2d 34 (1941), when sledding and skiing were permitted on the same hill without adequate barriers to prevent participants in each activity from colliding with each other, the court held that the state was liable for negligence.

Supervision

Children are entrusted by parents to recreation, health, and physical education programs, and it is expected that adequate supervision will be provided in order to reduce to a minimum the possibility of accidents.

Questions of liability in regard to supervision pertain to two points: (1) the extent of the supervision and (2) the quality of the supervision.

Regarding the first point, the question would be raised as to whether adequate supervision was provided. This is a difficult question to answer becuase it would vary from situation to situation. However, the answers to these questions: "Would additional supervision have eliminated the accident?" and "Is it reasonable to expect that additional supervision should have been provided?" will help to determine this.

In regard to the quality of the supervision, it is expected that competent personnel will handle specialized programs in health, physical education, and recreation. If the supervisors of such

---

*National Education Research Division for the National Commission on Safety Education, op. cit., pp. 18-20.

†Begley, R. F.: Legal liability in organized recreational playground areas, Safety Education Digest, 1955.

Gen. No. 1 100M-1-54-3181   **WAIVER FORM**   Long Beach, California
LONG BEACH PUBLIC SCHOOLS   Date_____

We,_____, are the parents or guardians
of_____, and in consideration of the special benefits
of the extracurricular activity being afforded the student by the Long Beach Board of Education and
the school districts whose school the aforementioned child attends, hereby permit_____
_____to participate in_____

_____

and we hereby release and discharge the said Long Beach Board of Education, the said school district,
and each and all their agents and employees from any liability whatever to the undersigned resulting from or in any manner arising out of any injury or damage which may be sustained by
the said_____, on account of his participation in

_____or in the transportation in connection therewith.
We further agree that in case of any action being brought for, or on behalf of the aforementioned child on account of any injury received during his participation in the above mentioned
events, or in the transportation connected therewith, that we will be personally responsible to the
school district, the Board of Education, and any of its officials or agents concerned, and will repay
to them and hold them harmless against any judgment recovered in any such action against them
or either of them.
Signed this_____day of_____, 195____

_____   _____
Signature of Parent or Guardian   Address

_____   _____
Signature of Parent or Guardian   Address
NOTE: Parents or Guardians, read the reverse side of this form.

---

activities do not possess proper training in such work, the question of negligence can be raised.

Waivers and consent slips

Waivers and consent slips are not synonymous. A waiver is an agreement whereby one party waives a particular right. A consent slip is an authorization, usually signed by the parent, permitting a child to take part in some activity.

In respect to a waiver, a parent cannot waive the rights of a child who is under 21 years of age. When a parent signs such a slip, he is merely waiving his or her right to sue for damages. A parent can sue in two ways, from the standpoint of his rights as the parent and from the standpoint of the child's own rights that he has as an individual, irrespective of the parent. A parent cannot waive the right of the child to sue as an individual.

Consent slips offer protection from the standpoint of showing that the child has the parent's permission to engage in an activity.

THE COURTS AND ELIGIBILITY RULES

Traditionally, when eligibility regulations have been challenged, courts have been reluc-

tant to substitute their judgment for the judgments of school athletic associations. In recent years, however, federal judges have been finding eligibility rules unconstitutional and administrators and physical educators should note this change in court rulings.

Recent court decisions where eligibility rules have been found to be segregationist in nature have been consistently found unconstitutional. A recent ruling found that the common practice in Alabama of having racially based athletic associations was unconstitutional, and a specific ruling of the United States Circuit Court ordered the Louisiana High School Athletic Association to admit a private Negro high school.

Other significant rulings concerning eligibility include a recent federal court order voiding the Indiana High School Athletic Association rule that prohibited married students from athletic participation. Another significant decision involved the Iowa High School Athletic Association and their suspension of a student athlete because he was riding in a car that was transporting beer. The student was not drinking, athletic training was not taking place, and the event occurred in the summer when school was not in session. In addition, no state or federal law was broken. The eligibility law was found to be unreasonable and the student was reinstated.

WOMEN IN SPORTS AND THE COURTS

Recent years have found the media reporting on numerous cases involving discrimination against women in sports. For example, a 1974 ruling by the State Division on Civil Rights of New Jersey requires Little League baseball teams to permit girls to play. New Jersey was the first state in the nation to have such a ruling. The order also requires that both boys and girls be notified of team tryouts and that both sexes be treated equally.

A recent amendment to the Education Law of New York State provides that no one may be disqualified from school athletic teams because of sex, except by certain regulations of the state commissioner of education. These regulations conclude that there may be mixed competition for men and women in interschool athletic teams except for the sports of baseball, basketball, field hockey, football, ice hockey, lacrosse, soccer, softball, speedball, team handball, power volleyball, and wrestling.

A federal court in Minnesota, recently overruled the Minnesota State High School Leagues' rule that prohibited girls from participation in certain interscholastic sports traditionally reserved for boys. Court decisions like this one support a new tendency in decisions to substitute judgmental rule for that of the association officials, especially in eligibility cases.

Another case involved two women coaches who were denied admittance to the North Carolina Coaching Clinic because of their sex. A lawsuit was instituted by the women against the all-male coaching association.

In Indiana, the Indiana Supreme Court ruled that it was discriminatory for a high school to sponsor a boy's team and not a girl's team. A girl was allowed to play on the boy's golf team because of this ruling.

Another interesting case involved the participation of a Teaneck, New Jersey girl on a boy's tennis team where no girl's team existed. New Jersey Interscholastic Athletic Association (NJSIAA) had a rule prohibiting girls from competing with boys in noncontact interscholastic sports. The suit against the NJSIAA charged that the rule was in violation of the equal-protection clause of the fourteenth amendment.

SAFETY

It is important to take every precaution possible to prevent accidents by providing for the safety of students and other individuals who participate in programs of health education, physical education, and recreation. If such precautions are taken, the likelihood of a lawsuit will diminish and the question of neligence will be eliminated. A few of the precautions that the leader or teacher should make provision for are as follows:

1. Instructor should be properly trained and qualified to perform specialized work.

2. Instructor should be present at all organized activities in the program.

3. Classes should be organized properly according to size, activity, physical condition, and other factors that have a bearing on safety and health of the individual.

4. Health examinations should be given to all pupils.

5. A planned, written program for proper disposition of students who are injured or become sick should be followed.

6. Regular inspections should be made of such items as equipment, apparatus, ropes, or chains, placing extra pressure upon them and taking other precautions to make sure they are safe. They should also be checked for deterioration, looseness, fraying, splinters, and so on.

7. Overcrowding athletic and other events should be avoided, building codes and fire regulations should be adhered to, and adequate lighting for all facilities should be provided.

8. Protective equipment such as mats should be utilized wherever possible. Any hazards such as projections or obstacles in an area where activity is taking place should be eliminated. Floors should not be slippery. Shower rooms should have surfaces conducive to secure footing.

9. Sneakers should be worn on gymnasium floors and adequate space provided for each activity.

10. Activities should be adapted to the age

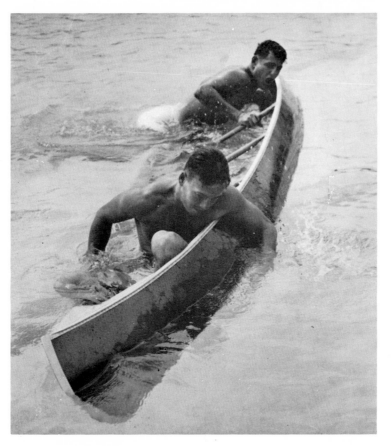

Every precaution should be taken to prevent accidents. Students learn to handle a canoe in water safety course. (University of Florida, Gainesville, Fla.)

and maturity of the participants, proper and competent supervision should be provided, and spotters should be utilized in apparatus and other similar activities.

11. Students should be instructed in the correct methods of using apparatus and performing in physical activities. Any misuse of equipment should be prohibited.

12. The buildings and other facilities used should be inspected regularly for safety hazards such as loose tiles, broken fences, cracked glass, and uneven pavement. Defects should be reported immediately to responsible persons and necessary precautions be taken.

13. In planning play and other instructional areas the following precautions should be taken:

a. There should be sufficient space for all games.

b. Games that utilize balls and other equipment that can cause damage should be conducted in areas where there is minimum danger of injuring someone.

c. Quiet games and activities that require working at benches, such as arts and crafts, should be in places that are well protected.

14. Truesdale lists certain questionable practices in which teachers, coaches, nurses, and trainers sometimes engage:

1. Supply "pills" for headaches or as laxatives or for menstrual discomfort.
2. Examine and diagnose by the stethoscope.
3. Prescribe anticold pills or capsules.
4. Strap joint injuries under supposition of sprain without expert assessment for possible fracture.
5. Permit return to play of a player with a head injury.
6. Play injured players not medically certified.
7. Permit return of students without medical certification to class, or particularly to activity, after illness.
8. Prescribe gargles or swabs for sore throats.

9. Use cutting tools (knives or razor blades) on calluses, corns, blisters, ingrown nails, etc.
10. Administer local anaesthesia to permit play after injury.
11. Employ physical forces such as heat or electric current to produce tissue change and decongestion and repair without medical order, or by unqualified persons.
12. Possibly further damage unconscious players by dashing water in the face, by slapping the face or by unwarranted use of aromatic spirits of ammonia to "bring them to."*

Truesdale also points out that "it is the duty of adults engaged in education not only to know of and be skillful in the proper techniques for protecting persons against injury, or protecting injured persons against aggravation, but also to know the limits beyond which the untrained or the partially trained person may not go."

15. In the event of accident the following or a similar procedure should be followed:

a. The nearest teacher or leader should proceed to the scene of the accident immediately, notifying the person in charge and nurse, if available, by messenger. Also, a doctor should be called at once if one is necessary.

b. A hurried examination of the injured person will give some idea as to the nature and extent of the injury and the emergency of the situation.

c. If the teacher or leader is well versed in first aid, assistance should be given (a qualified first-aid certificate will usually absolve the teacher of negligence). Every teacher or leader who works in these specialized areas should and is expected to know first-aid procedures. In any event everything should be done to make the injured person comfortable and reassure the injured until the services of a physician can be secured.

d. If the injury is serious, an ambulance should be called.

e. After the injured person has been provided for, the person in charge should fill out the accident forms and take the statements of witnesses and file for future reference. Reports of accidents should be prepared promptly and sent to proper persons. They should be accurate as to detail and complete as to information. Among other things they should contain information about:

Name and address of injured person
Activity engaged in
Date, hour, and place
Person in charge
Witnesses
Cause and extent of injury
Medical attention given
Circumstances surrounding incident

f. There should be a complete followup of the accident, an analysis of the situation, and an eradication of any hazards that exist.

Herman Rosenthal, Assistant to the Law Secretary, City of New York, in addressing a health education conference in New York City, pointed up the following remarks in respect to reporting accidents:

Reports should be complete, full and in detail. He advised that where a case does go into litigation, there is a delay in the court calendar of 2 to 3 years before the case is tried. A complete and detailed report is always better than a teacher's or a child's memory. He pointed out that the completion of accident reports was the function and duty of the teacher and in no case should a child be expected to prepare the report. Reports in the handwriting of children, he said, should be limited only to the statements and signatures of the injured and of the witnesses to the accident. He emphasized that should an injured child at the time of the accident be unable to prepare a written statement or affix his signature to a report, the teacher should prepare the necessary statement and signature and indicate the reasons for so doing. He further focused attention on the fact that teachers should not attempt to color or distort facts in order to protect the school or the child, because such a practice does more harm than good. An extremely important point, he said, was the need to report where the teacher was at the time of the accident, the extent of the supervision, and the teacher control of the activity at the time of the accident. Also, he said that with few exceptions reports should be submitted within 24 hours of the time of the accident. He explained that in some cases this might not be possible, but in such cases no report need be delayed more than 48 hours.*

g. Thelma Reed, Chairman of Standard Student Accident Report Committee of the National Safety Council, listed the reasons why de-

*Truesdale, J. C.: So you're a good samaritan! Journal of the American Association for Health, Physical Education, and Recreation **25:**25, 1954.

*Proceedings of the City Wide Conference with Principals' Representatives and Men and Women Chairmen of Health Education, City of New York Board of Education, Brooklyn, N. Y., 1953, Bureau of Health Education.

(check one)		RECOMMENDED		(check one)
☐ School Jurisdictional		**STANDARD STUDENT ACCIDENT REPORT**		Recordable ☐
☐ Non-School Jurisdictional		(See instructions on reverse side)		Reportable Only ☐

School District:

City, State:

General

1. Name	2. Address		
3. School	4. Sex Male ☐ Female ☐	5. Age	6. Grade/Special Program

7. Time Accident Occurred

Date: Day of Week: Exact Time: AM ☐ PM ☐

Injury

8. Nature of Injury

9. Part of Body Injured

10. Degree of Injury (check one)

Death ☐ Permanent ☐ Temporary (lost time) ☐ Non-Disabling (no lost time) ☐

11. Days Lost

From School: From Activities Other Than School: Total:

12. Cause of Injury

Accident

13. Accident Jurisdiction (check one)

School: Grounds ☐ Building ☐ To and From ☐ Other Activities Not on School Property ☐

Non-School: Home ☐ Other ☐

14. Location of Accident (be specific)	15. Activity of Person (be specific)
16. Status of Activity	17. Supervision (if yes, give title & name of supervisor) Yes ☐ No ☐
18. Agency Involved	19. Unsafe Act
20. Unsafe Mechanical/Physical Condition	21. Unsafe Personal Factor

22. Corrective Action Taken or Recommended

23. Property Damage

School $ Non-School $ Total $

24. Description (Give a word picture of the accident, explaining who, what, when, why and how)

Signature

25. Date of Report	26. Report Prepared by (signature & title)
27. Principal's Signature	

This form is recommended for securing data for accident prevention and safety education. School districts may reproduce this form adding space for optional data. Reference: *Student Accident Reporting Guidebook*, National Safety Council, 425 N. Michigan Avenue, Chicago, Illinois 60611. 1966. 34 pages.

(over)

Accident report form recommended by National Safety Council.

GROVER CLEVELAND HIGH SCHOOL
HIMROD & GRANDVIEW AVE.
Ridgewood, New York

STATEMENT BY WITNESS
(Write in Ink)

Witness..Address..

Age..Rank..Class..................................

Name of one injured..Injured's Official Class.................Age of Injured....................

Date of accident..Time....................................Day of week................................

A. Circumstances of Accident

1. Locate the position from which you witnessed the accident, using such phrases as, in front of, as I entered, standing on the, in back of, etc...

....

....

....

2. Locate the position where the accident occurred, using such phrases as, on the landing, exit 8 up, on the horizontal bar, etc...

....

....

3. Tell what you saw...

....

....

....

B. Additional remarks, if any...

....

....

C. Signature of Witness..

Statement by witness to accident. (Grover Cleveland High School, Ridgewood, N. Y.)

tailed injury reports are important for school authorities:

1. Aid in protecting the school personnel and district from unfortunate publicity and from liability suits growing out of student injury cases;

2. Aid in evaluating the relative importance of the various safety areas and the time each merits in the total school safety effort;

3. Suggest modifications in the structure, use, and maintenance of buildings, grounds, and equipment;

4. Suggest curriculum adjustments to meet immediate student needs;

5. Provide significant data for individual student guidance;

6. Give substance to the school administrators' appeal for community support of the school safety program;

7. Aid the school administration in guiding the school safety activities of individual patrons and patrons' groups.

Some suggestions to help reduce injuries on the gridiron

Approximately 700 American boys have been killed directly or indirectly playing football in the last quarter century. Studies show that football is by far the most dangerous part of the educational program. According to the National Safety Council, in a recent year football accounted for one out of every five accidents occurring under the school's jurisdiction to students in the sophomore year, one out of every four to junior-year students, and one out of every three to seniors. By contrast baseball accounted for one out of twenty-six to sophomore students, one out of twenty-nine to the juniors, and one of thirty-three to the seniors.

Football can be made a much safer game. Many times chances are taken, players are urged to participate when not in the best of physical condition, the safest type of uniforms and equipment are not used, and the necessary precautions are not taken. In some cases there is negligence on the part of school authorities. Some suggestions to help make football a safer game are as follows:

1. A qualified coaching staff and a qualified trainer should be hired.

2. The best equipment that money can buy should be purchased.

3. Qualified officials should be present for all games and scrimmages.

4. Safe facilities, such as good turf, adequate space, and elimination of all hazards should be required.

5. A doctor should be present at all games and at all scrimmages.

6. A thorough physical examination before the season starts and again at midseason is a *must*. It should include a detailed study of the health history of each player. If health history shows heart abnormalities or other defects that might be aggravated, the boy should not be permitted to play.

7. Provisions should be available for such essentials as an x-ray study, encephalogram, physical therapy, and bandaging.

8. Accident insurance to cover full cost of diagnosis and treatment of all injuries should be obtained.

9. No boy should be allowed to return to a game after a head injury until an x-ray film has been taken and a doctor has approved return to action. If the injury is diagnosed as severe concussion, he should never be allowed to participate in gridiron activities again.

10. The temptation to send in the star who insists that he is not hurt and wants to return to play should be resisted. Decision to return to play should not be permitted unless approved by the doctor in writing.

11. Each school should play only schools of its own size and teams of its own stature.

12. More stress should be placed on training and conditioning: at least twenty practices spaced over a 3-week period before the first game for each player, longer warmups for reserves sitting on the bench and for all players at halftime of the game, and greater emphasis on fundamentals, such as blocking, tackling, and techniques of play.

13. If the rules could be changed as follows, injuries could be reduced:

a. Eliminate second-half kickoff.

b. Increase the penalty for piling on. Ban from the game the player who persists in ignoring this rule.

c. Allow for substitutions to the extent that exhausted players will not be in the game.

d. Provide 5 minutes longer between halves of the game, with specific stipulation that this time is to be used for warmup.

Safety code for the physical education teacher

The following safety code should be followed by the physical education teacher:

1. Have a proper teacher's certificate in full force and effect.
2. Operate and teach at all times, within the scope of his employment as delimited and defined by the rules and regulations of the employing board of education and within the statutory limitations imposed by the state.
3. Provide the safeguards designed to minimize the dangers inherent in a particular activity.
4. Provide the amount of supervision for each activity required to ensure the maximum safety of all the pupils.
5. Inspect equipment and facilities periodically to determine whether or not they are safe for use.
6. Notify the proper authorities forthwith concerning the existence of any dangerous condition as it continues to exist.
7. Provide sufficient instruction in the performance of any activity before exposing pupils to its hazards.
8. Be certain that the task is one approved by the employing board of education for the age and attainments of the pupils involved.
9. Do not force a pupil to perform a physical feat which the pupil obviously feels incapable of performing.
10. Act promptly and use discretion in giving first aid to an injured pupil, but nothing more.
11. Exercise due care in practicing his profession.
12. Act as a reasonably prudent person would under the given circumstances.
13. Anticipate the dangers which should be apparent to a trained, intelligent person (a legal principle known as "foreseeability").*

INSURANCE MANAGEMENT

There are three major types of insurance management that school districts utilize to protect themselves against loss. The first type is insurance for *property,* owned by the school district. The second type is insurance for *liability protection,* where there might be financial loss arising from personal injury or property damage for which the school district is liable. The third type is insurance for *crime protection* against a financial loss that might be incurred as a result of theft or other illegal act. This section on insurance management is primarily concerned with the second type of insurance, namely, liability protection.

A definite trend can be seen in school districts toward having some form of school accident in-

*Munize, A. J.: The teacher, pupil injury, and legal liability, Journal of Health, Physical Education, and Recreation **33:**28, 1962.

surance to protect students against injury. School administrators and boards of education in many communities feel this is one additional and important way of giving service to its school population. Along with this trend can be seen the impact upon casualty and life insurance companies that offer insurance policies for school children and staff. The premium costs of school accident policies vary from community to community and also in accordance with age of insured and type of plan offered. The area of interscholastic athletics has been responsible for the development of many state athletic protection plans as well as the issuance of special policies by commercial insurance companies. When it is realized that accidents are the chief cause of death among students between the ages of 5 and 18, it can readily be seen that some protection is needed.

Common features of insurance management plans

Some common features of insurance management plans across the United States are as follows:

1. Premiums are paid for by the school, by the parent, or jointly by the school and parent.
2. Schools obtain their money for payment of premiums from the board of education, general organization fund, or a pooling of funds for many schools taken from gate receipts in league games.
3. Schools place the responsibility upon the parents to pay for any injuries incurred.
4. The blanket type coverage is a very common policy for insurance companies to offer.
5. Insurance companies frequently offer insurance coverage for athletic injuries as part of a package plan that also includes an accident plan for all students.
6. Most schools have insurance plans for the protection of athletes.
7. Most schools seek insurance coverage that provides for benefits whether x-ray films are positive or negative.
8. Hospitalization, x-ray films, and medical fees and dental fees are increasingly becoming part of the insurance coverage in schools.

Some school boards have found it a good policy to pay the premium on insurance policies because the full coverage of students provides peace of mind for both parents and teachers. Furthermore, it has been noted by some educators that many liability suits have been avoided in this manner.

Other school officials investigate the various insurance plans available and then recommend a particular plan and the parents deal directly with the company. Such parent-paid plans are frequently divided into two options: (1) they provide coverage for the student on a door-to-door basis (to and from school, while at school, and in school-sponsored activities) and (2) they provide 24-hour accident coverage with premiums usually running to four times higher than the "school only" policy. The "school only" policy rates are based upon age with rates for children in the elementary grades less than those in the higher grades. These policies also usually run only for the school year.

Student accident insurance provides coverage for all accidents regardless of whether the insured is hospitalized or treated in a doctor's office. Such medical plans as Blue Cross and Blue Shield are limited in the payments they make. Student accident insurance policies, as a general rule, offer reasonable rates and are a good investment for all concerned. Parents should be encouraged, however, to examine their existing family policies before taking out such policies to avoid overlapping coverage.

A survey of nine school districts in Ohio a few years ago indicated some practices and problems concerned with answering the question: "What to look for in selecting an insurance policy for athletics?"* These facts were disclosed by this survey:

1. The chief school administrator was the person who usually selected the insurance company from whom the policy would be purchased.

2. Medical coverage on policies purchased ranged from $30 to $5,000 and dental coverage from nothing to $500.

3. The claims collected for one particular type of injury ranged from nothing to $792.30.

4. Companies did not follow through at all times in paying the amount for which the claim was made.

5. Most insurance companies writing athletic policies have scheduled benefit plans.

6. Catastrophe clauses were absent from all policies.

7. Athletes covered ranged from 80% to 100%.

8. In most cases part of each athlete's premium was paid for from a school athletic fund.

9. Football was covered in separate policies.

As a result of this survey the following recommendations were made:

1. Some person or group of persons should be delegated to explore insurance policies and, after developing a set of criteria, to purchase the best one possible.

2. Where feasible, cooperative plans with other schools on a county or other basis should be encouraged in order to obtain less expensive group rates.

3. Criteria for the selection of an insurance policy should, in addition to cost, relate to such important benefits as maximum medical, excluded benefits, maximum dental, hospital, death or dismemberment, surgical, and x-ray.

4. The greatest possible coverage for cost involved should be an important basis for the selection of policy.

5. In light of football programs especially, the catastrophe clause should be investigated as possible additional coverage.

6. Deductible clause policies should not be purchased.

7. Dental injury benefits are an important consideration.

8. Determine what claims the insurance company will and will not pay.

9. The school should insist on 100% enrollment in the athletic insurance program.

10. Schools should have a central location for keeping insurance records, and there should be an annual survey to ascertain all the pertinent facts about the cost and effectiveness of such coverage.

Procedure for insurance management

Every school should be covered by insurance. There are five types of accident insurance that can be used: "(1) commercial insurance policies written on an individual basis; (2) student medical benefit plans written on a group basis by

---

*Rockhold, J.: How to buy athletic insurance, The Ohio High School Athlete **23:**169, 1964.

commercial insurers; (3) state high school athletic association benefit plans; (4) medical benefit plans operated by specific city school systems; and (5) self-insurance.''* Before adoption by any school each type of insurance should be carefully weighed so that best coverage is obtained for the type of program sponsored.

A suggested procedure to be followed as a guide for the administration of an insurance program follows:

(1) the entire school should be organized to study the insurance problems and needs, (2) a survey should be made to ascertain the need for insurance before it is purchased, (3) after the need has been established, specifications should be constructed indicating the kind and amount of insurance needed, (4) the specifications should be presented to several insurers to obtain estimates of coverage and costs, (5) the plans presented to the school by the several insurers should be studied, and the one best suited to that particular situation should be selected, (6) parents should be given full information about the insurance, (7) workable and harmonious relations should be established with the insurer selected, (8) continuous evaluation of the insurance program should be carried out, and (9) records should be carefully kept of costs, accidents, claims payments, and other pertinent data.

School administrators should insist upon the following conditions and requirements when purchasing accident insurance: (1) the coverage should include all school activities and provide up to $500 [more today] for each injury to each pupil, (2) the medical services should include (a) cost of professional services of physician or surgeon, (b) cost of hospital care and service, (c) cost of a trained nurse, (d) cost of ambulance, surgical appliances, dressings, x-rays, etc., and (e) cost of repair and care of natural teeth, (3) the policy should be tailor-made to fit the needs of the school, (4) the coverage should be maximum for minimum cost, (5) all pupils as well as all teachers, should be included, (6) a deductible clause should be avoided unless it reduces the premium substantially and the policy still fulfills its purpose, (7) blanket rather than schedule type coverage should be selected, and (8) claims payment must be simple, certain, and fast.†

School athletic insurance‡

According to Grimes, prior to 1930 there was very little accident insurance carried by school

districts to protect their athletes, and there was little activity on the part of commercial insurance companies in this area. Only a very few schools were self-insured, and if they were it was primarily for football. Grimes further relates that the Wisconsin High School Athletic Association provided the first movement in school athletic insurance coverage when it established its plan in 1930 and made it available to member schools. Thereafter, many other states followed the example set by Wisconsin, and athletic associations established their own athletic insurance plans. The practice grew and by the 1940's, twenty-five states had such plans. By the 1950's commercial insurance companies, recognizing the possibilities in this area, started to enter the high school athletic field and provided special policies to cover athletes in various sports. The commercial insurance companies became so competitive that they made deep inroads into the nonprofit state athletic association plans. Also, according to Grimes, as a result of the commercial insurance company inroads, insurance plans became more comprehensive and coverage was extended to pupils for all school activities for all grades. Today, only eight high school athletic associations sponsor their own insurance plans. These plans stay in business largely because they have adopted many of the features of commercial insurance plans, such as nonallocated benefits, catastrophic coverage, group coverage, nonduplication of benefits, and varying premium rates.

Athletic protection funds usually have these characteristics: they are a nonprofit venture, they are not compulsory, a specific fee is charged each person registered with the plan, and there is provision for recovery for specific injuries. Generally the money is not paid out of tax funds but instead is paid either by the participants themselves or by the school or other agency.

In connection with such plans, it should be recognized that an individual, after receiving benefits, could in most states still bring action against the coach or other leader whose negligence contributed to the injury.

In respect to paying for liability and accident insurance out of public tax funds, the states vary as to their practices. Some states do not permit

---

*Joint Committee: Administrative problems in health education, physical education and recreation, Washington, D. C., 1953, American Association for Health, Physical Education, and Recreation, p. 105.

†Joint Committee. op. cit., p. 106.

‡From Grimes, L. W.: Trends in school athletic insurance. In Secondary school athletic administration—a new look, Washington, D. C., 1969, The American Association for Health, Physical Education, and Recreation.

CLAIM NO.			

REQUEST FOR ACCIDENT BENEFIT

INTERSCHOLASTIC

To be filled in by School

SPORT_____

Dr._____

X-Ray_____

Total_____

DO NOT WRITE
IN ABOVE SPACE

1. School _____   4. Grade_____

2. Name _____   5. Age_____

3. Date and Time of Injury _____   6. No. of years of competition _____

7. Game_____	8. Type of play at time of injury	9. Boy activity at time of injury
Practice _____	Offense _____ Run _____	Block _____
Scrimmage _____	Defense _____ Pass _____	Tackle _____
Skills _____	Rebound _____ Kick _____	Shooting _____
Night Football Game _____	Etc. _____	Etc. _____

10. Explain exactly where and how the injury occurred _____

_____

_____

11. Name of the doctor who first attended or examined your injury_____

Date and hour?_____**STATE DATES** of treatment _____

12. After the injury I returned to the squad on _____ (date), was not in school for _____ days.

13. Does the parent have other Insurance to cover this expense_____

I, Principal of_____High School, have examined the above statements, and the statements of the Doctor or Dentist who attended this student. The statements are true to the best of my knowledge and I believe this claim to be just.

_____   _____
(Date)   (Principal)

(Signature of Claimant)

This boy was given a Physical Examination on **(DATE)** _____ at the beginning of **THIS SPORTS SEASON,** which was recorded on the regulation Physical Examination Card which is on file in the school.

_____
(Signature of Coach present at time of injury)

AFFIDAVIT OF ATTENDING PHYSICIAN

1. Date of first treatment _____   2. Diagnosis _____

(Here state the nature, character and extent of injury to claimant)

3. **X-RAY READING REPORT MUST ACCOMPANY ALL CLAIMS FOR INDEMNITY FOR FRACTURE OR DISLOCATION.**

_____

4. In your opinion was there any predisposing factor contributory to the injury? _____

5. Give name of any consulting or assistant physician _____

6. Describe your treatment and **State Dates** of examination or treatment _____

_____

_____

7. Prognosis and General Remarks_____

Facsimile of Physician's Fees

(   ) Office Calls @ $3.00 _____ $_____

(   ) Home Calls @ $4.00 _____ $_____

(   ) Operation _____ $_____

(   ) X-ray _____ $_____

_____ $_____

Total_____ $_____

X-RAY not taken by you — attach official copy of report and statement for charge.

SINCE THE PROTECTION PLAN IS A NON-PROFIT ORGANIZATION ESTABLISHED TO SERVE THE SCHOOLS, THE MAXIMUM SCHEDULED INDEMNITY IS NOT TO BE CLAIMED UNLESS ITEMIZED PROFESSIONAL SERVICES JUSTIFY THAT AMOUNT AS LISTED ON REVERSE SIDE.

8. The above named student is again able to PARTICIPATE in athletics and physical education on _____
date

9. Patient discharged from my care on _____
date

I, a Duly Licensed Physician, personally performed the above services.

Signature of Physician: _____ M. D.

Address _____

Form No. 2
25M—5-62

PHYSICIAN: RETURN FORM TO SCHOOL WITH STUDENT ON LAST VISIT
All Bills Must Be Presented Within 90 Days of Accident If Claims Are To Be Paid

Request for accident benefit form. (New York State High School Athletic Protection Plan, Inc.)

tax money to be used for liability or accident insurance to cover students in physical education activities. On the other hand, the state legislature of Oregon permits school districts to carry liability insurance. This section is stated as follows in the revised code, O.R.S.:

332.180 Liability insurance; medical and hospital benefits insurance. Any district school board may enter into contracts of insurance for liability coverage all activities engaged in by the district, for medical and hospital benefits for students engaging in athletic contests and for public liability and property damage covering motor vehicles operated by the district, and may pay the necessary premiums thereon. Failure to procure such insurance shall in no case be construed as negligence or lack of diligence on the part of the district school board or the members thereof.

Some athletic insurance plans in use in the schools today are entirely inadequate. These plans indicate a certain amount of money as the maximum that can be collected. For example, a boy may lose the sight of an eye. According to the athletic protection fund, the loss of an eye will draw, say, $1,500. This amount does not come even remotely close to paying for such a serious injury. In this case a hypothetical example could be taken by saying that the parents sue the athletic protection fund and the teacher for $30,000. In some states if the case is lost, the athletic fund will pay the $1,500 and the teacher the other $28,500. It can be seen that some of these insurance plans do not give complete and adequate coverage.

In many states teachers need additional protection against being sued for accidental injury to students. Legislation is needed permitting school funds to be used as protection against student injuries. In this way a school would be legally permitted to and could be required to purchase liability insurance to cover all pupils.

Questions and exercises

1. Consult the legal files in your local governmental unit to determine any court cases on record that have implications for the fields of health education, physical education, and/or recreation. Describe the circumstances surrounding each.
2. Arrange a mock trial in your class. Have a jury, prosecutor, defendant, witnesses, and other features characteristic of a regular court trial. Your instructor will state the case before the court.
3. Why is it important that leaders in health, physical education, and recreation have knowledge in respect to legal liability?
4. Define and illustrate each of the following: (a) liability, (b) tort, (c) negligence, (d) *in loco parentis,* (e) plaintiff, (f) nuisance, (g) misfeasance, (h) *respondeat superior,* and (i) proximate cause.
5. What are the defenses against negligence? Illustrate each.
6. What is the difference between governmental and proprietary functions? Illustrate each.
7. How does the charging of fees affect liability?
8. What is the extent of liability of (a) municipality, (b) school district, (c) board member, and (d) coach?
9. Discuss some of the legal aspects of women in sports. Are you familiar with a legal case concerning women and athletic programs? If so, briefly explain the situation.
10. Why is it so important that adult fitness programs be competently conducted? Explain the principles involved in the possible legal liability of instructors who teach adult fitness classes.
11. What are some safety procedures that should be followed by every physical education teacher?
12. What are the advantages of waivers and consent slips?

Reading assignment in *Administrative Dimensions of Health and Physical Education Programs, Including Athletics:* Chapter 14, Selections 77 to 82.

Selected references

American Association for Health, Physical Education, and Recreation: Secondary school athletic administration—a new look, Washington, D. C., 1969, The Association.

Appenzeller, H.: Bench and bar, Kendal Sports Trail **28:**12, 1973.

Bird, P. J.: Tort liability, Journal of Health, Physical Education, and Recreation **41:**38, 1970.

Bucher, C. A.: Football can be made safer, New York World-Telegram and Sun, Saturday Feature Magazine, Sept. 1, 1956.

Casey, L. M.: School business administration, New York, 1964, The Center for Applied Research in Education, Inc. (The Library of Education).

Chambless, J. R., and Mangin, C.: Legal liability and the physical educator, Journal of Health, Physical Education, and Recreation **44:**42, 1973.

Foraker, T., and others: School insurance, School and Community, p. 28, October, 1967.

Garber, L. O.: Tort and contractual liability of school districts, Danville, Ill., 1963, The Interstate Printers & Publishers, Inc.

Garber, L. O.: Yearbook of school law, Danville, Ill., 1963, The Interstate Printers & Publishers, Inc.

Gauerke, W. E.: School Law, New York, 1965, The Center for Applied Research in Education, Inc. (The Library of Education).

Grieve, A.: Legal aspects of spectator injuries, The Athletic Journal **47:**74, 1967.

Grieve, A.: State requirements for physical education, Journal of Health, Physical Education, and Recreation **42:**19, 1971.

Guenther, D.: Problems involving legal liability in schools,

Journal of the American Association for Health, Physical Education, and Recreation **20:**511, 1949.

Hamilton, R. R.: School liability, Chicago, 1952, National Safety Council.

Jensen, G. O.: State requirements in health and physical education, The Society of State of Health, Physical Education and Recreation, July, 1973.

Johnson, T. P.: The courts and eligibility rules: is a new attitude emerging, Journal of Health, Physical Education, and Recreation **44:**34, 1973.

Kurtzman, J.: Legal liability and physical education, The Physical Educator **24:**20, 1967.

Liebee, H. C.: Liability for accidents in physical education, athletics, recreation, Ann Arbor, Mich., 1952, Ann Arbor Publishers.

National Education Association, Research Division: School laws and teacher negligence: summary of who is responsible for pupil injuries, National Education Association Research Bulletin **40:**75, 1962.

National Education Association: The pupil's day in court: review of 1968, Washington, D. C., 1969, The Association.

National Education Association: Tort liability and liability insurance, School Law Summaries, NEA Research Division, March, 1969.

Proceedings of the City Wide Conference with Principals' Representatives and Men and Women Chairmen of Health Education, City of New York Board of Education, Bureau of Health Education, 1953.

Rosenfield, H. N.: Liability for school accidents, New York, 1940, Harper & Row, Publishers.

Shroyer, G. F.: Coach's legal liability for athletic injuries, Scholastic Coach **34:**18, 1964.

State school laws and regulations for health, safety, driver, outdoor, and physical education, Washington, D. C., 1964, Department of Health, Education, and Welfare.

The coaches and the courts: Journal of Health, Physical Education, and Recreation **41:**10, 1970.

Truesdale, J. C.: So you're a good samaritan! Journal of the American Association for Health, Physical Education, and Recreation **25:**25, 1954.

Van Der Smissen, B.: Legal aspects of adult fitness programs, Journal of Health, Physical Education, and Recreation **45:**54, 1974.

Van Der Smissen, B.: Legal liability of cities and schools for injuries in recreation and parks, including physical education and athletics, Cincinnati, 1968, suppl. 1973, W. H. Anderson Co., Legal Publishers.

Curriculum development and revision

Curriculum development and revision are essential to meeting educational objectives. The best possible education can only be provided if curriculums are carefully developed and continuously evaluated by both students and teachers. Student involvement is an essential factor in curriculum development and change. Education must be relevant to the students, and to be relevant the students' opinions must be elicited.

Each subject matter field must relate to and help each student approach self-realization and effective social behavior through an involvement of pertinent ideas, people, and activities. Individual differences must be provided for. Each school system's program must reflect the fact that learning is a continuous and individual process that proceeds at various rates and to various degrees in the attainment of each student's maximum potential.

The curriculum in health education or physical education represents the experiences that are provided children and young people so that the objectives of the profession may be met. The curriculum functions as the vehicle for achieving such objectives as organic development, motor development, cognitive development, and social development. It provides for experiences in terms of courses, subject matter, and

activities that will best approach those goals. It creates the environment that will enable sound and meaningful education to take place. The experiences provided are means to an end—that end being the realization of the broad goals that we have established as a profession and that enrich human living. Each student is, through the experiences provided, helped to develop his or her abilities and to realize his or her full potential.

IMPORTANCE OF CURRICULUM DEVELOPMENT AND ROLE OF ADMINISTRATION

Curriculum development is important as a service to the student. It should be concerned with matching the experience and the student; it must meet the needs of boys and girls. Since no two students are exactly alike, there is great need for flexibility and for a wide range of experiences that meet the requirements of all pupils. Continuous curriculum development is a way of determining what needs to be learned and of providing the means for seeing that it is accomplished.

The administration plays a very important part in curriculum planning. The end result of all administrative effort is to provide better instructional services, better programs, better learning situations, and better experiences to achieve the objectives that have been established. Since new problems constantly arise and since unmet needs continue to exist or go unrecognized, there is an urgent need for continuous curriculum planning. It is the administrator who provides the required leadership. The educational philosophy that represents the foundation of curriculum development should reflect faculty thinking as determined by their study of pupil needs. If an administrator possesses what he or she considers to be a better philosophy, this should be discussed with the faculty, bringing forth facts, good reasoning, and logic to support his or her concept. If it is then accepted by the faculty, it can be utilized. Otherwise, it will not receive extensive practical application because it is not understood or accepted.

Curriculum construction requires the selection, guidance, and evaluation of experiences in the light of both long-term and more immediate goals. It provides for an orderly periodic evaluation of the total program, both the inclass and the out-of-class, with changes being made whenever necessary. It takes into consideration such factors as students, total community, existing facilities, personnel, time allotments, national trends, and state rules and regulations. It sets up a framework for orderly progression from the kindergarten through college. It offers a guide to health education and physical education teachers so that they are better able to achieve educational goals.

Curriculum development is very important and school administrators have the responsibility for making the necessary provisions to see that it is accomplished.

CATALYSTS THAT BRING ABOUT CURRICULUM CHANGE

Changes occur in health education and physical education curriculums as they do in other areas of the school offering. There is usually a continuous list of myriad proposals for change. Each proposal should be considered on its own merits and put to the test of whether or not it has value.

What are the influencing factors in regard to change? A few associations, agencies, and individuals who produce change in health and physical education are discussed in the following paragraphs.

Student opinion

Student opinion is often the first step toward curriculum revision. Students want to be involved and should be consulted about the curriculum and suggested changes. It is important to find out what they have on their minds and the types of programs they need and desire. Recently, the District of Columbia public schools engaged in a project designed to restructure and improve the physical education curriculum for its junior and senior high schools. Besides meeting with consultants, staff members, and persons from other areas, an interest survey was taken among all students in grades seven through twelve in order to ascertain the activities and programs they desired. The interest survey included both team and individual sports that students might be interested in. They were asked to indicate those they would like to see offered. In addition, they were given an opportunity to indicate other activities they would like offered, select those activities that they thought should be coeducational, and indicate the number of periods they thought physical education classes should meet. A similar survey was prepared for health education. This type of survey is essential if curriculum revision is going to be relevant to the students.

National associations and agencies

The President's Council on Physical Fitness and Sports is an outstanding example of one national governmental agency that brought about much change in programs of health, physical education, and recreation throughout the United States and the world. Through their speakers, publications, and communication media pronouncements, many changes have taken place in the schools and colleges of this nation. Physical fitness in some communities has become the overriding purpose of programs of health education and physical education, sometimes at the expense of the other objectives of these fields and a well-balanced program of activities.

Examples of other national associations and agencies that play a part in curriculum change are the National Education Association, the American Alliance for Health, Physical Education, and Recreation, the United States Office

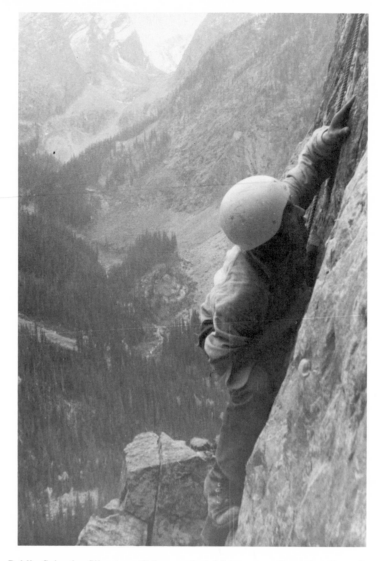

In the Silverton Public Schools, Silverton, Colo., students' interests and opinions have been taken into consideration with the result they engage in many outdoor activities peculiar to the area. (Courtesy George Pastor.)

of Education, the Association for Supervision and Curriculum Development, and The American Medical Association.

State associations and agencies

As national organizations influence the curriculums of our schools and colleges, so do state organizations. State boards of education or departments of public instruction, state bureaus, departments or divisions of health and physical education, state education associations, citizens committees, teachers associations, and associations for health, physical education, and recreation are a few examples of organizations that influence curriculums. Through the publication of syllabuses, sponsorship of legislation, enactment of rules and regulations, exercise of supervisory powers, allocation of funds, and initiation of projects, organizations promote certain ideas and programs that initiate changes in schools and colleges.

Research

Research brings about change. As new knowledge is uncovered, more information is known about the learning process, new techniques are developed, and other research is conducted. Change eventually ensues if the research is significant, but the change may be slow in coming. It usually takes a long period of time for the creation of knowledge to penetrate to the grass roots, where it becomes part of an action program.

In the fields of health education and physical education, research on motor learning, the relationship of health and physical fitness to academic achievement, movement education, cognitive learning, physiologic changes that occur in the body through exercise and smoking, ecology, and the relationship of mental health and physical activity represent a few examples of research that has or will have a bearing upon programs of health education and physical education throughout the country.

College and university faculties

The leaders in education from the campuses of this nation who serve as consultants, write textbooks, make speeches, and are active in professional associations, help to bring about changes in education in general and in the special fields of health education and physical education.

Social forces

Such social forces in the American culture as the civil rights movement, automation, mass communication, student activism, black studies, sports promotion, and collective bargaining through unions are a few of the movements sweeping the nation that have implications for curriculum change in schools and colleges. In addition, the social trends of the times involving attitudes toward sex, driving, alcohol, tobacco, and narcotics also bring about curriculum change. Times change, customs change, the habits of people change, and with such change the role of educational institutions and their responsibilities to their society frequently change.

THE HEALTH EDUCATOR AND PHYSICAL EDUCATOR AND CURRICULUM CHANGE

Since there are so many factors that continually influence curriculums, it is important for the health educator and physical educator to assess the recommended changes so that informed and wise decisions may be made. Four questions that administrators and teachers might ask themselves in rationalizing the importance of suggested changes are as follows:

1. *What are the functions of the schools and colleges?* To what extent is the suggested change in conformance with the philosophy and purpose of education in the American society? How will it better help the students?

2. *Am I sufficiently well informed so that I can make an intelligent decision?* Teachers and administrators will need to be knowledgeable about the learning process, the patterns of human growth and development, current program needs, and such matters as the needs and interests of the people in the local community who are served by the educational institution. The responsibility rests with administrators and teachers to be well informed in the areas pertinent to the decisions that need to be made.

3. *How does the change relate to staff, plant, budget, and other important administrative items?* The change must be practical to implement, and the best use of staff, plant, and other items must be taken into consideration in making the decision.

4. *What do the experts say?* What is the thinking of professionals who have done research, studied the problem intensively, and tested the proposal on a wide scale? Expert opinion may be of help as an additional source of information for making a wise curriculum decision.

PROCEDURAL CONSIDERATIONS FOR CURRICULUM CHANGE

Curricular revision cannot occur without taking into consideration an investigation into such procedural matters as the following:

1. *Students.* The number of students, their characteristics and needs, and their socioeconomic backgrounds and interests need to be considered prior to initiating any pertinent curriculum change.

2. *Faculty.* The members of the staff play a key role in curricular revision. For example, the attitude of faculty toward change, present teaching loads, comprehension of goals of the school, attitudes toward inclass and out-of-class programs, competencies in areas of curriculum re-

vision, and past training and experience are a few important considerations. Change in curriculum might well mean new members being added to the faculty or a different type of competency being represented on the staff.

3. *Physical plant*. Information in regard to the adequacy of the physical plant for present and future programs must be considered. Information should be available on capabilities and limitations of the present plant. There may be new demands placed upon facilities through a curricular revision that brings about changes in such matters as class size.

4. *Budget*. The financial plan is another important consideration in curriculum change. What will the new program cost? What are the sources of support? Before the faculty expends large amounts of time and effort in a study of curriculum change, there should be a reasonable assurance that proposed changes are economically feasible. In school systems utilizing PPBS, budgets are formulated taking the objectives of curriculum planning into consideration. PPBS also provides for evaluation techniques that require curriculum change if educational goals are not being met.

5. *Curriculum*. Since any new curricular proposal is likely to reflect present practices to some degree, it seems logical that the present curriculum needs careful scrutiny to determine what has happened over the years, the degree to which the faculty has brought about change, and the general direction in which the institution is moving.

6. *Administration*. It is important for the faculty to take a hard look at the administrative leadership of the school or college, including the principals, superintendents, deans, and presidents, as well as the boards of education and boards of trustees. The philosophy of the administration and its views toward change should be carefully weighed. Administrators will need to approve budgetary allocations and necessary expenditures as well as, in many cases, pass upon the proposed changes.

PEOPLE INVOLVED IN CURRICULUM DEVELOPMENT

Curriculum planning should be characterized by broad participation on the part of many peo-ple. The consideration of administrators, teachers, state groups, students, parents, and other individuals in important.

Administrators

Administrators—whether the college president in the field of higher education, the superintendent of schools or principal of an elementary, middle, junior high, or senior high school, or the chairperson or director of the health and physical education department—are key personnel in curriculum planning. These individuals serve as the catalytic forces that set curriculum studies into motion; as the leadership that encourages and stimulates interest in providing better learning experiences for students; as the obstacle clearers who provide the time, place, and materials for doing an effective job; and as the implementors who help to see that the appropriate results of such studies are actually put into practice.

Teachers

Teachers, because they are the persons representing the grass-roots level of the curriculum enterprise, are the ones who actually know what is feasible and what will or will not work. They mingle daily with the pupils, and they play a key role in curriculum planning. In smaller school systems each member of the health education and physical education staff should take part in curriculum planning. In larger school systems volunteers or representatives from the various schools might make up the study group.

The teacher's role in active curriculum development can involve contributing his or her experiences and knowledge and presenting data to support recommendations of desired changes. An effective way to utilize faculty groups is the committee system. Committees can be established for the study of such considerations as school philosophy, specific instructional areas, pertinent case studies, immediate and specific objectives for each grade level, needs of children, student readiness for various activities, experiences to satisfy the needs of children, means of implementing curriculum changes, and the program of evaluation.

Each teacher in the school should be regarded as a curriculum planner in regard to his or her

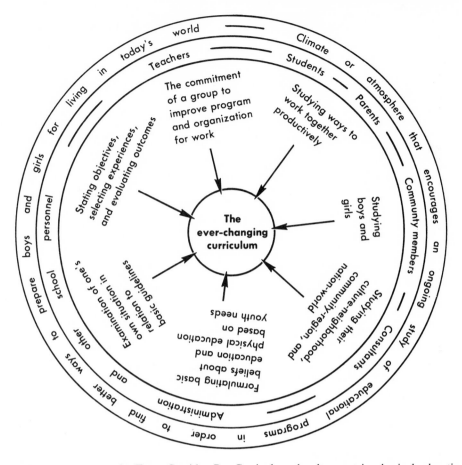

The curriculum merry-go-round. (From Cassidy, R.: Curriculum development in physical education, New York, 1954, Harper & Row, Publishers.)

own instructional offering and, in addition, as a contributor to the total departmental and all-school educational program.

State groups

Throughout most states are located many people and agencies that can help in health and physical education curriculum planning. These include the state department of public instruction or education, the state department of health, colleges and universities, and voluntary health agencies. These groups may provide curriculum guides, courses of study, advice, teaching aids, other materials, and help that will prove invaluable in curriculum planning.

Students

Students can play a part in curriculum development. As a result of an indication of their thinking in regard to such items as their interests, significant learning experiences, obstacles to desirable learning, and learning experiences recommended in the out-of-class program, guides may be provided that will help in curriculum development. The suggestions and ideas of students can be taken and evaluated by adults, in the light of their own thinking; it may be that the adults will find much merit and substance in the thinking of students.

Parents and community leaders

Discussions with parents and other interested citizens can sometimes help in curriculum development. Since the home plays such an important part in a child's learning and since parents are in essence one-half of the teaching team, there is an opportunity present, in group planning, to communicate to the public what the

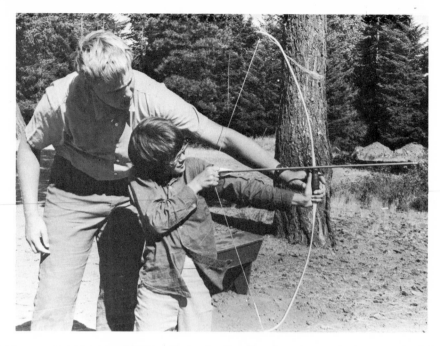

The curriculum must take into consideration the needs of each student. A camp junior counselor helps a special education (handicapped) student with a bow and arrow. Archery is one of many activities offered the special education students during a week-long summer camp near Ellensburg, Wash., as part of the Broadfront Program.

school is trying to achieve and how it can best be accomplished. Mothers and fathers and other community-minded people can also make significant contributions in evaluating students' behavior in terms of desired outcomes, as established and delineated by the schools.

Other individuals from specialized areas

Curriculum development should utilize the services of individuals who are interested and who can make a worthwhile contribution. For example, such persons as doctors, nurses, and recreation leaders should not be overlooked. It is desirable to look at the curriculum from all sides and all angles, to look at it from the student's as well as the teacher's point of view, and from the parent's as well as the administrator's point of view. Desirable results will flow from a continuous appraisal of the curriculum, made by many persons whose efforts, resources, qualifications, and interests are utilized in a meaningful manner.

STEPS IN CURRICULUM DEVELOPMENT

The major steps involved in curriculum planning include: (1) determining the objectives of education, (2) analyzing the objectives in terms of a total educational program, (3) analyzing the objectives in terms of subject matter areas, (4) providing instructional aids and important curriculum guides and other resource materials, and (5) assessing the effectiveness of the teacher-learning process. The following paragraphs discuss these steps in greater detail.

Determining the objectives of education

This step involves studying the various factors that contribute to and result in the formulation of objectives, such as the nature of society, the learning process, and the needs of children and youth. After consideration has been given to such important factors by a faculty or presentations have been made by curriculum specialists,

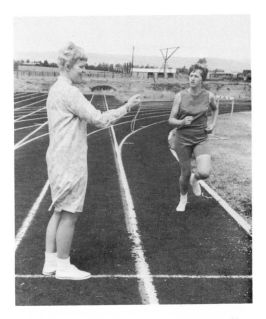

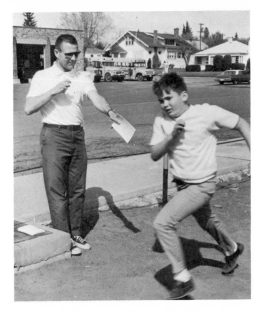

High school physical education instructor Sherry Ortman checks the stopwatch as a student finishes a jog around the track, as part of the Broadfront Program.

Broadfront Program physical education specialist Clyde Buehler times a sixth-grade student in a 50-yard dash, one of the physical fitness test items administered in the fall and spring.

educational objectives can be more clearly formulated.

Analyzing objectives in terms of a total educational program

Having determined the objectives of education as a whole and knowing the characteristics of children of different grade levels, those persons developing a curriculum can focus attention on outlining and analyzing broad categories of learning experiences and assigning relative emphases to the various phases of the educational process. The specialized fields of health and physical education should be viewed as part of the total educational program. Consequently, their specific objectives should relate to the overall educational objectives.

Analyzing objectives in terms of subject matter areas

The next step is to focus attention on subject matter and the activities of the teaching-learning process. Relating this to one phase of the physical education program, for example, it is obvious that the physiologic needs of children would

necessitate provision of ample opportunities for a wide range of physical movements involving the large muscles. Growth and development characteristics of children, physical capacities and abilities, and other considerations also would need to be studied.

Providing curriculum guides and instructional aids

Curriculum guides and instructional aids such as textbooks, visual aids, and other materials are an important consideration in curriculum development. An opportunity is presented here to utilize educationally sound materials that will assist the teacher in exploiting the educational environmental situation most effectively so that desirable learnings will take place and objectives will be accomplished.

Assessing the effectiveness of the teaching-learning process

This step represents the culmination of the curriculum development process—what actually takes place in the classroom, gymnasium, playfield, or swimming pool. The effectiveness with

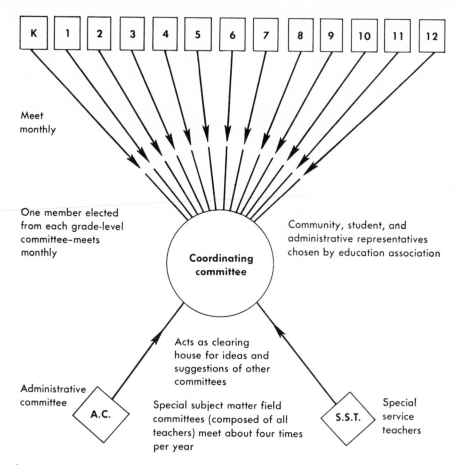

Grade-level committees. Purpose of program is to ascertain the needs of children and to devise means of meeting those needs. (From Oliver, A. I.: Curriculum improvement—a guide to problems, principles, and procedures, New York, 1965, Dodd, Mead & Co.)

which learning takes place, the aids and materials utilized, the excellence of methods used, and the desirable outcomes accomplished determine the success or the failure of curriculum development.

From the point of view of physical education the most effective factors in curriculum building in the process of cooperative program planning include:

1. A group of individuals committed to work cooperatively in the study and organization of curriculum-related materials
2. Formulation of a philosophy of physical education that is related to today's youth, their needs and goals
3. A thorough understanding of the objectives of education in general, and physical education in particular
4. Analysis of the students and the community in reference to their needs, attitudes, values, and objectives in terms of programs and facilities
5. Statement of objectives that are consistent with student needs and general principles of the formulating group
6. Selection of activity units that satisfy the statement of objectives
7. Development of instructional aids and resource material
8. Development of evaluation techniques and provisions for continuous program assessment

A CONCEPTUAL APPROACH TO PHYSICAL EDUCATION

The goal of education is to help boys and girls to become mature adults, possess ability to make wise decisions, and be capable of intelligent self-direction.

Physical education, as a part of education, should provide each boy and girl with carefully planned experiences that result in knowledge about the value of physical activity, essential motor skills, strength, stamina, and other essential physical characteristics and about the social qualities that make for effective citizenship.

Over the years physical educators in many of our schools have attempted to achieve these goals in a dedicated and conscientious manner. However, most physical educators will agree there is still much room for improvement. Those persons who advocate change cite educational systems where there is lack of progression, sequential treatment of subject matter, and an orderly developmental pattern for teaching motor skills. Furthermore, they say, physical education curriculums vary from school to school and state to state without any degree of uniformity. As a result of these conditions, they lament, students are not becoming as physically educated as they could be, and, also, physical education is not gaining the respectability in the educational process it justly deserves.

A development that has won the acclaim of educators is the concept approach to curriculum planning. This approach has possibilities for helping physical education to achieve a more important and respected place in the schools of this nation.

Each subject matter field has objectives toward which teaching is directed and that represent the worth of the field for the students. Physical education has advocated the objectives of physical development, cognitive development, and social development. These goals have proved valuable as targets toward which both the teacher and student strive. At the same time, they are rather general in nature and may not provide the best basis for the most effective structural organization of physical education.

The student should be aware of the general objectives of physical education but, in addition, as a result of school experiences, should be sensitive to and understand, and know the framework that constitutes the field of physical education. He or she should be aware of the unity, the wholeness, and the interrelatedness of the many activities in which he or she engages from kindergarten through college. He or she should even think at times as a physical educator might think, particularly from the standpoint of recognizing the importance and value of such course experiences to human beings. He or she should understand what constitutes the master plan of education and the structure of physical education as it fits into this master plan.

In creating this structure of physical education, one might draw an analogy between this field and the construction of a house. Just as there are key pillars and beams that give the house form and support, so the key unifying elements within physical education that give it a strong foundational framework and hold it together as a valuable educational experience for every boy and girl should be identified. These unifying threads would tie together the various parts of the discipline into a meaningful and cohesive learning package.

These unifying threads would be the *concepts* and, as such, would represent the basic structure of physical education in the school program. They would be the *key ideas, principles, skills, values,* or *attitudes* that represent points upon which we as physical educators should focus our efforts throughout the school life of the child. They would be part of both the teacher's and student's thinking and would range from very simple ideas to high-level abstractions. They would start with simple, elementary, fundamental experiences and in a sequential, progressive, and developmental pattern gain depth and comprehensiveness over the years as schooling progresses and the student matures. They would as unifying threads define the domain of physical education.

Concepts in physical education would not be memorized by the students. Rather, they would be ideas—analytic generalizations that would emerge and be understood by the student as a result of his school experiences in physical education. They would also provide him or her with a reservoir of information, skills, and understandings that would help him or her to meet new problems and situations.

The concepts, of course, would need to be carefully selected according to acceptable criteria and be scientifically sound. Furthermore, after the concepts had been identified, there would be need for extensive testing of their validity by many experts, including teachers in the field and specialists in curriculum development.

To implement the concepts within the physical education structure, there would be a need to delineate the identified concepts into meaningful units and topics that would be progressive in nature and reinforce the concepts that had been identified. The subdivisions of concepts in the structure would represent basic elements needed to develop a meaningful course of study and bring about desirable behavior. Furthermore, they would emanate and flow from the key concepts and would help to give greater meaning and understanding to them. As the conceptual, unifying threads were developed at each ascending grade and educational level, the student would be provided with new challenges, where the information, skills, and understanding acquired could be applied. The result would be that finally the student would reach a point where he or she could arrive at valid answers and make wise decisions in the area of physical education.

As a result of the concept approach, students would have a greater mastery of the field of physical education, increased understanding and power in dealing with problems related to their physical self that are new and unfamiliar, and motivation to want to become physically educated in the true sense of the term. The approach would provide a stable system of knowledge and provide guideposts for thinking intelligently about physical education.

The concept approach would have particular value to physical education because of such things as the great breadth of skills, knowledge, and values that make up this field of endeavor. It would provide a logical and systematic means for identifying among the many elements those that give form and structure to the type of phys-

ical education program professionals want taught in schools. The identified concepts would have permanence, and as the explosion of knowledge takes place in the years ahead through the efforts of scholarly researchers, this new information can become part of the structure, wherever applicable. Finally, the concept approach would be readily adaptable to individual differences that exist among students as well as sufficiently flexible to provide for the many geographic types of facilities and other factors that differentiate one community or school from another.

Some physical educators might say that the subject matter, skills, and other elements of physical education are the same under the concept approach as under the traditional approach. It may be that the facts will be the same in some cases but the approach will be different. For example, in the new mathematics, as developed by one professional group in grade nine, there is still concentration upon algebra, but the emphasis is not on the solving of algebraic equations but, instead, on the behavior of numbers—a verbalization of concepts.

Under the traditional approach, the organization of courses involved topics and activities, but without sufficient regard to the relationship of the topic and activity to what had gone on previously for the student and what lies ahead. This new method would still discuss topics and conduct activities, but topics and activities would be related to key concepts that the topic and activity are designed to elaborate upon, contribute more understanding, and make the area of learning more meaningful in the life of the student.

Physical education needs a curriculum study with careful consideration being given to the concept approach. At a time when the curriculum reform movement is very evident, physical education can no longer be apathetic about what it teaches and how it teaches. The concept approach is one that should be very carefully weighed for the *new physical education*.

CURRICULUM DEVELOPMENT IN PRACTICE

A noteworthy example of practical curriculum planning was the work of leaders in the

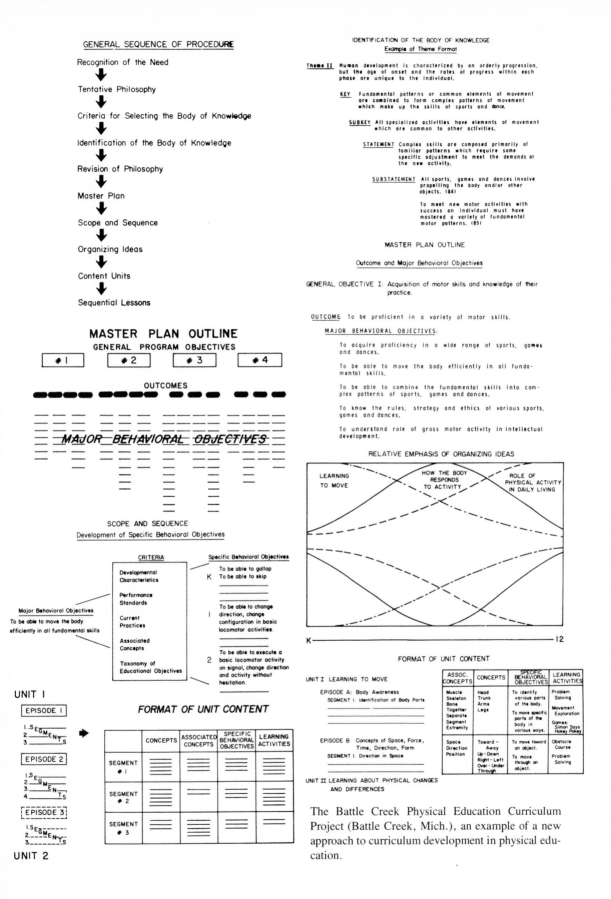

The Battle Creek Physical Education Curriculum Project (Battle Creek, Mich.), an example of a new approach to curriculum development in physical education.

Columbus, Ohio, public schools,* who developed a curriculum guide for a school health science course. The procedures for curriculum development were formulated by a committee consisting of a supervisor of health education, six health teachers, two advisory committee members, a school physician, and a director of public information. This committee consulted with curriculum authorities in health education and read literature on curriculum research. The plan involved the following eight-point process:

1. *Study of the existing program.* A review of course offerings, teaching guides, textbooks, and other curriculum materials was made.

2. *Collection and review of pertinent literature.* Thirty cities, counties, states, and professional health associations were canvassed and thirty health textbooks reviewed.

3. *Aims and objectives of guide determined.* The basic philosophy of health education as viewed by the committee was formulated.

4. *Needs and interests identified.* The needs and interests of the students who would represent the consumer of the teaching were studied.

5. *Judgments obtained from selected individuals.* The thinking of administrators, health teachers, nurses, counselors, parents, and health authorities was sought on problem areas of health education.

6. *Available resources screened.* Resources within the school system, within the community, and out-of-town resources were surveyed relating to selected health problem areas and what was available to help in solving problems.

7. *The organization of resource units.* After problem areas had been identified and resources screened, resource units were developed for teaching.

8. *Experimental use of guide.* The guide was used experimentally for 2 years in the Columbus schools. Evaluations were done and changes made where it was thought they were needed.

An example of one community of more than 50,000 people that made a curriculum study is White Plains, New York. The methods and materials utilized by this community have been described elsewhere* and may be of help to other communities or school districts.

The study was initiated by the director of health and physical education for the public schools after a discussion with several faculty members. The board of education allocated $750 for the study, and these funds enabled the staff to secure, as a consultant, a university professor who was well versed in the field of physical education.

The consultant and the director prepared the outline for the study group that consisted of the physical education staff. The board of education allowed the experience to be credited toward in-service education credit that was recognized on the salary increment scale. The workshop experience required that staff members meet one evening each week as a group. All administrative arrangements were handled by the director and leader. During the actual deliberations, however, the director remained in the background, allowing the staff to act on its own.

The physical education staff was divided into committees according to school level—elementary, junior high school, and senior high school. Each committee prepared its recommendations, worked with the study leader, and presented its findings to the staff as a whole. The entire faculty discussed and made suggestions to each committee. In the light of these deliberations each group then reworked its recommendations into final form.

The curriculum guide that was developed as a result of these deliberations contains the following:

1. A general statement of philosophy in regard to the curriculum guide
2. A statement of objectives for each educational level
3. A grouping of activities to meet objectives
4. The time requirement for each grade
5. The percentage of total time used for each grade activity at each grade level
6. A statement on evaluation—its purposes and its use as a basis for grading
7. A cumulative record card

---

*Cauffman, J. G.: How to develop a curriculum guide for a school health science course, Journal of Health, Physical Education, and Recreation **33**:19, 1962.

*Bucher, C. A., and Koenig, C.: Methods and materials for secondary school physical education, St. Louis, 1974, The C. V. Mosby Co.

The White Plains curriculum guide placed the physical education program in a more favorable light among the students, administrators, and teachers and in the community. Most important, it helped to ensure that the right experiences were provided each school child as part of his or her education.

EVALUATION OF THE CURRICULUM

Once a curriculum has been developed, evaluation is essential. The major purpose of such an evaluation is to determine the extent to which the experiences provided are reflected in desirable learnings on the part of the students. Unless the educational outcomes are desirable and acceptable to educators, the curriculum cannot be considered successful. Essential characteristics of an evaluation program include:

1. The relationship between curriculum planning and evaluation is essential and should be understood by all individuals involved in the program.
2. All curricular changes should be based on evaluation techniques.
3. All learning experiences should include evaluative programs for both students and teachers.
4. Evaluation should be primarily concerned with: (a) meeting student's needs, (b)

SUGGESTED OUTLINE OF A CURRICULUM EVALUATION CHECKLIST

The following evaluation checklist for physical education programs suggests methods of assessing curriculum development in this area.

	Yes	No
1. Does the physical education curriculum meet the established objectives?		
2. Does the physical education curriculum provide for the keeping of records to show student progress?		
3. Is evaluation used to help each student in the physical education program find out where he or she is in relation to the program objectives?		
4. Are objective as well as subjective measures used to determine the progress of students in attaining program objectives?		
5. Are the students protected by periodical medical examinations to see if they are subject to health deficiencies?		
6. Does the physical education curriculum provide for the administration of physical fitness tests to evaluate the degree of fitness of each student?		
7. Does the physical education program provide for the testing of skills and utilize specific ability tests?		
8. Does the physical education curriculum provide for cognitive testing of students to see how much knowledge was obtained?		
9. Does the physical education curriculum provide for the testing of the social adjustment of each student?		
10. Are the attitudes and interests of the students evaluated?		
11. If scientific methods of testing are not feasible, does the physical education curriculum provide for teacher-made tests?		
12. Does the physical education program utilize tests results in planning and assessing units of activity?		
13. Does the physical education curriculum provide for mobility of students based on evaluation results?		
14. Does the physical education curriculum provide for student evaluation as well as teacher evaluation?		
15. Does the physical education program provide for the recognition of curriculum problems and then try to bring about change?		
16. Once change in the curriculum is recognized, is it easy to bring about change?		
17. Is the physical education staff receptive to change?		
18. Is there a provision for ongoing evaluation of programs in reference to satisfying objectives according to an established schedule?		

meeting the objectives of the program, (c) considering the requirements of parents, teachers, and community members.

Curriculum evaluation to date has used four means of determining whether or not a new program has worth.* One method is through observations of students who have been exposed to the new program and the progress they have made. A second method is systematic questioning of teachers and students involved in the program. A third procedure involves testing of students periodically to determine their progress. A fourth method is the comparative testing of students under the "new" and under the "old" programs to determine progress under each.

PRINCIPLES TO CONSIDER IN CURRICULUM DEVELOPMENT

In summary, it can be pointed out that although curriculum development will vary from school to school and from community to community, some general principles are applicable to all situations:

1. Learning experiences should be selected and developed that will be most helpful in achieving educational outcomes.

2. Curriculum development is a continuous effort rather than one that is accomplished at periodic intervals.

3. The leadership in curriculum development rests primarily with the administration and supervisory staffs.

4. The administration should utilize (wherever possible and practicable) the services of teachers, laymen, students, state consultants, and other persons who can contribute to the development of the best curriculum possible. The work should not, however, place an unreasonable demand on any person's time and effort.

5. Curriculum development is dependent upon a thorough knowledge of the needs and characteristics, developmental levels, capacities, and maturity levels of the students, as well as an understanding of the environments in which those students live.

6. Curriculum development should permit teachers to exploit sound principles of learning in the selection and development of learning experiences.

7. Curriculum development should take into account out-of-school learning experiences and integrate them with school experiences.

8. The main value of curriculum development is determined by the degree of improved instruction that results.

EDUCATIONAL INNOVATIONS AFFECTING CURRICULUM DEVELOPMENT

There are many new developments that affect the curriculum, both from the standpoint of administrative innovations that affect school organization and scheduling and what is taught and from the standpoint of new teaching techniques that influence how the subject matter is taught and the degree to which learning takes place.

Developments affecting methods and techniques of teaching

New approaches to the presentation of subject matter and other educational experiences have gained widespread recognition. These innovations have implications for the teacher, by utilizing special talents and saving time, and for the student, by promoting learning and recognizing individual differences and abilities. A few of the innovations that have special implications for health education and physical education are briefly cited here since they are of concern to all teachers, administrators, and leaders in these special fields.

Creativity. Creativity is a process whereby the student or individual formulates and produces new ideas, patterns of thinking, products, or something entirely new. Since creativity is designed to help each person reach his or her fullest development, it should be encouraged on the part of students and teachers. The teacher is a very important factor in encouraging creativity among students. By being interested in seeking new and better ways of creativeness among his or her students, he or she recognizes its value and nurtures it constantly.

Environment also plays an important part in creativity. The school must be characterized by a congenial and friendly atmosphere. Freedom

---

*Goodlad, J. I.: School curriculum in the United States, New York, 1964, The Fund for the Advancement of Education, p. 59.

must be afforded the student since creativity does not occur during a particular period or time of day. Also, the physical environment should be conducive to creativity by being cheerful, colorful, and challenging.

Courses in health education and physical education should encourage boys and girls to explore, investigate, express themselves, and experiment. Each student should be recognized for his or her uniqueness. Movement education, gymnastics, dance, and many other activities in physical education, as well as such experiences as problem-solving in health education, offer opportunities for creativity. Independent study programs are an excellent method of encouraging creativity.

Teachers of health education and physical education should try to think up new and different approaches to subject matter presentation. By being creative in the teaching process itself, the instructor may stimulate new interests among the students in the subject matter being taught and the experiences being provided.

Movement education. Movement education is primarily concerned with the teaching of physical education through a sound understanding and application of the basic and scientific fundamentals of movement. Movement educa-

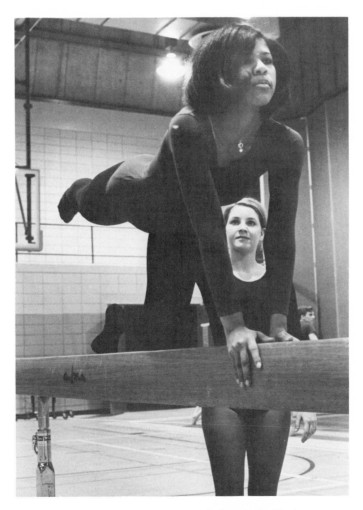

Physical education classes at Florissant Valley Community College in St. Louis encourage students to explore as this girl is doing on the balance beam. (Photograph by LeMoyne Coates.)

tion had its origin in England, where Rudolf Laban gave it considerable thought, emphasis, and impetus. It can be the basis for teaching all forms of physical activity.

Movement education is based upon the concept that movement involves time, space, force, and flow. All sports and activities in the physical education program require basic movements for accomplishment. The student attempts to determine what he or she can achieve through problem-solving situations. Students try to discover why they move in a particular way, how they move differently than other persons, where they may move, and with what and with whom they may move. They become aware of body movements and how they affect not only the activities in physical education but also daily living.

Movement education may be utilized in physical education in different ways. In some cases it represents a different and separate course, whereas in other situations it may represent the basic philosophy underlying the entire program.

Team teaching. Team teaching usually refers to an arrangement in which two or more teachers cooperatively work together in planning, instructing, and evaluating one or more class groups in order to utilize the special competencies and qualifications of the team members. In some team teaching projects, the team is

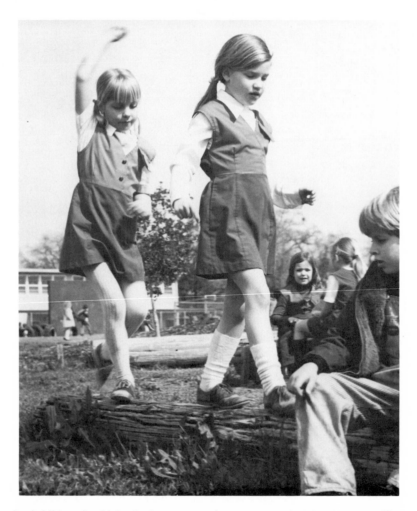

Elementary school children developing body awareness in movement education program. (Courtesy AAHPER and Charles Holbrook.)

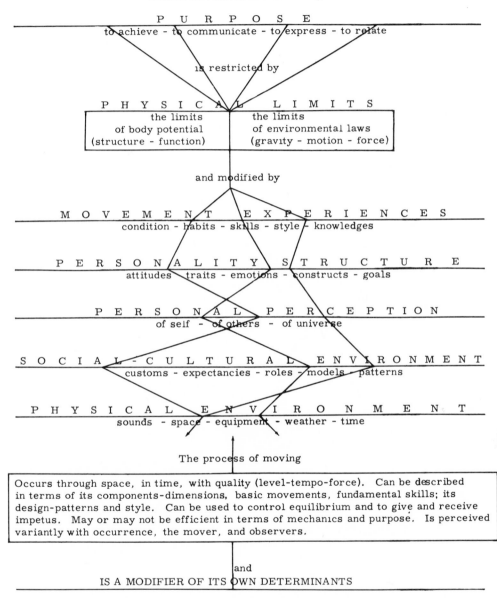

Human movement is initiated by

P U R P O S E

to achieve - to communicate - to express - to relate

is restricted by

P H Y S I C A L   L I M I T S

the limits of body potential (structure - function)	the limits of environmental laws (gravity - motion - force)

and modified by

M O V E M E N T   E X P E R I E N C E S

condition - habits - skills - style - knowledges

P E R S O N A L I T Y   S T R U C T U R E

attitudes - traits - emotions - constructs - goals

P E R S O N A L   P E R C E P T I O N

of self - of others - of universe

S O C I A L - C U L T U R A L   E N V I R O N M E N T

customs - expectancies - roles - models - patterns

P H Y S I C A L   E N V I R O N M E N T

sounds - space - equipment - weather - time

The process of moving

Occurs through space, in time, with quality (level-tempo-force). Can be described in terms of its components-dimensions, basic movements, fundamental skills; its design-patterns and style. Can be used to control equilibrium and to give and receive impetus. May or may not be efficient in terms of mechanics and purpose. Is perceived variantly with occurrence, the mover, and observers.

and

IS A MODIFIER OF ITS OWN DETERMINANTS

Movement education—an approach to the study of observable movement. (From Abernathy, R., and Waltz, M.: Toward a discipline: first steps first, Quest, monograph II, p. 3, April, 1964.)

made up of two or more experienced and inexperienced teachers, a student teacher, a master teacher, teacher aids, consultants, and secretary.

The purpose of team teaching is to involve the talents of many teachers and specialties. As a team they formulate the program of study and plan a schedule that consists of lecture sessions for large groups of students, small study group classes for practice, review, and discussion, and independent study time or individual projects to meet the individual needs and interests of students. A student might find himself following a schedule that consisted of 40% of his or her time in large group instruction, 40% in smaller group discussions, and 20% in individual study or research.

Differentiated staffing, previously discussed, has been a great aid to both teachers and students. By making it possible for teachers to instruct in the areas in which they are specialists, both teachers and students derive greater benefits from the learning process. In addition, when the teacher's additional responsibilities (clerical work, supervision, and care of supplies and equipment) are taken over by the staff members,

the teacher has more time to spend with individual students.

Educational television. Teaching with the aid of television has been introduced into health and physical education programs with considerable success. Areas of first aid and instruction in many health problems and various forms of physical activities have been successfully brought to large groups viewing televised lectures or demonstrations by specialists. Furthermore, such a technique has also permitted questions and answers on the part of students, with the entire audience benefiting from such an exchange.

One of the most impressive studies in educational television was performed by the Board of Education, Washington County, Hagerstown, Maryland, where this medium was used on a closed-circuit basis for 8 years. The results showed that pupil achievement was enhanced, the teacher's professional growth was accelerated, the curriculum was enriched and upgraded more readily, more pupils were reached, and the team teaching concept with the studio teacher and the classroom teacher was enhanced.

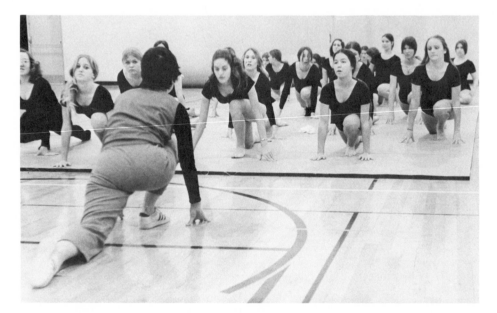

Differentiated staffing enables teachers to instruct in areas in which they are specialists. Here is a teacher instructing in her area of specialty at El Camino Real High School in Los Angeles. (Los Angeles Unified School District, Student Auxiliary Services Branch. Courtesy Gwen R. Waters.)

Programmed instruction. Programmed instruction was introduced by B. F. Skinner, a psychologist at Harvard. It is a process that arranges materials to be learned in a series of small steps designed to help the student educate himself or herself by progressing from what he or she actually knows to areas of learning that are new and more complex. The student is usually checked as he or she progresses to determine mastery of the material to be learned. If successful, the student proceeds to the next material, but if not correct, goes back and reviews the material missed. The learning program represents an orderly, sequential route to the mastery of the subject.

Programs are found in two major forms—the teaching machine and the programmed textbook. However, both forms operate on the basic principles outlined in the previous paragraph. Both techniques have proved of value in supplementing classwork and in meeting individual differences.

The fields of health education and physical education are fertile territory for programmed instruction. New materials are starting to appear on the market for programmed teaching. Much more will be available in the months and years ahead. Obvious advantages to such teaching are that students will be able to learn much more on their own outside of class, the student who is absent because of illness will have a medium for making up what has been missed, and large classes may be broken down, with some of the students doing programmed instruction.

RESEARCH IN HEALTH EDUCATION AND PHYSICAL EDUCATION

There is an urgent need to advance the frontiers of knowledge in the fields of health education and physical education. There have been too many unsupported claims for the value of physical education and health in education. There is a need to determine their worth through valid research findings—basic research that will advance knowledge and also applied research that will determine the best ways of applying this knowledge to these fields of endeavor.

There are many questions left unanswered. A few problems that need considerable investiga-

tion include the following: Why do school accidents happen? Why are health practices not followed? How much can retarded children learn? What is the value of programmed learning materials? What are the attitudes toward physical education? What should be the place of international studies in education? What are the biomechanics of human movement? What do we know about exercise physiology? What is the scientific basis for human movement? What is the relationship of personality development to motor performance? What is the relationship of scholastic achievement to physical fitness? What are the best ways to develop creativity? What social changes take place through outdoor education and camping? What is the therapeutic value of recreational activity? What are the qualities of leadership needed for working with mentally disturbed patients?

Research can help physical education and health to develop a better understanding of the accepted body of knowledge, skills, attitudes, and practices that should be imparted through educational means and how they can best be transmitted. In so doing the status of these professions will be enhanced.

Graduate schools in particular should sponsor and encourage research. They should extend a student's range of knowledge and understanding of his or her field of special interest, as well as provide opportunities to engage in creative research.

There is a need for effective channels for the communication of research findings to the practitioners in the field. The *Research Quarterly* of the American Alliance for Health, Physical Education, and Recreation is one good outlet but offers an opportunity for only comparatively few research studies. One estimate points out that the field of medicine has more than 400 journals published monthly, as well as some published weekly, such as the *Journal of the American Medical Association*.

There is a need for the professions of health, physical education, and recreation to more clearly delineate the answers to such questions as the following:

1. What areas need research in health, physical education, and recreation?
2. What questions does research raise about

present programs in health, physical education, and recreation?

3. How can research findings be disseminated and used most effectively in our professional programs?
4. What constitutes a desirable program of research for health, physical education, and recreation?
5. What are some of the problems concerning financing, misconceptions, and poor techniques in research in the professional fields of health and physical education?

STATE AND FEDERAL LEGISLATION—FINANCIAL AID TO EDUCATION PROGRAMS

State and federal legislation, philanthropic foundations, and other agencies are becoming increasingly interested in education and are providing financial help to schools and colleges.

Education and the pursuit of learning are becoming major points of emphasis in the American culture. At the turn of the century the population was approximately 76 million and only about 6% of the nation's 17 year olds graduated from high school, and only approximately 4% of the college-age persons went to college. Today, better than 70% of the 17 year olds are graduating from high school and about 30% of the college-age population is on campus. The bill for education is more than $50 billion a year and going up. There are approximately 125,000 schools, 100,000 administrators, and 2 million teachers in America's largest industry.

With the explosion in knowledge playing such a prominent role in American life, there are many concerns for the types of programs to be offered and individuals to be served. Consequently, dollars are being poured into facilities, personnel, programs, and other essentials.

The health educator and physical educator need to be conscious of these grants-in-aid monies that are being given to educational pursuits. Many of the sources of funds can be tapped for programs in the special fields of health education and physical education. Furthermore, it may be possible for specialists in these fields to influence legislation at the state or national level so that the bills passed include allocations for these special fields in the wording of the legislation.

Some of the specific ways in which the professions of health education and physical education may use this money might be to correct weak spots in the lack of facilities, sponsor research, hire additional personnel, offset low salaries, and purchase equipment.

A sampling of suggested projects, activities, and programs that might receive funds for research and grants-in-aid at the federal level in programs of health, physical education, recreation, and safety are as follows:

1. Employment of specialists to help in developing and implementing programs in adapted physical education
2. Inservice education programs for teachers
3. The development of curriculum guides
4. The purchase of special types of equipment, supplies, and facilities
5. The employment of specialists to work with underprivileged children who have special health problems
6. The employment of consultants who are specialists on various health and physical education problems
7. The development of health guides
8. The conduct of research for more effective teaching and better meeting the needs of children
9. The conduct of workshops
10. Immunization programs
11. The development of programs for physically underdeveloped children

Questions and exercises

1. Outline the steps you think should be followed in curriculum planning by a chairperson of a health and physical education department.
2. What is the relationship between curriculum planning and objectives?
3. What is the relationship between curriculum development and PPBS? Do you think that a school utilizing PPBS is better able to evaluate its curriculum? Explain.
4. Examine the health and/or physical education curriculum of three high schools. What are their strong and their weak points?
5. What are three references that the teacher can use for curriculum planning?
6. Do you think that students should be involved in curriculum development? Explain your answer. Write a brief survey that you might distribute to senior high school

students regarding physical and health education curriculums.

7. How can community resources be used effectively in curriculum planning?

8. Prepare what you consider to be an outstanding curriculum for health and/or physical education at the elementary, junior high school, or senior high school level. Analyze the steps you followed in constructing this curriculum.

Reading assignment in *Administrative Dimensions of Health and Physical Education Programs, Including Athletics:* Chapter 15, Selections 83 to 86.

Selected references

Association for Supervision and Curriculum Development: Assessing and using curriculum content, Washington, D. C., 1965, The Association.

Brameld, T.: A cross-cutting approach to the curriculum: the moving wheel, Phi Delta Kappan, March, 1970, p. 346.

Bucher, C. A.: Administrative dimensions of health and physical education programs, including athletics, St. Louis, 1971, The C. V. Mosby Co.

Bucher, C. A.: Dimensions of physical education, St. Louis, 1974, The C. V. Mosby Co.

Bucher, C. A.: Physical education for life, New York, 1969, McGraw-Hill Book Co., Inc.

Bucher, C. A., and Reade, E.: Physical education and health in the elementary school, New York, 1971, The Macmillan Co.

Bucher, C. A., and Koenig, C.: Methods and materials for secondary school physical education, ed. 4, St. Louis, 1975, The C. V. Mosby Co.

Crosby, M.: Who changes the curriculum and how? Phi Delta Kappan, March, 1970, p. 385.

Curriculum for people, Today's Education 60:42, 1971.

Daniels, A. S.: The potential of physical education as an area of research and scholarly effort, Journal of Health, Physical Education, and Recreation 36:32, 1965.

Eichhorn, D. H.: The middle school, New York, 1966, The Center for Applied Research in Education, Inc. (The Library of Education).

Goodlad, J. I.: School curriculum reform in the United States, New York, 1964, The Fund for the Advancement of Education.

Goodlad, J. I., and Anderson, R. H.: The nongraded elementary school, rev. ed., New York, 1963, Harcourt, Brace & World, Inc.

Grieve, A.: Try it; you'll like it: Journal of Health, Physical Education, and Recreation 43:34, 1972.

Kidd, F. M., and others: Guidelines for secondary school physical education, Journal of Health, Physical Education, and Recreation 42:47, 1971.

Koopman, G. R.: Curriculum development, New York, 1966, The Center for Applied Research in Education, Inc. (The Library of Education).

Lloyd, F. V.: Curricular responsibilities of today's school board, Administrator's Notebook, vol. 14, October, 1965.

Metcalf, L. E., and Hunt, M. P.: Relevance and the curriculum, Phi Delta Kappan, March, 1970, p. 358.

Meyers, K.: Administering the curriculum, The Clearing House 39:145, 1964.

Nixon, J. E., and Jewett, A. E.: Physical education curriculum, New York, 1964, The Ronald Press Co.

Oliver, A. I.: Curriculum improvement—a guide to problems, principles, and procedures, New York, 1965, Dodd, Mead & Co.

Report of the Second National Conference on Curriculum Projects: Assessing and using curriculum content, Washington, D. C., 1964, Association for Supervision and Curriculum Development.

School Health Education Study: Health education: a conceptual approach, New York, 1965, sponsored by the Samuel Bronfman Foundation of New York City.

Shane, J. G., and Shane, H. G.: Cultural change and the curriculum: 1970-2000 A.D., Educational Technology, April, 1970, p. 13.

Silberman, C. E.: Crisis in the classroom—the remaking of American education, New York, 1971, Random House, Inc.

Sliepcevich, E.: A conceptual approach to curriculum development in health education, Journal of Health, Physical Education, and Recreation 36:12, 1965.

The University of the State of New York, The State Education Department, Bureau of Secondary Development: Physical education in the secondary schools, Albany, 1964, State Department of Education.

The University of the State of New York, The State Education Department: Final report on the workshop on the concept of "redesign" for New York State physical educators, Stamford, New York, October 11-13, 1970, Albany, November 20, 1970.

Toffler, A.: Future shock, New York, 1970, Random House, Inc.

Van Til, W.: Curriculum: quest for relevance, New York, 1971, Houghton-Mifflin Co.

Willgoose, C. E.: The curriculum in physical education, Englewood Cliffs, N. J., 1969, Prentice-Hall, Inc.

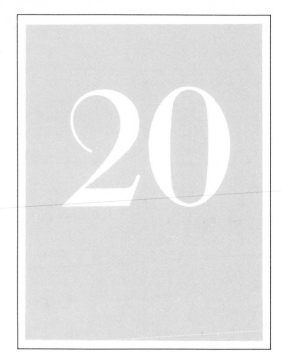

Professional and public relations

In this day and age when educational budget cutbacks are affecting physical education and health programs, a sound public relations program is needed to interpret to the public the worth of physical and health education. For example, it has been estimated that over half of all school bond issues were defeated in recent years.* Such bond issue defeats produce revenue losses that frequently result in cutbacks of physical and health education programs.

Sometimes when the terms *public* or *professional relations* are used, the reader, administrator, physical educator, or other person frequently associates the term with radio, television, and other communications media. However, one should not forget that the most effective avenues of public and professional relations include: (1) relations with students, (2) relations with parents of students, (3) personal contacts with the public at large, (4) the leadership role exerted by physical educators and health educators in their communities, (5) contacts established with various groups in the community, and (6) communications media such as correspondence, records, and telephone conversations.

*COMPASS (Competitive Athletics in Service to Society), 1973, Chicago, Illinois.

PUBLIC RELATIONS DEFINED

Public relations is a much-defined term. Some of the common definitions for this term as given by experts in this specialized field are as follows: Philip Lesly speaks of it as comprising the activities and attitudes that are used to influence, judge, and control the opinion of any individual, group, or groups of persons in the interest of some other individuals. Professor Harwood L. Childs defines it as a name for those activities and relations with others that are public and that have significance socially. J. Handly Wright and Byron H. Christian, experts in public relations, refer to it as a program that has the characteristics of careful planning and proper conduct, which in turn will result in public understanding and confidence. Edward L. Bernays, who has written widely on the subject of public relations, lists three items in his definition: first, information that is for public consumption, second, an attempt to modify the attitudes and actions of the public through persuasion, and third, the objective of attempting to integrate the attitudes and actions of the public and of the organization or people who are conducting the public relations program. Benjamin Fine, a specialist in educational public relations, defines public relations as the entire body of relationships that go to make up our impressions of an individual, an organization, or an idea.

These selected definitions of public relations

help to clarify its importance for any organization, institution, or group of individuals trying to develop an enterprise, profession, or business. Public relations takes into consideration such important factors as consumer's interests, human relationships, public understanding, and good will. In business, it attempts to show the important place that specialized enterprises have in society and how they exist and operate in the public interest. In education, it is concerned with public opinion, the needs of the school or college, and acquainting constituents with what is being done in the public interest. It also concerns itself with acquainting the public with the educational problems that must be considered in order to render a greater service.

Some of the purposes of school public relations include: (1) serving as a public information source concerning school activities, (2) aiding the promotion of confidence in the schools, (3) gathering support for school funding and programs, (4) stressing the value of education of all individuals, (5) improving communication between students, teachers, parents, and community members, (6) evaluating school programs, and (7) correcting misunderstandings and misinformation concerning the aims and objectives of the school.

Public relations means that the opinions of the populace must be taken into consideration. Public opinion is very powerful, and individuals, organizations, and institutions succeed or fail in terms of its influence. Therefore, in order to have good public relations, the interests of human beings and what is good for people in general must be considered.

The practice of public relations is pertinent to all areas of human activity: religion, education, business, politics, military, government, labor, and other affairs in which individuals engage. A good public relations program is not hit-and-miss. It is planned with considerable care, and great amounts of time and effort are necessary to produce results. Furthermore, it is not some-

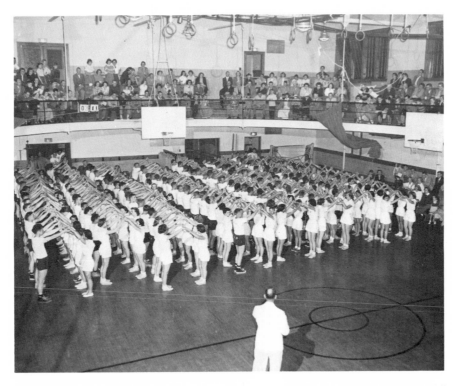

Wisconsin State College at LaCrosse utilizes a physical education demonstration to inform the public about its work.

thing in which only the "top brass," management, executives, or administrative officers should be interested. In order for any organization to have a good program, all members must be public relations–conscious.

The extent to which interest has grown in the field of public relations is indicated by the number of individuals specializing in this area. The *Public Relations Directory and Yearbook* lists personnel who specialize in this work. A recent edition of this publication listed more than 800 individuals who are doing work in this area on an independent basis, approximately 4,500 who were directors of public relations with business firms, approximately 1,900 who were associated with trade and professional groups, and nearly 700 who were with social organizations. In a recent Manhattan telephone directory there were over 500 names listed under the heading of "Public Relations." In contrast, in 1935, there were only ten names.

The importance of public relations is being in-creasingly recognized for the part it can play in educational, business, or social advancement. All need public support and understanding in order to survive. Public relations helps in obtaining these essentials.

PLANNING THE PUBLIC RELATIONS PROGRAM

Public relations programs are much more effective when they are planned by many interested and informed individuals and groups. Such individuals and groups as school boards, teachers, administrators, and citizens' committees can provide valuable assistance in certain areas of the public relations program. These people, serving in an advisory capacity to health and physical education departments, can help immeasurably in fulfilling the following specific steps that should be followed in planning a public relations program, which have been identified by McCloskey:

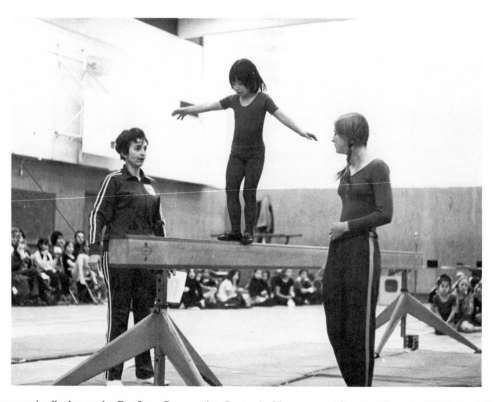

A gymnastic display at the Renfrew Community Center in Vancouver. (Courtesy Board of Parks and Public Recreation, Vancouver, B. C.)

1. Establish a sound public-communications policy.
2. Determine what educational services and developments benefit pupils.
3. Obtain facts about what citizens do and do not know and believe about educational values and needs.
4. Decide what facts and ideas will best enable citizens to understand the benefits children obtain from good schools and what improvements will increase these benefits.
5. Make full use of effective teacher-pupil planning techniques to generate understanding and appreciation.
6. Relate cost and tax facts more closely to opportunity for boys and girls to achieve.
7. Decide who is going to perform specific communication tasks at particular times.*

---

*McCloskey, G.: Planning the public relations program, National Education Association Journal **49**:17, 1960.

McCloskey further suggests that after putting the public relations plan into operation, it is important to test and evaluate its results and then improve the educational program accordingly.

PUBLIC RELATIONS MEDIA

There are many media that can be utilized in a public relations program. Some have more significance in certain localities than others. Some are more readily accessible than others. Health and physical education persons should survey their communities to determine media that can be utilized and will be most effective in their public relations program.

It should be pointed out, however, that the *program* and the *staff* represent the best media

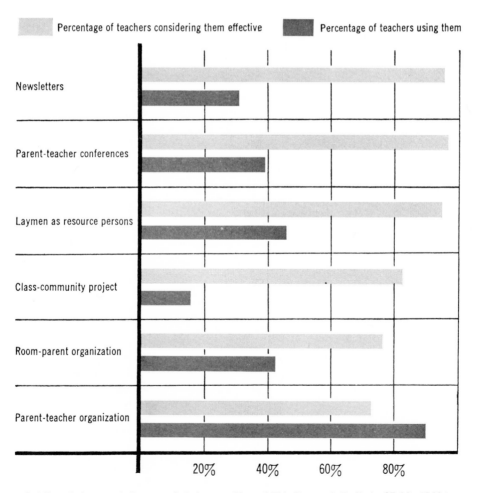

Public relations techniques and their use. (From NEA Research Bulletin **37**:39, 1959.)

for an effective public relations program. Through the activities and experiences provided and the leadership given, much good will may be built for any school, or college, department or profession. This should never be forgotten.

Another important consideration is that the most effective public relations is carried on through the person-to-person medium. This might be teacher to student, student to parent, or teacher to citizen. In all cases the child is a very important consideration, indeed the most important means of communication between the school and the home. What is accomplished in school or college, the effectiveness of a teacher's work, and the material learned become subjects of conversation around the dinner table and other places in the home. The attitudes developed in students often become those of the parents as well.

Newspapers

The newspaper is one of the most common and useful media for disseminating information. It reaches a large audience and can be very helpful in interpreting health and physical education to the public at large. Some questions that might be asked to determine what makes a good news story are: Is the news of interest to the public? Are the facts correct? Is it direct in style, written in the third person in a layman's vocabulary, and well organized? Does it include news on individuals who are closely related to the schools or colleges? Does the article have a plan of action, and does it play a significant part in interpreting the school or college program?

When a story is submitted to a newspaper, there are certain standard rules that apply in the preparation of copy:

1. Prepare all copy in typewritten form as neatly as possible, double spaced, and on one side of the paper only.

2. The name, address, and telephone number of your organization should be on page one, in the upper left-hand corner. Also at the top of page one, but below the address, should be the headline and release date for the story.

3. Paragraphs should be short, and if the story necessitates more than one page, write the word "More" at the end of each page. At the top of each additional page, list the name of the story in the upper left-hand corner. The symbols # # # should be placed at the end of the article to indicate the end.

One expert on newspapers has pointed out that the most common reasons for rejecting material include limited reader interest, poor writing, inaccuracies, and insufficient information.

Pictures and graphic materials

Pictures represent a very effective medium for public relations. Two words should be kept in mind by the persons who take and select the pictures for publication. These words are "action" and "people." Pictures that reflect "action" are much more interesting and appealing than "still" pictures. Furthermore, pictures that have people in them are much more effective than ones that do not possess this essential ingredient. It should also be recognized that usually a few people are better than many persons. Finally, such considerations as good background, accuracy in details, clearness, and educational significance should not be forgotten.

Educational problems, such as budgets, statistical information in regard to growth of school population, information about participation in various school or college activities, and many other items can be made more interesting, intelligible, and appealing if presented through colorful and artistic charts, graphs, and diagrams.

Magazines

There are thousands of popular magazines, professional journals, trade publications, and other periodicals published today.

Such national magazines as *Newsweek, U. S. News and World Report, McCalls,* and *Reader's Digest* are excellent for publicity purposes. It is, however, very difficult to get stories in such publications because of their rigid requirements and the fact that the editors like to cover the stories with their own staff. Many times it is better to suggest ideas to them rather than to submit a manuscript. There are other methods that may be used. One can attempt to interest the editors in some particular work being done and have them send a staff writer to cover the story. It might be possible to get a free-lance writer interested in the organization and have him or her develop a story. Someone on the department staff who possesses writing skill can be assigned to write a piece for magazine consumption and then submit it to various periodicals for consideration.

Public speaking

Public speaking can be a very effective medium for public relations. Through public addresses to civic and social groups in the community, public affairs, gatherings, professional meetings, and any organization or group that desires to know more about the work that is being performed, a good opportunity is afforded for interpreting one's profession to the public. However, it is very important to do a commendable job or the result can be disadvantageous rather than good public relations.

In order to make an effective speech, one should observe many fundamentals. A few that may be listed are mastery of the subject, sincere interest and enthusiasm, interest in putting thoughts across to the public rather than in putting the speaker across, directness, straightforwardness, preparation, brevity, and clear and distinct enunciation.

If the organization is of sufficient size, a speakers' bureau may be an asset. This may be utilized if there are several qualified speakers within an organization. Various civic, school, college, church, and other leaders within a community can be informed of the services that the organization has to offer along this line. Then, when the requests come in, speakers can be assigned on the basis of qualifications and availability. The entire department or organization should set up facilities and make information and material available for the preparation of such speeches. If desired by the members of the organization, inservice training courses could even be worked out in conjunction with the English department or some experienced person in developing this particular phase of the public relations program.

Discussion groups

Discussion groups, forums, and similar meetings are frequently held in various communities. At such gatherings, representatives from the community, which usually include educators, industrialists, businessmen, physicians, lawyers, clergymen, union leaders, and others, discuss topics of general interest. This is an excellent setting to clarify issues, clear up misunderstandings, enlighten civic leaders on particular fields of endeavor, and discuss the pros and cons of community projects. Health and physical education persons should play a larger role in such meetings than has been the case in the past. Much good could be done for these specialized fields through this medium.

Radio and television

Radio and television are powerful media of communication because of their universal appeal. These public relations media are well worth the money spent for the purpose, if this is the only way they are available. First, however, the possibilities of obtaining free time should be thoroughly examined. The idea of public service will influence some radio and television station managers to grant free time to an organization. This may be in the nature of an item included in a newscast program, a spot announcement, or a public service program that utilizes a quarter, half, or even a full hour.

There are some radio and television stations that are reserved for educational purposes. This possibility should be examined carefully. Many schools and colleges have stations of their own that may be utilized.

Sometimes one must take advantage of these media on short notice; therefore, it is important for an organization to be prepared with written plans that can be put into operation immediately. This might make the difference between being accepted or rejected for such an assignment. The organization must also be prepared to assume the work involved in rehearsals, preparation of scenery, or other items that are essential in presenting such a program.

Radio and television offer some of the best means of reaching a very large number of people at one time. As such, organizations concerned with specialized work of health and physical education should continually utilize their imaginations to translate the story of their professions into material that can be utilized effectively by these media.

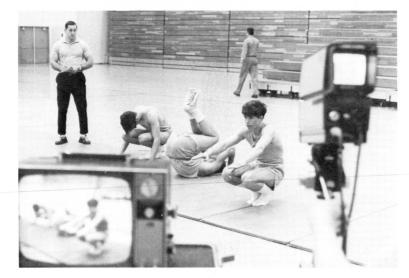

Omaha Public Schools utilize television in the physical education classes.

Films

Films can present dramatically and informatively such stories as an organization's services to the public and highlights in the training of its leaders. They constitute a most effective medium for presenting a story in a short period of time. A series of visual impressions will remain long in the minds of the audience.

Since such a great majority of the American people enjoy movies today, it is important to consider them in any public relations program. Movies are not only a form of entertainment but also an effective medium of information and education. Films stimulate attention, create interest, and provide a way of getting across information not inherent in printed matter.

Movies, slides, slidefilm, educational television, and other phases of these visual aids have been utilized by a number of departments of health and physical education to present their programs to the public and to interest individuals in their work. Voluntary associations, professional associations, and official agencies in these fields have also used them to advantage.

Posters, exhibits, brochures, demonstrations, miscellaneous media

Posters, exhibits, and brochures should be recognized as playing an important part in any public relations program concerned with health and physical education. Well-illustrated, brief, and attractive brochures can visually and informatively depict activities, facilities, projects, and services that a department or organization has as part of its total program.

Drawings, paintings, charts, graphs, pictures, and other aids, when placed upon posters and given proper distribution, will illustrate activities, show progress, and present information visually. These media will attract and interest public thinking.

Exhibits, when properly prepared, interestingly presented, and properly located, such as in a store window or some other prominent spot, can do much to demonstrate work being done by an organization.

Demonstrations that present the total program of an organization or profession in an entertaining and informative manner have a place in any public relations program. The main reasons for a physical education demonstration include: (1) informing the public and providing an outlet for interest in physical education programs by community members, (2) providing an opportunity for students to work together toward a common goal, and (3) demonstrating the need and benefit of physical education to all students. The objectives of physical education demonstrations should include the following: (1) providing opportunities for the general public to see the physical education program in action, (2) contributing to the overall educational objectives of the school, (3) including all students, (4) reflecting the needs of students in the present and in the future, and (5) contributing to the health, social, and emotional wellbeing of participants and spectators.

Other miscellaneous media, such as correspondence in the forms of letters and messages to parents, student publications, and reports, offer opportunities to develop good relations and favorable understanding in respect to schools and colleges and the work they are doing. Every opportunity must be utilized in order to build good public relations.

PPBS AND PUBLIC RELATIONS

School systems utilizing PPBS have found it easier to take their budget problems to the public and gain positive support. Where taxpayers are given a clear picture of the budget in terms of overall educational objectives, they can see the need for funding requirements and therefore will be more likely to support bond issues and other funding programs. PPBS budgets can be expressed in unsophisticated terms that the layman can easily understand. Areas of the school program that are suffering from funding inadequacies can more easily be appreciated in terms of PPBS.

THE PEPI PROJECT

The Physical Education Public Information (PEPI) Project is designed to educate the public regarding the vital contribution of physical education to children and youth. Through the project emphasis is given to the use of local media—press, radio, and television—as a means of gaining greater public understanding.

In its initial phase the project identified a local PEPI coordinator for each of the nation's 100 largest metropolitan (listening and viewing) areas. (There are now more than 600 PEPI coordinators.) The PEPI coordinator's responsibility is to organize and report PEPI activity in his or her area. This means such things as arranging with local radio and television stations for programming.

PEPI was developed by the Physical Educa-

tion Division of the American Alliance for Health, Physical Education, and Recreation and funded by AAHPER, a national affiliate of the National Education Association. The President's Council on Physical Fitness and Sports also provides both technical and material support for PEPI.

The basic concepts of the PEPI program include: (1) physical education is a form of health insurance, (2) physical education contributes to academic achievement, (3) physical education contributes to lifetime sports' skills, and (4) physical education helps in developing a positive self-concept and an ability to both compete and cooperate with others.

The PEPI Action Corps (PAC) was recently organized to aid PEPI coordinators with public information and media contact. PAC consultants were selected on the basis of their enthusiasm and outstanding achievements in behalf of physical education. Many of the consultants have their own television and radio programs and all act in an advisory position to further the objective of publicizing the benefits of physical education.

THE COMPASS PROGRAM

COMPASS (Competitive Athletics in Service to Society) is a recently organized program to recognize and give support to the role of competitive athletics in schools and in community recreation. The objectives of COMPASS are as follows:

1. To inform parents and taxpayers of the benefits of competitive athletics as deterrents to crime, drug abuse, and school dropouts
2. To reaffirm the traditional character-building traits that are a part of competitive athletics
3. To create greater public awareness of competitive athletics in an effort to gain support of such programs
4. To promote competitive athletics at the community level to help children develop physically, emotionally, mentally, and socially

The COMPASS program was formed by the Athletic Institute and the Sports Foundation, Inc. to direct attention to the positive aspects of competitive sports. COMPASS recognizes that school physical education programs, particularly extracurricular activities have suffered because of austerity budgets. These budgets are often the result of the defeat of bond issues for school funding. There is a widespread and very definite need for groups like COMPASS to publicize the funding problems inherent in physical education activities and to change public attitudes through public relations.

THE MANY PUBLICS

In order for any public relations program to be successful, accurate facts must be presented. To establish what facts are to be given to the public, the particular public at which the program is directed must be known. Contrary to general belief there is no *one* public. There are an infinite number of publics varying according to interests, problems, and other factors that make individuals different.

A public is a group of people who are drawn together by common interests, who are located in a specific geographic area, or who are characterized by some other common feature. There are over 230 million people in the United States composing hundreds of different publics—farmers, organized laborers, unorganized workers, students, professional people, and veterans. The various publics may be national, regional, and

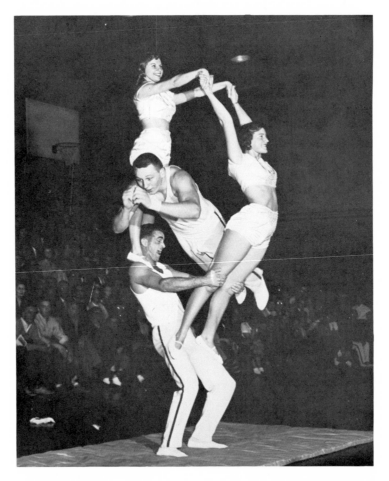

Demonstrations as part of a public relations program. Gamma Phi gym circus. (Illinois State University, Normal, Ill.)

local in scope. They can be classified according to race or nationality, age, religion, occupation, politics, sex, income, profession, economic level, or business, fraternal, and educational backgrounds. As one can readily see, there are many publics. Each organization or group that has a special interest is a public. The public relations–minded person must always think in terms of the publics with which he or she desires to promote understanding and how they can best be reached.

In order to have a meaningful and purposeful public relations program, it is essential to obtain some facts about these various publics. It is necessary to know their understanding of the professions, their needs and interests, their health practices and hobbies, and other essential information.

Public opinion decides whether a profession is important or not, whether it meets an essential need, whether it is making a contribution to enriched living. It determines the success or failure of a department, school, institution, or profession. Public opinion is dynamic and continually changing. Public opinion results from the inter-

action of people. Public opinion has great impact, and any group of individuals or organization that wants to survive should know as much about it as possible.

To get information on what the public thinks, why it thinks as it does, and how it reaches its conclusions, various techniques may be used. Surveys, questionnaires, opinion polls, interviews, expert opinion, discussions, and other techniques have proved valuable. Anyone interested in public relations should be acquainted with these various techniques.

Public opinion is formed to a great degree as a result of influences in early life, such as the effect of parents, home, and environment; on the basis of people's own experiences in everyday living, what they see, hear, and experience in other ways; and finally by media of communication such as newspapers, radio, and television. It is important not only to be aware of these facts but also to remember that one is dealing with many different publics, each requiring a special source of research and study in order to know the most effective way to plan, organize, and administer the public relations program.

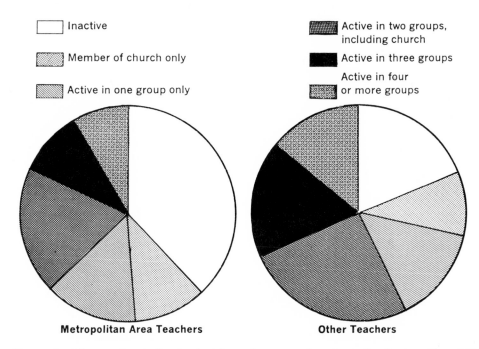

Metropolitan area teachers are less inclined to be joiners than are teachers in smaller districts. (From NEA Research Bulletin **40:**73, 1962.)

PUBLIC RELATIONS IN PRACTICE

A survey was conducted among eleven school systems to determine the nature and scope of their professional and public relations programs. Several questions were asked of health and physical education personnel through the personal interview technique. The information gained from these interviews is highlighted in the following paragraphs.

In respect to policies

1. The director of health and physical education was directly responsible for all public relations releases to the press.

2. All printed matter needed the approval of the director of health and physical education and the superintendent of schools before being released.

3. The coaches of interscholastic athletics were responsible for preparing all releases in regard to their programs.

4. Each staff member in the health and physical education program was urged to recognize that his or her activities were part of the professional and public relations programs of the school.

In respect to communication

In respect to communications media, the following were utilized:

Total physical education program
Newspaper
Posters
Films
Public speaking
School publications
Newsletter
Letters to parents
Demonstrations and exhibits
Personal contact
Pictures
Radio
Television
Window displays
Brochures
Sports days
Bulletin boards

The five media found to be most effective in their professional and public relations programs were (1) the total physical education program and the total health education program, (2) personal contact, (3) newspapers, (4) public speaking, and (5) demonstrations and exhibits.

All of the directors of health and physical education indicated that athletics received more publicity than any other phase of the physical education program. When asked why they thought this was so, some typical comments were: "The public demands it," "It is required because of public interest," and "The newspapers will only accept and print releases on athletics."

In respect to the message that was desired to be communicated to the public

When the directors were asked, "What message are you trying to convey to the public?" the following are typical answers that were given:

1. The value of the total physical education and health program

2. The importance of the program to the student

3. Recognition and achievement of all students in all areas of health and physical education, not just athletics

4. Efforts and energies being expended to give each child a worthwhile experience in health and physical education

5. The role of the health and physical education program in enhancing the health and welfare of the student

6. The aims and objectives of the total health and physical education programs

Guiding principles

In summary, the professional and public relations programs in the eleven school districts were conducted in light of the following principles:

1. Each physical education and health department recognized the importance of an active public relations program.

2. Definite policies guided the program.

3. Responsibility for public relations was shared by all members of the department, with the central authority residing with the director.

4. Many different communications media were used to interpret the program to the numerous publics.

5. The total health and physical education program was recognized as being the most effective medium of professional and public relations.

6. Efforts were made to interpret accurate facts about physical education and health to the public.

7. Considerable planning was needed for the effective utilization of public relations media.

Limitations of program of professional and public relations

Some obvious limitations of the professional and public relations programs surveyed were as follows:

1. Information had not been gained through research on how various publics thought and felt about health and physical education—what they did and did not know concerning these special fields.

2. There was a lack of budgetary allocations to carry on a professional and public relations program.

3. No specific plans had been established to evaluate the professional and public relations programs in the various schools.

4. Communications media overemphasized the role of athletics in the total physical education program.

5. Information had not been gained through research on what services most benefited pupils and what facts best enabled the public to understand the benefits children derive from such programs.

6. There was a lack of effective pupil-teacher planning techniques.

PRINCIPLES OF PUBLIC RELATIONS

A few of the principles that should be observed in developing a public relations program are listed:

1. Public relations should be considered internally before being developed externally. The support of everyone within the organization, from the top administrator down to the last worker, should be procured. Furthermore, such items as purpose of program, person or persons responsible, funds available, media to be utilized, and tools to carry on the program should be primary considerations.

2. A public relations program should be outlined and put in writing, and every member of the organization should become familiar with it.

The better it is known and understood, the better chance it has of succeeding.

3. The persons directly in charge of the public relations program must have complete knowledge of the professional services that are being rendered; the attitudes of those who are members of the profession and of the organization represented; and the nature, background, and reactions of the consumers and of all the "publics" that are directly or indirectly related to the job being performed.

4. After all the information has been gathered, a program should be developed that meets the needs as shown by the research that has been done.

5. There should be adequate funds available to do the job. Furthermore, the person or persons in charge of the public relations program should be given freedom in spending this money in whatever ways they feel will be most helpful and productive for the organization.

6. The formation of a public relations staff will be determined by the needs of the organization, the amount of money available, the attitude of the administration, and the size of the organization. If additional staff is available, special talents should be sought to provide effectively for a well-rounded program.

7. Individuals assigned public relations work should stay in the background instead of seeking the limelight, keep abreast of the factors that affect the program, develop a wide acquaintance, and make contacts that will be helpful.

8. In developing a public relations program, such items as the following should be checked: Is there a handbook or a newsletter to keep members of the organization informed? Is there a system for dispensing information to local radio and press outlets? Is there a booklet, flyer, or printed matter that tells the story of the organization? Do members of the organization participate regularly in community affairs? Is there provision for a speakers' bureau where civic clubs and other organizations may procure speakers on various topics? Does the organization hold open house for parents and interested persons? Does the organization have a film or other visual material that can be shown to interested groups and that explains and interprets the work?

9. A good public relations program will uti-

lize all available resources and machinery to disseminate information to the public in order to ensure adequate coverage.

PUBLIC RELATIONS AND EDUCATION

Education is recognized as essential in present-day society. In order that knowledge and experience may be transmitted from generation to generation, education is necessary. This is the essential that gives continuity to any culture.

A major obstacle to education today is in the area of public relations. Unless the public understands the work being performed by the schools, educators cannot expect support. Today a great segment of the American public does not understand and appreciate the work that is being performed in the schools and colleges.

The need for a broad public relations program is evidenced by many facts in American life. The American people spend more for tobacco each year than they do for education and twice as much for liquor. Schools and colleges are overflowing and there is a need for $10 to $20 billion for new buildings alone. Schools and colleges must absorb thousands of pupils a year, yet the necessary provisions have not been made. There is need for greater financial support, increased teachers' salaries, more buildings, and better teacher training. The necessary improvements cannot be obtained without public understanding and public support.

The National Education Association conducted a survey several years ago that included the factor of teachers' salaries. Of the persons surveyed, 33% felt that teachers' salaries were satisfactory, 2% thought they were high, and most of the remaining did not have sufficient information on which to base an opinion.

A Gallup poll showed that 87% of the American people are satisfied with the schools their children attend.

Elmo Roper conducted a poll that showed that 71.6% of the people in this country are either very satisfied or fairly well satisfied with the public school system. Less than one-half indicated that teachers were underpaid and yet the poll showed that teachers received the highest percentage when the public was asked to "rank the order of importance to the community of public school teachers, clergymen, public officials, merchants, and lawyers."

The public in general is not informed in respect to education. What is true of education in general is even more true of health and physical education, which are important phases of the educational program. This has important implications for a well-organized and long-term public relations program.

Bernays, in addressing the American Association of School Administrators, listed some pertinent remarks that he felt were essential to public understanding and action on the part of the American people.

He pointed out that three forces are responsible for social change: namely, public opinion, voluntary groups, and the law, which is dependent upon public opinion. In the light of this principle, voluntary groups are needed to aid in informing the public about education. These voluntary groups should consist of leading civic leaders, professional educators, and students. Lay and professional groups must coordinate their programs closely and gear their campaigns to everyone, from kindergarten to college, throughout the entire country. One of the most important considerations is that a unified front be presented to the public. All should agree on the issues and present them in the same light. If the various professional associations that are now organized and exist on national, district, state, and local levels and the various lay organizations could speak with one voice and with unison and similarity of purpose, much could be accomplished.

Bernays also recommended that a central board of strategy establish policy and goals and iron out problems so that a unified approach would be followed. Through such a board, research could be conducted to ascertain and reach a common agreement at the various levels on what the needs of education are. It could also determine the reasons for the apathy, indifference, and misunderstanding on the part of the public. It could wage a unified battle against enemies of public education.

Another step in the overall public relations program would be a clear-cut operational program. Such a program would provide for a continuous campaign, personnel, money, utilization of mass communications media, close cooperation between school, college, and parents and between the school, college, and community in general, and a more active role for teachers in community activities.

The American Association of School Administrators lists various principles that it considers essential to school public relations:

> School public relations must be honest in intent and execution.
> School public relations must be intrinsic (school program should be recognized as worthwhile in itself).
> School public relations must be continuous.
> School public relations must be positive in approach.
> School public relations should be comprehensive.
> School public relations should be sensitive to its publics.
> The ideas communicated must be simple.*

Through such a public relations program, all the people would have a better understanding of education in this country.

PUBLIC RELATIONS IN SCHOOL HEALTH AND PHYSICAL EDUCATION PROGRAMS

A definition of public relations heard some time ago stated: ''Public relations is getting the *right facts* to the *right people* at the *right time* and in the *right way*.''

Some of the facts that we need to get across to the public are these:

1. Physical education, health education, and recreation are closely allied but not the same. Each is separate and distinct; each needs its own specialists and deserves its own place in the educational program.

2. The professional fields of physical education, health education, and recreation are more than muscle and perspiration. Skills are not performed in a vacuum. Something happens to behavior, ethics, and cognitive development.

3. Athletics are an integral part of physical education, but physical education is not just athletics.

4. A well-rounded health program is an essential and integral part of modern education.

Some of the right people we must reach are the following:

1. Superintendents of public instruction,

school administrators, presidents and deans of colleges and universities, mayors, and others. They are the ones who make the decisions, determine the main points of emphasis, and decide how funds will be allocated. They can help us to grow into that dynamic force for good that we are capable of becoming.

2. Other members of the faculty. The teachers of English, mathematics, industrial arts, and other disciplines are very important in the educational system. We should not isolate ourselves from them. They can help us and we can help them. We are all in this business together, working toward common goals.

3. Consumers of our products and services. Let's reach those for whom we exist. And let's get to more than just the star player—let's contact the novice as well as the skilled, the girl as well as the boy, the oldster as well as the youngster.

The right time is now. Now is the time when:

1. There is a great interest in education, America's largest industry.

2. There is interest in the *whole* individual. The theory of dualism of mind and body has been exploded. We are interested in the physical as well as the cognitive, emotional, and social aspects of human beings.

3. Research is pointing up the importance of our fields of endeavor. This research shows the importance of exercise, the value of hobbies, the need for health instruction and recreation, and the contribution that sports can make in helping conquer physical and mental problems.

4. The President of the United States is interested in fitness. He places a high priority on our fields of endeavor.

5. The automation era is at hand, with its increased hours of leisure. Education also consists of knowing what to do when you have nothing to do.

6. The interest in such areas as obesity, drugs, ecology, sports, sex education, alcohol, and smoking is at an all-time high.

The right facts, the right people, and the right time will lose effectiveness unless we *act in the right way:*

1. Since close national-community relationships are important, keep the lines of communication constantly open from the national organi-

*American Association of School Administrators, op. cit., pp. 16-33.

zations down to the grass roots programs. There should be a constant flow of ideas that can be translated into action.

2. Develop the best possible programs of health and physical education. Have satisfied children and youth go out from your programs.

3. Utilize every opportunity available to sell someone else on the worth of your professional field of endeavor. If you yourself are sold, it will not be difficult to sell someone else.

4. Exploit every medium of communication to get your message across.

5. Think in positive terms—think *success*, and our chances of achieving it will be better assured.

Questions and exercises

1. Outline what you consider to be an effective public relations plan for a school program of health or physical education.
2. Prepare a news release on some event or phase of the department program. Follow through with it for publication or broadcast.
3. How can PPBS interpret budget requirements to the public? If your school utilizes this system, do some research to find out how the system is used in public relations. Write a brief report on your findings.
4. Discuss the PEPI and COMPASS programs. Does your area have an active PEPI or COMPASS program? If so, write a brief report on their activities.
5. What is meant by the fact that we are dealing in public relations with not just one but many "publics"?
6. Why is a knowledge of public relations important to teachers and administrators alike?
7. Discuss the potentialities of five public relations media in promoting physical education, health education, and recreation.
8. Prepare a speech that is to be given before a lay audience on the importance of physical education and health education to community welfare. Give the speech before class.
9. Prepare a bibliography of films that could be utilized effectively to interpret your profession to the public.
10. What qualifications would you need to become a full-time public relations person in your field?
11. List and discuss some principles that should be observed in public relations.
12. To what extent have the schools done a good public relations job?

Reading assignment in *Administrative Dimensions of Health and Physical Education Programs, Including Athletics:* Chapter 16, Selections 87 to 90.

Selected references

American Association for Health, Physical Education, and Recreation: PEPI-GRAMS, a series of communications on the Physical Education Public Information Project, 1972.

American Association for Health, Physical Education, and Recreation: Physical education—an interpretation, Washington, D. C., The Association.

Baughman, M. D.: The school's role in community life, School and Community **51**:9, 1969.

Bucher, C. A.: Back to school—what kind of education is relevant? (syndicated newspaper column), Washington, D. C., September, 1972, President's Council on Physical Fitness and Sports.

Bucher, C. A.: Play and your child's report card (syndicated newspaper column), Washington, D. C., May, 1972, President's Council on Physical Fitness and Sports.

Caldwell, S. F.: Toward a humanistic physical education, Journal of Health, Physical Education, and Recreation **43**:31, 1972.

Chester, E. B.: School district in trouble, American School Board Journal **150**:17, 1965.

Dapper, G.: Public relations for educators, New York, 1964, The Macmillan Co.

Douglas, H. R.: Trends and issues in secondary education, New York, 1962, The Center for Applied Research, Inc. (The Library of Education).

Geyer, C.: Physical education for the electronic age, Journal of Health, Physical Education, and Recreation **43**:32, 1972.

Healey, W.: Physical education demonstrations, Journal of Health, Physical Education, and Recreation **42**:43, 1971.

Humphrey, J. W.: Educators at your service, The Clearing House **38**:556, 1964.

Jones, J. J.: School public relations, New York, 1966, The Center for Applied Research, Inc. (The Library of Education).

Lepke, P.: PR for PE: Journal of Health, Physical Education, and Recreation **44**:10, 1973.

McCloskey, G.: Planning the public relations program, National Education Association Journal **59**:17, 1970.

PEPI-GRAM #9—A report of progress: Journal of Health, Physical Education, and Recreation **44**:10, 1973.

Scherer, D. J.: How to keep your district in the public eye, School Management **10**:22, 1966.

Torpey, J.: Interpreting physical education for the public, The Physical Educator **24**:131, 1967.

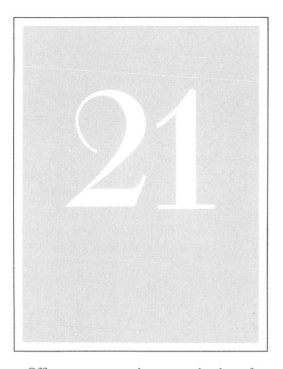

Office management

Office management is an area that has often been neglected by health and physical educators and administrators. Efficient office management often indicates a well-run department that has good student-teacher rapport. The office is the place for first impressions, communication between student and teacher, the focus of administrative duties, and a point of contact for administration and staff.

IMPORTANCE OF OFFICE MANAGEMENT

Colleagues, pupils, visitors, and other persons frequently have their initial contacts with departments of health and physical education in the central office. Their reception, the courtesies they are shown, the efficiency with which the office work is carried out, and other operational details leave a lasting impression upon their minds. Friends are often made or lost at this strategic point.

Center for communications

Office work, broadly conceived, is the handling and management of information. The office is usually the place where schedules are arranged and distributed, telephone calls made and received, reports typed and mimeographed, bulletins prepared and issued, conferences arranged and held, appointments made and confirmed, and greetings voiced and exchanged. The office represents the setting for a hub of activity around which revolves the efficient functioning of the work of health and physical education personnel. Unless these communications are carried out with dispatch, accurately and courteously, the entire administrative process breaks down.

Focus of administrative duties

The chief administrative personnel, secretarial assistants, and clerical help comprise the office staff. The filing system, key records, and reports are usually housed in the office. When inventories need to be examined, letters pulled from files, or the chairperson of the department consulted on important matters, the office is frequently the point of contact. Administrative responsibilities are carried out in the office, making this space a central point or focus for the entire organization.

Point of contact for administration and staff

Staff members visit the office regularly. Mailboxes are located there, and telephone calls may be taken in the office. Conferences and appointments with pupils and visitors often bring the teacher to the office. Constant communication takes place between administration and staff in this setting. High staff morale, efficiency, a friendly climate, and a feeling of working toward common goals can be imbued to a large degree through the atmosphere that exists in the office.

OFFICE SPACE

The central office for the health and/or physical education department, in accordance with its clearinghouse activities, should be located in a readily accessible position in the school or college plant. This office should be as near the entrance of the building as possible and at the same time have ready accessibility to health service offices, gymnasiums, locker rooms, athletic fields, and other facilities of the department.

Most central offices for health and physical education should consist of at least three divisions: general reception area, clerical space, and private office. Other desirable features to be considered are a bathroom, storage room, and conference room for staff and other meetings.

General reception area

The general reception office is that part of the office layout used by visitors as a waiting room or information center, for teachers and pupils who desire to get their mail, have appointments, or wish information, and for office services in general. It should be attractive, with some pictures on the wall, comfortable chairs, bulletin boards, and other items essential to carrying out the necessary administrative routines and creating a warm, friendly climate. A counter or railing should separate the general waiting room from the rest of the office facilities. This helps to ensure greater privacy and more efficient conduct of office responsibilities.

Clerical space

The clerical space should be separated from the general waiting and reception room. It should be equipped with such necessary materials as typewriters, files, tables, and telephones. It is often desirable to have a private alcove or office for one or more of the secretaries, depending upon the size of the depart-

ment and office. Privacy is often needed for the typing of letters, the preparation of reports, or the convenience of visitors and other personnel. There should be ample lighting, freedom of movement, and sufficient space for the various administrative duties to be carried out with a minimum of confusion and of difficulty.

Private offices

The chairperson of the department and possibly other personnel, depending upon the size of the department, should have private offices. The offices should be such that the persons in charge of administration can concentrate on their work without interruptions, have private conferences with students, faculty members, or visitors, and in general carry out their duties in the most efficient way possible. The offices should be decorated and equipped in an appropriate manner. There should be desks of sufficient working size that are neat in appearance, with calendars, schedule pads for appointments and conferences, and other essential materials. Filing cases, storage cabinets, and other equipment should be provided as needed. Faculty should also be provided with offices whenever possible.

OFFICE PERSONNEL

The number of office personnel will depend upon the size of the department. The staff could consist of secretaries, stenographers, transcribing machine operators, a receptionist, switchboard operator, and typists in a large department in a school or college. However, the usual office will probably consist of one secretary. In some small schools, student help may be all the personnel available.

The *secretary* should be a "good right arm" to the chairperson and to the department as a whole. To be most helpful, he or she will be a typist, a stenographer, and a public relations representative, will operate a dictaphone and mimeograph machine, and will see that the office runs smoothly. The secretary will help the chairperson and other staff members to remember facts, appointments, and other important information. He or she should know where materials are filed and be able to obtain them on a

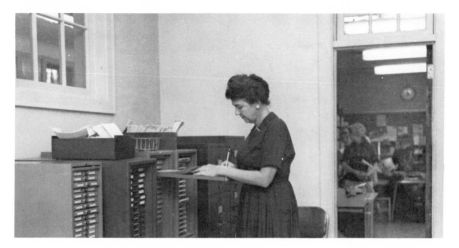

The secretary should be a "good right arm" to the administrator. (Office in senior high school, Mamaroneck, N. Y.)

moment's notice, relieve the supervisor of minor details, and see that reports are sent out on time and that accurate records are kept.

A *stenographer* is a typist who can also take shorthand. A stenographer, however, differs from a secretary. The stenographer usually takes dictation and types letters and other material but does not have the personal relationship and confidential duties that a secretary has. Large departments frequently have stenographic "pools" wherein individuals are on call to do work for any faculty member having work to be done.

A *transcribing operator* takes correspondence and other material that has been dictated and listens to a dictaphone or other playback mechanism upon which such information has been recorded. Using earphones, he or she sits at a typewriter and listens and types in accordance with the instructions that have been given.

A *receptionist's* position will vary with the department. In some departments a receptionist is a "greeter" who presents an attractive appearance and is polite, courteous, and helpful to callers. Some departments also assign to this person certain typing, filing, and telephone duties, in addition to the reception of callers.

Large departments frequently have *switchboard operators* who cover the phones for many faculty members and other personnel. Fre-quently staff members are not in, and messages are then relayed by the switchboard operator through the prescribed channels.

Office personnel should be selected very carefully. Experience, character, personality, appearance, and ability should play important roles in the selection process. The secretary should have, as a minimum of education, a high school diploma. The achievements of an individual who has been through the commercial course and who has a good background in typewriting, bookkeeping, English, and secretarial practice will be of value to the department.

The chairperson of the department and other faculty members should treat a secretary and other office personnel with respect and make them feel that they are very important parts of the work being accomplished. The staff should be patient and see that clerical help know the details of their jobs, recognize the importance of each, and appreciate the responsibilities that rest with their positions.

In smaller high schools, elementary schools, and colleges, the administrator may have to rely partially or entirely upon *students* to get some of the clerical work accomplished. Probably, senior students who have particular inclinations along this line will be most successful. Inservice education should take place for these students to see that acceptable precedures are followed in filing, typing, mimeographing, maintaining records, and performing other office duties.

EQUIPMENT AND SUPPLIES

Whether or not an office is efficient in its clerical and other responsibilities will depend upon the equipment and supplies available. It must be recognized that the materials needed will vary with the size of the school or college. In smaller schools and colleges such equipment as adding machines might readily be available in the central office but not in departmental offices. Following are some of the items that should be considered:

Adding machine	Paper cutter
Bookcases	Paste
Bulletin boards	Pencil sharpeners
Buzzers	Pencils and pens
Calendars	Reproducing machines
Chairs	Rulers
Clips	Safe
Cloak racks	Scissors
Clock	Scrapbooks
Desk baskets	Stamps
Desk lights	Stapling machine
Desk pads	Stationery and paper
Desks	Tables
Dictionaries	Telephone
Ditto machine	Typewriters
First-aid cabinet	Umbrella rack
Letter trays	Wardrobe cabinets
Magazine racks	Wastebaskets

In some large offices where many, many details are handled, data processing equipment should be available.

OFFICE WORK AND AUTOMATION

The rapid progress made in recent years begs the question as to whether or not new automated equipment should be installed in the office. The way this question is answered will depend upon such factors as the extent of the program the office serves, the amount of clerical work that needs to be done, and the size of the allocated budget.

Automation as used here refers to the processing of data by some mechanical device or system other than typewriters, adding machines, calculators, and photocopiers. Automation can be used in respect to handling such items as accounts payable, cumulative records, health records, inventories, personnel records, schedules, work requests, and transcripts.

Automation can be utilized by an organization either by installing its own machines or by working through some business organization that processes educational data for a fee. Also, the procedure of joining with several other school or college systems for such a service will work very well in some situations. Depending upon the size of the operation, it may be that a job can be done better, the hiring of additional personnel can be eliminated, and the cost will be less with automation.

REFERENCE MATERIALS

An area that high school and college offices should not overlook is the area of reference materials. The elementary, high school, and college offices will find it valuable to develop professional libraries that contain some of the outstanding professional books, periodicals, and standard references for their professional fields. In addition, there should be such references as books and periodicals; bulletins of the state department of education, state department of health, state and national professional organizations; facility references; and catalogues of athletic equipment and supplies.

Although there may be such material in the school library, it may be of value in many locations to have such references in the central office. In this way faculty members utilize them to a greater extent and thus keep up to date with their professional fields.

ADMINISTRATIVE ROUTINE

The administrative routine or manner in which the day-to-day business of the department is carried out by the office represents the basic reason why such a facility exists. Therefore, this matter should receive very careful consideration.

Hours

The office should be open during regular school hours. This usually means from 8 or 9 A.M. to 4 or 5 P.M. During this time there should always be someone present to answer the telephone, greet visitors, and answer students' questions. There may be some exceptions to these hours in a small school, but even in these cases there should be regular office hours that have been publicized as widely as possible.

Teachers should also have regular office hours at which they will be accessible to students, colleagues, and other persons who would like to see them. These office hours should be posted, office personnel informed, and the schedule carefully observed so that requests for information and assistance can be properly handled.

Assignments

All assignments, whether for office personnel or faculty, should be made very clear, be in writing, and be properly publicized. Office personnel may be required to ring electric bells to signal a change in periods, set clocks, take messages, mimeograph daily or weekly bulletins, distribute minor supplies, check the calendar of school events, provide messenger service to teachers and pupils, or assist in the health examination. These details should be clearly understood and carried out at the proper time. Specific responsibilities should be fixed and a schedule of duties prepared to prevent any misunderstanding.

Correspondence

Correspondence represents a most effective public relations medium. Letters can be written in a cold, impersonal manner or they can carry warmth and help to interpret what a program expects and is trying to do for a student or other person. Letters should be prepared carefully, using proper grammar and a neat manner that meets the highest standards of secretarial practice. If a health or physical education teacher has to do his or her own letters, these same standards should be met. Letters should convey the feeling that the department is anxious to help and to be of assistance wherever possible. Letters should be answered promptly, not placed in a drawer and left for weeks or months. Carbon copies of letters should be made and filed for future reference.

Files and filing

The office should contain steel filing cases for vertical filing. The filing system used will depend upon the number of personnel involved and the person doing the filing, but in any case it should be simple and practical. Files will usually consist of correspondence and informa-

tional material. For ease of finding material some form of alphabetical filing should usually be utilized, although numerical filing may at times be practical. The alphabetical files can be done on a name or subject basis, such as "Brown, Charles A.," or "Health Examinations," using a manila folder for all the material to be filed under the name or subject. Cross references should be included to facilitate finding material. Guide cards can be used to show which divisions of the file pertain to each letter of the alphabet, thus making the search for material much more rapid.

A visible filing system for any records and reports that are used currently and constantly will prove helpful. These are usually prepared on cards, and the visible filing case contains flat drawers that at a moment's notice will show the names or index numbers when pulled outward.

Office files should be kept very accurately. The person filing should be careful to see that the letter or other material gets into the proper folder and that folder into its correct location. Filing should also be kept up to date. A periodic review of the files should be made in order to weed out material that is no longer pertinent to the department. Files that for any reason are removed from the cabinet should be returned. If they are to be kept out for any length of time, an "out" sign should be substituted, showing where they are.

Telephone

The use of the office telephone is a major consideration for good departmental public relations. A few simple rules that should be observed are indicated below.

Promptness. The telephone should be answered as promptly as possible. It should not be allowed to ring for some length of time before the receiver is taken off the hook. Answering promptly reflects efficient office practice and consideration for the person calling.

Professional purposes. The telephone is installed in an office for professional purposes. Secretaries or other office personnel should not be permitted to talk for long periods of time about personal matters that have no relationship to departmental affairs. The telephone should be kept clear for business that is of importance to the achievement of professional objectives.

Courtesy, friendliness, and helpfulness. The person answering the phone should be pleasant in manner and courteous in approach and should desire to be of assistance to the caller. This should be the procedure not only when one is feeling his or her best but at all times. Such a telephone manner represents a professional responsibility that should be carried out with regularity.

Messages. At times faculty or staff members who are being called will not be available. A pencil and telephone pad should be kept at hand for recording calls in such cases, a definite procedure should be established for relaying these messages to the proper person.

Appointments

Appointments should not be made unless it is believed that they can be kept. Furthermore, all appointments should be kept as nearly at the time scheduled as possible. Many times the person making an appointment has arranged his or her day with the understanding that the conference will be at a certain time. If this time is not adhered to, it means the schedule has to be altered, and complications frequently arise as a result of such a procedure. The secretary should keep an accurate list of appointments. If no secretary is available, the staff member should keep his or her own schedule of appointments and check it regularly to see that it is met.

RECORDS AND REPORTS

At times, records and reports are not prepared and maintained accurately because the directions given by the chairperson of the department or the teachers are not clear and definite. When complicated reports are to be prepared, oral instructions, by themselves, will usually not be sufficient. Instead, directions should be written, typed, and distributed. The preparation of a sample will also help to ensure better results.

Administrators are often responsible for poorly kept records, inaccurate reports, and late submissions. There should be clear directions, announcements at regular intervals, reminders of when reports are due, and a prompt checking of reports to see if they are all in and whether there are omissions or other inaccuracies.

A survey was conducted of twenty-one school systems to determine the types of records that were kept in departmental files for health and physical education personnel. The result of this survey showed that some of the schools were very conscientious in regard to record keeping; others were not. In general, most of the department heads and teachers admitted they should put more time and effort into this phase of health and physical education administration.

In the school systems surveyed, the boys' departments usually kept more records and forms than the girls' departments. This can be explained partially by the fact that athletic programs for boys have many more records associated with them.

The survey showed that in some schools records were kept in the department of health and physical education, whereas in other schools these same records were kept in another department. For example, in some schools attendance records were kept by the health and physical education department, whereas in other schools an attendance officer had complete control. In some schools the health and physical education department kept records on health, while in other schools these records were kept by the school nurse. The same was true in regard to budgetary and inventory records. Some heads of health and physical education departments kept these records, while the business administrator and principals kept them in other schools.

Examples of reports and records that are maintained by the health and/or physical education departments include the following:

Health records and reports

    Health consultation request
    Medical examination record
    Health history
    Growth records
    Excuse forms
    Exercise card
    Height and weight card
    Body mechanics inspection form
    Films and visual aids list
    Health habits record form
    Accident records

B = Boys
G = Girls

School	Accident	Adapted program	Application for participation in interscholastic sports	Attendance	Cumulative class record	Equipment	Extracurricular activities	Game reports	Health	Interscholastic sports	Intramurals	Inventory	Medical form for interscholastic sports	Medical form for physical education	Parental permission sports	Physical fitness
School 1	B-G			B-G	B-G				B-G	B-G	B-G					B-G
School 2	B-G	B-G			B-G					B-G	B	B-G			B-G	B-G
School 3	B-G			B-G				B	B-G						B-G	B-G
School 4	B-G	B-G		B-G		B-G				B		B-G	B	B-G	B	B-G
School 5		B-G		B-G	B-G								B		B	B-G
School 6	B-G			B-G	B-G			B	B-G	B	B-G		B		B-G	B-G
School 7	B-G		B	B-G	B-G							B-G				B-G
School 8	B-G			B-G			B-G				G	G		B-G	B-G	B-G
School 9	B-G		B	B-G						B			B-G			
School 10	B-G	B-G		B-G	B-G				B-G		B-G				B-G	B-G
School 11	B-G			B-G						B	B-G	B-G			B	
School 12	B-G			B-G		B-G				B-G	B-G	B-G				B-G
School 13	B-G	B-G		B-G		B-G	B-G				B-G	B-G			B-G	
School 14	B-G	B-G		B-G						B-G	B-G					B-G
School 15	B-G		B	B-G					B-G					B	B-G	
School 16				B		B		B	B							
School 17					B							B-G			B	B-G
School 18				B-G					B-G					B-G	B-G	B-G
School 19			B-G	B-G												B-G
School 20	B-G			B-G	B-G	B-G	B-G		B-G	B-G	B-G		B		B-G	B-G
School 21	B-G												B		B-G	B-G

Physical education records used in twenty-one schools.

*Physical education activity, skill, and
squad records and reports*

  Basket card
  Physical education record
  Field event report card

*Physical education test and
achievement forms*

  Physical fitness record
  Report to parents
  Résumé of personality traits
  Citizenship guide sheet
  Athletic report

*Physical education attendance and
excuse records and reports*

  Squad card attendance record
  Appointment slip
  Absence report
  Change of program

Physical education equipment forms

  Padlock record
  Equipment record
  Equipment inventory and condition report
  Lost property report

CHECKLIST OF SOME IMPORTANT CONSIDERATIONS FOR OFFICE MANAGEMENT

Space and working conditions   Yes   No

 1. Does the reception room provide ample space for waiting guests? ____ ____
 2. Is the clerical space separated from the reception room so that office work is not interrupted by the arrival of guests? ____ ____
 3. Are there private offices for the Director of Health and Physical Education and as many of the staff as possible? ____ ____
 4. Is there an up-to-date health suite that provides an office and other essential facilities for the school nurse? ____ ____
 5. Is there adequate space and equipment for filing? ____ ____
 6. Are file drawers arranged so that papers can be inserted and removed easily and with space for future expansion? ____ ____
 7. Is the office arranged so that as many workers as possible get the best natural light with glare from sunlight or reflected sunlight avoided? ____ ____
 8. Has the office space been painted in accordance with the best in color dynamics? ____ ____
 9. Have provisions been made so that unnecessary noise is eliminated, distractions are kept to a minimum, and cleanliness prevails? ____ ____
10. Is there good ventilation, appropriate artificial lighting, and satisfactory heating conditions? ____ ____

Personnel

11. Is a receptionist available to greet guests and answer queries? ____ ____
12. Is there a recorded analysis of the duties of each secretarial position? ____ ____
13. Are channels available for ascertaining causes of dissatisfaction among secretarial help? ____ ____
14. Do secretaries dress neatly and conservatively? ____ ____
15. Do secretaries maintain a desk that has an orderly appearance and clear their desks of working papers each day? ____ ____
16. Do secretaries concern themselves with the efficiency of the office? ____ ____
17. Are secretaries loyal to the department and staff members? ____ ____
18. Do staff members have regular office hours? ____ ____
19. Are appointments kept promptly? ____ ____

Procedures

20. Is up-to-date reading material furnished for waiting guests? ____ ____
21. Does the office help continually pay attention to maintaining offices that are neat, with papers, books, and other materials arranged in an orderly manner? ____ ____

CHECKLIST OF SOME IMPORTANT CONSIDERATIONS FOR OFFICE MANAGEMENT—cont'd

Procedures—cont'd	Yes	No
22. Are the secretaries knowledgeable about departmental activities so that they can answer intelligently queries about staff members and activities?		
23. Do secretaries wait upon guests promptly and courteously?		
24. Are letters typed neatly, well placed on the sheet, properly spaced, free from erasures, smudge, and typographic errors?		
25. Is correspondence handled promptly?		
26. Is the filing system easily learned and is the filing done promptly so that the work does not pile up?		
27. Is the office routine efficient of human time and energy with the elimination of duplicate operations or forms?		
28. Are the most effective and efficient office methods utilized?		
29. Is the clerical output satisfactory, with work starting promptly in the morning and after lunch, breaks taken according to schedule, and work stoppage taking place as scheduled?		
30. Has a streamlined procedure been developed so that telephones are answered promptly, guests are courteously treated, and personal argument and gossiping eliminated?		
31. Are are essential records properly maintained and kept up to date?		
32. Have procedures for typing and duplicating course outlines, committee reports, examinations, bulletins, fliers, letters, announcements, etc., been developed to eliminate uncertainty or confusion on the part of staff members?		
33. Are regular office hours for staff posted and known so that office staff can make appointments as needed?		
34. Are secretaries acquainted with such details as securing films and other visual aids, obtaining reference material, helping in registration, duplicating material, and obtaining additional forms and records?		
35. Is the office covered continuously during working hours?		

Questions and exercises

1. Why is good office management essential for good public relations? What are some important reasons why office management is important to a department of physical and/or health education?
2. What three main divisions should office space include? Discuss the physical layout of each of these three divisions.
3. What office personnel should be available in a small high school, in a large high school, and in a college or university?
4. List the equipment and supplies that should be readily available in the average physical education office.
5. What importance can be attributed to a professional list of references in an office? Prepare a list of outstanding references for both the fields of health and physical education.
6. Prepare rules for effective administrative routine in respect to (a) hours, (b) assignments, (c) records and reports, (d) correspondence, (e) files and filing, (f) telephone, and (g) appointments.

Reading assignment in *Administrative Dimensions of Health and Physical Education Programs, Including Athletics:* Selections 16 and 71.

Selected references

American Association of School Administrators: Profiles of the administrative team, Washington, D. C., 1971, The Association.

Castetter, W. B.: The personnel function in educational administration, New York, 1971, The Macmillan Co.

Courtesy in correspondence, The Royal Bank of Canada Monthly Letter **46:**1, 1965.

Duryea, E. D. and others: Faculty unions and collective bargaining, San Francisco, 1973, Jossey-Bass Publishers.

Fawcett, W.: Policy and practice in school administration, New York, 1964, The Macmillan Co.

Ford, K.: The development of our office copying processes, The Office, June, 1973, p. 18

Pittman, J.: Office may become a leader of management, The Office **67:**110, 1968.

Shiff, R. A.: Satellite administrative service centers, Administrative Management **30:**26, 1969.

Siegel, G. B.: Management development and the instability of skills: a strategy, Public Personnel Review **30:**15, 1969.

Van Zwoll, J. A.: School personnel administration, New York, 1964, Appleton-Century-Crofts.

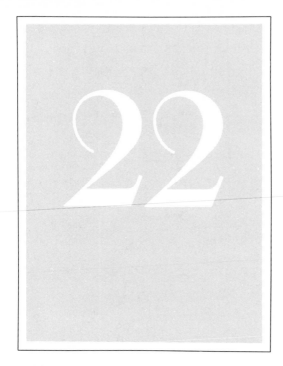

Measurement
of pupil
achievement*

Measurement techniques and evaluation procedures have seen many changes in recent years. The progress of students in such areas as physical fitness, social development, cognitive achievement, and skill improvement are some of the areas where change has taken place. Grading based on performance objectives, individualized learning, and contract grading will be discussed in detail later in this chapter.

The term *measurement* is used here to refer to the use of techniques to determine the degree to which a trait, ability, or characteristic exists in an individual.

During the last 35 years many measurement techniques have been developed in the fields of health and physical education. Some of these have been carefully constructed in a scientific manner, but many fall below acceptable standards. The administration should focus its attention on the materials that give valid and reliable results. Furthermore, all interested persons should be encouraged to construct new techniques in areas where shortages exist.

There are measurement techniques other than tests. Some of these are rating scales, checklists, photographic devices, controlled observation, and various measuring instruments.

The Joint Committee on Health Problems in

Education of the National Education Association and the American Medical Association†
states that the most common instruments or procedures used by health teachers are (1) observations, (2) surveys, (3) questionnaires and checklists, (4) interviews, (5) diaries and other autobiographic records kept by students, (6) health and growth records, (7) other records of health conditions or improvements, (8) samples of students' work, (9) case studies, and (10) health knowledge tests.

PURPOSES OF MEASUREMENT

Many purposes exist to support the utilization of measurement techniques in the administration of school health and physical education programs. A few of these will be discussed.

Measurement helps to determine the progress being made and the degree to which objectives are being met. It aids in discovering the needs of the participants. It identifies strengths and weaknesses of students and teachers, aids in curriculum planning, and shows where emphasis should be placed. It also gives direction and

---

*See also Chapter 11, Administering Physical Fitness Programs, for information on physical fitness tests.
†Joint Committee on Health Problems in Education of National Education Association and American Medical Association: Health education, Washington, D. C., 1961, National Education Association, p. 343.

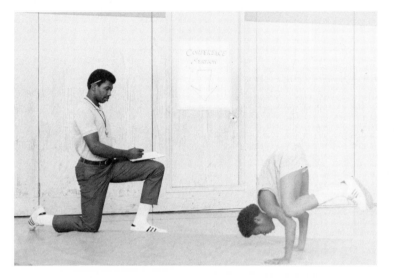

Grading based on performance objectives in Omaha Public Schools.

Table 22-1. Extent of use of pupil evaluation techniques*

Techniques used†	Percent of 38 city school systems	Percent of 44 county school systems
Tests	100.0	100.0
Cumulative records	92.0	77.0
Interviews	89.5	71.0
Case studies	84.2	57.0
Case conferences	81.6	55.0
Group discussion	68.4	68.0
Anecdotal records	63.2	32.0
Observation	60.5	73.0
File of sample materials	57.9	48.0
Questionnaires	53.3	30.0
Rating scales	44.7	11.0
Checklists	36.8	21.0
Inventories	31.6	18.0
Logs or diaries	13.2	16.0
Sociograms	10.5	2.0

*From Bonney, M. E., and Hampleman, R. S.: Personal-social evaluation techniques, New York, 1962, The Center for Applied Research in Education, Inc. (The Library of Education), pp. 4-5.
†Other techniques mentioned only once by either city, county, or both are the following: followup studies, autobiographies, clinics, case work, stenographic reports, films, recordings, psychiatric consultation, parental interviews, graphs of pupils' progress, interaction content records, and photographs.

helps to supply information for guidance purposes.

Measurement helps in determining where emphasis should be placed in teaching and the procedures that are effective and ineffective. It also has use in aiding pupils to determine their own progress in respect to health and physical education practices, as a basis for giving grades, and as a means of interpreting programs to administrators and the public in general.

The information provided by measurement techniques can also be utilized in other ways. In the area of measurement, findings can be used for such purposes as grouping individuals according to similar mental, physical, and other traits that will ensure better instruction. Measurement yields information that can be used as an indication of a person's achievement in various skills and activities. It provides information that can be used to predict future performance and development. It affords data on attitudes that determine whether or not the participant has proper motivation, and it focuses attention on future action that should be taken in the program.

THE COMPUTER
AND MEASUREMENT

The computer has many implications for the management of data concerned with pupil achievement in health and physical education programs. It enables the teacher and the administration to reduce the amount of time devoted to the analysis of data. The computer permits the analysis of test scores for thousands of students with comparative ease. It enables the physical educator to identify differentiating characteristics of students, such as scores that are high or low. The computer enables a battery of test items on such characteristics as speed, strength, or power to be analyzed item by item. It is an aid in scheduling in light of the results of measurement, for example, for purposes of grouping students with similar deficiencies into the same class. The computer makes it possible to prepare a profile of each student on the various health and physical education tests that are administered. Test scores of one class of students can be compared with other classes within the same school or with other schools where national norms are available.

These represent only a few examples of how the computer can be of value in the administration of a pupil measurement program. The uses of this device for the imaginative and creative administrator and teacher are limitless. The nation and world are rapidly being run on an electronic basis. Physical education and health education, if they desire to make their measurement programs most effective and meaningful, should examine the possibilities of the computer for their programs.

CRITERIA FOR TEST
CONSTRUCTION AND SELECTION

Criteria refer to those particular standards that may be used to evaluate measurement and evaluation materials in the field of education. Such criteria as validity, reliability, objectivity, norms, and administrative economy provide the scientific basis for the selection and construction of tests. Administrators should be particularly concerned that the tests they utilize meet these criteria. If they do, properly interpreted results should aid considerably in developing adequate school health and physical education programs.

Definitions and questions relating to the criteria mentioned previously are given in the following paragraphs.

Validity. Validity may be defined as how well a test measures what it claims to measure. In order to determine validity, an instructor should ask some of the following questions:

1. Does the test cover the content area for which it was designed?
2. Is it applicable to the grade level for which it was designed?
3. Is the criterion with which the material was correlated acceptable, and is the correlation coefficient also acceptable?
4. Does the test give insight into course objectives?
5. Is the sampling sufficiently representative and random?
6. Does evidence support whether the test is a classification, achievement, diagnostic, or prognostic technique?
7. Has the technique been tested in the appropriate area?

Reliability. Reliability may be defined as the consistency of measurement on the same individual or group, under the same conditions, and by the same person. Some questions relating to reliability include:

1. What are conditions under which reliability has been determined?
2. Is the size of the coefficient correlation acceptable?
3. What are the means of the two tests?
4. What is the method used for determining reliability? Is it valid?
5. Is the sample sufficient, random, and representative?
6. Has reliability been determined by using a similar group to the group for which the technique has been designed?

Objectivity. This is the degree to which the technique can be given to the same individual or group and obtain the same results. Questions that may be asked include:

1. Are the instructions simple and complete?
2. Is objectivity determination valid?
3. Is the sample sufficient, representative, and random?
4. Are the means indicated? Is there a difference in mean scores?
5. Are the procedures easily understood by examiner and subject?
6. Are alternate test forms available if needed?

Norms. The level of group performance or a statistical average may be defined as a norm for a group. Some questions concerning norms include:

1. What basis is used for norm construction—chronologic age, grade level, skill achievement?
2. Is the sample sufficient, random, and representative?
3. Are the norms based on local or national statistics?
4. Are the norms tentative, arbitrary, or experimental?
5. Are all important extraneous factors eliminated?
6. Are the statistics sufficiently refined?
7. Is the appropriate statistical tool utilized?

Administrative economy. The procedures involved with conducting the program may be defined as administrative economy. Questions concerning this area of testing criteria include:

1. What is the time allotment for technique administration?

2. What are the costs involved in administrating the technique?
3. Is the technique easy to administer, and does it require much training on the part of the examiner?
4. Are the objectives of the technique and the program compatible?
5. How many examiners are necessary, and is the technique within the scope of the health and/or physical education training?

TECHNIQUES AND INSTRUMENTS FOR OBTAINING DESIRED INFORMATION ABOUT STUDENTS

There are many techniques and instruments that can be utilized to obtain the various types of classification, achievement, diagnostic, and prognostic information about students. A few examples are listed for each category.

Classification information

An example of an instrument that would yield classification information is McCloy's Classification Index I.* This classification index takes into consideration such items as age, height, weight, and athletic skill, with a simple formula developed for the calculation of the index.

Another example of an instrument that could prove helpful for classification purposes is the Wetzel Grid.† This is valuable in either school health or physical education programs since it takes into consideration such elements as physique, developmental level, and nutritional progress with respect to weight, age, and height.

Achievement information

An example of an instrument that reflects achievement information would be the Indiana Physical Fitness Text.‡ This instrument involves such test items as straddle chins, squat-thrusts, push-ups, and vertical jumps. Norms have been developed for boys and girls.

---

*McCloy, C. H., and Young, N. D.: Tests and measurements in health and physical education, ed. 3, New York, 1954, Appleton-Century-Crofts, pp. 59-60.
†Wetzel, N. C.: Grid for evaluating physical fitness, Cleveland, 1948, National Education Association Service, Inc.
‡State of Indiana Department of Public Instruction: High school physical education course of study, Bulletin 222, Indianapolis, 1958, The Department.

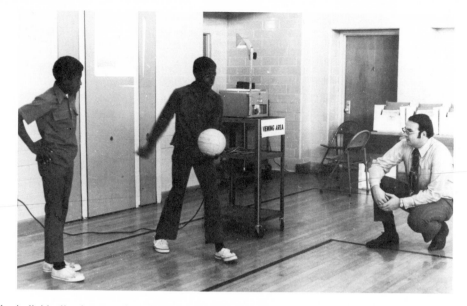

With the individualized approach to learning in Omaha Public Schools, each student meets with teacher for evaluation of prescribed task. (Courtesy Omaha Public Schools.)

FRAMEWORK FOR MEASUREMENT PROCEDURES

To give the reader a clearer knowledge of some of the types of information that can be measured concerning some of the objectives of health and physical education, a partial framework is listed on the following pages. It is presented for the purpose of giving an indication of the vast scope of measurement and how it can influence these specialized programs. Objectives and terms used in the framework are defined for purposes of clarification.

Objectives

1. *Organic development objectives* refer to the activity phase of the program that builds physical power in an individual through the development of the various organic systems of the body.
2. *Skill development objective* deals with the phase of the program that develops coordination, rhythm, and poise, through which some particular act may be performed with proficiency.
3. *Cognitive development objective* deals with the phase of the program that develops a comprehensive knowledge of principles, historical background, rules, techniques, values, and strategies.
4. *Human relations development objective* refers to the phase of the program that aids an individual in making personal and group adjustments and in developing desirable standards of conduct essential to good citizenship.

Definitions

1. *Classification information* refers to those elements that can be used as a basis for segregating individuals into homogeneous groups for which they are reasonably well suited mentally, physically, emotionally, and socially.
2. *Achievement information* refers to those elements that can be measured to determine the scope and magnitude of an individual's achievement in organic development, skills, knowledge, and adaptability.
3. *Diagnostic information* refers to those elements that can be used to determine the causal factors of development and performance.
4. *Prognostic information* refers to those elements that can be used as valid forecasters of development and performance.
5. *Basic element* is an aspect of organic, neuromuscular, or mental growth that is a foundation for, and makes possible the development of, a skill.
6. *Fundamental skill* refers to a basic skill that is common to, and essential for participation in, most forms of activity.
7. *Activity skill* refers to a skill that is pertinent to successful participation in a particular activity.

FRAMEWORK FOR MEASUREMENT PROCEDURES—cont'd

Types of information concerning the objectives

1. *Organic development objective*
   a. Classification information
      (1) Age, weight, height
      (2) Strength
      (3) Posture
      (4) Sensory capacity
      (5) Physical fitness
      (6) Anthropometric measurements
      (7) Mental capacity
      (8) Power
      (9) Energy
      (10) Cardiac efficiency
   b. Achievement information
      (1) Strength
      (2) Endurance
      (3) Speed
      (4) Sensory capacity
      (5) Physical fitness
      (6) Power
      (7) Energy
      (8) Posture
      (9) Cardiac efficiency
      (10) Nutrition
   c. Diagnostic information
      (1) Age, weight, height
      (2) Strength
      (3) Endurance
      (4) Nutrition
      (5) Speed
      (6) Sensory capacity
      (7) Physical fitness
      (8) Power
      (9) Energy
      (10) Cardiac efficiency
      (11) Posture
   d. Prognostic information
      (1) Age, weight, height
      (2) Posture
      (3) Speed
      (4) Endurance
      (5) Sensory capacity
      (6) Physical fitness
      (7) Power
      (8) Energy
      (9) Cardiac efficiency

2. *Skill development objective*
   a. Classification information
      (1) Basic elements (concerned mainly with physical activity—would need development for other types)
         (a) Age, weight, height
         (b) Endurance
         (c) Strength
         (d) Native motor ability
         (e) Motor educability
         (f) Reaction time
         (g) Motor interest
         (h) Sensory capacity
      (2) Fundamental skills (mainly concerned with physical activity—other aspects would need to be developed)
         (a) Running
         (b) Throwing
         (c) Kicking
         (d) Jumping
         (e) Dodging
         (f) Leaping
         (g) Vaulting
         (h) Climbing
         (i) Skipping
         (j) Accuracy
         (k) Objective body control
         (l) Agility
         (m) Timing
         (n) Balance
         (o) Spring
         (p) Hand-eye, foot-eye, arm-eye coordinations
      (3) Activity skills (would need to be broken down into the various components affecting the development of each skill)
   b. Achievement information
      (1) Basic elements (similar to basic elements under classification information)
      (2) Fundamental skills (similar to fundamental skills under classification information)
      (3) Activity skills (would need to be broken down into the various components affecting the development of each skill)
   c. Diagnostic information
      (1) Basic elements
         (a) Nutrition
         (b) Health habits such as sleep, rest, and mental state
         (c) Cardiac efficiency
         (d) Sensory capacity
         (e) Motor interest
         (f) Reaction time
         (g) Motor educability
         (h) Native motor ability
         (i) Strength
         (j) Endurance
         (k) Age, weight, height
      (2) Fundamental skills (similar to fundamental skills under classification information)

Continued.

FRAMEWORK FOR MEASUREMENT PROCEDURES—cont'd

    (3) Activity skills (would need to be broken down into the various components affecting the development of each skill)

  d. Prognostic information

    (1) Basic elements (similar to basic elements under diagnostic information)

    (2) Fundamental skills (similar to fundamental skills under classification information)

    (3) Activity skills (would need to be broken down into the various components affecting the development of each skill)

3. *Cognitive development objective*

  a. Classification information

    (1) Mental capacity

    (2) Health education, physical education, and recreation background

    (3) Academic background

    (4) Moral background

    (5) Home environment

  b. Achievement information—such knowledge, attitudes, and practices as:

    (1) Rules of games

    (2) First-aid procedures

    (3) General health, health habits, proper living, health knowledge

      (a) Personal   (d) Social

      (b) Community   (e) Emotional

      (c) Mental

    (4) Rules of safety

    (5) Proper forms in games, athletic events, swimming, dancing, and other physical activities

    (6) Etiquette in certain game situations

    (7) Team play

    (8) Strategy in games and events

    (9) Regulations governing meets, tournaments, and other athletic events

    (10) Duties of officials

    (11) Physical activities

    (12) Values of health and physical education

    (13) Techniques

    (14) Historical background of games and activities

    (15) Principles of hygiene and sanitation

    (16) Effect of exercise on body

    (17) Best kind of exercise to take under certain circumstances

  c. Diagnostic information

    (1) Mental capacity

    (2) Health and physical education background

    (3) Academic background

    (4) Interest

    (5) Home environment

    (6) Physical fitness

    (7) Achievement records

    (8) Health records

  d. Prognostic information

    (1) Mental capacity

    (2) Interest

    (3) Physical fitness

    (4) Achievement records

    (5) Health records

4. *Human relations development objective*

  a. Classification information

    (1) Character

    (2) Personality

    (3) Mental health

    (4) Social attitudes

    (5) Conduct

    (6) Habits

    (7) Citizenship

    (8) Emotions

    (9) Drives

    (10) Appreciations

    (11) Interests

    (12) Capacity for leadership

    (13) Ability to transfer training

    (14) Group living

    (15) Sportsmanship

    (16) Service to community

  b. Achievement information

    (1) Character and personality

      (a) Honesty

      (b) Loyalty

      (c) Fair play

      (d) Good sportsmanship

      (e) Courage

      (f) Unselfishness

    (2) Leadership

      (a) Initiative

      (b) Cooperation

      (c) Quickness of decision

      (d) Fairness and judgment

      (e) Vision and imagination

      (f) Executive ability

      (g) Ability to get along with others

      (h) Personal magnetism

    (3) Transfer of training

      (a) From game situations to other situations in life

      (b) Motor transfer—capacity to solve motor situations and to make a new coordinated movement accurately

    (4) Habits and practices

      (a) Health (eating, sleeping, bathing, and so on)

      (b) Exercise and recreation

    (5) Attitudes and appreciations

      (a) Value of health

      (b) Value of physical recreation

      (c) Good sportsmanship

FRAMEWORK FOR MEASUREMENT PROCEDURES—cont'd

(d) Team play
(e) Value of acquiring certain skills
(f) Appreciation of recreation and exercise
(g) Appreciation of health and practicing health habits
(h) Attitude toward cheating
(i) Attitude toward winning
(j) Attitude toward intraschool versus interschool competition
(k) Appreciation of playing with a novice
(l) Appreciation of training for competition
(m) Appreciation of ways of spending leisure time
(n) Appreciation of awards and rewards
(6) Social attitudes
    (a) Toward individuals of different race, color, and creed
    (b) Toward good citizenship
(7) Emotions
(8) Service to community
c. Diagnostic information
    (1) Health and physical education background
    (2) Mental capacity
    (3) Character

(4) Family background
(5) Companions
(6) Personality
(7) Emotional control
(8) Drives
(9) Interests
(10) Group living
(11) Sportsmanship
(12) Physical fitness
d. Prognostic information
    (1) Sportsmanship
    (2) Character
    (3) Personality
    (4) Mental capacity
    (5) Group living
    (6) Leadership
    (7) Emotional control
    (8) Habits
    (9) Attitudes and appreciations
    (10) Physical fitness
    (11) Interests
    (12) Personal ambitions
    (13) Home environment
    (14) Parental influence

There are many achievement tests available that can be utilized by school and college programs of health and physical education. Some excellent tests are listed in a later section of this chapter.

Diagnostic information

Examples of diagnostic techniques for a school or college health program would be the health examination, audiometer, and vision tests. These techniques or instruments yield information on an individual's health, including heart, lungs, teeth, hearing, vision, and posture.

An example of a diagnostic instrument in physical education would be the Dyer Backboard Test* for tennis. This test evaluates general tennis ability. It does not analyze the various strokes and elements of the game. It merely consists of volleying a tennis ball as rapidly as possible against a backboard.

---

*Dyer, J. T.: The backboard test of tennis ability, Supplement to the Research Quarterly **6**:63, 1935; Revision of backboard test of tennis ability, Research Quarterly **9**:25, 1938.

Prognostic information

An example of a prognostic instrument would be a sociometric test, which reflects a person's ability to get along with others. Another instrument would be a test of mental capacity to forecast academic achievement. Also, it could be a health record to forecast certain aspects of mental health essential to success in various endeavors. It could be a test of general motor ability to forecast achievement in specific skills. Several types of measurement instruments yield information that would forecast future performance in many of life's activities.

TECHNIQUES AND INSTRUMENTS FOR OBTAINING INFORMATION ABOUT OBJECTIVES

In addition to gaining classification, achievement, diagnostic, and prognostic information about students, it also is necessary to identify particular instruments, materials, resources, and methods for evaluating pupil status in respect to organic, neuromuscular, cognitive, and social development.

YORKTOWN HEIGHTS ELEMENTARY SCHOOLS

PHYSICAL EDUCATION Progress Record	Grade Weight Height	3				4				5				6			
Name		Dec. 196	Grade Average	June 196	Grade Average	Dec. 196	Grade Average	June 196	Grade Average	Dec. 196	Grade Average	June 196	Grade Average	Dec. 196	Grade Average	June 196	Grade Average
CHIN-UPS (Arm strength)																	
JUMPING ROPE - number of jumps completed in 30 seconds (Endurance, leg strength, coordination)																	
STANDING BROAD JUMP (Body movement forward) (feet)																	
JUMPING FOR HEIGHT (Jump - Reach - Body movement upward) (inches)																	
CLIMBING 20-FOOT ROPE (General strength & coordination) (feet)																	
TRAVEL HORIZONTAL LADDER (Arm strength & coordination) (feet)																	
SIT-UPS* (Abdominal strength)																	
50-YARD DASH (Speed) (seconds)																	
SOFTBALL THROW 30 FEET, 10 THROWS (Accuracy)																	

* Maximum sit-ups:
   3rd - 20
   4th - 30
   5th - 50
   6th - 50

FOUR YEAR FITNESS REPORT CARD

Fitness report card reflects growth and progress. Parents in Yorktown Heights, N. Y., know just how their children did in every phase of the semiannual physical fitness test because they receive fitness report cards twice each year and can check progress and growth. (From Klappholz, L., editor: Successful practices in teaching physical fitness, New London, Conn., 1964, Croft Educational Services. Reprinted by permission.)

Organic development objective

A medical examination is a valuable technique for obtaining information about the organic development of the pupil. Such an examination should be given at least once a year by a competent physician.

Physical fitness tests will be helpful in determining student status in regard to this objective. Several excellent tests are listed in Chapter 11.

Other tests that should be reviewed as possible instruments for determining the organic development status of pupils are as follows*:

Circulatory-respiratory tests

Cureton All-Out Treadmill Test
Henry Tests of Vasomotor Weakness
MacCurdy-Larson Organic Efficiency Test
Schneider Cardiovascular Test
Turner Test of Circulatory Reaction to Prolonged Standing
Tuttle Pulse-Ratio Test

Anthopometric, posture, and body mechanics measurements

Cureton Technique for Scaling Postural Photographs and Silhouettes
Cureton Tissue Symmetry Test
Cureton-Grover Fat Test
Cureton-Gunby Conformateur Test of Antero-Posterior Posture
Cureton-Holmes Tests for Functional Fitness of the Feet
Cureton-Nordstrom Skeletal Build Index
Cureton-Wickens Center of Gravity Tests

Muscular strength, power, and endurance tests

Anderson Strength Index for High School Girls
Carpenter Strength Test for Women
Cureton Muscular Endurance Tests
Larson Dynamic Strength Test for Men
MacCurdy Test of Physical Capacity
McCloy Athletic Strength Index
Rogers Physical Capacity Test and Physical Fitness Index
Wendler Strength Index

Flexibility tests

Cureton Flexibility Tests
Leighton Flexometer Tests

Neuromuscular development objective

Physical skills represent a major part of the physical education program; therefore, appro-priate valid tests of physical skills should be utilized. Such qualities as *motor educability, motor capacity, physical capacity, motor ability, and motor efficiency* are terms frequently utilized in connection with neuromuscular development.

Tests have been developed for skills in sports such as archery, badminton, soccer, basketball, bowling, football, golf, handball, field hockey, and ice hockey. Descriptions of these tests are given in some of the source books listed at the end of this chapter. These suggested tests should be studied carefully to determine their suitability or adaptability to a particular school situation. Some of the instruments that should be explored in measuring this objective in students are as follows:

Motor fitness tests

Bookwalter Motor Fitness Tests
Cureton-Illinois Motor Fitness Tests
O'Connor-Cureton Motor Fitness Tests for High School Girls

General motor skills tests

Brace Test of Motor Ability
Carpenter Test of Motor Educability for Primary Grade Children
Cozens Test of General Athletic Ability
Humiston Test of Motor Ability for Women
Iowa Revision of the Brace Motor Ability Test
Johnson Test of Motor Educability
Larson Test of Motor Ability for Men
Metheny Revision of the Johnson Test
Powell-Howe Motor Ability Tests for High School Girls
Scott Test of Motor Ability for Women

Sports skills tests

Borleske Touch Football Test for Men
Cureton Swimming Endurance Tests
Cureton Swimming Tests
Dyer Backboard Test of Tennis Ability
Johnson Basketball Test for Men
Lehsten Basketball Test for Men
Rodgers-Heath Soccer Skills Tests for Elementary Schools
Russell-Lange Volleyball Test for Girls
Schmithals-French Field Hockey Tests for Women
Young-Moser Basketball Test for Women

One of the most significant new developments in the area of skill measurement has been encouraged under the sponsorship of the American Alliance for Health, Physical Education, and Recreation. Their Research Council has worked to devise tests and norms for effective evaluation of boys and girls, grades five through

---

*These tests may be found in copies of Research Quarterly, American Alliance of Health, Physical Education, and Recreation, or in one of the measurement and evaluation texts listed in the selected references at the end of this chapter.

twelve, in physical education programs across the United States. This total project includes skill tests for such activities as:

Archery	Football	Softball
Badminton	Golf	Swimming
Baseball	Gymnastics	Tennis
Basketball	Lacrosse	Track and field
Field hockey	Soccer	Volleyball

Administrators should obtain the sports skills test manuals that have been developed. They will be most helpful not only for testing purposes but for instructional suggestions as well. Sample class composite record forms, data, and profile forms are also available from the Alliance.

Cognitive development objective

In the field of health education there are several tests for measuring health knowledge and attitudes. Solleder* has compiled a list of several of these instruments for each educational level. Such tests could be used to evaluate the effectiveness of teaching procedures, weaknesses in the instructional program, and health knowledge of students and for the purpose of grouping students in health classes. They could also be used to determine the impact of health instruction on health knowledge and the attitudes and practices of students, as well as to grade students.

In order to illustrate the types of tests available in health education, one test is listed for each educational level as taken from Solleder's compilation of health evaluating instruments:

Elementary school—Dzenowagis, J. G.: Self-Quiz of Safety Knowledge. This test has been developed to measure safety preparedness of pupils at the fifth- and sixth-grade levels. Available from the National Safety Council, School and College Department, 425 N. Michigan Ave., Chicago, Ill.

Junior high school—Kilander, H. F.: Nutrition Information Test. This test is designed for students in junior high school through college. Norms are available from Dr. H. F. Kilander, Wagner College, Staten Island, N. Y.

Senior high school—Thompson, C. W.: Thompson Smoking and Tobacco Knowledge Test. This test includes the most important physiologic, psychologic,

and socioeconomic facts relating to smoking and tobacco. For more information on this test see Thompson, C. W.: Thompson Smoking and Tobacco Knowledge Test, Research Quarterly **35**:60, 1964.

Junior college—Junior College Health Knowledge Test. This multiple-choice test covers eleven areas of health instruction. For more information write to Supervisor of Health Education, P. O. Box 3307, Terminal Annex, Los Angeles, Calif. 90054.

College or university—Dearborn, T. H.: College Health Knowledge Test. For more information write to Stanford University Press, Stanford, Calif.

In the field of physical education, several standardized tests are available for written tests in various sports. Also, some tests may be found in rule books and source books. Some knowledge and understanding tests in physical education that should be explored are the French Tests for Professional Courses in Knowledge and Sports, Hewitt Comprehensive Tennis Knowledge Tests, Scott Badminton Knowledge Test, Scott Swimming Knowledge Test, and Scott Tennis Knowledge Test.

Teachers may devise their own tests appropriate to the subject and age level being taught. When teachers develop their own tests, however, they should keep in mind the following principles of test construction:

1. The items selected should stress the most important aspects of the material.
2. The length of the test should be determined in relation to the time available for testing.
3. The test should be appropriately worded and geared for the age level to be tested.
4. Questions or test items should be worded to avoid ambiguity.
5. Statements should be simple and direct, not tricky or involved.

Social development objective

There have been several tests developed in the school and college health program to indicate pupil attitudes and behavior. Solleder* has listed several of these in her publication. A sampling of these behavior and attitude instruments are as follows:

Elementary school—Yellen, S.: Health Behavior Inventory, 1963. Designed for grades three to six and covers

---

*Solleder, M. K.: Evaluation instruments in health education, Washington, D. C., 1965, American Association for Health, Physical Education, and Recreation.

---

*Solleder, M. K., op. cit.

COMPARISON OF ESSAY AND OBJECTIVE TESTS

Characteristic	Essay test	Objective test
Preparation of test item	Items are relatively easy to construct	Items are relatively difficult to construct
Sampling of the subject matter	Sampling is often limited	Sampling is usually extensive
Measurement of knowledges and understandings	Items can measure both; measurement of understanding is recommended	Items can measure both; measurement of knowledges is emphasized
Preparation by pupil	Emphasis is primarily on larger units of material	Emphasis is primarily on factual details
Nature of response by pupil	Pupil organizes original response	Except for supply test items, pupil selects response
Guessing of correct response by pupil	Successful guessing is minor problem	Successful guessing is major problem
Scoring of pupil responses	Scoring is difficult, time-consuming, and somewhat unreliable	Scoring is simple, rapid, and highly reliable

From Ahmann, J. S.: Testing student achievements and aptitudes, New York, 1962, The Center for Applied Research in Education, Inc. (The Library of Education), p. 35.

such items as health habits, nutrition, safety, rest, and disease prevention. For more information on this test write to California Test Bureau, Monterey, Calif.

Junior high school—Colebank, A. D.: Health Behavior Inventory, 1963. Designed for grades seven to nine and covers various health information items through a 100-item test. For more information write to California Test Bureau, Monterey, Calif.

Senior high school—Johns, E. B., and Juhnke, W. L.: Health Practice Inventory, 1952. Covers thirteen health areas. Manual of directions and norms also available for senior high students. For more information write to Stanford University Press, Stanford, Calif.

College or university—Leonard, M. L., and Horton, C. W.: An Inventory of Certain Practices in Health, 1949. Instrument can be used to study health behavior of college students. For more information write to California State Department of Education, Sacramento, Calif.

General tests of social adjustment have also been developed, such as the Bell Adjustment Inventory, Science Research Associates Inventory, Minnesota Multiphasic Personality Inventory, and Bernreuter Personality Inventory. The guidance department in almost any school or college would be a good source of information for many tests of social adjustment.

Attitudes may be measured in different ways. Three techniques utilized in this area are teacher evaluation (observation of students with an anecdotal record being kept by the teacher), opinion polls, and rating scales. The physical education teacher should ask for the assistance of other teachers, particularly of the guidance personnel, in this type of testing.

Sociometrics is being used extensively for measurement of social relationships as determined by use of a sociogram. The sociogram points out the natural leaders in the groups and the outsiders trying to become members. When used more than once with the same group, a comparison of the results indicates social growth or change. A sociogram may be taken, for example, by asking all members of a team to list two people whom they would like to have as their friends, with their choices limited to a given group or team. Results may be pictured with arrows pointing to the names listed.

MINIMUM AND DESIRABLE STANDARDS

A minimal program of measurement must include the following points:

1. A *health examination* should be conducted by a physician; as a minimum it would be given to all first-year students. It should be

given at the start of every school year, if possible. A posture screening test should be given at the same time.

2. *Neuromuscular skills* should be tested after the final period of instruction for each new motor activity. This provides the teacher and student with information concerning skill mastery and may also be used later for classification purposes.

3. *Cognitive testing* enables the teacher to ascertain knowledge and information gained from activity programs.

4. *Attitude testing* may be based on observation and evaluation techniques. Students asked to evaluate the activity program will also express their general attitudes concerning the content and instruction of the program. Observation of students on a daily basis can give the instructor a good idea of student attitudes toward the class.

5. *Physical fitness tests* should be conducted annually to determine the progress of the student in this important area.

6. *Self-evaluation* by the instructor is essential to the program as well as professional, personal, and social growth of the teacher.

KEEPING RECORDS AND USING TEST RESULTS

There are many clerical duties associated with the measurement program. For most effective use, records should be kept up-to-date and new test results constantly analyzed in terms of student progress and program planning. In some school districts teacher aides and community volunteers have been used to do the clerical work. Also, in today's automation era some schools and colleges have found it advantageous to use IBM cards to record test results. It may also be helpful to maintain a record file of measurement instruments used, adding comments concerning possible success or problems involved in their administration. This would prevent repetition of testing with unsuitable instruments.

The purpose of testing is to help the student and improve the educational program. As pointed out earlier in this chapter, tests can yield classification, achievement, diagnostic, and prognostic information. Therefore, after the testing has been accomplished, the results should be used appropriately.

NEED FOR A STANDARDIZATION OF MEASUREMENT MATERIALS

There are at least three reasons why the need is great for a standardization of measurement materials for the fields of health and physical education.

In the first place, many of the techniques being used today have been developed by individuals who have failed to use or interpret cor-

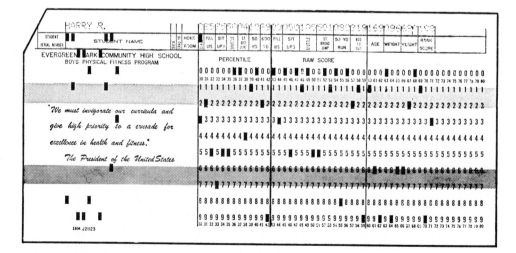

IBM card for recording test results. (From Bucher, C. A., and Koenig, C. R.: Methods and materials for secondary school physical education, ed. 4, St. Louis, 1974, The C. V. Mosby Co.)

rectly scientific methods of construction. As a result, there are materials being used in our schools and colleges that have either failed to be scientifically evaluated or else have fallen below acceptable standards. In light of these conditions, it is necessary to ensure that only materials that meet acceptable criteria will be used. Standardization would make such a practice possible.

In the second place, it is impossible to make comparisons between individuals of different localities because of the different techniques being used in each section. When a student transfers from one geographic locality to another, the instructor is at a loss to analyze his or her status, because of the lack of standards for all sections

of the country. As a result, the instructor must start from the beginning in determining an individual's physical condition, traits, or characteristics. Standardization would make it possible for records to be interpreted intelligently, regardless of who administers the technique or the locality in which it is administered.

In the third place, it is difficult to measure progress on a national basis without the use of standards. It is imperative that measurement materials be standardized so that the professions can know whether they are meeting the objectives that have been set, can evaluate the various types of programs and instruction, and can know what they are achieving through these programs. Standardization would make it possible to better

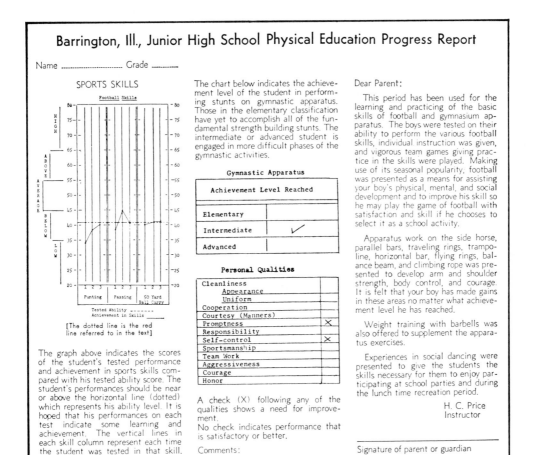

Physical education progress report, Barrington, Ill., Junior High School. (From Bucher, C. A., and Koenig, C. R.: Methods and materials for secondary school physical education, ed. 4, St. Louis, 1974, The C. V. Mosby Co.)

determine individual and program weaknesses, quality of instruction, and progress achieved. Furthermore, standardization would serve as a means of motivation and comparison.

GRADING

The giving of grades in most school programs of health and physical education represents an administrative necessity. The purposes for grading include the following:

1. It serves as a means of indicating student achievement in the areas for which the course or experience is offered.

2. It serves as a means of informing such persons as parents, employers, colleges and universities, honorary societies, and other groups of the quality of a pupil's work.

3. It serves as a motivational device for some students.

4. It serves as a guide to program planning and for the grouping of students (grades identify areas of strength and weakness in the curriculum and in the students) and as a basis for counseling students (abrupt changes in a student's grades might be indicative of problems).

Since grading is an established custom in the

PHYSICAL EDUCATION REPORT CARD
NASHVILLE CITY SCHOOLS

Pupil_____ School_____

Homeroom_____ Classroom _____ Year 19____ 19____

GRADE LEVEL	FALL					SPRING					YEAR'S AVERAGE
	1	2	3	Ex	Av	4	5	6	Ex	Av	

Items checked (✔) below need improvement

	1	2	3	4	5	6
Develops co-ordination						
Shows knowledge of rules						
Develops physically						
Strength						
Endurance						
Weight						
Participates						
Dress						
Playing						
Shower						
Attendance (Days absent from class)						
Conduct						

CODE
(Teacher may add plus or minus if she wishes)

A=90 - 100—Consistently does excellent work

B =82 - 89—Does good work

C=75 - 81—Does fair work

D=70 - 74—Low, but passing

F =Below 70—Failing

Comments enclosed   Date_____ Date_____ Date_____
                     Date_____ Date_____ Date_____

Teacher_____

Physical education report card, Nashville city schools. (From Bucher, C. A., and Koenig, C. R.: Methods and materials for secondary school physical education, ed. 4, St. Louis, 1974, The C. V. Mosby Co.)

educational system of this country, physical education must conform and grant grades or utilize some other method of denoting the progress that has been achieved.

Grades have been issued in physical education in several ways, ranging from granting letter or numeral grades to ranking in a class. These grades have also been based on many factors, many of which have questionable value. Some present practices base grades on such factors as attendance, punctuality, effort, dress, achievement, general attitude, initiative, hygiene, skill, knowledge of rules, and coopera-

tion. Nationally, there seems to be no set formula or procedure. Each individual instructor establishes the basis on which grades should be granted.

The following recommendations represent some of the more advanced thinking among educators in general. At the elementary level especially, the feeling is increasing that it is not wise to issue a single grade or numerical rating. It is felt that a descriptive paragraph telling in more detail what progress is being made by the pupil is much better. Discussing such items as a student's strengths and weaknesses and where

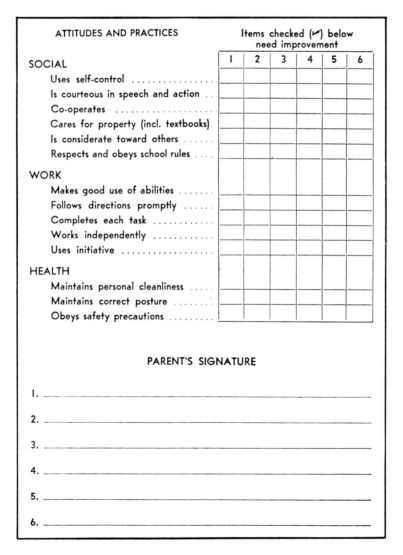

For legend see opposite page.

PASSING OR FAILING IN PHYSICAL EDUCATION*

In response to numerous inquiries from school officials, the following is intended to clarify the statement that boards of education may not refuse graduation or promotion because of failure in physical education.

Physical education is required for all pupils by Education Law and Regulations of the Commissioner of Education. It is expected that each pupil will participate in such classes and that he will exert sufficient effort to enable him to achieve his optimal progress toward all program objectives. If a pupil refuses to attend physical education classes and otherwise does not fulfill course requirements approved by the board of education, and prompt and appropriate notification is given to all concerned, a failing mark may be given and graduation withheld until such time as the deficiency has been removed.

On the other hand, a pupil who fulfills all the requirements and has exhibited acceptable evidence of satisfactory progress in terms of his abilities but who has been unable to meet minimal standards of physical performance may not be given a failing mark in physical education.

Pupils who act in ways deemed undesirable as good school citizens while participating in physical education classes, such as disobeying the teacher, refusing to exert reasonable effort or deliberately violating stated policies and procedures, should be treated as disciplinary cases.

Physical education is an integral part of the school curriculum. It is recognized that achievement of the program's major goals including physical fitness, skills, knowledge, social qualities and attitudes will help provide valuable assets for each pupil. Therefore, every effort should be made to insure that physical education is a meaningful and profitable experience for each boy and girl, particularly for those who possess lower levels of physical ability. One of the most valuable outcomes of a physical education program is the inculcation of a strong appreciation of, desire for and interest in participation in physical activities which will endure throughout life. Would failing in physical education help to reach this goal?

Reviewed and Approved by Division of Law,
State Education Department,
January, 1969

*From New York State Education Department: Curriculum guide: physical education in the secondary school, 1964, p. 21.

---

he or she needs to improve is much more meaningful and purposeful. This type of report and talks with parents will better achieve the purpose of showing to what degree educational objectives are being attained and what needs to be accomplished in the future. This method also has implications for grading above the elementary level.

When grades are given, they should be based on the achievement of objectives—the degree to which the student has achieved the desired outcomes. These objectives should be clear in the instructor's and students' minds at the outset of the course so that the desired direction will be known. The individuals getting the best grades would be those students most nearly achieving the objectives that have been listed as desirable goals for the course. In physical education the physical, motor, cognitive, and social objectives would all be kept in mind.

A further recommendation is that, as far as possible, the degree to which desired objectives

are achieved should be determined objectively rather than subjectively. This means that wherever possible scientific evaluation and measurement techniques should be utilized. Since there is a dearth of such techniques, some subjective judgments will have to be made.

Grades should be understood by the student. He or she should know how they are arrived at and how the factors that go into the grades are weighed. The grades should also be easily understood by parents, particularly how they relate to the objectives of the course the student is taking. As far as possible, the grades should be expressed in the same manner as grades in other subject matter areas throughout the school. This not only facilitates record keeping and transfer of credits but also places health and physical education on the same level as other subjects.

Table 22-2 outlines a proposed plan by Dr. Lynn McCraw for grading as a means of assessing the various objectives in an objective manner.

Student ....

....   **19**............ - **19**......

Grade

RICHWOODS COMMUNITY HIGH SCHOOL

Progress Report in Physical Education

....
Teacher   Counselor

1st pd.	2nd pd.	3rd pd.	Sem. exam	Sem. avg.	4th pd.	5th pd.	6th pd.	Sem. exam	Sem. avg.	Units crdt.

EXPLANATION OF MARKING SYSTEM

Achievement—Grading for actual work done by the student

A—94-100—Excellent   D—70-77—Below Average
B—86- 93—Above Avg.   F—Below 70—Failure
C—78- 85—Average   E—Conditional
                      Inc.—Incomplete

ACTIVITIES INCLUDED IN GRADING PERIODS

ACTIVITIES	PERIOD 1	2	3	4	5	6
Flicker Ball						
Flag Football						
Soccer						
*Field Hockey						
*Speed Ball						
*Campcraft						
Basketball (beginning) (advanced)						
Volleyball (beginning) (advanced)						
Tumbling (beginning) (advanced)						
Apparatus (beginning) (advanced)						
Wrestling (beginning) (advanced)						
Handball						
Badminton						
Recreational Games						
*Fundamental Rhythms—Modern Dance						
Track and Field						
Softball						
Archery						
Golf						
Co. P.E. Social Dance						
Co. P.E. Square Dance						
Co. P.E. Volleyball & Rec. Games						
Driver Training (Classroom)						
Health Education (Classroom)						
*Indicates Girls' Activity Only						

GRADING PROCEDURE

The six week grade is evaluated in the following areas:
1. Performance of Skills
2. Knowledge of Skills and Physical Fitness
3. Social Attitudes including cooperation, sportsmanship, and leadership
4. Hygiene conditions (uniforms, showers), and attendance.

PHYSICAL FITNESS TESTS
(Based on National Norms)

	Trial 1 (Fall) Score	% ile	Trial 2 (Spring) Score	% ile
Pull-Ups (Boys) (shoulder strength)				
Modified Pull-Ups (Girls) (shoulder strength)				
Sit-Ups (abdominal strength)				
Shuttle Run (agility)				
Standing Broad Jump (leg power)				
50-Yard Dash (speed)				
Softball Throw (arm power)				
600-Yard Run-Walk (endurance)				

The National Norms and Scores are based on Age, Weight, and Height.

PARENT'S SIGNATURE

Your signature means only that you have seen this report.

1st Period...

2nd Period..

3rd Period..

4th Period..

5th Period..

Each absence, however short, interferes with the student's progress.

Progress report in physical education, Richwoods Community High School, Peoria Heights, Ill. (From Bucher, C. A., and Koenig, C. R.: Methods and materials for secondary school physical education, ed. 4, St. Louis, 1974, The C. V. Mosby Co.)

Table 22-2. Proposed plan for grading*

Components	Weightings	Instruments
Attitude in terms of Attendance Punctuality Suiting out Participation	5% to 25%	Attendance and other records Teacher observation
Skills in terms of Form in execution of skill Standard of performance Application in game situation	20% to 35%	Objective tests Teacher observation Student evaluation
Physical fitness with emphasis on Muscular strength and endurance Cardiovascular-respiratory endurance Agility Flexibility	20% to 35%	Objective tests Teacher observation
Knowledge and appreciation of Skills Strategy Rules History and terms	5% to 25%	Written tests Teacher observation
Behavior in terms of Social conduct Health and safety practices	5% to 25%	Teacher observation Student evaluation

*From McCraw, L. W.: Principles and practices for assigning grades in physical education, Journal of Health, Physical Education, and Recreation **35:**2, 1964.

Contract grading

Contract grading is an innovation in the grading system that permits the student to choose a standard of performance established by the instructor (sometimes with student participation) and work toward satisfying the contract in order to receive a certain specified grade. Different grades (A, B, C) require different contract items to be satisfied. In order to receive an A in a course, the student would have to complete all the A requirements, as well as satisfactorily complete an examination in that area.

John is in the twelfth grade at Ft. Pierce, Florida and is scheduled to take golf as part of his physical education requirement. Before taking the course, he signed a contract with his teacher, which spells out in detail the work in golf that he must complete in order to earn a grade of his choice. For example, John knows he can earn 10 points as part of the contract if he learns to swing a club properly, demonstrate proper technique to the instructor, and write a short report that analyzes the sequence of movements to be followed in using the club effec-

tively. Another part of the golf contract that is valued at 20 points requires John to read a book on golf and then write a summary and critique of the publication. There are other contract options that permit John to earn additional points. In order to get a grade of A in golf, John must earn a minimum of 125 points. If he wants a B, he needs 100 points; a C, 90 points; and a D, 80 points. No completed contract receives a failing grade. If the quality is not acceptable, the contract time is extended.

Contract learning is an innovation that some school teachers are utilizing in various subjects in order to individualize learning and provide for students who have different interests and motivations. These teachers have described the contract-for-grade system as a way in which they can interact with students and both have the opportunity to indicate their expectations for the course.

What the student accomplishes in the contract system depends entirely upon individual effort. In physical education at Ft. Pierce, Florida, the sports contracts are designed to be utilized

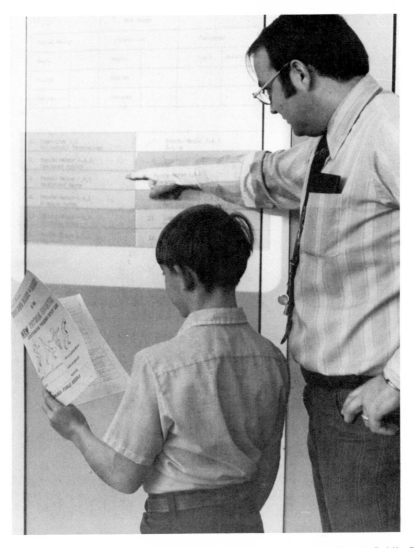

Teacher of physical education discussing Phy-Pak contract with student in Omaha Public Schools.

by students working at their own pace on an individual basis. The goal is not necessarily to create super-skilled players, but instead, to have each boy and girl learn the fundamentals, rules, and etiquette of the sport and be able to participate in the activity with some degree of understanding and enjoyment.

In order to fulfill contract requirements, students frequently use as resources the school library, programmed texts and other supplemental materials, teacher-student discussions, visual aids, the community, and consultants who are familiar with the subject. The teacher

is on call to advise students during and after school hours. The sources of information for the students are as unlimited as their imagination and ingenuity. Attendance in class is not always required. In some schools the students check in to class daily but thereafter are free to go where their resources are located.

Student reaction to contract learning has been favorable. For example, at Madison Consolidated High School in Indiana, students were asked to express their opinions. About 80% said they enjoyed contract better than traditional learning and wanted to use it again. Three out of every four students felt they learned more under the contract system than under methods that had been in use in past years. Nearly nine out of every ten students liked the independent method of work, the opportunity to earn the grade they wanted, and have the teacher state exactly what must be done to be awarded a specific grade. Some representative student comments include: "You get the grade you want," "It gives the student a change," "The system helped me more than the teacher," "I knew exactly what was required in order to get a certain grade," "It permitted me an opportunity to work at my own pace," "It places the responsibility upon the student and this is as it should be."

Contract learning is an innovation that school systems will want to consider as a possible method to personalize and motivate student learning.

Performance objectives

Performance objectives can also be used as a grading method. Glenbrook North High School in Glenview, Illinois began this project a few years ago. The performance objectives were written by a group of physical educators and were based on general organic, neuromuscular, emotional, social, and cognitive goals. For example, a performance objective unit in gymnas-

tics for freshmen was divided into a 10-day introductory unit and a 3-week advanced unit. A lecture and a demonstration of the 40 selected gymnastic stunts was presented to the students, followed by the introductory unit of instruction and practice. The grading system was as follows, based on satisfactory performance as predetermined by the instructor:

16 to 28 stunts—A
10 to 15 stunts—B
6 to 9 stunts—C
3 to 5 stunts—D
0 to 2 stunts—F*

The advanced unit required a 3-week instruction-demonstration period with the students continuing from the introductory unit. A student who satisfactorily completed 29 to 40 stunts received an A, 16 to 27 stunts a B, and 10 to 15 stunts a C. A performance objective unit was also prepared for sophomores required to take a 3-week unit in soccer.

The committee wrote performance objectives for all activities in the 4-year high school curriculum. The freshmen and sophomores started in the program with those teachers who desired to

---

*Sherman, W.: Performance objectives, Journal of Health, Physical Education, and Recreation **42**:37, 1971.

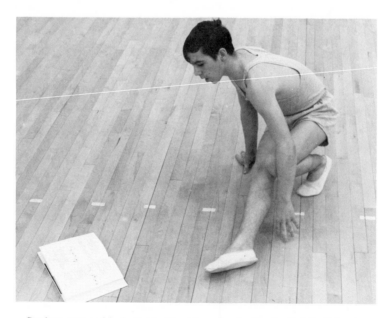

Student engaged in individualized learning in Omaha Public Schools.

work with the performance objective concept. The initial evaluation was very positive for both students and teachers involved in the performance-objective units.

Individualized learning

Individualized learning has had a great impact on education in recent years. Grading concepts have also changed in schools that have adopted the concept of individualized learning. In student-centered learning the following processes are included:

1. Performance objectives are based on psychomotor and cognitive tasks.
2. The individual is allowed to regulate his or her own progress.
3. The teacher is an aid in learning rather than a demonstrator.
4. The gymnasium becomes a resource center that includes areas for audiovisual aids, discussions, practice, and evaluation.
5. Students help in directing each other as well as themselves.
6. Grading is eliminated and replaced by a progress reporting system.

According to this system, the teacher is an evaluator and determines each student's success in meeting the established educational objectives. The student consults with the teacher concerning his or her progress and comes to the teacher when prepared for the final evaluation consisting of satisfactory completion of tasks, acknowledgment by other students, teacher approval, and recording progress on a record card. If a student has not completed the tasks successfully, alternative approaches are suggested by the teacher. This one-to-one contact has had very positive results in schools that have adopted the individualized learning concept.

Questions and exercises

1. Define the term *measurement*. Why is it important to the successful administration of any program of health, physical education, or recreation?
2. List as many measurement techniques as possible that are utilized in the schools. Take three of these and describe their use in detail.
3. What is the relationship of measurement to objectives?
4. Why is it important to have classification, achievement, diagnostic, and prognostic information about each individual participating in the program of health, physical education, and/or recreation?

5. What are some general guides in respect to the measurement program that should be known by every administrator and teacher?
6. List and describe the various criteria essential to the construction and selection of scientific tests.
7. How would the standardization of measurement materials contribute to better programs of health, physical education, and recreation?
8. What are the minimum and desirable standards for a measurement program?
9. Develop what you consider to be a satisfactory and practical measurement program for a health, physical education, and/or recreation program.
10. Discuss contract grading in detail. Develop a contract grading system for one unit in the physical education and/or health program.
11. Explain how performance objectives can be used as a basis for grading. Develop a performance-based grading system for a unit of the physical education program.
12. How can individualized learning techniques be applied to changes in the grading system? Report on any such learning technique and its effect on grading that you have personally observed.

    Reading assignment in *Administrative Dimensions of Health and Physical Education Programs, Including Athletics:* Chapter 17, Selections 91 to 93.

Selected references

American Association of Health, Physical Education, and Recreation: Sports skills test manuals (archery, basketball, football, softball), 1966, 1967, The Association.

American Association for Health, Physical Education, and Recreation: Grading in physical education, Journal of Health, Physical Education, and Recreation **38:**34, 1967.

Bonney, M. E., and Hampleman, R. S.: Personal-social evaluation techniques, New York, 1962, The Center for Applied Research in Education, Inc. (The Library of Education).

Boyd, C. A., and Waglow, I. F.: The individual achievement profile, The Physical Educator **21:**3, 1964.

Clarke, H. H.: Application of measurement to health and physical education, ed. 4, Englewood Cliffs, N. J., 1967, Prentice-Hall, Inc.

Fabricius, H., and others: Grading in physical education, Journal of Health, Physical Education, and Recreation **38:**5, 1967.

Fast, B.: Contracting, Journal of Health, Physical Education, and Recreation **42:**31, 1971.

Herman, W. L.: Teaching attitude as related to academic grades and athletic ability of prospective physical education teachers, The Journal of Educational Research **61:**40, 1967.

Jensen, C.: Evaluate your testing program, The Physical Educator **21:**49, 1964.

Jorndt, L. C.: Point systems—motivational devices, The Physical Educator **23:**1, 1966.

Latchaw, M., and Brown, C.: The evaluation process in health education, physical education, and recreation, Englewood Cliffs, N. J., 1962, Prentice-Hall, Inc.

Lawrence, T.: Appraisal of emotional health at the secondary school level, The Research Quarterly **37:**2, 1966.

Liba, M. R., and Loy, J. W.: Some comments on grading, The Physical Educator **22:**4, 1965.

Link, F. R.: To grade or not to grade, The PTA Magazine **62:**10, 1967.

Mathews, D. K.: Measurement in physical education, ed. 2, Philadelphia, 1963, W. B. Saunders Co.

Meyers, C. R., and Blesh, T. E.: Measurement in physical education, New York, 1962, The Ronald Press Co.

National Education Association: Reports to parents, National Association Research Bulletin **45:**2, 1967.

Oxendine, J. B.: Social development—the forgotten objective? Journal of Health, Physical Education, and Recreation **37:**5, 1966.

Piscopo, J.: Quality instruction: first priority, The Physical Educator **21:**4, 1964.

Sherman, W.: Performance objectives, Journal of Health, Physical Education, and Recreation **42:**37, 1971.

Shrader, R.: Individualized approach to learning, Journal of Health, Physical Education, and Recreation **42:**33, 1971.

Smith, B., and Lerch, H.: Contract grading, The Physical Educator **29:**80, 1972.

Smithells, P. A., and Cameron, P. E.: Principles of evaluation in physical education, New York, 1962, Harper & Row, Publishers.

Solleder, M. K.: Evaluation instruments in health education, Washington, D. C., 1965, American Association for Health, Physical Education, and Recreation.

Trump, C.: Meaningful grading, Scholastic Coach **35:**44, 1966.

Weber, L., and Paul, T.: Approaches to grading in physical education, The Physical Educator **28:**59, 1972.

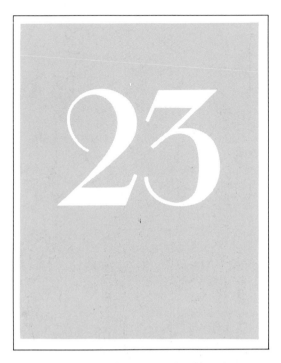

Teacher and program evaluation

Teacher and program evaluations have received much attention in recent years. Accountability has become almost a household word; some communities insist that accountability become a part of a teacher's contract. Accountability and other innovations in teacher evaluation, as well as a discussion of program evaluation, are included in this chapter.

FRAMEWORK FOR EVALUATION PROCEDURES

There are many items that can be evaluated in terms of the process of administration. These include an evaluation of various aspects of each category: in administration, this might include policies, finance, publicity, community relationship, and records; in leadership, performance, results, training, and qualifications; in facilities, the various factors that pertain to effective construction, use, and maintenance; in equipment, supply, use, cost, number, and maintenance; in activities, time, facilities, participation, and conduct; and in participation, utilization of facilities, and amount of time permitted.

MEANS FOR EVALUATION

Various means of evaluating educational programs have been devised. These range from very elaborate and detailed checklists, rating scales, and score cards to a list of questions that the administration should ask to determine the relative merits of certain administrative practices and programs. For example, score cards such as the LaPorte Score Cards have been developed to rate health and physical education programs; Score Card 1 relates to the evaluation of health and physical education programs in the elementary school, and Score Card 2 is used for junior and senior high schools and the 4-year high schools. These score cards cover such items as program of activities, class program, and intramural and interschool athletics. Each area can be rated according to a possible score that would represent an excellent program. The score cards have been successfully applied to several thousands of schools. Norms have been developed for purposes of comparison. Also some states, such as Ohio and Indiana, have developed program score cards that are pertinent to their respective states.

Many aspects of evaluation are discussed in this text in chapters that relate to such specific items as facilities, equipment and supplies, class program, health services, and a healthful environment. Therefore, this chapter is designed to cover the broad field of evaluation and to pay particular attention to teacher evalu-

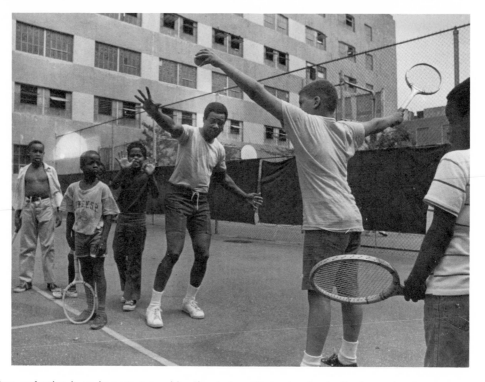

Teacher evaluation is an important consideration today. Here a teacher in the inner city demonstrates proper form in tennis to a youngster as part of the National Summer Youth Sports Program. (Courtesy President's Council on Physical Fitness and Sports.)

ation, which is of considerable concern to administration today. Recent advances in education have necessitated development of sound methods of rating teachers and their abilities.

TEACHER EVALUATION

In recent years, administrators, parents, teachers, and communities have been concerned with developing ways and means of establishing methods to measure teacher effectiveness for the purpose of making sound decisions for retention, salary adjustments, and promotion, as well as to help teachers to improve.

The administration has an important role to play in the evaluation of teachers. Leadership should be provided in this area to establish a planned program of evaluation. Teachers need to be helped to improve their own effectiveness. Records should be kept to determine progress.

Some guidelines for the evaluation of teachers are as follows:

1. *Appraisal should involve the teachers themselves.* Evaluation is a cooperative venture, and teachers should be involved in the development of the criteria for evaluation and need to understand the process.

2. *Evaluation should be centered on performance.* The job that is to be accomplished should be the point of focus with other extraneous factors omitted.

3. *Evaluation should be concerned with helping the teacher to grow on the job.* The purpose of evaluation is to help the teacher evaluate himself or herself and maintain strengths and reduce weaknesses.

4. *Evaluation should look to the future.* It should be concerned with developing a better health program, a better physical education program, and a better school system.

5. *Evaluation of teachers should be well organized and administered,* with the step-by-step approach clearly outlined.

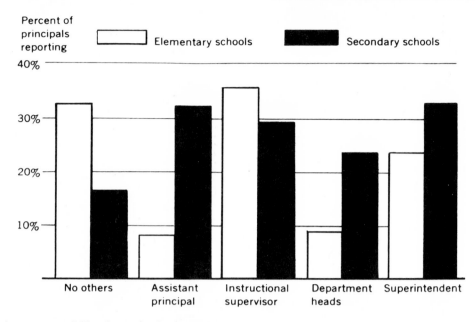

Who shares responsibility for evaluating probationary teachers with the school principal (limited to systems with written evaluations)? (From NEA Research Bulletin **42:**85, 1964.)

Fawcett* suggests the following outline, which includes some of the broad areas in which a teacher might be evaluated, as a means of initiating an evaluation program.

Interpersonal relations

Teacher-teacher
Teacher-students
Teacher-parents
Teacher-community
Teacher-administrators

Classroom management

Setting of classroom goals and individual learning goals for each student
Assignment and acceptance of individual responsibility by each student in the class
Confirmation of desired behavior of students and re-direction of undesirable behavior
Exercise of authority to secure necessary decisions in the classroom
Research behavior of the teacher to keep goals and activities of the classroom consistent with the culture
Record-keeping behavior of the teacher essential to the conduct of the classroom
Coordination of the instruction in the classroom not only with other instructional activities of the school

but with out-of-school learning experiences of the students
Inclusion of each student in the learning activities of the class
Communication in the classroom not only to make the teacher understand, but to make it possible for each person to share in classroom activities
Judgment in the allocation of time and resources to different activities in the classroom

Teacher-learning

1. Analysis of students:
   Skills
   Attitudes
   Knowledge
2. Presentation of subject matter through:
   Lectures
   Group discussions
   Student research
   Programmed learning
3. Utilization of instructional material and resources:
   Libraries
   Books
   Machines
   Television
   Radio
   Films
   Supplementary materials, organizations, and people of the community
4. Creation of an efficient learning environment through organization of the physical surroundings in the classoom

---

*Fawcett, C. W.: School personnel administration, New York, 1964. The Macmillan Co., pp. 58-59.

Some methods of evaluating teachers are:

1. *Observation of teachers in the classroom or in the gymnasium.* The National Education Association Research Division, in studying this method, reported that the median length of time for the most recent observation was 22 minutes, about 25% of the teachers were notified 1 day in advance that the observation would take place, and about 50% of the teachers reported that a conference followed up the observation with the teacher's performance being discussed and evaluated. Nearly one-half of the teachers reported that the observation was helpful to them.

2. *Student progress.* With this method standardized tests are used to determine what progress the student has made as a result of exposure to the teacher.

3. *Ratings.* Ratings vary and may consist of an overall estimate of a teacher's effectiveness or consist of separate evaluations of specific teacher behaviors and traits. Self-ratings may also be used. Ratings may be conducted by the teacher's peers, by students, or by administrative personnel and may include judgments based on observation of student progress. In order to be effective, rating scales must be based on such criteria as objectivity, reliability, sensitivity, validity, and utility.

At college and university levels the evaluation of teacher performance is sometimes more difficult than at precollege levels because of the unwillingness of the faculty to permit members of the administration, or other persons, to observe them. Various methods have been devised in institutions of higher learning to rate faculty members, including statements from department heads, ratings by colleagues, ratings by students, and ratings by deans and other administrative personnel.

A question that frequently arises in the development of any system of teacher evaluation is: what constitutes effectiveness as it relates to a teacher in a particular school or college situation? Several studies have been conducted with some interesting findings. For example, there is only a slight correlation between intelligence and the rated success of an instructor. Therefore, the degree of intelligence a teacher has, within reasonable limits, seems to have little value as a criterion. The relation of knowledge of subject matter to effectiveness appears to relate most in particular teaching situations. A teacher's demonstration of good scholarship while in college appears to have little positive relationship to good teaching. There is some evidence to show that teachers who have demonstrated high levels of professional knowledge on National Teachers Examinations are more effective teachers. However, the evidence here is rather sparse. The relationship of experience to effectiveness also seems to have

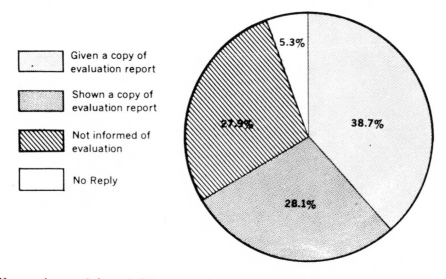

How teachers are informed of their evaluations. (From NEA Research Bulletin **42:**86, 1964.)

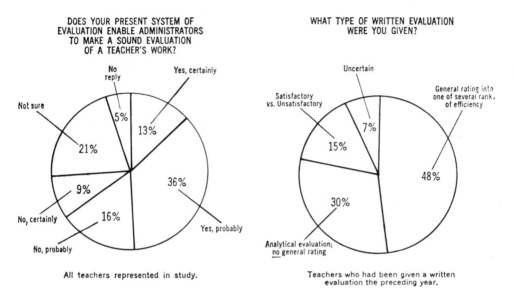

What teachers say about evaluation of teachers. (From NEA Research Bulletin **54**:38, 1965.)

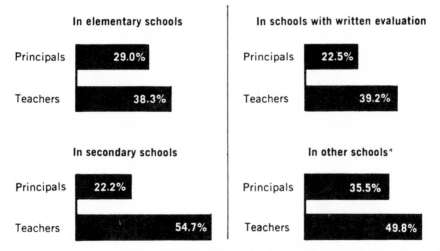

ᵃ Where there was no written evaluation in the school systems, or teachers did not receive a written evaluation in 1961-62, or were employed in a different school system in 1961-62, or who did not know whether there was written evaluation.

Principals and teachers express doubt or a negative opinion on the system of teacher evaluation. (From NEA Research Bulletin **42**:111, 1964.)

questionable value. Experience during the first 5 years of teaching seems to enhance teacher effectiveness but then levels off. There is little, if any, relationship between effectiveness and cultural background, socioeconomic status, sex, and marital status. Finally there is little evidence to show that any specified aptitude for teaching exists. The studies indicate that more research needs to be done in order to establish what constitutes teacher effectiveness on the job.

Innovations in teacher evaluation

With schools plagued by austerity budgets, an excess of teachers, community relations problems, and rural and minority group controversies, the era of teacher accountability has come of age. The community wants to know what the teachers are doing and how well they are doing it. Administrators, students, and parents are demanding standards of teacher performance. Accountability and other new concepts of teacher evaluation are discussed in the following sections.

Accountability. Accountability may be simply defined as a means of holding the teacher (and other school or college staff members) responsible for what the students learn. Articles are frequently appearing in newspapers, which cite high school students reading at grade levels far below their present grade. Many persons feel that the teachers and administrators should be held accountable for such situations.

"The emphasis behind accountability must be learning on the part of the students rather than teaching on the part of the teachers."* When the subject matter or method of teaching has become useless, relevant learning cannot take place. In order for accountability to be valid, curriculum revision must take place to allow for the best possible student progress. Once this has been accomplished (continuous program evaluation is essential), the teacher can direct his or her time and energy towards learn-

---

*Field, D.: Accountability for the physical educator, Journal of Health, Physical Education, and Recreation **44**:37, 1973.

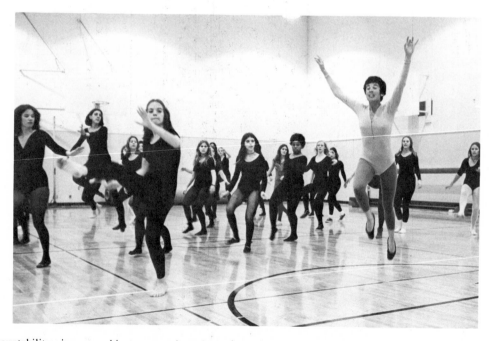

Accountability aims at making sure students learn from their educational experiences. A teacher instructing jazz dancing at El Camino Real High School in Los Angeles. (Los Angeles Unified School District, Student Auxiliary Services Branch. Courtesy Gwen R. Waters.)

ing motivation. When an atmosphere of enjoyment is created, learning comes more naturally.

How can accountability be assessed? The first obstacle that must be overcome in order to have a valid accountability program is the acceptance by educators that certain student objectives must be met. This can usually be accomplished by developing performance objectives. Such tests as the AAHPER Cooperative Physical Education Tests for major students, distributed by the Educational Testing Service in Princeton, for example, are very helpful. Once objectives have been developed, both the student and teacher know what is expected of them. Accountability can be based on how well the students satisfy the stated performance objectives for each unit. Some persons have suggested that student performance should be a basis for teacher bonuses. This is one method of accountability that has many pros and cons.

Student evaluations are another method of assessing teacher accountability. This area is discussed in the following section.

Student evaluations. The student is the individual who is most exposed to the teacher and his or her methodology. Therefore, the student should have some say about whether the teacher is doing a satisfactory job of teaching. Harristhal's study,* devoted exclusively to women physical educators at the college level, was designed to obtain information concerning the desirable characteristics of teachers in a given subject area. The following factors were found to be related to teacher effectiveness based on student responses in this study:

1. Subject familiarity
2. Interest in individuals
3. Fairness
4. Patience
5. Leadership that was amicable but firm
6. Enthusiasm
7. Skill in activities

Many teachers are using instruments for teacher evaluation. The student is asked to respond to certain multiple choice questions that

indicate such items as: (1) interest level in activity, (2) skills learned, (3) time spent outside of class on activity, (4) knowledge gained, and (5) rating of instructor in regard to understandability of his or her instructions, organization of presentation, enthusiasm; knowledge, skill, and interest in students. There is often a space left for the student to express himself or herself in paragraph form concerning changes in curriculum or teaching methods.

Self-evaluation. An area of evaluation often overlooked is self-evaluation. Self-evaluation is often the key to self-improvement. One should ask himself or herself some of the following questions:

1. Have I been innovative?
2. Do I alter my teaching to meet the different ability levels I encounter?
3. Are my classes planned well in advance to be sure of teaching space, equipment, and facility use?
4. Do I involve all my students in activities?
5. Do I stress cognitive, social, and behavioral objectives?
6. Do I change my activities from year to year and try new concepts such as contact grading, performance objectives, self-directed learning, and resource centers?
7. Do I continually evaluate my activity programs?
8. Do I try to improve myself by continuing my education?

Such questions as these can help the teacher to begin to evaluate himself or herself. Self-evaluation is not easy, but can be very valuable in improving one's teaching.

Independent evaluators. In recent years there has been a trend toward using independent evaluators since they may be more objective in assessing a teacher's abilities. Independent evaluators should be thoroughly trained and familiar with the subject area they are evaluating and should have teaching and administrative background. Often the evaluators are drawn from education consultant groups, education specialists in civil service positions, or university or college professors.

Evaluating the prospective teacher. The competence of the prospective teacher is a very important facet of the total educational evalua-

*Harristhal, J.: A student reaction inventory for rating teachers in the college women's physical education Service program (an unpublished doctoral thesis), Eugene, Oregon, 1962.

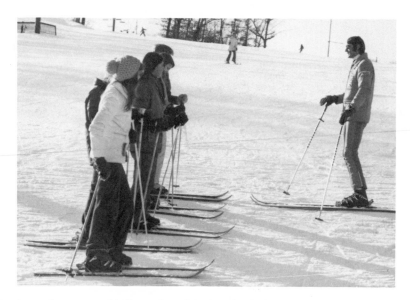

Paraprofessionals are also accountable for students learning physical education skills. Here a paraprofessional is teaching skiing in an off-campus course at Regina High School, Minneapolis. (Photograph by Rollie Baird, Dellarson Studios.)

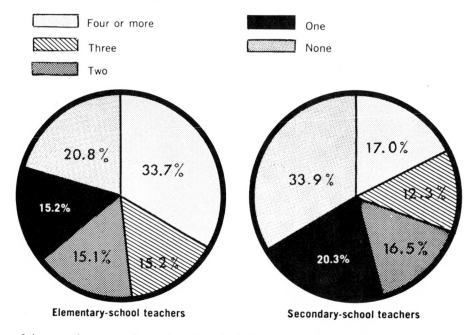

Number of times teachers were observed teaching in their classroom for 5 minutes or more, as reported by teachers from beginning of 1962-1963 term to February 1, 1963. (From NEA Research Bulletin **43:**14, 1965.)

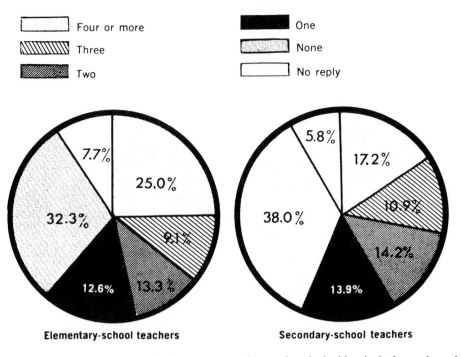

Number of individual conferences of 10 minutes or more that teachers had with principals or other school system official, as reported by teachers from beginning of 1962-1963 term to February 1, 1963. (From NEA Research Bulletin **43:**17, 1965.)

tion system. Traditionally the undergraduate education major was evaluted in terms of grade-point average, completion of required course work, and a minimum grade level in major-area subjects. Obviously, such evaluation techniques are not sufficient to produce quality teachers. New criteria of assessment must be established and should include such factors as: (1) comprehensive testing to ascertain mastery of both general and specific knowledge as well as teacher-education objectives, (2) performance testing based on teaching task analysis, and (3) internship to develop teaching skills.

The prospective teacher should be ''field oriented'' with much of his or her four years spent in school or doing school-related tasks. During undergraduate years, the individual should have experience in grading papers, keeping records, individual tutoring, and actual classroom teaching. The teacher who has graduated from such a program and has satisfied the assessment criteria previously mentioned will be a better teacher and will also have an easier and more enjoyable adjustment to the first few years of teaching.

Performance based teacher education

The trend today, as has been pointed out earlier in this text, is toward performance based teacher education. Under this plan the prospective teacher is evaluated, not in terms of courses taken, but in regard to certain competencies (skills, knowledge, abilities) that have been determined as essential to doing a satisfactory job of teaching. The prospective teacher is evaluated by scientific assessment techniques, and the stress is on his or her performance. A major consideration is whether this prospective teacher can change student behavior through his or her teaching.

EVALUATING SCHOOL AND COLLEGE HEALTH PROGRAM ADMINISTRATION

Evaluation of the school or college health program represents a major undertaking.

Checklists and other forms have been developed to rate the health instruction, health services, and healthful school or college environment aspects of the total program.

To give the reader a clearer understanding of what a checklist for health education is like, a very abbreviated one developed in the state of Colorado is included below.

Other means of evaluating school and college health programs that have been utilized in addition to checklists and score cards in various parts of the nation are *questionnaires* that have been developed and sent to parents, students, and other individuals; *surveys* of interested groups of people; *expert evaluations* by authorities, such as sanitarians or curriculum specialists; *analysis of health records; tests and inventories;* and *interviews and conferences.*

Evaluation is a continuous process to determine if the program is accomplishing the purposes for which it exists.

Johns* points out an evaluation experience with selected schools and colleges in the Los Angeles area where there was a concerted effort to determine the answers to such ques-

tions as: How good is the school health program? How well is it being carried out? How well does it compare to what should be done? Evaluations were carried out through self-appraisal as well as by outside consultants and resource persons. Three approaches to evaluation were utilized: (1) appraisals of the health education program, (2) appraisals of behavior changes in pupils as a result of exposure to the program, and (3) appraisals of the process of evaluation. Such procedures were followed as formulating, classifying, defining, and suggesting situations in which the achievement of objectives could be evaluated, tryout of different evaluation methods, developing and evaluating appraisal methods, and interpreting results in light of a more effective health program. A handicapping condition in the study was the lack of available valid appraisal instruments for the total health program. The findings of this study were used to justify the significance of health education in the curriculum.

---

*Johns, E.: An example of a modern evaluation plan, Journal of School Health **32:**5, 1962.

CHECKLIST FOR HEALTH EDUCATION*

	Yes	No
1. *Sanitary, safe, and wholesome environment*		
a. Are the state-approved medical certificates required for all personnel?	_____	_____
b. Is there a written plan for first-aid care of illness and accidents?	_____	_____
c. Do the buildings and grounds meet state or local sanitary standards?	_____	_____
d. Are cases of communicable disease detected and excluded promptly according to state policy?	_____	_____
e. Are the state policies for busses being followed?	_____	_____
f. Are the state policies for lunchrooms being followed?	_____	_____
2. *Graded health and safety education*		
a. Is there a written plan of health instruction throughout all the grades?	_____	_____
b. Is physical education a regular part of the program for all pupils?	_____	_____
c. Are pupils prepared to understand the health services offered in the school and community?	_____	_____
d. Are first-aid courses offered in the high school?	_____	_____
3. *Detection of health problems that may diminish effectiveness of the educational program*		
a. Is vision of all pupils periodically checked?	_____	_____
b. Is hearing of all pupils regularly checked?	_____	_____
c. Are you using the new state bulletin on testing vision and hearing?	_____	_____

*From the Colorado Education Association's Journal, October, 1956.

CHECKLIST FOR HEALTH EDUCATION—cont'd

	Yes	No
d. Is attention paid to periodic growth measurements?		
e. Are children screened regularly for dental health?		
f. Are medical evaluations of all pupils made peridocially?		
g. Are cumulative health records maintained on all pupils?		

4. *Guidance on these health problems of individual pupils, including counsel with parents and others*
   a. Is professional follow-up given to known health problems?
   b. Are the community health facilities known and used?
   c. Are these community facilities adequate for pupil needs?
5. *Special facilities for physically, mentally, and emotionally exceptional children who are educable*
   a. Are these pupils accurately classified for their learning potential?
   b. Are special programs available for all exceptional children?

Such an experiment has implications, it seems, for other schools and colleges throughout the United States.

Following is a list of pertinent questions compiled by Smolensky and Bonvechio to evaluate the total school health program:

School health and safety education

1. Which curriculum areas should be emphasized at the various grade levels?
2. What are the most significant present, future, and contemplated health and safety needs of the school-age population?
3. Where and how does health and safety instruction best fit into the crowded school curriculum?
4. What should be the scope and sequence of the health and safety units in the curriculum?
5. What experiences are most conducive to developing health-educated pupils and communities?
6. How can health instruction be best integrated through experiences in the school environment?
7. How can health services be made educational in nature and scope?
8. What instructional techniques and materials are needed?
9. How can in-service staff education be practically accomplished?

School health services

1. How can health appraisal of pupil and school personnel best be accomplished?
2. What is the most effective way to counsel pupils, parents, teachers, and others in interpreting the findings of health appraisal?
3. What can be done to encourage the correction of remediable health defects in children?
4. What is the most effective way to identify, health educate, and generally educate handicapped children?
5. How can the school best control and prevent the spread of disease?
6. What kinds of service, policies, and procedures best meet the needs for emergency services for school children?
7. How can school health service be made educational in nature?
8. What are the responsibilities of the home, school, family physicians, and public health organization for health services?
9. What is the most effective way to ensure communication and coordination between all persons and groups interested in improving child health?
10. Are the duties of the school health team well defined?

Healthful school living (environment)

1. Are all educational programs of the school contributing to the health and safety of the pupils and school employees?
2. Do school administrative policies and procedures contribute to the physical and emotional health of pupils, teachers, and school employees?
3. Is the school's physical and emotional environment conducive to effective learning?
4. Is the school lunch program contributing to nutritional education and good nutrition?
5. How can school sanitation be best maintained, improved, and promoted?
6. Are regular and continuous sanitary inspections made by qualified personnel?

Administration

1. Does the school administrator help to formulate, clarify, and evaluate the goals of the school health program?
2. Does the school administrator coordinate the efforts of all school personnel who work in the school health program?
3. Does he (school administrator) assign the most qualified

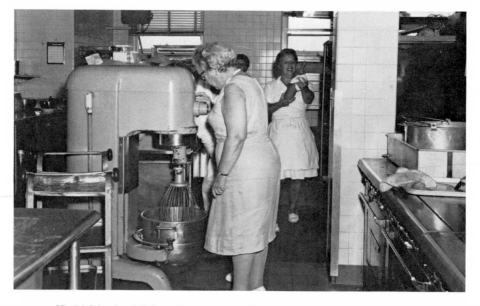

Healthful school living. (Mamaroneck High School, Mamaroneck, N. Y.)

personnel to the various tasks in the school health program?

4. Does the school make the best possible use of local health resources?
5. Does he (school administrator) adapt the school health program to local needs and interests?
6. Does he (school administrator) motivate others in the school health program through leadership?
7. Does the school have an effective school health council?
8. Does the school district have an effective school health committee?*

EVALUATING SCHOOL AND COLLEGE PHYSICAL EDUCATION PROGRAM ADMINISTRATION

Evaluation of student achievement in physical education represents only part of the evaluation responsibility. Evaluation of program administration is also important. Such phases of the program as classes, intramurals, interscholastics, intercollegiates, and adapted physical education activities should be evaluated in terms of activities, leadership, equipment, facilities, participation, records, research, and budgetary allotment.

---

*Smolensky, J., and Bonvechio, L. R.: Principles of school health, Boston, 1966, D. C. Heath & Co., pp. 101-102 As adapted from Davis, R L: Quality in school health administration, National Elementary Principal **39:**8, 1960.

The following are sample questions such as might be formulated for use in evaluation of program administration. They might either be answered with ratings of poor, fair, good, or excellent or be scored on a numerical basis of 1 to 10.

Class program

1. Does the teaching program devote equitable time to team sports, individual sports, rhythms and dance, and gymnastic activities?
2. Are the equipment and facilities adequate to allow maximum student participation?
3. Are reasonable budgetary allotments made for the class teaching program?
4. Are accurate evaluation procedures carried out and worthwhile records kept?
5. Are minimal participation requirements met by all students?
6. Are students meeting proper physical education requirements in regard to dressing and showering?
7. Are proper safety measures taken in all activities?
8. Are opportunities for developing student leadership being afforded in the class program?

Adapted program

1. Do adequate screening procedures determine all possible participants in this program?
2. Are adequate facilities, equipment, time, and space made available to the program?
3. Are proper supervision and instruction afforded each individual participant?

4. Is medical approval obtained for each individual's regimen of activity?
5. Do participants engage in some of the regular class work, as well as remedial classes, when advisable?
6. Are careful records and progress notes kept on each student?
7. Is the financial allotment to the program adequate?
8. Does student achievement indicate the value of the program?

Intramural and extramural programs

1. Are intramural and extramural sports offered to all students in as many activities as possible?
2. Has participation in these programs increased during the past year?
3. Is maximum coaching supervision available to players?
4. Is adequate financial assistance given to this phase of the program?
5. Are accurate records maintained concerning the participants, their honors, awards, and electives?
6. Does the reward or points system emphasize the joys of participation rather than stress the value of the reward?
7. Is equipment well cared for and properly stored to gain the most use from it?
8. Are competitive experiences wholesome and worthwhile for all participants?

Interscholastic program

1. Is financial support for this program provided by the physical education budget?
2. Is there equitable financial support for all sports in the interscholastic or intercollegiate program?
3. Are interscholastic and intercollegiate sports available to all students, boys and girls alike?
4. Are adequate health students being met in respect to amount of practices, number of games, fitness of participants, and type of competition?
5. Is competition provided by schools and colleges of a similar size?
6. Is the program justifiable as an important educational tool?
7. Are academic standards for participants maintained?
8. Are good public relations with the community furthered through this program?

Administration

1. Is the teaching staff well qualified and capable of carrying out the program?
2. Is the program run efficiently with little loss of teaching time or space, and is maximum use made of facilities?
3. Are professional standards maintained as to class size and teacher assignment?
4. Is the departmental organization on a democratic basis, with all members sharing in the decisions?
5. Do members of the staff have a professional outlook, attend professional meetings, and keep up with the latest developments in the field?
6. In what areas have scientific tests and research been made for contribution to the profession?*

These sample questions represent only a few that can be used in the evaluation process. The key to successful evaluation of this type lies in the followup steps taken for improvement.

CHECKLIST OF SELECTIVE ITEMS FOR EVALUATING A PHYSICAL EDUCATION PROGRAM'S RELEVANCE TO THE MODERN SCHOOL

At the present time many changes are taking place in education, as well as in physical education, in the schools of this country. These changes mean that the administration of education and physical education programs must also change if it is to be relevant to what is happening in our society. In order to aid the administrator in evaluating his or her program on its relevance to the changes that are occurring in education today, a checklist of selected items

---

*Bucher, C. A., and Koenig, C.: Methods and materials for secondary school physical education, ed. 4, St. Louis, 1974, The C. V. Mosby Co.

CHECKLIST OF SELECTIVE ITEMS FOR EVALUATING A PHYSICAL EDUCATION PROGRAM'S RELEVANCY TO THE MODERN SCHOOL

Educational philosophy	*Yes*	*No*
1. The educational philosophy of the school encourages innovation.		
2. Close school-community relationships are encouraged.		
3. The educational program is relevant to the times and to society.		
4. Faculty and students are actively involved in the total educational process.		
5. Education is individualized for each student, including the culturally disadvantaged, physically handicapped, mentally retarded, and other atypical conditions.		

Continued.

CHECKLIST OF SELECTIVE ITEMS FOR EVALUATING A PHYSICAL EDUCATION PROGRAM'S RELEVANCY TO THE MODERN SCHOOL—cont'd

Educational philosophy—cont'd   *Yes*   *No*

6. The worth of a physical education program is recognized and supported.   _____   _____
7. A clear written statement of educational philosophy exists with general education and physical education objectives enumerated.   _____   _____

Administration

1. The administration represents a means to an end—an excellent educational program—rather than an end in itself.   _____   _____
2. The administrative structure enhances the implementation of the educational program.   _____   _____
3. The school, including the physical education program, has a meaningful and accurate system of keeping records.   _____   _____
4. The school and physical education records are accurate and up to date.   _____   _____
5. The school is open to the community.   _____   _____
6. The school utilizes community resources.   _____   _____
7. Adequate facilities, supplies, and equipment exist.   _____   _____
8. Equipment and supplies are checked periodically to ensure they are in good condition and that adequate amounts are readily available as needed.   _____   _____
9. The school building is utilized to its maximum potential.   _____   _____
10. Facilities are designed to meet program needs, permit effective instruction, and ensure pupil safety.   _____   _____
11. School facilities are utilized on a 12-month basis.   _____   _____
12. Sufficient teaching stations exist to carry on a meaningful physical education program.   _____   _____
13. The administration of the school and physical education department is carried out in a democratic manner.   _____   _____
14. Meetings are held regularly with the faculty to share new ideas and methods and discuss common problems.   _____   _____
15. Students have representation at important administrative and faculty meetings.   _____   _____
16. The administration is receptive to innovative teaching techniques.   _____   _____
17. Channels of communication are readily available to faculty and students.   _____   _____
18. Faculty and students play an important role in decision making and policy formation.   _____   _____
19. The community is kept informed of educational objectives.   _____   _____
20. The administration understands the needs of physical education and its contribution to the achievement of educational goals.   _____   _____
21. Office practice is efficient and represents a valuable service in carrying out educational objectives.   _____   _____
22. Scheduling is done in an effective and modern manner, including the utilization of flexible scheduling.   _____   _____

Students

1. The students play a role in curriculum planning.   _____   _____
2. The students are given an opportunity to evaluate the physical education and other school programs.   _____   _____
3. The students are assigned to physical education classes on the basis of their physical development, needs, and achievement.   _____   _____
4. The students pursue a program that meets their individual needs.   _____   _____
5. The students are properly grouped for each activity.   _____   _____
6. The students find school and physical education a pleasurable and worthwhile experience.   _____   _____
7. The students have a good rapport with their teachers.   _____   _____
8. The students have an opportunity to develop their leadership potential.   _____   _____
9. The students are permitted to pursue individual dress and hair styles providing they do not interfere with the rights of others and are not a deterrent to their health, safety, and performance in school activities.   _____   _____

CHECKLIST OF SELECTIVE ITEMS FOR EVALUATING A PHYSICAL EDUCATION PROGRAM'S RELEVANCY TO THE MODERN SCHOOL—cont'd

Teachers	Yes	No
1. Teaching assignments are made with regard to a teacher's interests, strengths, and experience.	___	___
2. Teachers are given the opportunity to experiment with new teaching methods and materials.	___	___
3. The beginning teacher is provided with proper orientation to school and to the role he or she will play in that school.	___	___
4. Teachers are evaluated objectively with a view to improving their teaching ability and service to students.	___	___
5. Teachers are accountable for outstanding teaching and service to students.	___	___
6. Teachers are paid according to the role they play in the educational process.	___	___
7. Teachers attend faculty meetings regularly.	___	___
8. Teachers provide leadership for the community in their specialty.	___	___
9. Teachers have excellent relationships with students.	___	___
10. Teachers utilize student leaders and paraprofessionals in order to develop leadership qualities in boys and girls and in order that they may devote more time to teaching and serving students.	___	___
11. Teachers are creative.	___	___
12. Teachers keep up to date with new developments in their special field.	___	___
13. Teachers work closely and harmoniously with other members of the faculty.	___	___
14. Teachers are active professionally.	___	___

Physical education program

	Yes	No
1. Innovative ideas are utilized.	___	___
2. Students participate in the development and the evaluation of the program.	___	___
3. Classes are of sufficient length to permit meaningful participation in scheduled activities.	___	___
4. The intramural program provides for the maximum participation of all students.	___	___
5. Transportation is provided for athletic events.	___	___
6. A close working relationship exists between the physical education and health education programs.	___	___
7. Provision is made for individual differences of students.	___	___
8. The program is progressive in nature with a smooth transition existing between elementary and junior high school and between junior high school and senior high school.	___	___
9. The physical education program represents an integral part of the total educational offering.	___	___
10. The physical education program is evaluated periodically with necessary changes being made as indicated by the evaluation.	___	___
11. The physical education program is relevant to the times, society, the student, and the role of education in present-day America.	___	___

is presented on the following pages. How does your program rate?

Questions and exercises

1. Survey five teachers to determine what they think constitutes the most objective method of evaluation of their performance on the job.
2. Should teachers of health education and of physical education be evaluated in the same way? Why? Why not?
3. What contributions can evaluation make to helping the teacher grow professionally?
4. Discuss teacher accountability in terms of how it can best be assessed.
5. Explain the concept of student evaluations and write a student evaluation instrument that you might give to students in a class you were teaching. Have the instrument include both program and teacher evaluation questions.
6. You are responsible for evaluating a school health program and/or a school physical education program.

Select the instrument for evaluation, conduct the evaluation, and report to the class on your findings.

7. What areas of school health and physical education programs, according to your observation and evaluation, need the most professional upgrading?

Reading assignment on *Administrative Dimensions of Health and Physical Education Programs, Including Athletics:* Chapter 18, Selections 94 to 97.

Selected references

Billet, R. E.: Evaluation: the golden fleece, New York State Education **55:**42, 1968.

Brian, G.: Evaluating teacher effectiveness, National Education Association Journal **54:**2, 1965.

Bucher, C. A., and Koenig, C.: Methods and materials for secondary school physical education, ed. 4, St. Louis, 1974, The C. V. Mosby Co.

Caldwell, S. F.: Evaluation in the elementary physical education program, The Physical Educator **22:**153, 1965.

California State Department of Education: Criteria for evaluating the elementary health program, Sacramento, 1962, The Department.

Fawcett, C. W.: School personnel administration, New York, 1964, The Macmillan Co.

Field, D.: Accountability for the physical educator, Journal of Health, Physical Education, and Recreation **44:**37, 1973.

Fisher, M.: Assessing the competence of prospective physical education teachers, The Physical Educator **29:**93, 1972.

Goldman, S.: The school principal, New York, 1966, The Center for Applied Research in Education, Inc. (The Library of Education).

Howsam, R. B.: Facts and folklore of teacher evaluation, The Education Digest **29:**7, 1964.

Johns, E.: An example of a modern evaluation plan, Journal of School Health **32:**5, 1962.

Jornat, L.: Self-appraisal check list for physical education teachers in high school, The Physical Educator **27:**160, 1970.

La Grand, L.: Better teaching through student evaluation, The Physical Educator **28:**201, 1971.

La Porte, W. A.: Health and physical education scorecard no. 1 and no. 2, College Book Store, 3413 S. Hoover Blvd., Los Angeles, Calif. 90056.

Little, M.: Evaluation of the teacher trainee in the health education methods course **30:**12, 1973.

Malone, W. C.: A checklist for evaluating coaches, Coach & Athlete **29:**3, 1966.

Michigan School Health Association: Appraisal form for studying school health programs, 1962, The Association.

National Education Association: Methods of evaluating teachers, National Education Association Research Bulletin **43:**1, 1965.

National Education Association: What teachers and administrators think about evaluation, National Education Association Research Bulletin **42:**4, 1964.

Roundy, E. S.: Are our physical education programs meeting todays needs? Journal of Secondary Education **41:**221, 1966.

Simpson, R. H., and Seidman, J. M.: Student evaluation of teaching and learning, Washington, 1962, American Association of Colleges for Teacher Education.

Vander Werf, L. S.: How to evaluate teachers and teaching, New York, 1960, Holt, Rinehart & Winston, Inc.

PART FIVE

Administration of recreation, club, environmental education, and camping programs

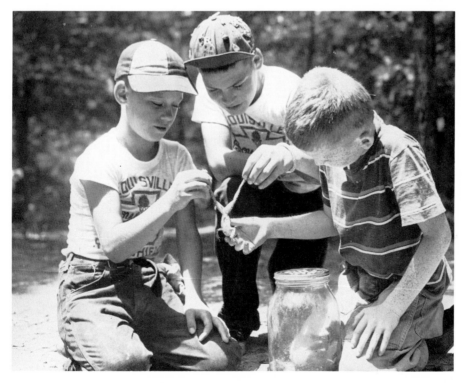

Louisville, Ky., City Division of Recreation.

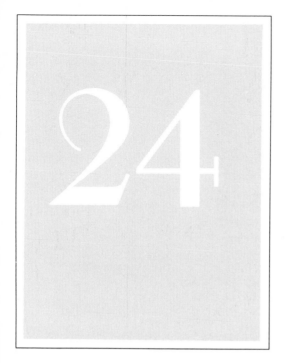

Community and school recreation, club, and activity programs

It has been estimated that the American worker has an average of 675 hours of free time annually. This does not include vacation time. When this is added, the net gain of free time is close to 800 hours annually or roughly 1 month out of every twelve.* With this much free time it is essential that recreation programs are developed to help people to fully enjoy their leisure hours in a constructive manner.

Recreation may be defined as that field of endeavor concerned with those socially acceptable and worthwhile activities in which a person voluntarily participates during leisure hours and through which he or she may better develop physically, mentally, emotionally, and socially.

The key concepts of any form of recreation advocated here are five in number. First, the activity must be conducted in hours other than work. It is a *leisure-time activity*. The activity must not be associated with productive labor that is aimed at profit or that is a regular part of one's daily routine as a means of making a living. Second, recreation is an *enjoyable activity*. It is something from which one gains

satisfaction, serenity, and happiness. Third, recreation is *constructive* in nature—it is *wholesome*. A person could become inebriated every night and say it is recreation. However, this is not the kind of recreation that is recommended. Recreation should do something to contribute to the individual's physical, mental, emotional, or social welfare. Fourth, recreation is *nonsurvival in nature*. Therefore, such things as sleep cannot be labeled as forms of recreation in the sense that it is discussed in this chapter. Finally, recreation is *voluntary*. The person engages in the activity because he or she has chosen to participate. There has been no compulsion. The choice has been made freely. These five criteria or concepts must be satisfied to be considered the type of recreation that this text is advocating for the benefit of people everywhere.

TYPES OF RECREATION

Some of the better-known kinds of recreation are community, industrial, hospital, school, family, and commercial. The kinds of recreation that will be considered primarily in this chapter are those concerned with community and school recreation.

Community recreation. Community recreation is that in which villages, towns, and cities sponsor a recreation program for their inhabitants. It is controlled, financed, and administered by the community.

---

*Hodgson, J. D.: Leisure and the American worker, Journal of Health, Physical Education, and Recreation **43**:38, 1972.

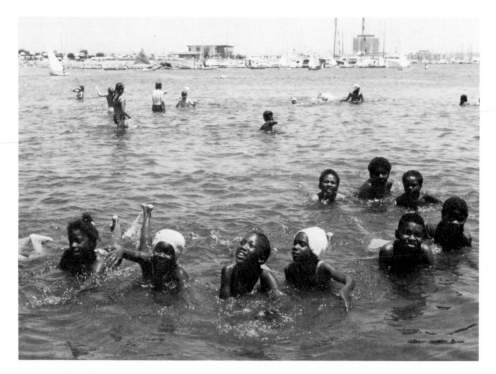

Inner-city youth in Los Angeles enjoy and benefit from recreational experiences. (Courtesy Youth Services Section, Los Angeles City Schools.)

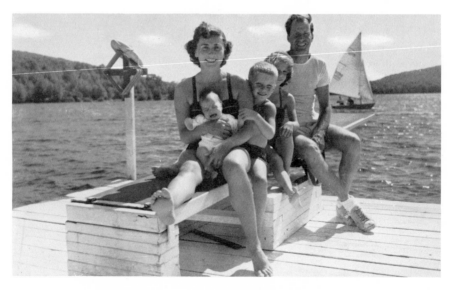

There is insufficient stress on family recreation today.

Industrial recreation. Industrial recreation is the type wherein an industrial concern or other business establishment, sponsors a recreation program for its own employees.

Hospital recreation. Hospital recreation refers to a program that is set up in a veterans, municipal, or other hospital for the benefit of the patients. It includes recreation for the ill and disabled. The therapeutic values of recreation are increasingly being recognized.

School recreation. School recreation refers to the program provided by a board of education for the students that attend a particular school system. Boards of education also provide recreation programs for the adult population of a community.

Family recreation. Family recreation means the activities that are engaged in by a family unit during their leisure hours and that have resulted from their own initiative.

Commercial recreation. Commercial recreation is the form of recreation that is found at amusement parks and that is conducted for profit.

GOALS OF RECREATION

Community recreation is a field of endeavor that deserves increasing recognition for the work that it is doing in enriching individual lives. The goals reflect this contribution. Many goals have been listed for the field of recreation. Some of those that have received attention are the following: physical, cognitive, emotional, and social health; happiness; satisfaction; balanced growth; creativeness; competition; learning; citizenship; socialization; and the development of one's talents.

Following are six goals for American recreation that have been stated by The Commission on Goals for American Recreation.* They represent one of the best professional statements on recreational goals.

1. *Personal fulfillment.* The democratic ideal is based on the concept that the individual is the most important consideration in society. To achieve one's place in our culture, each

---

*The Commission on Goals for American Recreation: Goals for American recreation, Washington, D. C., 1964, American Association for Health, Physical Education, and Recreation.

person needs to fulfill the basic need for adequacy or self-fulfillment. Each person wants to belong and to feel important. Each person should strive to become all that he or she is capable of becoming. Therefore, recreation should help each person to achieve full integration of total personality; contribute to mental, physical, social, and emotional development; and help to fill in the gaps that work and on-the-job activity do not provide. The many activities offered through a well-organized recreation program can contribute to the self-fulfillment of each person who participates.

2. *Democratic human relations.* The democratic society functions best through associated effort directed and channeled toward the accomplishments of those goals that are in the best interests of the majority. The recreation profession recognizes that its goals exist on the level of the individual as well as on the level of the democratic society of which it is a part. Recreation, therefore, constantly keeps in mind such important tenets as (a) each individual has worth and each personality must be respected, (b) the citizen in a democracy cooperates for the common good, (c) the citizen abides by the laws—rules that have been established to guard each individual's rights, and (d) the citizen living in a democracy guides his or her behavior by acceptable moral and ethical values.

3. *Leisure skills and interests.* Recreation is concerned with meeting the interests of those people who voluntarily participate in its programs, developing skills that will provide the incentive, motivation, and medium for spending free time in a constructive and worthwhile manner. As such, recreation must be concerned with a breadth and variety of interests, ranging from physical activities, social activities, and artistic activities to community service programs and learning activities.

4. *Health and fitness.* Recreation is cognizant of the nature of many individuals who live a sedentary existence with the implications this has for poor health and fitness. It also recognizes the importance of a vigorous and active life and seeks to meet the challenge of a society in which mental illness, stress, and inactivity prevail in many quarters.

5. *Creative expression and esthetic appreciation*. There is increased realization today of the need for each individual to give vent to personal expression, to creativity, and to the appreciation of the most beautiful and cultured activities in the various cultures of the world. Recreation seeks to contribute to each individual's desire for creative expression and esthetic appreciation by providing the environment, leadership, materials, and motivation for such experiences, recognizing that creativity can flourish only in a climate that has been properly prepared for its development and growth.

6. *Environment for living in a leisure society*. Recreation recognizes that the environment plays an important role in the determination of the quality and extent of the recreative experience. Therefore, recreation is particularly interested in preserving our natural resources; in the construction of parks, playgrounds, hobby centers, and other recreation centers; in seeing that recreation programs are taken into consideration in city planning; and in awakening the populace to the need for an appreciation of esthetic and cultural values.

Four objectives I have formulated for the recreation profession are:

1. *The health development objective*. The health development objective is important in the field of recreation. Health to a great degree is

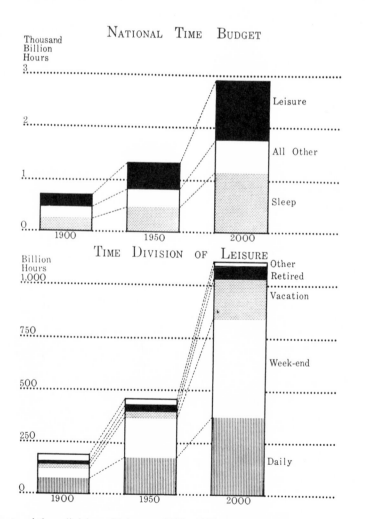

National time budget and time division of leisure—1900, 1950, and 2000. (From The American Academy of Political and Social Science: Leisure in America: blessing or curse? Philadelphia, 1964, The Academy.)

related to activity during leisure hours as well as during hours of work. The manner in which a person spends free time determines in great measure whether his or her physical, mental, emotional, and spiritual health is of high quality. Through recreation, adaptive physical activity is available that is conducive to organic, mental, emotional, and spiritual health. A range of activities exists that offers opportunities for every individual to promote his or her organic health. Activities are available in which the individual may relax, escape from the tensions of work, forget about problems, and thereby improve mental health. Activities are planned and conducted that provide individual enjoyment and pleasure and in this way contribute to emotional health. Activities requiring the participation of many individuals are included and are conducive to better social relations and higher standards of moral and spiritual values, thus promoting spiritual health. Public recreation programs are designed to provide activities that counteract the deteriorating effects of strenuous or routine work or study and thus comple-

ment the overall routine that an individual follows. They overcome many of the shortages that exist when the man or woman leaves the office, the child leaves school, or the family completes the housework. In this way they contribute to the integration and development of the whole individual.

2. *The human relations objective.* The human relations objective represents a major contribution of recreation to enriched living. Recreational programs develop many individual qualities that make for better adjustment. Such attributes as courage, justice, patience, tolerance, fairness, and honesty are only a few possible to develop while individuals are playing and recreating together in the many activities that comprise the total recreation program. Attitudes that promote good human relations are also developed. Wholesome attitudes of social cooperation, loyalty to the group, recognition of the rights of others, and the idea that one receives from a group in direct proportion to what one gives it are a few concepts that make for better relations and enable worthy

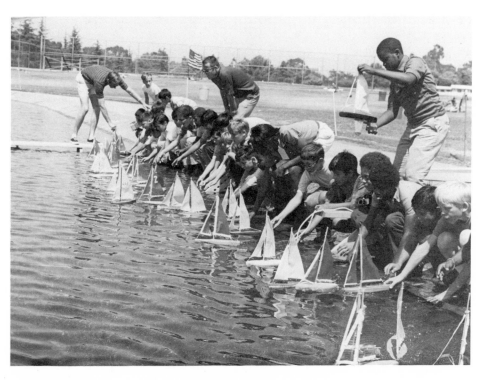

The annual regatta sponsored by the Youth Services Section, Los Angeles City Schools.

goals and projects to be accomplished. The growth of family recreation is a trend that also helps to make for a more unified home life. This is very important, since the family group represents the foundation on which good human relations are built. Furthermore, to develop good social traits, it is necessary to bring people together in a situation in which there is a feeling of belonging and in which each individual is recognized. There are innumerable opportunities for such interaction in the many recreational programs that exist throughout the country.

3. *The civic development objective.* The civic development objective is a noteworthy goal for recreation. Recreation contributes in many ways to the development of any community. It contributes to community solidarity by uniting people in common projects regardless of race, creed, economic status, or other discriminatory factors. It helps to build the morale of the members of the community. It is a contributing factor in alleviating crime since it provides settings and activities in which youth and other individuals may engage in constructive, worthwhile activities, rather than in destructive antisocial activities. It helps make the community a safer place in which to live through providing adequate playgrounds and other recreational centers that keep children and youth off the streets. It helps make the community more prosperous by contributing to the health of the individual, by cutting down on the dollar appropriation for crime, and by increasing the total work output of an individual. It helps the growth and development of the individual so that he or she becomes a more valuable citizen in the community and has more to contribute in its behalf.

4. *The self-development objective.* The self-development objective refers to the potentialities that participation in a program of recreational activities has for developing the individual to his or her capacity. Recreation does this through a variety of means. It contributes to the balanced growth of an individual. It allows for growth in ways other than in mere production of material things for utilitarian purposes. In other words, it satisfies the human desire for such things as creative music, art, literature, and drama. It allows an individual

to create things not for their material value but for the joy, satisfaction, and happiness that go with creating something through one's own efforts. It allows for the development of latent and dormant skills and abilities of the individual until they are aroused by leisure hours with proper settings and leadership. These skills help to make a better-integrated individual.

Recreation provides an avenue for the individual to experience joy and happiness through some activity in which he or she has the desire to engage. In this chaotic world where there are so many sorrows, heartbreaks, and frowns, it is essential for people to revitalize themselves through the medium of activities. These provide smiles and hearty laughs and release from the tension associated with day-to-day routine. They afford a place for many individuals to excel. Such an urge is many times not satisfied in one's regular job or profession. An opportunity is provided in recreation to satisfy this desire. It offers an educational experience. The participant learns new skills, new knowledge, new techniques, and develops new abilities.

TRENDS IN RECREATION

Innovations in recreation are happening all around us. The area of recreation is still in its early stages, and there are many concepts that must be tried and evaluated. Some innovations in this field are discussed in the following paragraphs.

Urban recreation

Urban recreation has a great challenge to meet. Inner-city areas are rapidly decaying, and there is a desperate need for excellence in recreation programs. In many inner-city areas, the community has responded to its recreational needs through such diverse programs as mobile recreation units and local recreation centers.

A recent survey* was taken of recreation and park administrators in eight major cities— Atlanta, Boston, Chicago, Detroit, Los Angeles, Philadelphia, San Francisco, and Washington, D. C.—and in 45 other cities with populations of over 150,000. The purpose of the

---

*Kraus, R.: Today's crisis in urban recreation, Journal of Health, Physical Education, and Recreation **44**:29, 1973.

survey was to determine how these cities have responded to the urban crises in recreation.

The results of this survey indicated that these urban areas had suffered from budget cutbacks. There was a marked decrease in new recreational facilities and in many cases there were freezes on hiring additional personnel. Other problems cited included: crime, vandalism, racial disconduct, and proverty.

Among the cities surveyed, some noted that additional financial aid was obtained through federal grants, special funding, and industrial sources. Programs had been introduced to develop ethnic or racial interests. Mobile recreation vans could easily move a swimming pool or small gymnasium into a given area. These vans also brought cultural programs such as drama, dance, and puppet shows. Youth programs attacking such problems as drug abuse and crime also become a part of the recreation program.

It was found that many cities were making an effort to hire more minority group workers in their programs and to have greater community involvement. Neighborhood centers were preferred to develop greater local participation, but city facilities were also used in certain phases of the program.

Community recreation programs

Community recreation programs are continuously growing. Many communities have year-round programs for persons of all ages that include: adult education classes, fitness programs, swimming pool—tennis court complexes, camp programs for children, and summer recreation programs for all residents.

An interesting 8-week summer program was recently conducted in Little Falls, New York. This city has a population of 8,000 people. Some of the events of the program included: (1) a trip to the Cooperstown Baseball Hall of Fame; (2) a trip to Yankee Stadium; (3) a trip to Mac Arthur Stadium in Syracuse, New York; (4) attendance at carnivals; (5) gymnasium activity days; and (6) full day programs that included an art festival, bike races, a field day, citywide picnic, and an all-city swimming meet.

Programs like the one described help the school and community to have a better understanding of each other. In addition, family recreation is also aided by the number of activities in which all age groups can participate.

Colleges can also participate in community recreation as recently exhibited by the physical education department of Brookdale Community College in Monmouth County, New Jersey. This college sponsored adult fitness programs, community athletic programs, and walk-in recreation activities where an individual could utilize certain facilities on a drop-in basis during the day. The implementation of such programs is invaluable to the community and enhances community-college relations.

Commercial recreation programs

Commercial recreation has grown rapidly in recent years. Such recreation attractions as Disneyland, Disney World, Sea World, and Cypress Gardens attract millions of visitors each year. The advantages of such attractions are numerous and include such factors as numerous recreational activities located in one central area, good weather and excellent locations, and an increase of tourism within the state where the complex is operated. However, there are certain disadvantages. Because of the energy crisis, many people have been unable to drive their cars to these recreation areas, money-tightening has reduced attendance, and frequently the local ecology has been disrupted.

GUIDING PRINCIPLES FOR PLANNING RECREATION PROGRAMS

Recreation programs should not be developed on a "hit-or-miss' basis. Instead, outstanding leaders in recreation have studied very thoroughly and carefully the types of programs that best serve the needs of people and have developed principles that can be used as guides for leaders who are engaged in program planning.

Brightbill* set forth his program principles, which, in adapted form, are as follows:

1. Individual interests, characteristics, needs, and capabilities should be taken into con-

---

*Langton, C. V., Duncan, R. O., and Brightbill, C. K.: Principles of health, physical education, and recreation, New York, 1962, The Ronald Press Co., pp. 251-261.

sideration in the planning of recreation programs.

2. The recreational interests and skills of individuals may be determined to some degree as a result of the cultural, economic, religious, and social phenomena that characterize them.

3. Recreation should be planned cooperatively, with the recreator taking into consideration interested individuals, departments, agencies, and organizations.

4. Program planning requires consideration of national standards modified to local conditions.

5. Program planning should take into consideration individual differences in skills and the progressive planning of skill experiences.

6. Creativity and self-expression are considerations in program planning.

7. Opportunities should be made available for individuals to be of service to others so that the personal satisfaction that comes from such service can be realized by such persons.

8. Recreation programs should provide for a wide spectrum of activities.

9. Leadership, financial means, and facilities are essential considerations in program planning.

10. Physical and human resources of the community should be mobilized for the recreation program.

11. The recreation program should seek to provide equality of opportunity for participation for all persons in the community.

12. Flexibility should be possible within a recreation program to provide for such exigencies as changed interests on the part of human beings and other conditions that affect program planning.

13. The health and safety of participants should always be a consideration in planning recreation programs.

14. The recreation program should seek to help each person exemplify acceptable standards of human behavior.

15. The participant in the recreation program should never be exploited for such means as raising money, personal glory, or other similar motives.

16. Recreation should be the object of continual evaluation to determine the measure to which the worthwhile goals are being achieved in light of the investment being made.

Brightbill's goals reflect recreation programs in general, with particular consideration for community recreation. The following principles developed for school recreation by a national conference of experts in this area* are much the same as those established by Brightbill:

1. The recreation program should be characterized by many different activities that are related to the needs and interests of the people they serve.

2. The welfare of the individual and group should be continually kept in mind when planning the recreation program.

3. The program should be planned so that each individual can realize some of the goals that have been established for recreation.

4. Opportunities should be provided for individuals to participate in the planning of the program. Also, the program should be adapted to local conditions.

5. The recreation program should take into consideration community mores and folkways.

RECREATION ACTIVITIES

The range of recreation activities is infinite in scope. Any activity that meets the criteria listed earlier in the chapter can be a recreational activity. This means that drama, music, art, crafts, games, sports, camping, literature, fairs, nature study, dance, and community work are possible avenues for millions of people to obtain the benefits that recreation can offer.

A list of a few of the possible activities for recreation purposes follows:

Arts and crafts	*Outdoor activities*
Ceramics	Campfires
Graphic arts	Camping
Leathercraft	Canoeing
Metalcraft	Conservation
Photography	Fishing
Plastics	Orienteering
Sewing	Outdoor cooking
Stenciling and block printing	Woodcraft

---

*National Conference on School Recreation: School recreation, Washington, D. C., 1960, American Association for Health, Physical Education, and Recreation.

Sports and games
  Archery
  Badminton
  Bowling
  Fencing
  Golf
  Hopscotch

Dramatics
  Clubs
  Festivals
  Plays

Dancing
  Folk

  Modern
  Social
  Square

Music
  Barber shop quartets
  Choral groups
  Community sings
  Instrumental
  Orchestral

Miscellaneous
  Cards
  Flowers
  Forums
  Hobby clubs

RECREATION AGENCIES

There are three major types of recreation agencies in the United States: (1) public recreation agencies, (2) private or voluntary agencies, and (3) commercial agencies. Some examples of each type are listed:

1. Public recreation agencies
   a. Municipal public agencies—the park department, recreation department, youth commission, education department, and other city or community departments that operate recreation programs
   b. State public agencies—state park departments, state conservation departments, and state education departments
   c. Federal public agencies—national parks, Forestry Service, Children's Bureau, Fish and Wild Life Service, and Tennessee Valley Authority
2. Private or voluntary agencies
   a. Youth-serving organizations—Boys' Clubs of America, Young Men's Christian Associations, Young Women's Christian Associations, Campfire Girls, Boy Scouts, and church centers
   b. Organizations serving an entire population—museums, libraries, athletic clubs, outdoor clubs, and granges
   c. Private voluntary agencies organized around special interests of certain groups—music specialties, photographic specialties, and sports specialties
3. Commercial agencies (operated for profit)— theaters, bowling alleys, art galleries, night clubs, and concert halls

National Recreation and Park Association

A major development in the field of recreation was the unification of five of the national organizations serving laymen and professional recreation. The American Institute of Park Executives, the American Recreation Society, the American Zoological Association, the National Council of State Parks, and the National Recreation Association were merged into a unified national organization known as the *National Recreation and Park Association.* Lawrence S. Rockefeller was elected as the first president of this association. The merger was designed to bring together a single organization supported by private citizens and professional groups and dedicated to helping all Americans to devote their free time to constructive and satisfying activities.

WAYS IN WHICH RECREATION PROGRAMS ARE ADMINISTERED

Recreation programs are not all administered in the same manner in this country. Government agencies, schools, business, and voluntary agencies play a role in many communities. Jenny* has listed five major types of administration of recreation programs in the United States that apply to community recreation.

The recreation board. A recreation board can be set up in any community where enabling legislation exists and permits such action. The board usually consists of five to nine members. The group is frequently composed of representatives of the city government, the school district, the recreation or park department, and the community at large. Terms of office usually run for varying periods of time depending upon the community, and the members usually serve without compensation. Members of the board are either elected or appointed to their positions.

The school board. In many communities the board of education, under a broad interpretation of its powers or under the provisions of state extension education law or enabling acts, conducts recreation programs. In some communities this responsibility is interpreted as

---

*Jenny, J. J.: Introduction to recreation education, Philadelphia, 1955, W. B. Saunders Co., pp. 31-35.

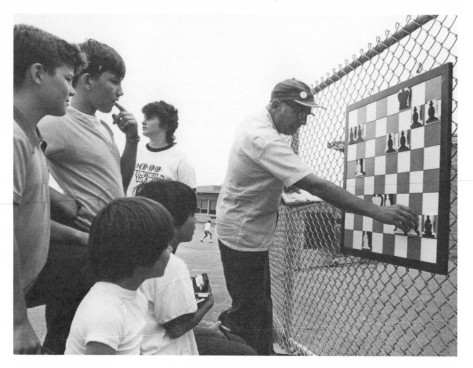

Chess as a recreational activity in Milwaukee. (Courtesy Division of Municipal Recreation and Adult Education, Milwaukee Public Schools.)

providing a program only for its children and youth, whereas other programs are provided for persons of all ages.

The park board. In such cities as Detroit and Seattle, the department of parks administers the recreation program. Since the community parks are used so extensively for recreation purposes, and to avoid duplication of facilities, budgeting, and planning, some citizens feel that the park board is the logical form of administration for community recreation programs. Those opposed to this arrangement, however, point out that recreation does not get priority under such an administrative setup.

The recreation board and the school board. In some communities the recreation board and school board cooperatively work together in administering the recreation program. The school board, for example, may provide the facilities and sometimes the funds, while the recreation board provides the personnel, equipment, and supplies. Regardless of how the responsibilities are shared, a close working relationship is developed between the two groups in providing a recreation program for the inhabitants of the particular geographic locality they serve.

The recreation association, nonprofit agency, and corporation. In villages and other communities where the park, recreation, or school board has not assumed the administration of the recreation program, sometimes recreation associations, clubs, and other organizations provide a program. The Boys' Clubs of America, Young Men's Christian Associations, and Recreation Promotion and Service Corporations are examples of this type of administrative organization. These organizations have made outstanding contributions in many communities.

THE SCHOOL AND RECREATION

The recommendations of the Second National Conference on School Recreation* included

---

*Report of the Second National Conference on School Recreation: Twentieth century recreation, re-engagement of school and community, Nov. 7-9, 1962, Washington, D. C., 1963, American Association for Health, Physical Education, and Recreation.

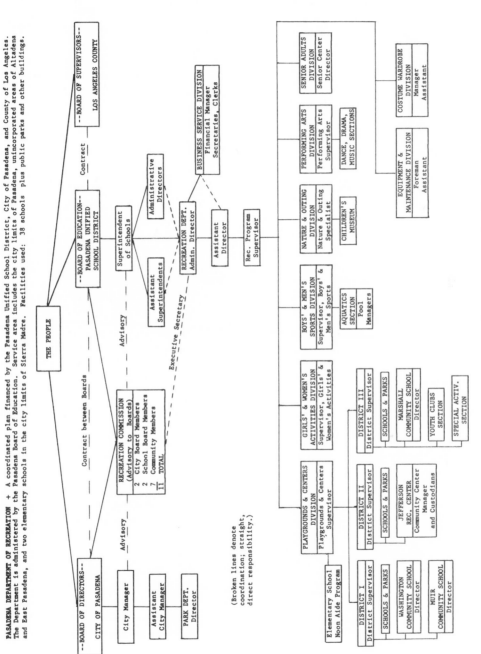

PASADENA DEPARTMENT OF RECREATION + A coordinated plan financed by the Pasadena Unified School District, City of Pasadena, and County of Los Angeles. The Department is administered by the Pasadena Board of Education. Service area includes the city limits of Pasadena, unincorporated areas of Altadena and East Pasadena, and two elementary schools in the city limits of Sierra Madre. Facilities used: 38 schools plus public parks and other buildings.

New organization chart of the Pasadena Department of Recreation, Pasadena, Calif.

setting forth a series of principles and statements regarding school-centered recreation and municipal-school recreation. These principles and statements are presented in adapted form:

Role of school

1. Schools should accept, as a major responsibility, education for leisure.

2. Schools and colleges should provide their students with opportunities for participation in wholesome, creative activities.

3. The facilities and resources of a school should be made available for recreation purposes when needed.

4. Where community recreation programs are missing or inadequate, the school should take the initiative and provide recreation programs for young and old alike.

5. The school should cooperate with community organizations and agencies interested in or sponsoring recreation programs.

6. The school should appoint a person to act as a community school director; he or she would be responsible for the recreation-education program in the school.

7. Recreation and education are not identical, but each has its own uniqueness and distinctive features.

8. The community-school director should provide inservice recreation education for his or her staff.

9. The federal level of government has a responsibility to stimulate recreation programs.

10. Recreation depends upon public understanding and support for its existence.

11. Recreation should be concerned with exploiting the interests of people.

12. The recreation program should consist of many varied activities.

13. Recreation should be concerned with contributing to the mental health of the individual.

Municipal-school recreation

1. The school should accept the responsibility to educate for the worthy use of leisure, contribute to recreation in the instructional program, mobilize community resources, and cooperatively plan facilities for recreation. The college and university should promote research

in recreation and provide professional preparation programs in this specialized area.

2. There should be joint planning of municipal school recreation based on stated principles and brought about by state departments of education and local boards of education.

3. School facilities should be available for recreational use.

Some recreation leaders have raised the question of whether or not recreation should be school centered. Hjelte and Shivers* list some arguments pro and con in respect to this issue.

School-centered recreation

The reasons that Hjelte and Shivers list *for* a school-centered program are as follows: The school possesses the facilities essential to a good recreation program, and duplicating these facilities results in waste and inefficiency. Schools are located within a community in much the same way as recreational centers are located—to meet the needs of the people within a particular geographic area. The school comes in contact with all the children and, therefore, the consumer of recreation can best be helped through this agency. The objectives of schools and the objectives of recreation are similar. The schools are a source of leadership for recreation programs.

Hjelte and Shivers' arguments *against* a school-centered recreation program are as follows: Education should restrict itself to intellectual training and not be concerned with experiences that are only indirectly related to intellectual training. Public schools have too many responsibilities without adding any more. Teachers are poorly paid and facilities are inadequate in many localities, and so a heavier burden should not be placed upon these resources. Recreation is hampered by the formality of the school environment and becomes regimented. Consequently, recreation is able to realize its potentialities to a greater extent through the establishment of a special agency. School facilities, equipment, and supplies are damaged through a recreation program and

---

*Hjelte, G., and Shivers, J. S.: Public administration of parks and recreational services, New York, 1963, The Macmillan Co.

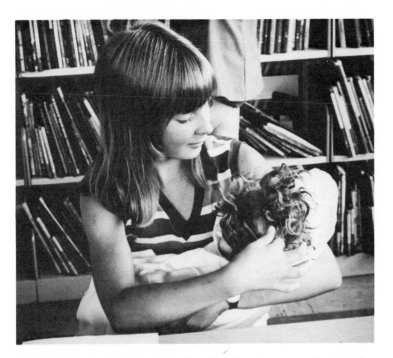

Babysitting as a recreational study activity—a 3-week series of sessions on caring for infants and young children sponsored by the North Castle County Department of Parks and Recreation, Wilmington, Del.

TEN GUIDELINES FOR THE ADMINISTRATION OF SCHOOL RECREATION *

1. The acceptance and commitment of the administration regarding the role of recreation in education.
2. The establishment of a representative ad hoc committee by the Board of Education to survey recreational needs and interests in the school district. Appropriate funds should be provided for the routine services for such a committee, including secretarial and consultant services.
3. The appointment of a qualified professional staff member, preferably the school district director of health, physical education, and recreation, to serve as coordinator of the study and liaison to the ad hoc committee.
4. The conduct of the study by the committee to determine the status of organized recreation in the school district. This should include: a review of the understanding and philosophy of people in the school district regarding recreation; existing recreational services available.
5. Arranging for technical, professional, consultant services in recreation through recognized agencies for the purpose of appraising the findings of the survey in terms of quality recreation for the school district.
6. Develop, in cooperation with the professional consultant, a proposed plan of recreation for the school district. Such a plan should include a statement of philosophy, principles, policies, procedures, and a financial plan.
7. A review of the ad hoc committee plan by the Board of Education and administration.
8. The acceptance or modification of the plan by the Board of Education.
9. The ratification of the plan and the adjustment of general school district administrative policies to appropriately provide for recreation.
10. The administrative implementation of recreation as officially adopted by the Board of Education, with emphasis on clear communication.

*New York State Department of Education, Albany, N. Y.

alterations are necessary, which raises the question of whether other facilities might not be provided more economically. Finally, in attempting to join the forces of education and recreation, difficulties are encountered in securing financial aid for both. Greater public support can be gained if recreation is not grafted onto the educational program.

Regardless of the arguments for or against school-centered recreation, the schools should play a vital part in the field of recreation. At the present time they are contributing staff and facilities. The program of studies in the schools, however, has a long way to go before it realizes

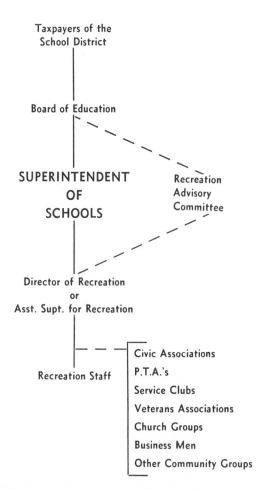

Recommended organization chart for school-operated recreation programs. (From School recreation, Report of the National Conference on School Recreation, copyrighted 1960.)

its potentialities for developing resources for leisure.

Contributions the regular school program can make

All subjects in the educational program have a contribution to make in developing resources for leisure. The school, with wide and varied educational offerings in such fields as science, art, music, physical education, and industrial arts, has infinite opportunities to develop many resources for leisure. During this age of mass production, application of atomic energy to industry, and increasing amounts of lesiure, the schools are being challenged to accept this responsibility.

Schools should help young people to adjust to the way of life that they will encounter after leaving school, aid them in solving the problems they will meet, and help them to become responsible citizens. Education most certainly must concern itself with leisure-time education. Leisure hours represent a challenge facing the nation's schools.

Contributions the out-of-class program can make

The school's job does not end when the 3 o'clock bell rings. Its influence extends into the child's life throughout the school day and is also reflected in those activities in which he or she engages after regular school hours. How the child spends free time after school and on Saturdays, Sundays, and holidays will influence his or her health and also success in life. During the school years the student may want to find out more about photography, choral singing, dramatics, or sports. The extracurricular program provides the opportunity to pursue these interests further. Probably one of the greatest values that out-of-school activities have for children is realized in later years. The interests they develop will carry over to adult life and supply them with many happy and profitable hours.

The school can help to enrich leisure

One of the best statements of how the school can help to enrich leisure of students was stated in an editorial by Joy Elmer Morgan, which is as true today as when it was written. He points out that the school can help to enrich leisure:

1. By introducing young people to a wide range of life interests.
2. By teaching the use of books and libraries and developing wholesome reading appetites closely related to each of the great objectives of education and life.
3. By developing appreciation of fine music and skill in singing, playing, and dancing.
4. By having children participate in games and sports which may be easily continued in after years.
5. By providing experience in pleasant social life through school activities.
6. By cultivating in children a love of the out-of-doors—appreciation of flowers, animals, landscape, sky, and stars.
7. By giving children an opportunity to develop hobbies in various creative fields—gardening, mechanics, applied arts, fine arts, architecture, city planning.
8. By making the school and its playfields the center and servant of a wholesome and satisfying neighborhood life.
9. By calling attention to various recreational agencies and the values which they serve—theaters, concerts, libraries, radio, periodicals and newspapers, museums, parks, playgrounds, travel. *

THE RECREATION LEADER

The recreation leader should have most of the qualifications of the health education and physical education specialists and in addition some that are pertinent especially to his or her field of work.

Qualifications

Various personal attributes are important for the recreation leader who is working with people so much of the time. These include such characteristics as integrity, friendly personality, enthusiasm, initative, organizing ability, and others that will aid in the achievement of recreation objectives.

Recreation leaders should possess a broad cultural background, with an understanding of the needs and problems facing society. This implies a fundamental knowledge of history, sociology, and anthropology. In addition, they should have the skills and competencies necessary for coping with such needs and problems. This would include the communicative arts,

knowledge of psychology, and other allied areas.

It is especially important that the recreation leader understand and appreciate human beings. He or she must have respect for the human personality; a broad social viewponit; the desire to inculcate a high standard of moral and spiritual values; a recognition of the needs, interests, and desires of individuals; an appreciation of the part that recreation can play in meeting these needs and interests; and a desire to serve humanity.

There is special need for an understanding and appreciation of community structure and the place of recreation at the "grass roots" level of this structure. The ability to utilize scientific survey techniques and other methods of social research is also an essential qualification.

There should be ability in the performance of skills in many of the areas with which recreation is concerned. These skills should not be limited to games and sports but in addition should branch out into such areas as arts and crafts, dramatics, camping and outdoor education, music, social recreation, and other important aspects of the total offering.

The philosophy of recreation, with the importance of constructive leisure-time activities to human beings, should be understood. In addition, there is the necessity for the special knowledge, attitudes, and skills concerned with methods and materials, safety, first aid, principles of group work, health, juvenile delinquency, and crime prevention.

Recreation positions and areas of recreation service

The following represent various types of recreation positions for which the aspiring student can prepare and the areas of recreation service:

Recreation positions

Superintendent of recreation
Assistant superintendent
Recreation director
Consultant
Field representative
Executive director
Hospital recreation supervisor
Campus recreation coordinator
Extension specialist

---

*Morgan, J. E.: Editorial, Journal of the National Education Association **19**:1, 1930.

Service club director
Girls' worker—boys' worker
District recreation supervisor
Recreation leader
Supervisor of special activities
Recreation therapist
Recreation educator

Areas of recreation service

Community recreation departments
Park departments
Schools
Service clubs for the armed forces
Churches and religious organizations
Hospitals
Institutions—public and private
Voluntary youth-serving agencies
Rural
Colleges and universities
Industry
State and federal agencies

SCHOOL CLUB AND ACTIVITY PROGRAMS

There are many out-of-class experiences that have educational value for students. Agricultural, cheerleading, music, camping, and journalism clubs and student government represent only a few of these experiences. In some cases these activities are run by the students themselves, whereas in other cases the faculty plays a significant role. The purpose of these programs, however, should be focused on helping the student to obtain a fuller and more total educational experience. Some of the objectives of such clubs are social, service, cultural, recreational, and exploratory in nature. They can provide students with opportunities for self-expression, leadership, constructive use of leisure time, creativity, responsibility, and practice skills.

The school club and activity programs should be planned as unified and integrated programs that dovetail with the curriculum. They should be organized and controlled in a manner that best serves the student's interests, develop special aptitudes and abilities, afford constructive use of leisure time, promote social assets, and provide intellectual and career information. The administration must also recognize that school activities cannot run themselves. They need continuous stimulation and guidance as well as financial support to be successful. The administration should be involved in the process by which the aims of a group are determined, its plans carried out, and the results evaluated to determine if the goals are being met. Problems can develop if the budget is not planned carefully, if qualified personnel are not available to give guidance to the activity, and if inadequate organization and control exist.

School club and activity programs can be a very important part of a well-balanced school program. They can provide opportunities for students to further their education in ways that the formal classroom situation does not permit. If properly administered, they can contribute to cutting down on dropouts, delinquency, and nonconstructive use of leisure hours.

The accompanying checklist highlights some of the important considerations for school club and activity programs.

CHECKLIST FOR SCHOOL CLUB AND ACTIVITY PROGRAMS

	Yes	No
1. Are club activity programs a normal outgrowth of the regular school program?	_____	_____
2. Are there clearly stated objectives for the club or activity program?	_____	_____
3. Does the club program supplement the formal curriculum by increasing knowledge and skills?	_____	_____
4. Are clubs organized in terms of educational value rather than administrative convenience?	_____	_____
5. Does the administration set adequate policies to guide the program?	_____	_____
6. Have the aims and objectives of the club or activity program been determined?	_____	_____
7. Can any student join a club?	_____	_____
8. Is a student limited to the number of clubs he or she may join?	_____	_____

CHECKLIST FOR SCHOOL CLUB AND ACTIVITY PROGRAMS—cont'd

	Yes	No
9. Does each club have a simple constitution and bylaws that can guide students in the conduct of the organization?		
10. Do the clubs prepare the student for democratic living?		
11. Do the activities help to develop school spirit?		
12. Does the school schedule club activities so that they do not conflict with regularly scheduled school activities?		
13. Does the school administrator ensure the program of adequate space and funds to carry on a worthwhile program?		
14. Can a student discover and develop special aptitudes and abilities through the club and activity program?		
15. Does the club and activity program offer opportunities for vocational exploration?		
16. Is the individual student able to develop socially acceptable attitudes and ideals through the club program?		
17. Does the club experience provide situations that will contribute to the formation of improved behavior patterns in the student?		
18. Do all club members actively participate in program planning?		
19. Are the projects and activities of the club initiated primarily by the students?		
20. Do the activities performed pertain to the club purposes?		
21. Are students allowed to select clubs and activities according to interests?		
22. Are students issued a calendar of events?		
23. Does the school library make available books and periodicals needed by club and activity groups?		
24. Does the club faculty adviser enlist the confidence of boys and girls?		
25. Is the club faculty adviser willing to give time and thought to making the club or activity program a success?		
26. Is the club faculty adviser able to find his or her chief satisfaction in pupil growth and not in appreciation of personal efforts?		
27. Does the administration of the school evaluate the club periodically?		
28. Does the club allow time for the evaluation of activities?		

Questions and exercises

1. Survey a community recreation program. In the light of this survey list the contributions the program makes to the community, its organization aspects, relation to schools, activities included in its program, and degree to which it is achieving professional objectives.
2. What are the objectives of recreation? Develop a group of guiding principles for the achievement of each of these objectives.
3. To what degree is recreation understood by the American public in general?
4. Discuss some innovations in recreation programs.
5. Discuss what you consider to be the outstanding accomplishments of the recreation profession during the last 50 years.
6. How can the recreation profession turn its shortcomings into accomplishments during the next 50 years?
7. Develop a plan whereby physical education, health education, and recreation can work together most productively in the community.
8. To what extent is your school achieving recreational objectives through its educational offering?
9. Read and critically review one article in *Recreation* magazine.
10. How can television be utilized most advantageously by the recreation profession?
11. Describe what you consider will be a community recreation program in the year 2000.

Reading asignment on *Administrative Dimensions of Health and Physical Education Programs, Including Athletics:* Chapter 19, Selections 98 to 100.

Selected references

American Association for Health, Physical Education, and Recreation: Leisure and the schools, Washington, D. C., 1961.

Bentz, C.: Operating a school swimming pool for the benefit of the total community, School Activities **39:** 12, 1968.

Bryant, A.: Activities program beginnings in a new junior college, School Activities **38:**5, 1966.

Bucher, C. A., editor: Methods and materials in physical education and recreation, St. Louis, 1954, The C. V. Mosby Co.

Bucher, C. A., and Bucher, R. D.: Recreation for today's

society, Englewood Cliffs, N. J., 1974, Prentice-Hall, Inc.

Bullock, N.: Aviation clubs in secondary schools, School Activities **39**:5, 1968.

Carlson, R., Deppe, T. R., and Maclean, J. R.: Recreation in American life, Belmont, Calif., 1971, Wadsworth Publishing Co., Inc.

Danford, H. G.: Creative leadership in recreation, Boston, 1964, Allyn & Bacon, Inc.

Donnely, K.: Current trends in commercial recreation, Journal of Health, Physical Education, and Recreation **44**:33, 1973.

Frederick, R. W.: Student activities in American education, New York, 1965, The Center for Applied Research in Education, Inc. (The Library of Education).

Heller, M. P.: School activities need an open door policy, Clearing House **40**:42, 1965.

Hjelte, G., and Shivers, J. S.: Public administration of park and recreational services, New York, 1963, The Macmillan Co.

Hodgson, J.: Leisure and the American worker, Journal of Health, Physical Education, and Recreation **43**:39, 1972.

Johnson, W. P., and Kleva, R. P.: The community dimension of college physical education, Journal of Health, Physical Education, and Recreation **44**:40, 1973.

Kraus, R.: Recreation and leisure in modern society, New York, 1971, Appleton-Century-Crofts.

Kraus, R.: Recreation today—program planning and leadership, New York, 1966, Appleton-Century-Crofts.

Kraus, R.: Today's crisis in urban recreation, Journal of Health, Physical Education, and Recreation **44**:29, 1973.

McKenzie, R. F.: Those extra curriculr activities, Texas Outlook **52**:35, 1968.

Nash, J. B.: Philosophy of recreation and leisure, St. Louis, 1953, The C. V. Mosby Co.

National Conference on School Recreation: School recreation, Washington, D. C., 1960, American Association for Health, Physical Education, and Recreation.

Report of the Second National Conference on School Recreation: Twentieth century recreation, re-engagement of school and community, Washington, D. C., 1963, American Association for Health, Physical Education, and Recreation.

Rodney, L. S.: Administration of public recreation, New York, 1964, The Ronald Press Co.

Shivers, J. S.: Leadership in recreational service, New York, 1963, The Macmillan Co.

Staffo, D.: A community recreation program, Journal of Health, Physical Education, and Recreation **44**:47, 1973.

The Commission on Goals for American Recreation: Goals for American recreation, Washington, D. C., 1964, American Association for Health, Physical Education, and Recreation.

Willgoose, C. E.: Recreation—obligation of the schools, Instructor **75**:39, 1966.

Yukic, T. S.: Fundamentals of recreation, New York, 1963, Harper & Row, Publishers.

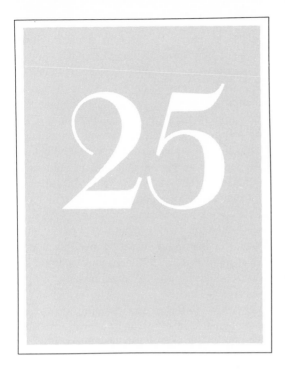

Outdoor environmental education and camping

A commitment to outdoor education has steadily increased in recent years. A variety of methods has been used to stimulate better use of the immediate school environment for education purposes. Some examples of this commitment are expressed in the following paragraphs.

In Ann Arbor, Michigan, the Forsythe Junior High School was developed for environmental education. The school site includes a courtyard with plantings and a waterfall. A greenhouse opens into the science classrooms.

In Berkeley, California, the Thousand Oaks School has created an extension of the school that includes a nature trail and a playground area with observation towers.

In an inner-city area of Washington, D. C., the students of the Madison Elementary School and local residents developed an abandoned lot and converted it into an outdoor environmental laboratory.

These are only a few of the projects that concerned citizens, teachers, and students have helped to develop. Both the urban and rural school offer numerous opportunities for outdoor education experiences.

The president* of the Minnesota Outdoor Education Association discussed in the *Journal of the National Education Association* how a kindergarten teacher takes her class outside to study the clouds in the sky, a third-grade class utilizes a compass to measure distances and determine directions preliminary to beginning a map for social studies, a sixth-grade class goes to a park and discovers fossils, and an eighth-grade class finds a spider web and relates it to what they were learning about conservation. Outdoor education is not just nature study but instead represents a vital part of the educational program at all education levels and in all subjects including art, social studies, mathematics, physical education, and industrial arts.

The out-of-doors is nature's laboratory. It is a setting that offers excellent opportunities to learn many knowledges and skills and to develop wholesome attitudes. Experiments and research have shown that boys and girls who use nature's classroom will learn more readily those things that directly relate to the out-of-doors and be more interested in doing so.

Outdoor education and school camping are not synonymous. Outdoor education includes school camping. The camp provides a laboratory by which many facets of the out-of-doors can be studied first hand. And the camp experi-

*Brinley, A.: Classrooms as big as all outdoors, NEA Journal **53**:45, 1964.

ence helps to develop qualities important to preparing young people for the lives they will live.

One hundred leaders in education, conservation, and recreation participated in a National Conference on Outdoor Education. This conference reaffirmed the importance of outdoor education and came to the following conclusions*:

1. There is an urgent need during the times in which we live for education in the out-of-doors.
2. There is a need to stress outdoor education in schools and colleges as well as in conservation, recreation, and other agency programs.
3. Those agencies and organizations involved in outdoor education should work cooperatively together to provide as many young people and adults as possible with experiences in this area.
4. The American Association for Health, Physical Education, and Recreation should make provision for outstanding leadership in this field of endeavor.

BEGINNINGS

In May, 1948, representatives of such well-known organizations and agencies as the

---

*Professional Report from the National Conference on Outdoor Education, Journal of Health, Physical Education, and Recreation 33:29, 1962.

American Association for Health, Physical Education, and Recreation; United States Office of Education; National Secondary School Principals Association; American Association of School Administrators; and the American Council on Education made recommendations that camping and outdoor education should be a part of every child's educational experience, that cooperative arrangements should be worked out with conservation departments and other agencies directly related to natural resources, and that experimental camping programs, as a phase of the educational program, should be established in Michigan and any other states that were interested in trying out this educational trend. Since 1948, camping and outdoor education have grown tremendously in this country.

Outdoor education and camping are rapidly being recognized as having an educational value that should be experienced by every boy and girl. Although there are comparatively few camps throughout the United States that are associated with school systems, the trend is more and more in the direction of required camping and outdoor education as part of the educational offering.

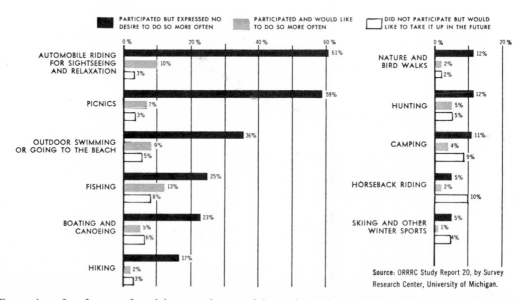

Expression of preference of participants and nonparticipants in outdoor activities. (From Action for Outdoor Recreation for America: A digest of the report of the Outdoor Recreation Resources Review Commission, with suggestions for citizen action, 1964.)

Many teacher education institutions preparing teachers of science, elementary education, health education, recreation, and physical education recognize the value of camping and its importance in education. Prospective teachers in some training programs are required to spend one or more sessions at a camp. The experience orients the student in camp living and in the organization and administration of a camp and emphasizes the value of oudoor education. It is also felt by some professional preparing institutions that the student should have a broad understanding of camping in education. This should include a study of the role of camping and outdoor education in the total educational process, the aims and objectives of camping and outdoor education, procedures essential in the conduct of a camp, qualifications and duties of the camp counselor in his or her relation to the director and to the campers, safety precautions and procedures, the program of activities for all types of weather conditions, and facilities.

SETTINGS FOR OUTDOOR ENVIRONMENTAL EDUCATION

A publication of the American Alliance for Health, Physical Education, and Recreation lists some of the significant settings for outdoor environmental education activities*:

1. *School sites and adjacent areas.* The trees, shrubs, streams, ponds, and outdoors in general offer many opportunities to develop outdoor laboratories that can be utilized for experiences related to such areas as science, social studies, arts and crafts, and physical education.

2. *Parks, forests, and farms.* Most communities have parks, farms, or other available outdoor areas nearby that can be utilized for outdoor education.

3. *School farms.* School farms are being developed in some communities and are providing agricultural experiences and a variety of learning situations that revolve around rural living. Such farms offer opportunities for studying birds, animals, conservation, gardening, milk

production, home management, care of farm machinery, and community life.

4. *School forests.* School forests or nearby municipal, county, state or national forests provide excellent outdoor education settings. School experiences relating to art, music, conservation, forestry, zoology, shop, archery, shelter construction, fire protection, camp crafts, and hiking can be provided.

5. *School and community gardens.* The opportunity to till the soil, see plants grow, and other similar activities can be provided for in school and community gardens.

6. *Museums and zoos.* An opportunity to study animals, collections of historic materials, works of art, and other important aspects of our culture is provided by museums and zoos.

7. *School camps.* The utilization of camps, either as a day camp or for an extended period of time, offers opportunities for group living, work experience, development of outdoor skills, and many other experiences important to the well-rounded education of every boy and girl.

VALUES OF OUTDOOR ENVIRONMENTAL EDUCATION AND SCHOOL CAMPING

The values of outdoor education and school camping are very much in evidence as a result of the many experiments that have been conducted throughout the United States. For purposes of discussion, it might be said that the values of such experiences are threefold: (1) they meet the social needs of the child, (2) they meet the intellectual needs of the child, and (3) they meet the health needs of the child.

A camping experience is an essential part of every child's school experience because it helps to develop the child socially. In a camp setting children learn to live democratically. They mix with children of other creeds or national origin, color, economic status, and ability. They aid in planning the program that will be followed during their camp stay; they assume part of the responsibility for the upkeep of the camp, such as making their own beds, helping in the kitchen, sweeping their cabins, and fixing the tennis courts; and they experience cooperative living. The children get away from home and

*American Association for Health, Physical Education, and Recreation: Leisure and the schools, Washington, D. C., 1961, The Association, p. 108.

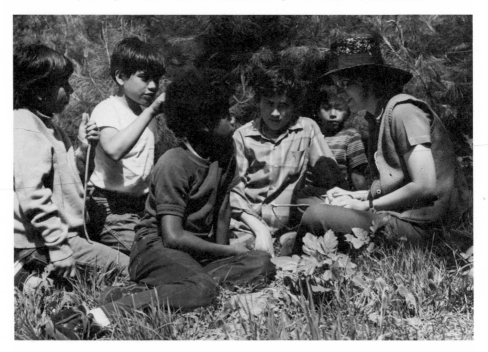

Outdoor environmental education experiences meet many needs of the child. Children in outdoor education program at Brea Canyon Camp sponsored by the Youth Services Section of the Los Angeles City Schools.

from their parents. They lose their feeling of dependency upon others and learn to do things for themselves. The child learns to rely on his or her own resources. The camp also provides an enjoyable experience for the child. A child is naturally active and seeks adventure. This experience provides the opportunity to release some of this spirit of adventure and to satisfy the "wanderlust" urge.

A camping experience is an essential part of every child's school experience because it helps to develop the child intellectually. While living in a camp, the child learns about soil, forests, water, and animal and bird life. He or she learns about the value of the nation's natural resources and how they should be conserved. He or she learns of ecology, the science concerned with the interrelationship between living organisms and their environment and between organisms themselves. He or she learns by doing rather than through the medium of textbooks. Instead of looking at the picture of a bird in a book, the child actually sees the bird chirping on the branch of a tree. Instead of reading about soil erosion in a textbook, he or she sees how it

actually occurs. Instead of being told about the four basic groups of food, he or she has the opportunity to live on a diet that meets the right standards. Instead of reading about the value of democratic living, he or she actually experiences it. The child experiences many new things that he or she cannot possibly do at home or within the four walls of a school building. Camping is also of special value to children who do not learn easily from books. In many cases the knowledge accumulated through actual experience is much more enlightening and beneficial.

Camping is an essential part of every child's school experience because it helps to meet the health needs of the child. Camps are located away from the turmoil, confusion, noise, and rush of urban life. Children experience having their meals at a regular time, obtaining sufficient sleep, and participating in wholesome activity in the out-of-doors. They wear clothing that does not restrict movement, that shields from the sun, and that they are not afraid to get dirty. The food is good. They are doing things that are natural for them to do. It is an

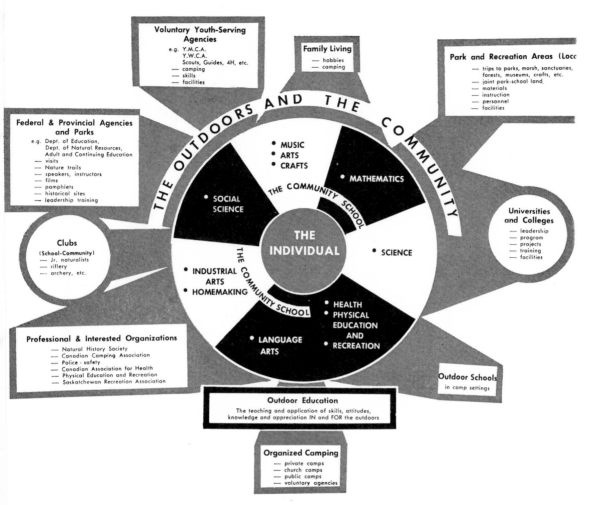

The world of outdoor education. (From MacKenzie, J.: Saskatchewan Community **14**:4, 1963-1964.)

outlet for their dynamic personalities. It is much more healthful, both physically and mentally, than living in a ''push-button'' existence with its lack of recreation, relaxation, and opportunity for enjoyable experiences. It is like living in another world, and children come away refreshed from such an experience.

THE FUTURE OF OUTDOOR ENVIRONMENTAL EDUCATION

Outdoor education holds great promise for the future. In the years to come it will become available to more people in such ways as adult education organizations, conferences, and seminars. As more children are educated to appreciate the outdoors, they will significantly increase their interest in outdoor programs.

There has been a veritable explosion in outdoor recreation areas attached to schools or used by schools. Regional recreation centers such as the Tennessee Valley Authority's YOUTH Station in Kentucky and the Cispus Center in Washington will probably increase in the next few years. These centers will be staffed with experts who will function as environment teachers conducting on-site activities and as in-service instructors providing educational resources to local school systems.

It is hoped that the community will become more involved in outdoor education and that government funding for special projects relating to this area will be increased.

In addition, schools in the near future will look to their staffs to develop outdoor education

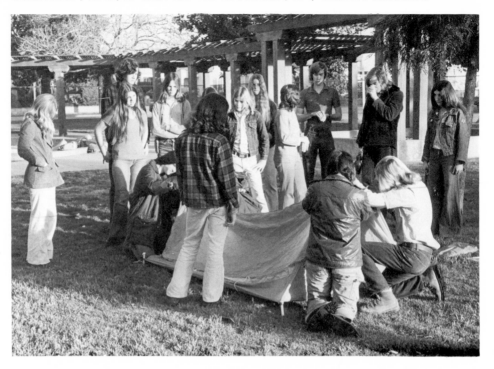

Students learning how to erect a tent. (Los Angeles Unified School District, Student Auxiliary Services Branch. Courtesy Gwen R. Waters.)

programs. Teachers should take in-service and outside courses that will help them in developing excellent outdoor education programs.

Outdoor education has numerous advantages; one of the most significant is providing a greater understanding of the environment and its problems. In this period of time when pollution, ecologic disruption, and the energy crisis are controversial problem areas, any understanding contributed by outdoor education programs will be invaluable to present and future generations.

THE SCHOOL CAMP PROGRAM

The program in most camps consists of such sports activities as swimming, boating, fishing, horseback riding, tennis, badminton, hiking, horseshoes, basketball, and softball; such social activities as campfires, frankfurter and marshmallow roasts, dancing mixers, and cookouts; and opportunities to develop skills and an appreciation in arts and crafts, photography, Indian lore, drama, music, and nature study.

The educational aspects can include a variety of experiences. Some of these are campfires,

outdoor cooking, woodcraft, camp sites, canoeing, conservation, astronomy, birds, animals, indoor and outdoor gardening, fishing, hiking, hunting, and orienteering.

SCHOOL CAMPS IN OPERATION

These are some outstanding examples of school systems that are using camping as an effective and worthwhile educational experience.

The sixth-grade children in the city of San Diego and San Diego County, California, have the opportunity to experience one week of camp life at Camp Cuyamaca. This is a former Civilian Conservation Corps Camp and is located in the nearby mountains. Year-round camping is included as part of the education of the boys and girls going to these schools. The staff is made up largely of school personnel, and the financial outlay is assured by the city council and county board of supervisors. From sixty to seventy children at a time experience all sorts of camp activities including arts and crafts, nature study, hikes, and care of living

OUTDOOR EDUCATION

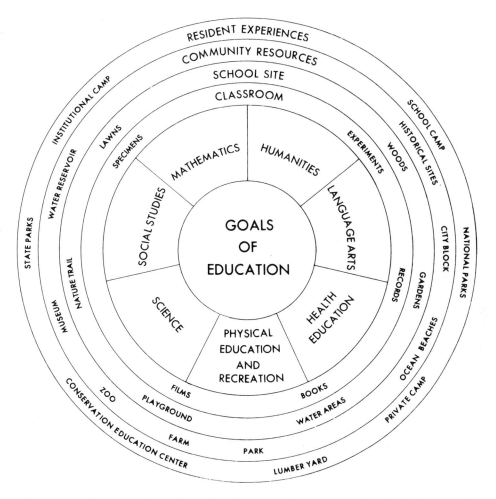

Outdoor Education in New York State. (From The University of the State of New York, The State Education Department: The great outdoors, Albany, 1970, State Education Department.)

quarters. Teachers accompany the children on camping trips. One main emphasis in the camp is to have children experience living together with other children in a democratic, healthful, and stimulating environment.

Another notable school camping experience takes place in the public school system of Battle Creek, Michigan, at Saint Mary's Lake Camp. As provided in the arrangements established in this educational setup, children have the opportunity of 2 weeks' camping experience, which may occur at any time during the year. The camp staff is made up of faculty

members of the Battle Creek schools. A novel feature of this camp is the banking experience that each child has. All boys and girls deposit their money in the camp bank, and a banking system is established analogous to that used by commerical banks. The campers also run their own post office. The only cost to each child for this valuable experience is the price of the food.

Long Beach, California, also offers a valuable camping experience to the children and faculties of its schools. Their camp, Camp Hi-Hill, is located about 50 miles from Long

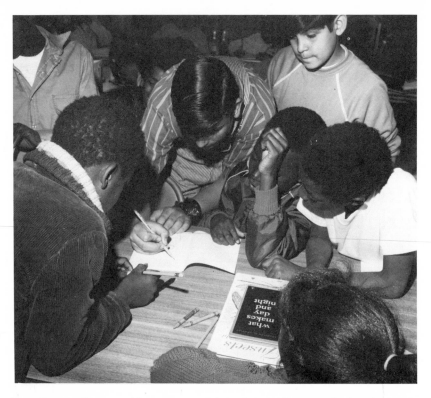

Students at Brea Canyon Camp working on a special outdoor environmental education project. (Courtesy Youth Services Section, Los Angeles City Schools.)

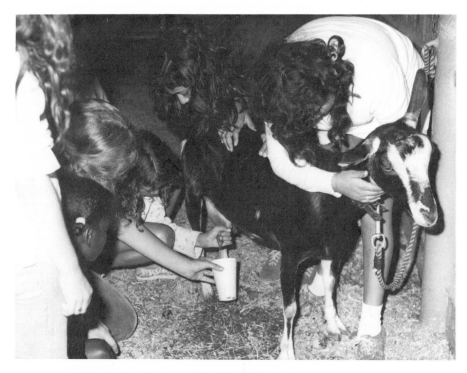

Students at Brea Canyon Camp milking a goat. (Courtesy Youth Services Section, Los Angeles City Schools.)

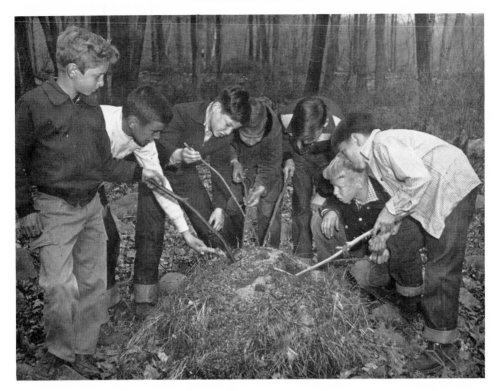

Education in the out-of-doors is meaningful.

Beach in the San Gabriel Mountains. This camp is primarily for sixth graders and faculty members, and the emphasis is on giving these children an opportunity to cope with various problems that arise when a group of individuals start living together in a democratic manner. This camp is also conducted on a year-round basis with winter activities playing just as important a role as summer activities.

Some states have passed legislation making tax money available to the schools for the support of camping provided for the public school children. This trend in state-level provision for camping in the public schools means that more and more opportunities are going to be made available for children to have this worthwhile experience. For example, in the state of Michigan a bill was passed providing that boards of education, with the exception of those in primary school districts, could operate camps independently or jointly with other boards of education or governing bodies for purposes of recreation and instruction. Provision was made

for the charging of fees, if necessary, to cover expenses incurred in maintaining the camp. However, these camps are to be run on a non-profit basis. Provisions were also made for boards of education to employ personnel to operate these camps, to maintain essential facilities, and to locate camps on property other than that owned by the board of education, provided that the consent of the owner of said property had been secured. Finally, a provision was made stipulating that the cost of operating a school camp should not be included in the determination of per capita costs of the regular school program.

In the state of New York legislation has provided that boards of education may operate camps on land secured by the school district for camp purposes. The legislature of the state of New York passed the Desmond School Camp Bill, which made it possible for school districts to appropriate funds for instructional programs deemed advisable for school children. Camping is one experience that is being recognized more and more as being an essential for all children of school age.

When historians look back at the twentieth century, there is a good possibility they will credit the school camping movement as the greatest educational innovation of the era and acclaim Michigan as one of the pioneer states in proving that nature's classroom helps to prepare the child much more effectively for living in today's world. The history of school camping in this state goes back some 25 years. In the early 1930's Tappan Junior High School in Ann Arbor utilized a camp setting for its junior high school students, and the Cadillac board of education developed a summer camp for its elementary school children. A little later, schools in Battle Creek, Decatur, and Otsego utilized camps in their educational programs. In 1945 the state government passed legislation making it possible for school districts to acquire and operate camps as part of their educational program. In 1946 their Departments of Public Instruction and Conservation, together with the W. K. Kellogg Foundation, joined forces to develop the program further. The late Lee M. Thurston, State Superintendent of Public Instruction, and P. J. Hoffmaster, State Director of Conservation, set as the goal for the state of Michigan: "A week of school camping for every boy and girl in the state."

The rapid development of camping in Michigan and other states has resulted to a great degree because of the educationally significant way in which the programs are operated. The groups going to camp usually include fifth- or sixth-graders on the elementary level, or home rooms and special subject matter areas on the secondary level. The camps are run by the teachers and students. Preplanning takes place in the classroom where such essentials as clothing needed, projects to be developed, and job assignments are arranged. The usual procedure is to have two teachers for the average classroom-size group, plus extra help for food preparation and camp maintenance. The parents assume the cost of food, with special provisions being made for those children whose families are unable to pay the expenses. Any child who wants to go to camp is given the opportunity. Schools assume the instructional cost. The school district or government agency bears the cost of the camp and its facilities.

Many educational systems include camping in their school programs at the present time in the state of Michigan. This state is pioneering in an educational movement that has many potentialities for furthering the social, mental, physical, and emotional growth of children. The fact that fewer than 10% of the children of camp age in America ever get any type of camp experience presents a challenge for other states to follow Michigan's lead.

The years ahead will undoubtedly find camping becoming more and more a part of the school program. Administrators, teachers, and educators in general should examine the potentialities that camping and outdoor education have for their own school systems.

Questions and exercises

1. Prepare a speech to be given to a parent-teacher's association on the importance of camping in education. Point up the values of camping to the children in the community.
2. What is the responsibility of professional preparing institutions in the field of camping and outdoor education?
3. Make a study of the program of camping and outdoor environmental education in the state of Michigan and give a report to the class.
4. Discuss some innovations in school outdoor environmental education programs.
5. How can outdoor education programs aid our understanding of environmental problems?
6. What should constitute some of the experiences provided in a camp setting?
7. Make a study of school camping in the fifty states and report to class on the progress that has been made during the last 5 years.
8. How can school camping contribute to the wise use of natural resources?
9. What is meant by enabling legislation? What type of enabling legislation is needed in your state to promote school camping? List a series of logical steps that should be followed to achieve such legislation.
10. Write an essay of 250 words on the subject: School camping is an extension of the classroom.

   Reading assignment in *Administrative Dimensions of Health and Physical Education Programs, Including Athletics:* Chapters 19 and 20, Selection 100 to 103.

Selected references

Adventures in environments: Morristown, N. J., 1971, Silver Burdett Company.

A guide to planning and conducting environmental study area workshops, Washington, D. C., 1972, National Education Association.

Brinley, A.: Classrooms as big as all outdoors, National Education Association Journal **53:**45, 1964.

Donaldson, G. W., and Donaldson, A.: Outdoor education: its promising future, Journal of Health, Physical Education, and Recreation **43:**23, 1972

Editorial: For these children: everything that camp should give, Michigan Education Journal **43:**26, 1965.

Freeberg, W. H.: Programs in outdoor education, Minneapolis, 1963, Burgess Publishing Co.

Fewer, R. D.: Administrative responsibilities for outdoor education, Illinois Journal of Education **55:**7, 1964.

Gabrielson, M. A., and Holtzer, C.: Camping and outdoor education, New York, 1965, The Center for Applied Research in Education, Inc. (The Library of Education).

Goldstein, J.: Environmental education for teachers, Journal of Health, Physical Education, and Recreation **44:**38, 1973.

Hammerman, D. R.: Research implications for outdoor education, Journal of Health, Physical Education, and Recreation **35:**89, 1964.

Hammerman, D. R., and Hammerman, W. M.: Teaching in the outdoors, Minneapolis, 1964, Burgess Publishing Co.

How to begin: Look at what we've got and then make it better, Journal of Health, Physical Education, and Recreation **44:**42, 1973.

Illinois State Superintendent of Public Instruction: Know about outdoor education. Springfield, Illinois, December, 1964, Journal of Education. (Available from Superintendent, Room 302, State Office Building, Springfield.)

Isenberg, R. M.: Education comes alive outdoors, National Education Journal **54:**24, 1967.

Shanklin, J. F.: Outdoor recreation land, Journal of Health, Physical Education, and Recreation **36:**19, 1965.

Shivers, J. S.: Camping-administration counseling, programming, New York, 1971, Appleton-Century-Crofts.

The University of the State of New York, The State Education Department: Outdoor education—a guide for planning resident programs, Albany, New York, 1972, The State Department of Education.

The University of the State of New York, The State Education Department: Outdoor education—experiences for emotionally handicapped children and youth, Albany, New York, 1972, The State Department of Education.

The University of the State of New York, The State Education Department: Outdoor education—the great outdoors, Albany, New York, 1970, The State Department of Education.

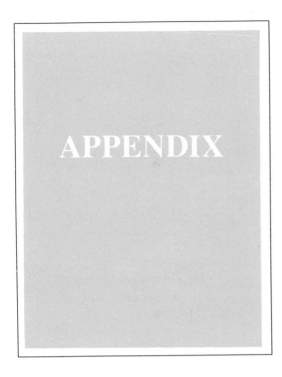

APPENDIX

Field and
court diagrams

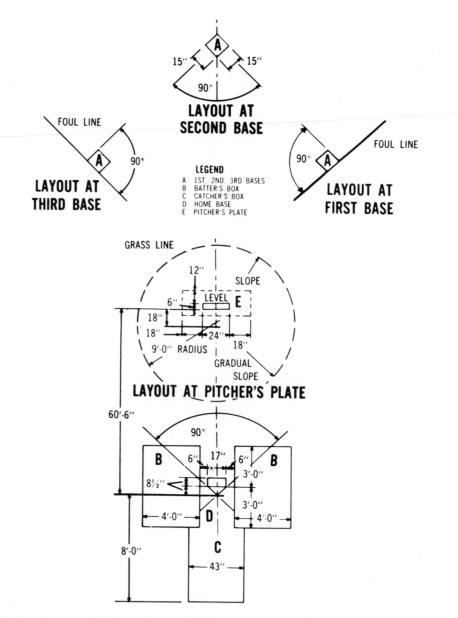

Reprinted courtesy McGregor-Consumer Division, Brunswick Company, Cincinnati, Ohio.

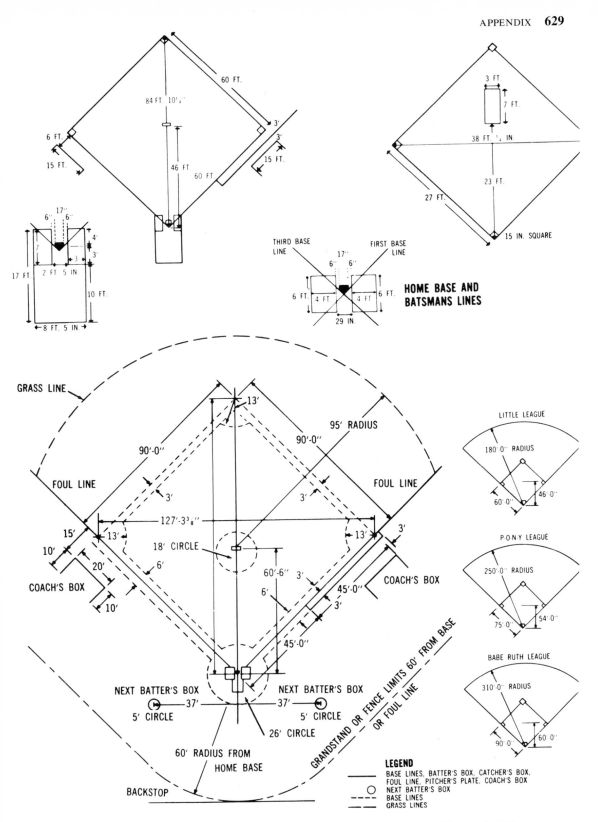

HOME BASE AND
BATSMANS LINES

LITTLE LEAGUE

P·O·N·Y LEAGUE

BABE RUTH LEAGUE

LEGEND
BASE LINES, BATTER'S BOX, CATCHER'S BOX,
FOUL LINE, PITCHER'S PLATE, COACH'S BOX
O NEXT BATTER'S BOX
BASE LINES
GRASS LINES

Reprinted courtesy McGregor-Consumer Division, Brunswick Company, Cincinnati, Ohio.

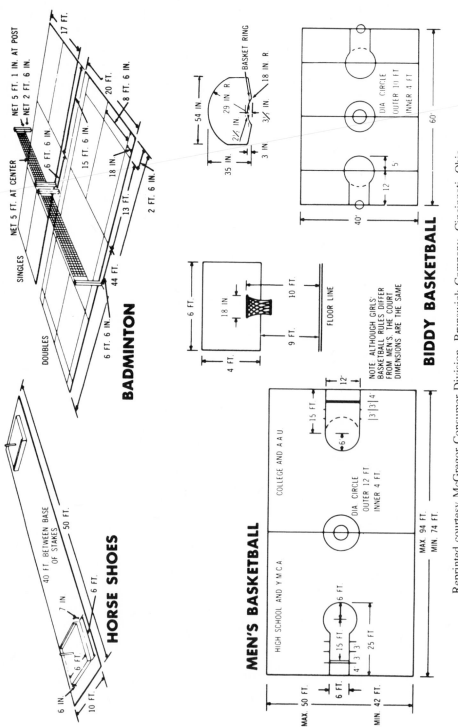

BADMINTON

HORSE SHOES

MEN'S BASKETBALL

BIDDY BASKETBALL

Reprinted courtesy McGregor-Consumer Division, Brunswick Company, Cincinnati, Ohio.

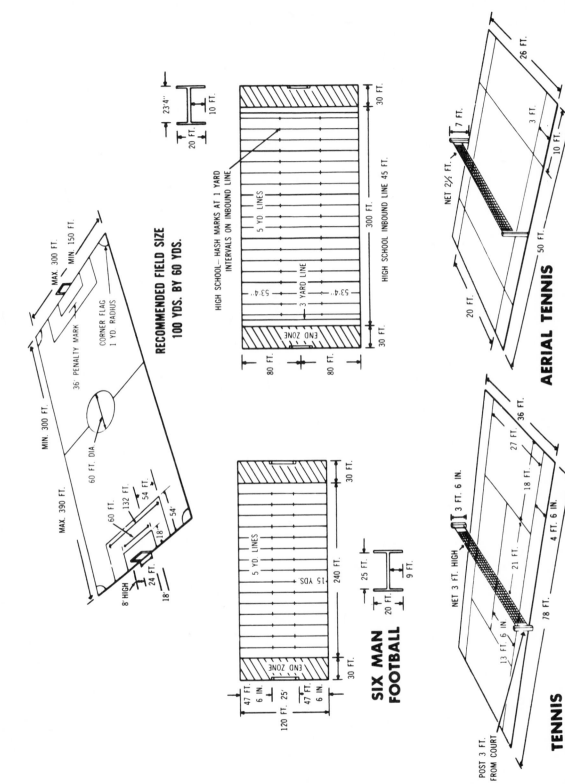

RECOMMENDED FIELD SIZE
100 YDS. BY 60 YDS.

HIGH SCHOOL— HASH MARKS AT 1 YARD
INTERVALS ON INBOUND LINE

SIX MAN
FOOTBALL

AERIAL TENNIS

TENNIS

Reprinted courtesy McGregor-Consumer Division, Brunswick Company, Cincinnati, Ohio.

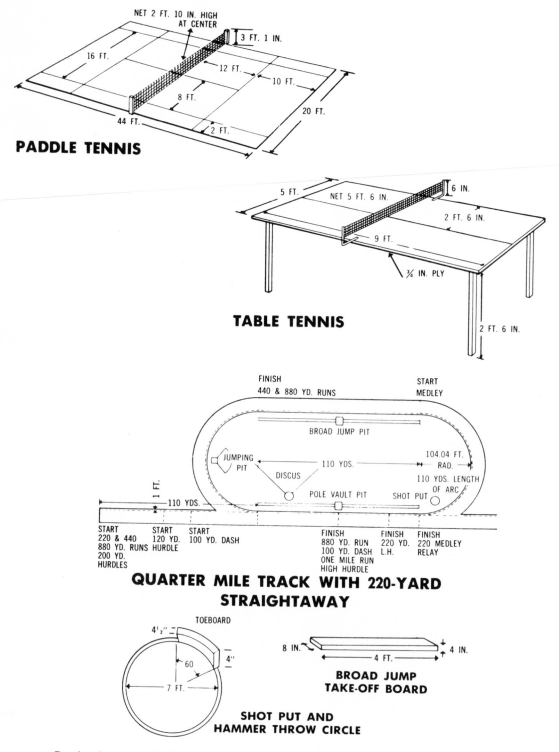

NET 2 FT. 10 IN. HIGH AT CENTER

3 FT. 1 IN.

16 FT.

12 FT.

10 FT.

8 FT.

20 FT.

44 FT.

2 FT.

PADDLE TENNIS

5 FT.

NET 5 FT. 6 IN.

6 IN.

2 FT. 6 IN.

9 FT.

¾ IN. PLY

2 FT. 6 IN.

TABLE TENNIS

FINISH
440 & 880 YD. RUNS

START
MEDLEY

BROAD JUMP PIT

JUMPING
PIT

104.04 FT.
RAD.

110 YDS.

DISCUS

110 YDS. LENGTH
OF ARC

POLE VAULT PIT

SHOT PUT

1 FT.

110 YDS.

START
220 & 440
880 YD. RUNS
200 YD.
HURDLES

START
120 YD.
HURDLE

START
100 YD. DASH

FINISH
880 YD. RUN
100 YD. DASH
ONE MILE RUN
HIGH HURDLE

FINISH
220 YD.
L.H.

FINISH
220 MEDLEY
RELAY

**QUARTER MILE TRACK WITH 220-YARD
STRAIGHTAWAY**

TOEBOARD

4½"

60

4"

7 FT.

8 IN.

4 FT.

4 IN.

**BROAD JUMP
TAKE-OFF BOARD**

**SHOT PUT AND
HAMMER THROW CIRCLE**

Reprinted courtesy McGregor-Consumer Division, Brunswick Company, Cincinnati, Ohio.

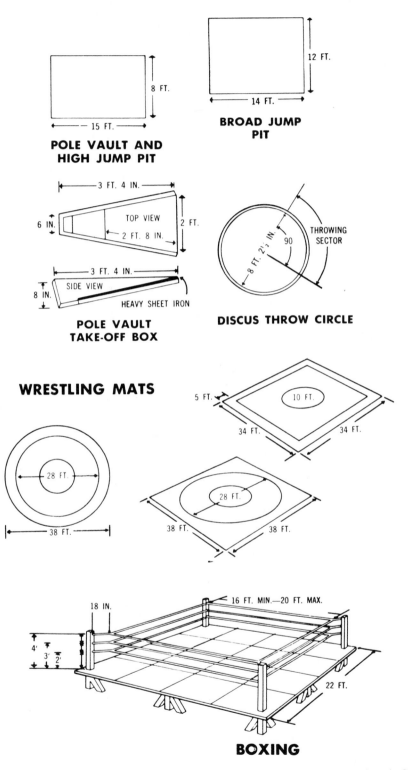

**POLE VAULT AND
HIGH JUMP PIT**

8 FT.

15 FT.

**BROAD JUMP
PIT**

12 FT.

14 FT.

**POLE VAULT
TAKE-OFF BOX**

3 FT. 4 IN.

TOP VIEW

2 FT. 8 IN.

2 FT.

6 IN.

3 FT. 4 IN.

SIDE VIEW

8 IN.

HEAVY SHEET IRON

DISCUS THROW CIRCLE

THROWING
SECTOR

90

8 FT. 2½ IN.

WRESTLING MATS

28 FT.

38 FT.

5 FT.

10 FT.

34 FT.

34 FT.

28 FT.

38 FT.

38 FT.

BOXING

16 FT. MIN.—20 FT. MAX.

18 IN.

4'

3'

2'

22 FT.

Reprinted courtesy McGregor-Consumer Division, Brunswick Company, Cincinnati, Ohio.

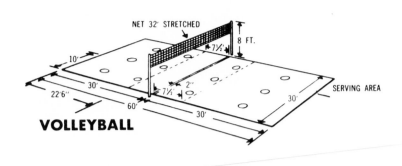

VOLLEYBALL

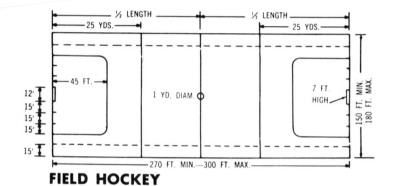

FIELD HOCKEY

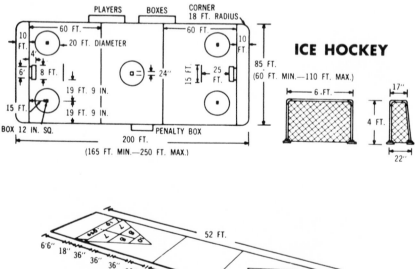

ICE HOCKEY

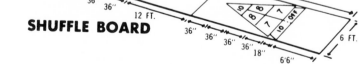

SHUFFLE BOARD

Reprinted courtesy McGregor-Consumer Division, Brunswick Company, Cincinnati, Ohio.

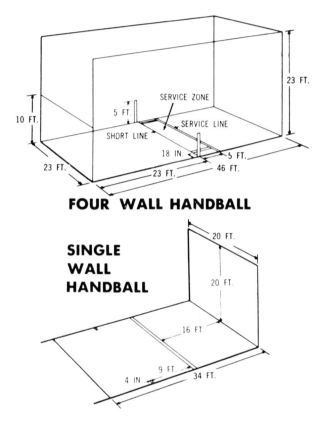

FOUR WALL HANDBALL

SINGLE WALL HANDBALL

Reprinted courtesy McGregor-Consumer Division, Brunswick Company, Cincinnati, Ohio.

Index

Pupil achievement, measurement of—cont'd
  techniques and instruments for, 559-567
    cognitive development, 566
    neuromuscular development, 565-566
    organic development, 565
    social development, 566-567
Purchasing supplies and equipment, 462-465

Q

Qualifications
  of administrator, 91-93
  of architect in facility planning, 396
  of health and physical educators, 97-102, 104
  of recreation leader, 611
  of student leaders in physical education, 118-119

R

Records
  in interschool athletics, 236-237
  in intramurals and extramurals, 218
  in physical education class, 152-153
Recreation, types of, 597-599; *see also* Community recreation
Recreation leadership, 115
Recruitment of athletes, 239
Reference materials in office, 550
Regina High School, 90, 128, 586
Remediable defects, correction of, 355-356
Repair of equipment, 467-469
Reporting of accidents, 500-503
Reports and records in the office, 552-554
Required physical education, 144
Research
  and curriculum change, 512-513
  in health education and physical education, 529-530
Responsibilities
  of business administrator, 78-80
  of general administrators, 105-106
  of health educators, 106-107
  of physical educators, 106-107
  for school health services. 339-341
  of students, 112-114
Rich Township High School, 116
Richwoods Community High School, 226, 372
Ridgewood High School, 145
Risk assumption, 489
Roll taking, 152

S

Safety
  code of, for physical education teacher, 504
  and football injuries, 503
  interschool athletics and, 230-232
  precautions for, 498-500
  reporting accidents and, 500-503
Satellite television, 476
Scheduling
  of adapted program, 187-189

Scheduling—cont'd
  of intramurals and extramurals, 203
  of physical education classes, 137-144
    and class size, 141-142
    and differentiated staffing, 142
    elementary and secondary levels and, 139-141
    and grouping, 143-144
    teaching loads and, 142
    time allotment for, 138-139
Scholarships, 239
School
  athletic insurance for, 506-508
  and college
    adapted physical education program in, 189-192
    administrator in health science instruction in, 300-301
    physical education programs in, 64-69
      evaluation of, 590-593
      in two-year college, 70-72
      and women, 57
    physician in health science instruction, 301
    structure of, 50-57
      administrative personnel, 53-57
      board of education, 52-53
      health programs, 57-64
      lay groups, 57
  and health services program, 338-339
  "lighted school" concept, 215-216
  and physical achievement, 267
  and role in physical fitness, 267-271
School administrative changes
  districts, 48-50
  organization patterns, 50
  state and federal control, 50
School board and administration of recreation programs, 605-606
School camp program, 620
School camps in operation, 620-624
School-centered recreation, 608-610
School club and activity programs and checklist for, 612-613
School-community health programs, coordination of, 321
School districts, 48-50
  liability of, 493
School health programs
  administrative problems of, 298-299
  evaluation of, 587-590
School health services, 97
School health team, 299-302
School laws and regulations for teaching health and physical education, 481-482
School, park, and recreation board members' liability, 493
School recreation, 599, 606-611
School vouchers, 24
Scouting in athletics, 240
Secondary school
  guidelines for basic instructional program in, 136-137
  health science instruction in, 315-318
  physical education class in, 156
    program for, 159-162
  teaching stations in, 406